# Natural
# Health Bible

# Other Books
# in THE NATURAL PHARMACIST Series

*The Natural Pharmacist Guide to Arthritis*

*The Natural Pharmacist Guide to Diabetes*

*The Natural Pharmacist Guide to Echinacea and Immunity*

*The Natural Pharmacist Guide to Feverfew and Migraines*

*The Natural Pharmacist Guide to Garlic and Cholesterol*

*The Natural Pharmacist Guide to Ginkgo and Memory*

*The Natural Pharmacist Guide to Heart Disease Prevention*

*The Natural Pharmacist Guide to Kava and Anxiety*

*The Natural Pharmacist Guide to Menopause*

*The Natural Pharmacist Guide to PMS*

*The Natural Pharmacist Guide to Reducing Cancer Risk*

*The Natural Pharmacist Guide to Saw Palmetto and the Prostate*

*The Natural Pharmacist Guide to St. John's Wort and Depression*

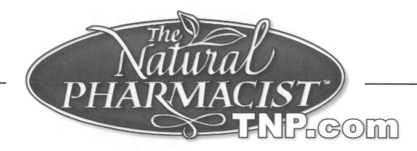

# Natural Health Bible

From the Most Trusted Source in Health Information,
Here Is Your A–Z Guide
to Over 200 Herbs, Vitamins, and Supplements

Edited by Steven Bratman, M.D. & David Kroll, Ph.D.

**Prima**
HEALTH

A Division of Prima Publishing

Visit us online at www.TNP.com

**Warning—Disclaimer**
**This book is not intended to provide medical advice and is sold with the understanding that the publisher and the author are not liable for the misconception or misuse of information provided. The author and Prima Publishing shall have neither liability nor responsibility to any person or entity with respect to any loss, damage, or injury caused or alleged to be caused directly or indirectly by the information contained in this book or the use of any products mentioned. Readers should not use any of the products discussed in this book without the advice of a medical professional.**

**The Food and Drug Administration has not approved the use of any of the natural treatments discussed in this book. This book, and the information contained herein, has not been approved by the Food and Drug Administration.**

PRIMA HEALTH and colophon are trademarks of Prima Communications, Inc.
THE NATURAL PHARMACIST™ is a trademark of Prima Communications, Inc.
TNP.com and TheNaturalPharmacist.com are trademarks of Prima Communications, Inc.

All products mentioned in this book are trademarks of their respective companies.

**Library of Congress Cataloging-in-Publication Data**

Bratman, Steven.
  Natural health bible : from the most trusted source in health information, here is your a–z guide to over 200 herbs, vitamins, and supplements / Steven Bratman and David Kroll.
    p.   cm.—(The natural pharmacist)
  Includes bibliographical references and index.
  ISBN 0-7615-2082-1
  1. Herbs—Therapeutic use.   2. Dietary supplements—Therapeutic use.   3. Naturopathy.
I. Kroll, David, pharmacist.   II. Title.   III. Series.
  RM666.H33B725 1999
  S15.5'35—dc21                                                        99-23813
                                                                          CIP

  00  01  02  DD  10  9  8  7  6  5
Printed in the United States of America

Visit us online at www.TNP.com and www.primahealth.com

# CONTENTS

# WHAT MAKES THIS BOOK DIFFERENT?

The interest in natural medicine has never been greater. According to the National Association of Chain Drug Stores, 65 million Americans are using natural supplements, and the number is growing! Yet it is hard for the consumer to find trustworthy sources for balanced information about this emerging field. Why? Frankly, natural medicine has had a checkered history. From snake oil potions sold at the turn of the century to those books, magazines, and product catalogs that hype miracle cures today, this is a field where exaggerated claims have been the norm. Proponents of natural medicine have tended to abuse science, treating it more as a marketing tool than a means of discovering the truth.

But there is truth to be found. Studies of vitamins, minerals, and other food supplements have been with us since these nutritional substances were first discovered, and the level and quality of this science has grown dramatically in the last 20 years. Herbal medicine has been neglected in the United States, but in Europe, this, the oldest of all healing arts, has been the subject of tremendous and ongoing scientific interest.

At present, for a number of herbs and supplements, it is possible to give reasonably scientific answers to the questions: How well does this work? How safe is it? What types of conditions is it best used for?

THE NATURAL PHARMACIST series is designed to cut through the hype and tell you what we know and what we don't know about popular natural treatments. These books are more conservative than any others available, more honest about the weaknesses of natural approaches, more fair in their comparisons of natural and conventional treatments. You won't find any miracle cures here, but you will discover useful options that can help you become healthier.

## WHY CHOOSE NATURAL TREATMENTS?

Although the science behind natural medicine continues to grow, this is still a much less scientifically validated field than conventional medicine. You might ask, "Why should I resort to an herb that is only partly proven, when I could take a drug with solid science behind it?" There are at least three good reasons to consider natural alternatives.

First, some herbs and supplements offer benefits that are not matched by any conventional drug. Vitamin E is a good example. It appears to help prevent prostate cancer, a benefit that no standard medication can claim. Also, vitamin E almost certainly helps prevent heart disease. While there are standard drugs that also prevent heart disease, vitamin E works differently and may be able to complement many of the other approaches.

Another example is the herb milk thistle. Studies strongly suggest that this herb can protect the liver from injury. There is no pill or tablet your doctor can prescribe to do the same.

Even if the science behind some of these treatments is less than perfect, when the risks are low and the possible benefit high, a treatment may be worth trying. It is a little-known fact that for many conventional treatments the science is less than perfect as well, and physicians must balance uncertain benefits against incompletely understood risks.

A second reason to consider natural therapies is that some may offer benefits comparable to those of drugs with fewer side effects. The herb St. John's wort is a good example. Reasonably strong scientific evidence suggests that this herb is an effective treatment for mild to moderate depression, while producing fewer side effects on average than conventional medications. Saw palmetto for benign enlargement of the prostate, ginkgo for relieving symptoms and perhaps slowing the progression of Alzheimer's disease, and glucosamine for osteoarthritis are other examples. This is not to say that herbs and supplements are completely harmless—they're not—but for most the level of risk is quite low.

Finally, there is a philosophical point to consider. For many people, it "feels" better to use a treatment that comes from nature instead of from a laboratory. Just as you might rather wear all-cotton clothing than polyester, or look at a mountain landscape rather than the skyscrapers of a downtown city, natural treatments may simply feel more compatible with your view of life. We can quibble endlessly about just what "natural" means and whether a certain treatment is "actually" natural or not, but such arguments are beside the point. The difference is in the feeling, and feelings matter. In fact, having a good feeling about taking an herb may lead you to use it more consistently than you would a prescription drug.

Of course, at times synthetic drugs may be necessary and even lifesaving. But on many other occasions it may be quite reasonable to turn to an herb or supplement instead of a drug.

To make good decisions you need good information. Unfortunately, while hundreds of books on alternative medicine are published every year, many are highly misleading. The phrase "studies prove" is often used when the studies in question are so small or so badly conducted that they prove nothing at all. You may even find that the "data" from other books comes from studies with petri dishes and not real people!

You can't even assume that books written by well-known authors are scientifically sound. Many of these authors rely on secondary writers, leading to a game of "telephone," where misconceptions are passed around from book to book. And there's a strong tendency to exaggerate the power of natural remedies, whitewashing them with selective reporting.

THE NATURAL PHARMACIST series gives you the balanced information you need to make informed decisions about your health needs. Setting a new, high standard of accuracy and objectivity, these books take a realistic look at the herbs and supplements you read about in the news. You will encounter both favorable and unfavorable studies in these pages and will learn about both the benefits and the risks of natural treatments.

THE NATURAL PHARMACIST series is the source you can trust.

Steven Bratman, M.D.
David Kroll, Ph.D.

# INTRODUCTION

So that you can easily access the information you need, the *Natural Health Bible* is divided into two parts. Part One, "Conditions," contains information about various illnesses and health problems, from acne to varicose veins. In each entry, you will find a description of the condition, as well as the various conventional treatments, herbs, supplements, and lifestyle changes that might help. Treatments that have fairly good evidence behind them or are widely used are called "Principal Natural Treatments"; the remainder are called "Other Natural Treatments."

If you're interested primarily in herbs, vitamins, minerals, and other supplements, then turn to Part Two, "Herbs and Supplements." This section covers over 150 of today's popular natural substances, from acidophilus to zinc. For each herb or supplement, I discuss its various uses, the scientific evidence behind those uses, and dosage information, as well as safety issues of which you should be aware. If there is considerable evidence for a substance's effectiveness for a given condition, or if it is widely used for that purpose, that condition is listed under "Principal Proposed Uses." Otherwise, it falls in the category of "Other Proposed Uses."

Throughout the book, you will see terms in boldface followed by a page number in parentheses. This means that there is a section about this subject in either Part One or Part Two to which you can turn for further information. For example, if you're reading about a condition and a treatment for it is listed in boldface, you can turn to the page mentioned in parentheses to learn more about that treatment in general, including its history, current uses, the scientific studies performed, and dosage and safety information.

## RESOURCES USED

The *Natural Health Bible* is based on science, not opinion, anecdote, or folk wisdom. To a considerable extent, it turns to European sources of scientific information, where the study of herbs and supplements is a part of mainstream medicine. For example, this book often quotes the opinions of Germany's Commission E, a branch of the German Federal Health Agency charged with evaluating the safety and efficacy of medicinal herbs. It also reports the conclusions of the European Scientific Cooperative on Phytotherapy (ESCOP). But even more than that, this book is based on a comprehensive survey of all the scientific evidence in world literature regarding the use of natural treatments. If there is evidence to report you will find it here; also, if there is little to no evidence backing a given treatment, that will be pointed out as well.

## DOSAGE INFORMATION FOR SUPPLEMENTS

There are two ways to take supplements: at a nutritional dose or a therapeutic dose. Because this is an issue that doesn't arise with standard medications (or with herbs), I want to take a moment to explain it here.

Your body needs a certain amount of various vitamins and minerals to maintain health. If you don't get enough in your diet, you may need supplements to avoid a form of malnutrition. When you take just enough of a nutrient to supply your body's needs, you are taking it at a *nutritional dose*. The exact quantity you need depends on your age, sex, and which authority you ask.

In the United States, the most important standard is the Recommended Dietary Allowance (RDA), which is now turning into the Recommended Daily Value (RDV). For some supplements, however, it has been impossible to determine the optimum intake, and a looser standard is used instead, the Estimated Safe and Adequate Daily Dietary Intake (ESADDI). To make matters more confusing, in Canada, the prevailing standard is the Recommended Nutrient Intake (RNI), and these figures often disagree with the U.S. RDA levels. Other standards have been set by the Food and Agricultural Organization and the World Health Organization of the United Nations, as well as by other individual countries, and again there is significant variation.

This book provides the U.S. RDA amounts when they're available; otherwise it uses the ESADDI guidelines.

But there is another, entirely different way of taking supplements. You can take them at a level that greatly exceeds your nutritional needs. This is described as a "therapeutic dosage" and it is listed under a heading separate from that for nutritional requirements.

For example, the estimated dietary requirement of vitamin E is about 10 to 15 IU (international units) daily. But when used as an antioxidant supplement to prevent heart disease or prostate cancer, the typical recommended dosage is 400 to 800 IU daily—25 to 80 times higher than nutritional needs. There is simply no way you could reasonably get this much from food. This is a *therapeutic dose,* not a nutritional dose.

It's hard to get too worried about the safety of supplements taken at or near your nutritional needs. However, when they are used in gigantic doses, it is always possible that new health risks are created. In this book, we carefully distinguish between nutritional and high-dose use of all supplements described. Each one has its own heading.

## TERMS YOU SHOULD KNOW

Throughout this book I refer to the various types of scientific studies used to evaluate the effectiveness of medical treatments. So that you will understand the nature of each one, and the level of confidence you can place in its results, I briefly describe these research methods here.

### Double-Blind Studies

The best and most reliable form of research is the double-blind placebo-controlled study. A treatment cannot really be said to be proven effective unless it has been examined in properly designed and sufficiently large double-blind studies.

In these experiments, one group of subjects receives the "real thing"—the active substance being tested. The other half receives a placebo designed to appear, as much as possible, like the real thing. The purpose of this kind of study is to eliminate the power of suggestion. It is true, although hard to believe, that placebo (fake) treatments can produce dramatic and long-lasting results in a majority of the people who are given them. The double-blind study keeps both doctors and participants in the dark as to who is receiving the placebo and who is receiving the real treatment. If the people in the real treatment group fare significantly better, it is a strong indication that the treatment really works.

A good double-blind study should enroll at least 100 people, preferably as much as 300. Dramatically effective treatments can prove themselves in somewhat smaller trials; however, research involving 30 or fewer people generally doesn't prove anything at all.

### Single-Blind Studies

If only the participants are kept in the dark, but the doctors know which group is which, the study is called single-blind. This type of study is a bit questionable as it allows for bias on the part of the doctors conducting the study. (Doctors can subtly convey confidence or a lack of it if they know who is receiving real treatment and who is not; they can also unconsciously bias their evaluation of the results.)

### Open Studies

If both the doctors and the participants know who is receiving a treatment and who is not, the procedure is called an open study. The results have to be taken with a handful of salt: Open studies are not at all reliable.

### Uncontrolled Studies

Sometimes a group of people are given a treatment and simply followed for a period of time to see if they improve. The results of such studies mean practically nothing at all. Due to the placebo effect, one can be sure from the outset that they will mostly improve; it is impossible to tell how much (if any) of this improvement is due to the effect of the treatment itself.

### Observational Trials Versus Intervention Trials

All of the studies just described involve giving participants a treatment; in other words, "intervening" in their lives. They all fall in the category of an "intervention trial."

Observational studies, on the other hand, simply follow large (sometimes gigantic) groups of people for years and keep track of a great deal of information about them, including diet. Researchers do not do anything to them; they just examine the collected data closely and try to identify which dietary and lifestyle factors are associated with better health and longer life.

Observational studies are often the only practical way to gain information about the long-term health effects of nutrition and lifestyle. Unfortunately, the results can be misleading. For example, if an observational study finds that people who drink green tea develop less cancer, it is not necessarily the green tea that deserves the credit. Green tea drinkers may also tend to exercise more and to eat more healthful foods in general. Maybe it is those habits, and not the tea, that plays the most important role. Researchers try to look closely at the data and eliminate such factors, but it can be very tricky to do so properly.

### In Vitro Studies

An in vitro study is a trial that tests a substance in a test tube. Such studies are really only spurs for further research, as they don't prove that a treatment is effective in real life. An herb or supplement taken by mouth must be absorbed into the bloodstream, survive processing by the liver, and still manage to be effective when diluted by the fluids of the body. It's a long leap from a test tube to a treatment that actually works.

### Animal Studies

Evidence from studies enrolling animals means more that from in vitro studies. However, because animals may process nutrients and even herbs differently than we do, the results can't be taken as completely reliable.

## STATISTICAL SIGNIFICANCE

For nearly all types of studies, there is one more step to take that is necessary to interpret the results. A mathematical analysis must be made to see if the results are meaningful.

It is always possible that an apparent result can be just due to chance. For example, if you flip a coin 20 times, and it comes up heads 14 times, does these mean that the coin is biased? Probably not. But if you flip it 4,000 times and it comes up heads 3,500 times, it probably is a trick coin.

Likewise, if a study only enrolls 20 people, the results might be due to chance alone. But results seen in larger studies are more likely to mean something.

Researchers use various statistical methods to analyze the outcome of a study and determine whether the results are meaningful. This analysis is called a *test for statistical significance*. You can't draw any conclusions from a study if the results are not statistically significant. In this book, unless stated otherwise, all results mentioned were found to be statistically significant according to the mathematical methods used by the researchers.

## THE LIMITATIONS OF THIS BOOK

Remember that no book can substitute for individualized medical care from a physician. Every person is different and has specific health needs only a doctor can assess. Furthermore, in many cases it is possible to use combinations of treatments—both natural and pharmaceutical—in sophisticated ways that cannot be described in a book of this type. The information contained in the following text should be regarded as an introduction, a suggestion for where to start.

P A R T

**ONE**

# Conditions

# ACNE

### Principal Natural Treatments
There are no well-established natural treatments for acne.

### Other Natural Treatments
Zinc, chromium, vitamin E, selenium, burdock, red clover, tea tree oil

---

The blackheads and sometimes painful pimples that we know as acne occur most commonly during adolescence, but they may persist into later life as well. There is much we still don't understand about what causes acne. We do know that during adolescence and other times of hormonal imbalance, such as around menopause, the oil-secreting glands in the skin increase their level of secretions. A combination of naturally occurring yeast and bacteria then breaks down these secretions, causing the skin to become inflamed and the pimples to eventually rupture. In severe cases, acne can lead to permanent scars.

Conventional treatment, which usually is quite successful, consists primarily of antibiotics, cleansing agents, and chemically modified versions of **vitamin A** (page 318).

## NATURAL TREATMENTS

While there are no dramatically effective alternative treatments for acne, there are a few options that may provide some help.

**Warning:** Do not rely on any of the treatments discussed in this section to treat severe acne where scarring is a consideration.

### Zinc

People with acne have been shown to have lower-than-normal levels of **zinc** (page 348) in their bodies.[1–5] However, this doesn't prove that taking zinc supplements will help acne. For example, it is possible that the factors that cause acne also affect zinc levels.

Double-blind studies involving a total of more than 300 people have tried to discover whether taking extra zinc can relieve the symptoms of acne. The results have been generally positive, indicating a definite but somewhat mild effect.

In one of these studies, 54 people were given either placebo or 135 mg of zinc as zinc sulfate daily. Zinc produced slight but measurable benefits.[6] Similar results have been seen in other studies using 90 to 135 mg of zinc daily.[7–11] In some studies, however, no benefits were seen.[12,13]

Two studies have compared zinc against a standard treatment for acne, the antibiotic tetracycline. One found that zinc was as effective as tetracycline,[14] but another found the antibiotic more effective.[15]

However, fairly high dosages of zinc (more than is completely safe) seem to be required to produce these benefits. See the chapter on zinc in Part Two for more information.

## Other Herbs and Supplements

Other commonly mentioned natural treatments for acne include **chromium** (page 161), **vitamin E** (page 337), **selenium** (page 297), **burdock** (page 145), and **red clover** (page 290). **Tea tree** (page 309) oil has antiseptic properties and has been suggested as an alternative to benzoyl peroxide for direct application to the skin. There haven't been any solid studies examining these treatments, however.

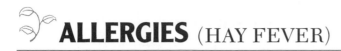

# ALLERGIES (HAY FEVER)

*(For Other Types of Allergies, see Asthma and Eczema)*

*Principal Natural Treatments*
There are no well-established natural treatments for allergies.

*Other Natural Treatments*
Nettle, quercetin, OPCs and other flavonoids, vitamin C, vitamin B$_6$, vitamin B$_{12}$, cat's claw, *Coleus forskohlii,* betaine hydrochloride, GLA, fish oil

About 7% of all Americans suffer from hay fever, an allergic condition that can cause runny nose, sneezing, and teary eyes. It is known officially as *allergic rhinitis, allergic sinusitis,* or *allergic conjunctivitis,* depending on whether symptoms manifest mainly in the nose, sinuses, or eyes, respectively. Hay fever usually peaks when particular plants are pollinating or when molds are flourishing. People who suffer from year-round hay fever may be allergic to ever-present allergens such as dust mites.

Here's how hay fever works. In response to the triggers noted above, an individual prone to allergies develops an exaggerated immune response. Substances known as IgEs flood the nasal passages, white blood cells called eosinophils arrive by the millions and billions, and inflammatory substances such as histamine, prostaglandins, and leukotrienes are released in massive amounts. The overall effect is the familiar one of swelling, dripping, itching, and aching.

The mechanism of allergic response is fairly well understood. Why allergic people react so excessively to innocent bits of pollen, however, remains a complete mystery.

Conventional treatment for hay fever consists of antihistamines (now available in forms that don't make you sleepy); decongestants, nasal steroids, or cromolyn sodium; and occasionally allergic desensitization ("allergy shots"). For most people, some combination of these treatments will be successful.

## NATURAL TREATMENTS

The following treatments are widely recommended for allergies, but they have not been scientifically proven effective at this time.

### Nettle Leaf

According to one preliminary double-blind placebo-controlled study, freeze-dried extract of stinging **nettle** (page 268) leaf can at least slightly help improve allergy symptoms.[1]

A typical dosage is two to three 300-mg capsules of nettle leaf. Nettle leaf has an extensive history of use in food and is believed to be safe. However, safety in young children, pregnant or nursing women, and those with severe liver or kidney disease has not been established.

For theoretical reasons, some researchers suggest that nettle may interact with conventional medications for diabetes and high blood pressure, but no actual problems of this type have been officially reported.

### Quercetin, OPCs, and Other Flavonoids

Test-tube studies suggest that flavonoids—biologically active compounds found in many plants—may help reduce allergy symptoms.[2–5] A particular flavonoid, **quercetin** (page 288), seems to be one of the most active.[6–10] Many texts on natural medicine claim that quercetin works like the drug cromolyn (Intal) by stopping the release of allergenic substances in the body. However, while we have direct evidence that cromolyn is effective, there have not been any published studies in which people were given quercetin and their allergic symptoms decreased. It is a long way from test-tube studies to real people. If you do wish to take quercetin, a particular form of the substance, *quercetin chalcone,* may be better absorbed than other forms.

**OPCs** (page 270) from grape seed or pine bark are also often said to be effective. But at the present time, we don't really know whether any of these treatments are really helpful for allergies.

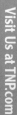

## Vitamin C

**Vitamin C** (page 331) is often suggested as a treatment for allergies, but the research results are very preliminary and somewhat contradictory.[11,12,13]

## Other Treatments

**Vitamin B$_6$** (page 326), **vitamin B$_{12}$** (page 329), **cat's claw** (page 154), *Coleus forskohlii* (page 166), **GLA** (page 210), **fish oil** (page 188), and **betaine hydrochloride** (page 134) are also sometimes recommended for hay fever, but there is as yet no significant evidence that they are effective.

# ALZHEIMER'S DISEASE
## (AND NON-ALZHEIMER'S DEMENTIA)

*Principal Natural Treatments*
   Ginkgo, phosphatidylserine, acetyl-L-carnitine

*Other Natural Treatments*
   Vitamin E, vitamin C, phosphatidylcholine in lecithin, zinc, magnesium, DHEA, inositol, vitamin B$_{12}$, NADH, pregnenolone, vitamin B$_1$

Alzheimer's disease is the most common cause of progressive mental deterioration (dementia) in the elderly. It has been estimated that 30 to 50% of people over 85 years old suffer from this disease.

Microscopic examination shows that nerve cells in the thinking parts of the brain have died and disappeared, particularly cells that release a chemical called acetylcholine. However, we do not know exactly what causes Alzheimer's disease.

Alzheimer's begins with subtle symptoms, such as loss of memory for names and recent events. It progresses from difficulty learning new information, to a few eccentric behaviors, to depression, loss of spontaneity, and anxiety. Over the course of the disease, the individual gradually loses the ability to carry out the activities of everyday life. Disorientation, asking questions repeatedly, and an inability to recognize friends are characteristics of moderately severe Alzheimer's. Eventually, virtually all mental functions fail.

Similar symptoms may be caused by conditions other than Alzheimer's disease, such as multiple small strokes (called multi-infarct dementia), alcoholism, and certain rarer causes. It is very important to begin with an examination to discover what is causing the symptoms of mental decline. Various easily treatable conditions, such as depression, can mimic the symptoms of dementia.

Once the diagnosis of Alzheimer's or non-Alzheimer's dementia has been made, treatment may begin with drugs such as Cognex or Aricept. These medications usually produce a modest improvement in mild to moderate Alzheimer's disease by increasing the duration of action of acetylcholine. However, they can cause sometimes severe side effects due to the exaggeration of acetylcholine's action in other parts of the body.

## PRINCIPAL NATURAL TREATMENTS

There are at least three natural treatments for Alzheimer's disease with significant scientific evidence behind them: ginkgo, phosphatidylserine, and acetyl-L-carnitine.

### Ginkgo: Strong Evidence It Improves Memory and Mental Function

The most well-established herbal treatment for Alzheimer's disease (and, indeed, one of the few herbs that probably deserves the description "proven effective") is the ancient herb *Ginkgo biloba*. **Ginkgo** (page 204), the oldest surviving species of tree, has been traced back 300 million years. Although it died out in Europe during the Ice Age, ginkgo survived in China, Japan, and other parts of East Asia. It has been cultivated extensively for both ceremonial and medical purposes, and some especially revered trees have been lovingly tended for over 1,000 years. Asian herbalists used ginkgo seeds to treat asthma and other conditions.

In Europe, researchers focused on ginkgo leaf, using standardized extracts of it rather than the whole herb. By 1995, ginkgo leaf extract had become the most widely prescribed herb in Germany. Today, German family physicians generally favor it above all drug treatments for dementia.[1]

Ginkgo is also used to treat normal age-related memory loss. Additionally, it may help **intermittent claudication** (page 83), tinnitus, **impotence** (page 77), **depression** (page 54), **macular degeneration** (page 85), and **PMS** (page 104) symptoms, although with much less evidence than for dementia.

### What Is the Scientific Evidence for Ginkgo?

The scientific record for ginkgo is extensive and impressive. According to a 1992 article published in *Lancet,* over 40 double-blind controlled trials had been performed by that date, evaluating the benefits of ginkgo in treating age-related mental decline.[2] Of these studies, which involved about 1,000 participants, eight were rated of good quality and all but one produced positive results. Most of these studies were performed prior to a full recognition of the identity of Alzheimer's disease, but they are presumed to have involved both Alzheimer's and non-Alzheimer's cases. The authors of the *Lancet* article felt that the evidence was strong enough to conclude that ginkgo extract is an effective treatment for severe age-related mental decline.

Studies since 1992 have provided additional evidence for this conclusion.[3,4] Interestingly, German physicians are so certain that ginkgo is effective that they find it difficult to perform scientific studies of the herb. To them, it is unethical to give a placebo to people with Alzheimer's when they could be taking ginkgo instead and have additional months of useful life ahead.[5] This objection does not apply in the United States, where physicians do not prescribe ginkgo.

A recent study published in the *Journal of the American Medical Association* reported the results of a year-long double-blind trial of ginkgo in over 300 people with Alzheimer's or non-Alzheimer's dementia.[6] Participants were given either 40 mg of the ginkgo extract or a placebo 3 times daily. The results showed that 27% of the treated group showed significant improvement on an overall rating scale that evaluates the severity of Alzheimer's disease, compared to only 14% in the placebo group. Also, 40% of those given placebo worsened over the course of the study, whereas only 19% of the treated participants worsened.

The study authors interpret these statistics to mean that in about 20% of cases, ginkgo may slow the development of Alzheimer's disease by 6 months to 1 year. These results do not make ginkgo out to be a miracle cure, but they do confirm that it is a useful treatment for dementia.

The results of one double-blind study suggest that ginkgo might be useful for ordinary age-related memory loss as well.[7]

### How Does Ginkgo Work?

In the past, scientists believed that dementia was caused by a reduced blood and oxygen supply to the brain. Because ginkgo appears to improve circulation (as described in the chapter on **intermittent claudication** [page 83]), European physicians assumed that ginkgo was simply getting more blood to brain cells and thereby making them work better. However, advances in the understanding of age-related mental decline have led scientists to move away from this theory. Ginkgo is now believed to function by directly stimulating nerve cell activity and protecting nerve cells from further injury.[8]

### Dosages

The standard dosage of ginkgo is 40 to 80 mg 3 times daily of a 50:1 extract standardized to contain 24% ginkgo-flavone glycosides.

### Safety Issues

Ginkgo appears to be very safe. Extremely high doses have been given to animals for long periods of time without serious consequences.[9]

In all the clinical trials of ginkgo up to 1991, which have involved almost 10,000 people, the incidence of side effects produced by ginkgo extract was extremely small. Only 21 cases of

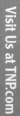

gastrointestinal discomfort were reported, and even fewer cases of headaches, dizziness, and allergic skin reactions.[10]

However, ginkgo is known to "thin" the blood, and highly regarded journals have reported cases of bleeding in the skull and the iris chamber associated with ginkgo use.[11,12] For this reason, ginkgo should not be combined with drugs that also thin the blood, such as Coumadin (warfarin), heparin, Trental (pentoxifylline), or even aspirin. In most German studies of ginkgo, participants were not allowed to take any blood thinners. There may conceivably be risks in combining ginkgo with natural substances that thin the blood as well, such as garlic and high-dose vitamin E, although there have been no reports of such problems. Ginkgo should also be used with caution, if at all, by those with bleeding disorders such as hemophilia, or during the periods before or after surgery and prior to labor and delivery.

Safety for pregnant or nursing women and those with severe liver or kidney disease has not been established.

## Phosphatidylserine:
## Good Evidence of Effectiveness

Like ginkgo, the supplement phosphatidylserine is widely used in Europe to treat various forms of dementia. Phosphatidylserine is one of the many substances involved in the structure and maintenance of cell membranes. While it is tempting to speculate that phosphatidylserine works by strengthening nerve cells against damage, we really don't know how this supplement works.

### What Is the Scientific
### Evidence for Phosphatidylserine?

**Phosphatidylserine** (page 280) appears to produce significant improvements in memory, mental function, and behavior in those with moderate to severe mental decline. The largest study of phosphatidylserine followed 494 elderly individuals in northeastern Italy over a course of 6 months.[13] The benefits produced by phosphatidylserine were roughly comparable to what has been seen with ginkgo.

Other double-blind studies performed over the last decade, involving a total of more than

500 people with age-related cognitive decline, have shown similarly positive results.[14–22]

### Dosages

The standard dosage of phosphatidylserine is 100 mg 2 to 3 times daily; however, some studies have used 200 mg twice daily. After full effects are achieved, a lower dosage of 100 mg daily may be sufficient to maintain good results.

### Safety Issues

Phosphatidylserine is generally regarded as safe. Side effects are rare and are typically limited to mild gastrointestinal distress. However, there are concerns that phosphatidylserine may interact with the blood-thinning drug heparin.[23] Maximum safe doses in young children, pregnant or nursing women, and those with severe liver or kidney disease has not been established.

## Acetyl-L-Carnitine:
## May Be Slightly Helpful

**Carnitine** (page 151) is a vitamin-like substance that is often used for **angina** (page 7), **congestive heart failure** (page 50), and other heart conditions. A special form of carnitine, acetyl-L-carnitine, sometimes called L-acetyl-carnitine, appears to be useful in Alzheimer's disease. Although we don't know precisely how it works, it may mimic the effects of the naturally occurring brain chemical acetylcholine, which is found in lower-than-normal levels in the brains of people with Alzheimer's disease.

### What Is the Scientific
### Evidence for Acetyl-L-Carnitine?

Numerous double- or single-blind studies involving a total of over 1,400 people have evaluated the potential benefits of acetyl-L-carnitine in the treatment of Alzheimer's disease and other forms of dementia.[24–35] Most have found at least mildly positive results. However, the benefits are slight at best, and one of the best studies found no benefit. One of these studies followed 130 people with the clinical diagnosis of Alzheimer's disease for 1 year.[36] The treated group showed a slower rate of deterioration in 13 of 14 measurements of dementia. However, one recent large study failed to find statistically significant benefit.[37] The probable explanation is that acetyl-L-carnitine is only slightly effective.

### Dosages

A typical dosage of acetyl-L-carnitine is 500 to 1,000 mg 3 times daily.

### Safety Issues

Acetyl-L-carnitine appears to be a very safe substance.[38] However, individuals on dialysis should not receive this (or any other supplement) without a physician's supervision. The maximum safe dosages for pregnant or nursing women and those with severe liver or kidney disease have not been established.

## OTHER NATURAL TREATMENTS

Preliminary evidence suggests that **vitamin E** (page 337) at the high dosage of 2,000 IU daily may slow the progression of Alzheimer's disease.[39] A physician's supervision is essential when taking this much vitamin E due to potential risks of bleeding complications.

**Vitamin C** (page 331), phosphatidylcholine in **lecithin** (page 243), **zinc** (page 348), **inositol** (page 231), **magnesium** (page 251), **DHEA** (page 176), **NADH** (page 267), **pregnenolone** (page 284), **vitamin B$_1$** (page 320), and **vitamin B$_{12}$** (page 329) have also been suggested as treatments for Alzheimer's disease. However, there has not yet been sufficient scientific investigation to confirm their effectiveness.

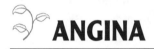

# ANGINA

*Principal Natural Treatments*
   L-carnitine and L-propionyl-carnitine

*Other Natural Treatments*
   Coenzyme Q$_{10}$, magnesium, hawthorn, khella, *Coleus forskohlii*

---

Essentially, angina is a muscle cramp in the heart—the one muscle that cannot take a rest. It develops when the heart muscle does not receive enough oxygen for its needs.

People usually experience angina as a squeezing chest pain, similar to a heavy weight or a tight band, accompanied by sweating, shortness of breath, and possibly pain radiating into the left arm or neck. Usually, angina is brought on by exercise—the more rapidly the heart pumps, the more oxygen it needs. Atherosclerosis (hardening of the arteries) is the most common cause of angina.

Conventional treatment for angina is very effective. Drugs that expand (dilate) the heart's arteries, such as nitroglycerin, can give immediate relief. Other drugs help over the long term by making the heart's work easier. Surgical treatments (such as angioplasty and coronary artery bypass grafting) physically widen the blood vessels that feed the heart.

To prevent heart attacks, current recommendations suggest that most people take daily doses of aspirin, make lifestyle changes such as diet and exercise to lower cholesterol, and reduce other factors that accelerate atherosclerosis.

## PRINCIPAL NATURAL TREATMENTS

Angina is a serious disease that absolutely requires conventional medical evaluation and supervision. No one should self-treat for angina. However, alternative treatments can provide a useful adjunct to standard medical care when monitored by an appropriate health-care professional. I intentionally do not give dosages in this section as they should be individualized by your physician; however, you can find general guidelines in the separate chapters on each substance later in this book.

## L-Carnitine

Double-blind studies suggest that the vitamin-like substance **L-carnitine** (page 151) can relieve angina symptoms. Carnitine plays a role in the cellular production of energy. Although carnitine does not address the cause of angina, it appears to help the heart produce energy more efficiently, thereby enabling it to get by with less oxygen.

In a double-blind study involving 200 participants, carnitine improved angina symptoms in people also taking standard medications.[1] Over the 6 months of the study, the carnitine-treated group showed significant improvement in exercise tolerance and a lower incidence of abnormal electrocardiogram readings. Side effects were negligible. A special form of carnitine known as L-propionyl-carnitine may be even more effective.[2] Consult with your physician regarding dosage and specific safety issues.

## OTHER NATURAL TREATMENTS

**Coenzyme $Q_{10}$ ($CoQ_{10}$)** (page 164) is best known as a treatment for congestive heart failure, but it may offer benefits in angina as well.[3] **Magnesium** (page 251) has also shown some promise.[4] **N-acetyl cysteine** (page 265) may be helpful when taken along with the drug nitroglycerin, but severe headaches may develop.[5,6]

The herbs **hawthorn** (page 222), khella, and *Coleus forskohlii* (page 166) may also be useful, but there is as yet little evidence that they work.

## Lifestyle Approaches

In the long term, restoring your heart's arteries back to normal is the best thing you can do for your angina. The famous Lifestyle Heart Trial, conducted by Dr. Dean Ornish, showed that people who adopt a lowfat vegetarian diet and other healthful lifestyle habits can actually reverse the level of blockage in their coronary arteries.[7]

Absolute vegetarianism is not essential for good results. In general, eating a diet low in red meat and high in whole grains and fresh fruits and vegetables seems wise. Olive oil and canola oil appear to be among the healthiest vegetable oils for use in cooking. For additional suggestions, see the discussion in the chapter on **atherosclerosis** (page 14).

# ANXIETY AND PANIC ATTACKS

*Principal Natural Treatments*
  Kava

*Other Natural Treatments*
  Valerian, skullcap, hops, lemon balm, GABA, selenium, flaxseed oil, general multivitamin, chamomile, passionflower, suma, 5-HTP, gamma oryzanol, inositol (for panic disorder)

As Kierkegaard pointed out long ago, we live in the age of anxiety. Most of us suffer from chronic anxiety to some extent because modern life is jagged, fast-paced, and divorced from the natural rhythms that tend to create a harmonious inner life. The calming cycles of farming, the instinctive satisfactions of hunting and gathering, and pure faith in religion gave our ancestors inner resources that few of us possess today.

People who suffer from the emotional illness called anxiety disorder, however, go a step beyond this common feeling. The quality of their lives is significantly diminished by the pervading presence of fear, which is often unrelated to any obvious cause. Even if a cause can be identified, the magnitude of anxiety they experience is greater than the actual degree of stress.

Typical symptoms of anxiety disorder include feelings of tension, irritability, worry, frustration, turmoil, and hopelessness, along with insomnia, restless sleep, grinding of teeth, jaw pain, an inability to sit still, and an incapacity to cope. Physical sensations frequently arise as well, including a characteristic feeling of being unable to take a full, satisfying breath; dry mouth; rapid heartbeat; heart palpitations; a lump in the throat; tightness in the chest; and cramping in the bowels. Anxiety can also give rise to panic attacks. These may be so severe that they are mistaken for heart attacks. The heart pounds and palpitates, the chest feels tight and painful, and the whole body tenses with unreasoning fear. Such attacks can be triggered by anxiety-provoking situations, but they may also come out of nowhere, perhaps even awakening you from sleep. When a person tends to suffer more from panic attacks than generalized anxiety, physicians call the illness *panic disorder.*

The medical treatment of anxiety involves mainly antianxiety drugs. Some, such as Xanax, are effective immediately; others, such as BuSpar, take a week or more to reach full effect. Antidepressant drugs may also be helpful. Panic attacks are generally more difficult to treat than other aspects of anxiety.

Medications are best used in the short term, and it is advisable to seek more permanent help through psychotherapy.

## PRINCIPAL NATURAL TREATMENTS

The herb **kava** (page 239) is widely used in Europe as a medical treatment for anxiety.

### Kava: Widely Used in Europe for Anxiety

In Europe, the herb kava is widely prescribed for anxiety. Kava is a member of the pepper family that has long been cultivated by Pacific Islanders for use as a social and ceremonial drink. The first description of kava came to the West from Captain James Cook on his celebrated voyages through the South Seas. Cook reported that when village elders and chieftains occasionally gathered for significant meetings, they would hold an elaborate kava ceremony at the beginning to break the ice. Typically, each participant would drink two or three bowls of chewed-up kava mixed with coconut milk. They also drank kava in less formal social settings as a mild intoxicant.

When European scientists learned about kava's effects, they set to work trying to isolate its active principles. However, it was not until 1966 that substances named *kavalactones* were isolated and shown to be effective on their own. One of the most active of these is the chemical dihydrokavain, which has been found to produce a sedative, painkilling, and anticonvulsant action.[1,2,3] Other named kavalactones include kavain, methysticin, and dihydromethysticin.

High doses of kava extracts cause muscular relaxation and, at very high doses, paralysis without loss of consciousness.[4–7] Kava is also a local anesthetic, producing peculiar numbing sensations when held in the mouth.

Germany's Commission E, that country's official herb-regulating body, has authorized the use of kava as a medical treatment for "states of nervous anxiety, tension, and agitation." It is also used for **insomnia** (page 80).

### What Is the Scientific Evidence for Kava?

According to double-blind studies involving a total of about 400 participants, kava appears to be an effective treatment for symptoms of anxiety. The best study was a 6-month double-blind trial that tested kava's effectiveness in 100 individuals with various forms of anxiety.[8] Over the course of the trial, they were evaluated with a list of questions called the Hamilton Anxiety Scale (HAM-A). The HAM-A assigns a total score based on symptoms such as restlessness, nervousness, heart palpitations, stomach discomfort, dizziness, and chest pain. Lower scores indicate reduced anxiety.

Although it took a while for results to develop, by 8 weeks participants who were given kava showed significantly improved HAM-A scores compared to the placebo group. These good results were sustained throughout the duration of the treatment. Interestingly, previous studies had showed a good response in 1 week, especially in menopause-related anxiety.[9,10,11] How fast does kava really work? We will need additional research to know for sure, but you should probably give it a couple of months before deciding whether it works for you.

Another study compared kava against standard antianxiety drugs. For a period of 6 weeks, 174 people with symptoms of anxiety were given either kava or one of two antianxiety medications (oxazepam or bromazepam).[12] Improvement in HAM-A scores was about the same in both groups. However, for technical reasons this study didn't actually prove that kava is equally effective as those standard medications.

Although we don't know exactly how kava functions in the body, its method of action seems to involve brain receptors for a substance known as gamma-aminobutyric acid (GABA).[13] This would make it similar to benzodiazepine drugs like Valium and Xanax. GABA is believed to play a role in anxiety that is somewhat similar to serotonin's role in depression, although there are many gaps in our knowledge.

### Dosages

Kava is usually sold in a standardized form for which the total dose of kavalactones per pill is listed. The dose used should supply about 40 to 70 mg of kavalactones 3 times daily. The total daily dosage should not exceed 300 mg of kavalactones. Be patient, because the benefits may take a while to develop (see What Is the Scientific Evidence for Kava?).

### Safety Issues

When taken appropriately, kava appears to be quite safe. Animal studies have shown that doses up to 4 times the normal dose cause no harm at all, and 13 times the normal dose causes only mild problems in rats.[14]

A study of 4,049 participants who took a rather low dose of kava (70 mg of kavalactones daily) for 7 weeks found side effects in 1.5% of cases.[15] These were mostly mild gastrointestinal complaints and allergic rashes. A 4-week study of 3,029 people, who were given a more realistic 240 mg of kavalactones daily, showed a 2.3% incidence of basically the same side effects.[16]

However, long-term use (months to years) of kava in excess of 400 mg kavalactones daily can create a very distinctive dry, scaly rash called "kava dermopathy."[17] It disappears promptly when the kava use stops.

Studies suggest that kava does not produce mental cloudiness or impair driving ability when used at normal doses;[18–21] however, I still would not recommend driving while taking it.

European physicians have not reported any problems with kava addiction.[22] However, one study in mice suggests that addiction might be possible.[23]

Because high doses of kava can cause inebriation, concern exists that it could become an herb of abuse. There have been reports of young people trying to get high by taking products that they thought contained kava. As it turned out, one of these products, fX, turned out to contain dangerous drugs but no kava at all.

Kava should not be combined with alcohol, prescription antianxiety drugs, sedatives, or other drugs that depress mental function. Reports suggest that the combination of kava and benzodiazepine drugs (in the Valium family) can lead to lethargy and disorientation.[24]

Germany's Commission E warns against the use of kava during pregnancy and nursing. Safety in young children and those with severe liver or kidney disease has also not been established.

### Transitioning from Medications to Kava

If you are taking Xanax or other drugs in the benzodiazepine family, switching to kava will be very difficult. You definitely must seek medical supervision because withdrawal symptoms can be severe and even life-threatening. Additionally, if you are taking Xanax on an "as needed" basis to stop acute panic attacks, kava cannot be expected to have the same rapidity of action.

It is easier to make the switch from milder antianxiety drugs, such as BuSpar, and antidepressants. Nonetheless, a physician's supervision is still strongly advised.

## OTHER NATURAL TREATMENTS

The following natural treatments are widely recommended for anxiety, but they have not been scientifically proven effective at this time.

### Valerian: May Provide Calming Effects

The herb **valerian** (page 315) is best known as a remedy for insomnia. However, according to one preliminary double-blind study, it also produces calming effects in stressful situations.[25] The standard dosage is 2 to 3 g twice daily.

Valerian is generally regarded as safe. However, safety in young children, pregnant or nursing women, and those with severe liver or kidney disease has not been established. At press time, there has been an unconfirmed report of severe withdrawal symptoms after extended use of valerian. (For other comments regarding dosage and safety, see corresponding chapter in Part Two.)

## Other Herbs and Supplements

Other herbs or supplements that are frequently recommended for anxiety include **skullcap** (page 300), **hops** (page 227), **lemon balm** (page 260), **chamomile** (page 156), **passionflower** (page 276), **suma** (page 307), **5-HTP** (page 191),

gamma oryzanol (page 196), and **inositol** (page 231) for panic disorder.

Supplementation with **selenium** (page 297) (200 mcg daily), **flaxseed oil** (page 193) (2 to 6 tablespoons daily), or a general multivitamin are all said to help relieve anxiety symptoms in some people.

## GABA: No Evidence That It Is Effective

Because GABA (gamma–aminobutyric acid) is known to play a central role in anxiety, some alternative practitioners suggest simply taking this amino acid as a supplement. However, no scientific evidence suggests that orally ingested GABA gets to where it can do any good.

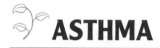

# ASTHMA

*Principal Natural Treatments*
  Tylophora, *Coleus forskohlii*, vitamin C, ephedra (unsafe)

*Other Natural Treatments*
  Vitamin B$_{12}$, quercetin, vitamin B$_6$, antioxidants (vitamin E, beta-carotene, selenium), essential fatty acids (fish oil, flaxseed oil, GLA from evening primrose oil), magnesium, licorice, grindelia, garlic, onions, marshmallow, mullein, *Lobelia inflata,* aloe, chamomile, damiana, elecampane, reishi, betaine hydrochloride, yerba santa

**P**eople who are having an asthma attack have real trouble taking a breath. Many people with stuffy noses from hay fever or colds say, "I can't breathe," but they retain the option of breathing through the mouth. Asthmatics, however, know what "I can't breathe" really means. Instead of their nasal passages, it is the bronchial tubes in their lungs that become swollen and clogged. Breathing can become frighteningly difficult.

Asthma involves two conditions: (1) contraction of the small muscles surrounding the bronchial tubes and (2) swelling of the lining of those tubes. Until recently, treatment usually addressed the first aspect of asthma; but in the last decade, it has become clear that tissue swelling is more fundamental.

Conventional medical treatment for asthma involves bronchodilators, which relax the bronchial muscles, and anti-inflammatory med-

ication, which helps relieve the swelling of tissue. The most effective treatments for reducing this inflammation are steroids, inhalable forms of which have been developed that do not cause as many side effects as oral drugs, such as prednisone. Nonsteroidal drugs, such as cromolyn (Intal), are also available.

The conventional treatment of asthma is highly effective in most cases.

## PRINCIPAL NATURAL TREATMENTS

Perhaps the most promising natural treatment for asthma is the herb tylophora. Another herb, *Coleus forskohlii,* may also be helpful, but it is really more like a drug than an herb. Vitamin C also appears to be somewhat helpful. The Chinese herb ma huang is definitely effective for mild asthma, but it isn't safe.

## Tylophora: A Promising Treatment for Asthma

The herb *Tylophora indica* (also called *Tylophora asthmatica*) appears to offer considerable promise as a treatment for asthma. It has a long history of use in the traditional Ayurvedic medicine of India. In a small 4-week, double-blind study, individuals who were given 40 mg of a tylophora alcohol extract daily for 6 days showed significant improvement, and this improvement only gradually faded away after use of the herb was stopped.[1] Other studies have shown similar results.[2,3] However, these studies are 20 years old or more, and they were not conducted according to modern scientific standards. Larger and better studies are necessary to discover whether tylophora is truly effective.

The typical dosage of tylophora leaf is 200 mg twice daily. Its safety has not been fully evaluated, and for this reason it should not be used by children, pregnant or nursing women, or those with severe kidney or liver disease. Whether tylophora interacts with any drugs is unknown. Tylophora occasionally causes mild digestive distress, mouth soreness, and altered taste sensation.

## *Coleus forskohlii*: May Be Effective, but More Like a Drug Than an Herb

Another herb often recommended for asthma also comes from India, *Coleus forskohlii* (page 166). However, I cannot give it a wholehearted recommendation. *Coleus forskohlii* contains a powerful substance called forskolin, which produces far-reaching effects in the body, perhaps relieving asthma symptoms. Unfortunately, we do not know the implications of all its other effects.

Natural *Coleus forskohlii* contains only small amounts of forskolin. However, manufacturers deliberately modify the herb to dramatically increase its forskolin content, making it more like a drug than an herb. Forskolin appears to be safe, but more studies need to be undertaken before it can be recommended for self-treatment.

## Vitamin C: Appears to Provide Some Benefits

Many studies have been conducted on the effects of **vitamin C** (page 331) in treating asthma.

When you put all the results together, it appears that the regular use of high-dose vitamin C provides some benefits.[4,5] A typical recommended dosage is 1 to 3 g daily, but taking more than 200 mg a day may not add any extra benefits.

Vitamin C has not been definitely associated with any significant harm. However, high-dose vitamin C can cause copper deficiency, so if you take more than 1 to 2 g per day of vitamin C, you should also take 1 to 3 mg of copper daily. Diarrhea is a common side effect at this dosage, but it usually goes away in a week or so. There is no direct evidence that vitamin C poses a risk for people with a history of kidney stones, but caution is recommended.

## Ma Huang: Effective, but Not Safe

The Chinese herb ma huang, also called **ephedra** (page 183), is definitely effective for mild asthma, because it contains the drug ephedrine. However, I cannot recommend using it because of safety concerns. This Chinese herb is a member of a primitive family of plants that look like thin, branching, connected straws. A related species, *Ephedra nevadensis*, grows wild in the American Southwest and is widely called Mormon tea. However, only the Asian species of ephedra contains the active compounds ephedrine and pseudoephedrine.

Ma huang was traditionally used by Chinese herbalists in the early stages of respiratory infections and for the short-term treatment of certain kinds of asthma, eczema, hay fever, narcolepsy, and edema. However, ma huang was not supposed to be taken for an extended period of time, and people with less than robust constitutions were warned to use only low doses or to avoid ma huang altogether.

Japanese chemists isolated ephedrine from ma huang at the turn of the twentieth century, and it soon became a primary treatment for asthma in the United States and abroad. Ephedra's other major ingredient, pseudoephedrine, became the decongestant Sudafed.

Although ephedrine can still be found in a few over-the-counter asthma drugs, physicians seldom prescribe it today. The problem is that ephedrine mimics the effects of adrenaline and causes symptoms such as rapid heartbeat, high blood pressure, agitation, insomnia, nausea, and loss of appetite. The newer asthma drugs are much safer and easier to tolerate. This is a situation in which synthetic drugs are less dangerous than a natural one. I do not recommend using ma huang for asthma.

## OTHER NATURAL TREATMENTS

The following natural treatments for asthma are often widely recommended, but they have not been scientifically proven effective at this time.

### Vitamin B$_{12}$

Supplementation with **vitamin B$_{12}$** (page 329) is said to be effective for asthma.[6] However, the scientific evidence in its favor consists almost entirely of open studies that did not attempt to eliminate the placebo effect.

### Quercetin

The flavonoid **quercetin** (page 288) is often recommended as a treatment for asthma on the basis of test-tube studies that show that it can inhibit the release of inflammatory substances from special cells called mast cells. Because the asthma drugs Intal and Tilade are believed to work in the same way, many natural medicine authorities have often recommended quercetin as an equivalent treatment. However, even though significant direct evidence exists that Tilade and Intal actually work, no such evidence yet exists for quercetin. Interestingly, Intal is derived from a Mediterranean herb named khella.

### Vitamin B$_6$

**Vitamin B$_6$** (page 326) is often mentioned as a treatment for asthma, but the evidence that it works is weak and contradictory. A double-blind study of 76 asthmatic children found significant benefit after 1 month.[7] Children in the treated group were able to reduce their doses of bronchodilators and steroids. However, a recent double-blind study of 31 adults who also used either inhaled or oral steroids did not show any benefit.[8]

The dosages of vitamin B$_6$ used in these studies were quite high, in the range of 200 to 300 mg daily. Because of the risk of nerve injury, it is not advisable to take this much without medical supervision.

### Antioxidants

Antioxidants, such as **vitamin E** (page 337), **beta-carotene** (page 131), and **selenium** (page 297), are frequently recommended for asthma on the grounds that they may protect inflamed lung tissue. However, there is little direct scientific evidence that they work at this time.

### Essential Fatty Acids

Essential fatty acids such as **GLA** (page 210) and those found in **fish oil** (page 188) and **flaxseed oil** (page 193) are suspected to inhibit inflammatory responses such as those that occur in asthma. However, most of the studies that tried fish oil as a treatment for asthma came up with negative results.[9–16]

### Magnesium

**Magnesium** (page 251) is frequently mentioned as a treatment for asthma, but no good studies have shown that oral magnesium is helpful. Some evidence exists that intravenous and inhaled magnesium may offer some short-term benefit,[17,18] but the relevance of these findings to taking magnesium supplements by mouth is unclear.

### Other Herbs and Supplements

Other commonly recommended asthma treatments include the herbs **licorice** (page 244), grindelia, **garlic** (page 197), onions, **marshmallow** (page 256), **aloe** (page 122), **chamomile** (page 156), **damiana** (page 173), **elecampane** (page 182), **reishi** (page 291), **yerba santa** (page 346), and **mullein** (page 264), as well as the supplement **betaine hydrochloride** (page 134). *Lobelia inflata* is a traditional herbal treatment for asthma; but according to traditional directions, it should be taken to the point of vomiting, a process I can hardly recommend.

# ATHEROSCLEROSIS AND HEART DISEASE PREVENTION

### Principal Natural Treatments

Vitamin $B_6$, folic acid, antioxidant supplements (vitamin E, vitamin C [in combination with vitamin E or alone], garlic, selenium, OPCs from grape seed or pine bark, lipoic acid, turmeric, resveratrol, coenzyme $Q_{10}$), lifestyle changes

### Other Natural Treatments

Omega-3 fatty acids (fish oil, flaxseed oil), aortic glycosaminoglycans, bilberry, ginger, ginkgo, hawthorn, chondroitin, astragalus, TMG, lutein, GLA, copper

### Not Recommended Treatments

Beta-carotene

A therosclerosis, or hardening of the arteries, is the leading cause of death in men over age 35 and all people over 45. Most heart attacks and strokes are due to atherosclerosis. Although the origin of this condition is not completely understood, we know that it is accelerated by factors such as high blood pressure or **hypertension** (page 75), high **cholesterol** (page 39), **diabetes** (page 60), smoking, and physical inactivity.

Current theories suggest that atherosclerosis begins with injury to the lining of arteries. High blood pressure physically stresses this lining, while circulating substances such as low-density lipoprotein (LDL) cholesterol, homocysteine, free radicals, and nicotine chemically damage it. White blood cells then attach to the damaged wall and take up residence. Then, for reasons that are not entirely clear, they begin to accumulate cholesterol and other fats. Platelets also latch on, releasing substances that cause the formation of fibrous tissue. The overall effect is a thickening of the artery wall called a fibrous plaque.

Over time, the thickening increases, narrowing the bore of the artery. When blockage reaches 75 to 90%, the person begins to notice **angina** (page 7) symptoms, specifically heart pain. In the lower legs, blockage of the blood flow leads to leg pain during exercise, a condition called **intermittent claudication** (page 83).

Blood clots can develop on the irregular surfaces of the artery and may become detached and block downstream blood flow. Fragments of plaque can also detach. Heart attacks are gener- ally caused by such blood clots, whereas strokes are more often caused by plaque fragments or gradual obstruction. Furthermore, atherosclerotic blood vessels are weak and can burst.

With a disease as serious and progressive as atherosclerosis, the best treatment is prevention. Conventional medical approaches focus on lifestyle changes, such as increasing aerobic exercise, reducing the consumption of saturated fats, and quitting smoking. The regular use of aspirin also appears to be quite helpful by preventing platelet attachment and blood clot formation. If necessary, drugs may be used to lower cholesterol levels or blood pressure.

Recently, conventional medicine has also begun to suggest keeping levels of homocysteine low by adding supplemental folic acid and vitamin $B_6$ to the diet. Consult with your physician for late-breaking information regarding the ideal dose of these supplements. At the time of this writing, recommendations suggest 400 to 800 mcg of folic acid daily along with 10 to 20 mg of vitamin $B_6$.

Because the following material is so complex, I have summarized this information in the section called Putting It All Together. You can skip to it now if you want just the conclusions.

## PRINCIPAL NATURAL TREATMENTS

In the field of preventing atherosclerosis, conventional and alternative approaches overlap. Natural medicine supports (indeed, it first championed) many of the lifestyle changes now encouraged by conventional medicine, and treatments such as **vitamin B$_6$** (page 326) and **folic acid** (page 194) are now widely recommended by physicians. Many other "alternative" approaches for preventing atherosclerosis are on the verge of acceptance into conventional medicine.

Numerous studies have been performed to determine precisely which nutrients are most helpful in preventing atherosclerosis. However, it is tricky to interpret the results of this research.

The most common and potentially most confusing type of study is the *observational study*. As described in the introduction, this type of study follows large groups of people for years and keeps track of a great deal of information about them, including diet. Researchers then examine the data closely and try to identify which dietary factors are associated with better health and longer life.

However, the results can be misleading. For example, if an observational study finds that people who take vitamin supplements live longer, it is not necessarily the vitamins that deserve the credit. Vitamin users also tend to exercise more and to eat more healthful foods, habits that may play a more important role than the vitamins. It is hard to tell.

A more reliable kind of study is the *intervention trial*. In these studies, some people are given a certain vitamin and then compared to others who are given a placebo (or sometimes no treatment at all). The best intervention trials use a double-blind design. The results of intervention trials are far more conclusive than those of observational studies. Unfortunately, they are very expensive to perform, and relatively few have been completed.

This section details the evidence that is available to date. Because this is such a rapidly changing field, new evidence will likely have been found by the time you read this book. Consult a health-care professional for the latest information.

(For other natural treatments that may reduce two important risk factors for atherosclerosis, see the discussions in the chapters on cholesterol and hypertension.)

## Antioxidants: Increasingly Accepted by Conventional Medicine

The body is engaged in a constant battle against damaging chemicals called *free radicals,* or pro-oxidants. These highly reactive substances are believed to play a major role in atherosclerosis, cancer, and aging in general.

To counter the harmful effects of free radicals, the body manufactures antioxidants to chemically neutralize them. However, the natural antioxidant system may not always be equal to the task. Sources of free radicals, such as cigarette smoke and smoked meat, may overwhelm this defense mechanism. In the not-too-distant future, tests of "antioxidant status" may join cholesterol and blood pressure as standard components of preventive medicine screening.

Certain dietary nutrients augment the body's natural antioxidants and may be able to help out when the primary system is under stress. Vitamins E and C and beta-carotene are the best known, but many other substances found in fruits and vegetables are also strong antioxidants.

It appears that antioxidants can help prevent atherosclerosis. However, precisely which ones are most effective remains an area of active study.

## Vitamin E: Dramatically Reduces Heart Attacks

**Vitamin E** (page 337) is the best-documented antioxidant supplement for the prevention of heart disease. Most of the evidence comes from observational studies, but a few intervention trials have shown this as well.

In a double-blind intervention trial of 2,002 people with proven coronary artery disease, 546 were given 800 IU of vitamin E daily, 489 were given 400 IU daily, and 967 were given placebo.[1] Participants were followed for an average of about 18 months. The treated individuals showed an almost 80% drop in nonfatal heart attacks. Curiously, fatal heart attacks were not reduced, for reasons that are unclear.

However, two other very large intervention trials (1,862 and 29,133 participants, respectively) found no benefit.[2,3] These trials involved smokers who were given only about 50 IU of vitamin E daily. It may be that vitamin E, especially at this relatively low dosage, cannot counter the powerful negative influence of smoking.

Observational studies have also given a strong indication that vitamin E can help prevent atherosclerosis. In one study of 11,178 people aged 67 to 105 years, those participants who were taking vitamin E supplements at the beginning of the study were found to have a 34% reduced likelihood of death from heart disease.[4] Vitamin C supplements alone did not seem to make a difference, but the combination of vitamins E and C produced a 53% reduction in risk. Long-term use of vitamin E appeared to be associated with an even greater risk reduction of 63%.

It makes sense that the combination of vitamin C and E would be especially beneficial because vitamin E fights free radicals that dissolve in fats while vitamin C fights those that dissolve in water. Together, the coverage would be expected to be very complete.

In another large observational study, 39,910 U.S. male health professionals were followed for 4 years.[5] Vitamin E supplementation of 100 IU or more daily was associated with a 37% reduced risk of heart disease.

Vitamin E seems to be helpful for women, too. An 8-year study of 87,245 female nurses aged 34 to 59 with no previously diagnosed heart disease found that women who took vitamin E supplements for at least 2 years had a 40% reduced risk of developing coronary disease.[6] Consumption of other antioxidants was not associated with much risk reduction.

Keep in mind, however, that observational studies are not completely reliable. As described previously, people who take supplements also tend to have healthier lifestyle habits, which makes it difficult to interpret the results. We need more, better intervention trials to know for sure.

It is not clear how vitamin E works. One theory points out that vitamin E protects fats and cholesterol from being converted by free radicals into unhealthy chemicals.[7] However, an animal study casts doubt on whether this is really significant.[8] Another possible explanation points to vitamin E's effects on the formation of dangerous blood clots. Like aspirin, which is known to help prevent heart attacks, vitamin E interferes with

the activity of platelets.[9] As mentioned earlier, platelets stick to the walls of blood vessels that have been damaged by atherosclerosis, forming blood clots that can then break off and cause obstructions downstream. Aspirin is believed to help prevent heart attacks and strokes by interfering with blood clots, and vitamin E may do the same.

The optimum dose of vitamin E is not known. A typical recommendation is 400 IU daily. This dosage is generally believed to be safe. However, in one study, vitamin E supplementation was associated with an increase in hemorrhagic stroke, the kind of stroke caused by bleeding.[10] This is not completely surprising considering vitamin E's ability to reduce blood clotting.[11] Certainly, vitamin E should not be combined with aspirin or prescription blood thinners except under a physician's supervision. On the other hand, some evidence exists that combination treatment with vitamin E and aspirin may offer additional benefits in preventing the more common kind of stroke caused by obstruction, so you may want to discuss this whole subject with your physician.[12] I definitely do not recommend taking more than 800 IU daily except on medical advice.

## Vitamin C: Best with Vitamin E

As noted earlier, **vitamin C** (page 331) may offer added benefit when it is combined with vitamin E. However the evidence that vitamin C supplements taken by themselves are helpful for atherosclerosis is weak.[13,14,15] There have been about as many positive as negative studies. Foods containing vitamin C do appear to be helpful, probably because they contain numerous other healthy substances as well.

## Beta-Carotene: Best in Food, Not As a Supplement

The study results involving **beta-carotene** (page 131) are interesting. Beta-carotene is one member of a large category of substances found in foods known as *carotenes*, which are found in high levels in yellow, orange, and dark-green vegetables.

Many studies suggest that eating foods high in carotenes can prevent atherosclerosis.[16] However, isolated beta-carotene in supplement form may not help and could actually increase your risk.

A huge double-blind intervention trial involving 29,133 Finnish male smokers found 11% *more* deaths from heart disease and 15 to 20% *more* strokes in those participants taking beta-carotene supplements.[17] This study was mentioned in the vitamin E section previously. Vitamin E was not found to be helpful, but at least it did not cause harm. Beta-carotene actually increased deaths from heart attacks and strokes. This certainly does not encourage one to take it.

Similar poor results with beta-carotene were seen in another large double-blind study in smokers.[18] Furthermore, beta-carotene supplementation was also found to increase the incidence of angina in smokers.[19]

What is happening here? Clearly, smoking presents a challenge to antioxidants. Vitamin E, so protective in other circumstances, seems to have a difficult time protecting smokers. However, the question remains: Why should beta-carotene not only fail to help but actually worsen the situation?

One possible explanation is that beta-carotene in the diet always comes along with other naturally occurring carotenes. It is quite likely that other carotenoids in the diet are equally or more important than beta-carotene alone.[20] Taking beta-carotene supplements may actually promote deficiencies of other natural carotenes,[21] and overall that may hurt more than it helps.

The moral of the story is that you should eat your vegetables but maybe not take beta-carotene supplements.

## Garlic: Lowers Cholesterol and May Provide Other Benefits

There is moderately strong evidence that **garlic** (page 197) can lower **cholesterol** (page 39), and some evidence indicates that it can reduce **hypertension** (page 75) as well. These two factors strongly suggest that garlic can reduce the risk of atherosclerosis. A few studies suggest that garlic can slow the development of atherosclerosis by other means as well. Garlic is a strong antioxidant, and this may explain some of its benefits.

Garlic preparations have been shown to slow the development of atherosclerosis in rats, rabbits, and human blood vessels, reducing the size of plaque deposits by nearly 50%.[22,23]

A recent observational study of 200 men and women suggests that garlic can do the same in humans as well.[24] Those who were taking 300 mg or more of garlic daily for 2 years showed a distinct improvement in the flexibility of the aorta, the main artery exiting the heart. This suggests a reduced level of atherosclerosis.

Significantly, there was no difference in cholesterol levels or blood pressure between those who regularly consumed garlic and those who did not. Therefore, it appears that garlic may also reduce atherosclerosis by other means besides affecting these two important risk factors.

Because garlic produces a blood-thinning effect, it should not be taken by those on blood thinners such as Coumadin (warfarin), heparin, Trental (pentoxifylline), and perhaps even aspirin except under medical supervision. Garlic might also conceivably cause bleeding problems if combined with other natural substances that mildly thin the blood, such as **ginkgo** (page 204) and high-dose **vitamin E** (page 337). Do not take garlic supplements immediately prior to or after surgery, or before labor and delivery.

## Other Antioxidants: May Be Helpful, but Little Direct Evidence

Many other antioxidant vitamins, supplements, and herbs have been suggested as preventive treatments for atherosclerosis. **Selenium** (page 297), **OPCs** (page 270) from grape seed or pine bark, **lipoic acid** (page 246), **turmeric** (page 311), **resveratrol** (page 292) from red wine and grape skins, and **coenzyme Q$_{10}$** (page 164) are commonly mentioned. However, although a number of interesting studies have suggested that these substances may be beneficial, the state of the evidence is still too preliminary to draw any conclusions.

## Lifestyle Approaches

This fact cannot be emphasized enough: The most important way to prevent atherosclerosis involves lifestyle changes such as quitting smoking, increasing exercise, and adopting a diet high in whole grains, fruits, and vegetables and low in animal products. Olive oil and canola oil are probably among the most healthful of vegetable oils. Heating oils to high temperatures (as in fried foods) can oxidize them and make them less healthful.[25]

It has been suggested that a high level of fish in the diet protects against atherosclerosis. However, doubt has been cast on this idea.[26] Strangely, like beta-carotene, fish appears to be connected with a higher incidence of heart disease in smokers.[27]

However, this subject is very tricky to study. The possible connection between fish and heart disease was so well publicized for a while that people with the worst heart health may have started eating fish on purpose. This may have led to a situation in which the sickest people were eating fish while healthy people were not, completely muddying the results of the studies! Much more remains to be learned on this subject.

The moderate use of alcohol, and specifically red wine, appears to help prevent atherosclerosis, although this is controversial as well.[28–31] Coffee may slightly increase cardiovascular risk,[32] although some studies have shown no effect when other factors, such as smoking and diets high in animal fats (often associated with coffee use), are taken into account.[33] It has been suggested that coffee may raise homocysteine levels.[34] Coffee probably does not have a significant effect on cholesterol levels, although this is debatable as well. See the chapter on cholesterol for further information.

## OTHER NATURAL TREATMENTS

Although the following treatments are widely recommended for atherosclerosis, they cannot be considered scientifically proven at this time.

### Omega-3 Fatty Acids

It has been suggested that omega-3 fatty acids, such as those found in **fish oil** (page 188), can prevent atherosclerosis.[35] However, the overall effects of omega-3 fatty acids are complex and include both positive and negative influences. They appear to significantly decrease serum

triglycerides (a good effect), leave total cholesterol alone (neutral), modestly raise LDL cholesterol (a bad effect), and even more modestly raise high-density lipoprotein, or HDL cholesterol (a good effect).[36] Fish oil may also lower blood pressure, help prevent blood clots, and lower homocysteine levels.[37] However, a recent large study involving more than 2,000 subjects found no effect on blood pressure.[38] The net effect regarding atherosclerosis is unclear.[39,40]

Even if its benefit is unproven, fish oil does appear to be safe. Contrary to some reports, it does not seem to increase bleeding or affect blood sugar control in people with diabetes.[41]

**Flaxseed oil** (page 193) has been suggested as an alternative to fish oil.[42] However, it doesn't lower triglycerides, which appears to be the primary benefit of fish oil.

## Aortic Glycosaminoglycans

**Aortic glycosaminoglycans (GAGs)** (page 125) are substances obtained from the inside lining of the arteries of cows.

According to a recent study, 200 mg per day of GAGs can significantly slow the rate of thickening of arteries.[43] After 18 months of treatment, the additional layering of the inside vessel lining was 7.5 times less in the group receiving GAGs than in the group that did not receive any treatment. Preliminary evidence suggests that this supplement may work in several ways: supplying material for repair of arteries, "thinning" the blood, and improving cholesterol levels.[44,45]

A typical dosage is 50 to 100 mg twice a day. Glycosaminoglycans are regarded as safe because they commonly occur in foods, although extensive safety studies have not been performed. However, if you are taking drugs that powerfully decrease blood clotting, such as Coumadin (warfarin) or heparin, do not use aortic GAGs except under physician supervision. Aortic GAGs interfere slightly with blood clotting, and there is at least a chance that the combination could cause bleeding problems.

### Other Herbs and Supplements

Many herbs appear to decrease platelet stickiness, including **bilberry** (page 135), **ginger** (page 202), **ginkgo** (page 204), **feverfew** (page

186), and **hawthorn** (page 222). Whether this translates into an actual benefit for preventing atherosclerosis remains unknown.

Other treatments sometimes mentioned for atherosclerosis include **chondroitin** (page 159), **astragalus** (page 129), **TMG** (page 310), **lutein** (page 248), **GLA** (page 210), and **copper** (page 169), although there is little evidence as yet that they are helpful.

For other natural substances that may help prevent atherosclerosis by lowering its major risk factors, see the discussions in the chapters on cholesterol and hypertension.

## PUTTING IT ALL TOGETHER

This section is so complicated that I'd like to summarize all the information here in one place.

Little doubt exists that regular exercise and a diet high in fresh fruits and vegetables and low in animal fats can help prevent atherosclerosis. Unheated olive oil and canola oil are probably among the most healthful sources of dietary fat.

Supplemental vitamin E at a dosage around 400 IU daily probably also helps prevent atherosclerosis, and adding vitamin C should provide additional benefit. Supplemental vitamin $B_6$ (10 to 20 mg daily) and folic acid (400 to 800 mcg daily) are probably also helpful because of their effects on homocysteine levels. Garlic, too, appears to be beneficial. The evidence for other herbs and supplements is promising but incomplete at present.

Finally, do not forget to take care of your cholesterol and blood pressure.

# ATTENTION DEFICIT DISORDER

*Principal Natural Treatments*
  There are no well-established natural treatments for attention deficit disorder.

*Other Natural Treatments*
  Calcium, zinc, magnesium, iron, trace minerals, blue-green algae, GABA, glycine, taurine, L-glutamine, L-tyrosine, St. John's wort, inositol, phenylalanine

O riginally, the term *attention deficit disorder* (ADD) referred to children who seemed incapable of concentrating at school. Today, however, the definition has broadened to include many adults as well. Characteristics of ADD include difficulty sustaining attention or completing tasks, easy distractibility, impulsive behavior, and hyperactivity (excessive movement and an inability to sit still). These problems make it difficult to succeed at work or at school.

Conventional treatment focuses on stimulants such as caffeine, Dexedrine, and Ritalin. These drugs produce a paradoxically calming effect in people with ADD, for reasons we don't understand. Certain antidepressants may also be useful.

## NATURAL TREATMENTS

There are no well-documented alternative treatments for ADD. Two authors sympathetic to natural medicine reviewed all the literature in print on a few widely recommended options: supplementation with niacin (or **vitamin B₃** [page 323]), **vitamin B₆** (page 326), and multivitamin and mineral tablets.[1] They failed to find any evidence of a positive effect.

Nonetheless, there are some supplements that certain alternative practitioners feel may be effective. These include **calcium** (page 146); **zinc** (page 348); **magnesium** (page 251); **iron** (page 234); **inositol** (page 231), trace minerals; blue-green algae, and the combined amino acids GABA, glycine, **taurine** (page 308), **L-glutamine** (page 215), **L-phenylalanine** (page 278), and **L-tyrosine** (page 312). **St. John's wort** (page 303) is also sometimes recommended.

# BENIGN PROSTATIC HYPERPLASIA
## (PROSTATE ENLARGEMENT)

*Principal Natural Treatments*
   Saw palmetto, pygeum, nettle root, sitosterol, grass pollen

*Other Natural Treatments*
   Pumpkin seeds, zinc, flaxseed oil

If you're a man, and you live long enough, you will almost certainly develop benign prostatic hyperplasia (BPH). Ninety percent of all men show signs of such prostatic enlargement by the age of 80. Symptoms include difficulty in starting urination, a diminished force of urinary stream, a sensation of fullness in the bladder after urination, and the need to urinate many times at night. Ultimately, the obstruction can become so severe that urination is impossible.

The most common treatment for BPH is surgery that removes most of the prostate gland. Although this surgery is fairly safe, it is traumatic. The drugs Cardura, Flomax, Hytrin, and Proscar can relieve symptoms of BPH. In addition, Proscar has been shown to shrink the prostate and cut by half the need for surgery.

For more information on BPH, see *The Natural Pharmacist Guide to Saw Palmetto and the Prostate.*

## PRINCIPAL NATURAL TREATMENTS

Men who suspect they may suffer from BPH should make sure to see a physician to rule out prostate cancer. After this has been done, many natural options are available that have good scientific backing. Indeed, it's hard to think of another condition for which so many natural therapies have been shown effective.

### Saw Palmetto: A Well-Documented Alternative to Prostate Medications

The best-documented herbal treatment for BPH is the oil of the berry of the **saw palmetto** (page 295) tree. Saw palmetto is a native of North America; although Europeans are the principal consumers of saw palmetto, it is still grown mainly in North America.

Historically, Native Americans used saw palmetto berries for the treatment of various urinary problems in men and for breast disorders in women. European and U.S. physicians took up saw palmetto as a treatment for BPH, but in the United States the herb ultimately fell out of favor.

European interest endured, and in the 1960s French researchers discovered that, by concentrating the oils of the saw palmetto berry, they could maximize the herb's effectiveness. Subsequently, a standardized version of saw palmetto oil became an accepted treatment for prostate enlargement in New Zealand, France, Germany, Austria, Italy, Spain, and other European countries.

This herb is so well accepted in Europe that conventional drugs are considered alternative therapy for BPH! In Germany, saw palmetto is the seventh most common single-herb product prescribed. Studies suggest that benefits will develop after about 4 to 6 weeks of treatment in two-thirds of men who try it.

Saw palmetto offers two potential advantages over conventional drug treatment. The most obvious is that it usually causes no side effects. Another advantage is that saw palmetto does not change protein-specific antigen (PSA) levels. Lab tests that measure PSA are used to screen for prostate cancer. However, the widely used drug Proscar can artificially lower PSA levels, which may have the unintended effect of masking prostate cancer.

Saw palmetto is also sometimes used for chronic prostatitis. However, there is no scientific evidence that it works for this problem.

### What Is the Scientific Evidence for Saw Palmetto?

The scientific evidence for saw palmetto in prostate enlargement is quite impressive, although not perfect.

At least seven double-blind studies involving a total of about 500 participants have compared the benefits of saw palmetto against placebo over a period of 1 to 3 months.[1–7] In all but one of these studies, the herb significantly improved urinary flow rate and most other measures of prostate disease.

A recent double-blind study followed 1,098 men who received either saw palmetto or the drug Proscar over a period of 6 months.[8] According to the results, the two treatments were about equally successful at reducing symptoms, and neither produced much in the way of side effects. However, Proscar lowered PSA levels, presenting a risk of masking prostate cancer (see the previous discussion under the heading Saw Palmetto). Saw palmetto did not cause this problem. On the other hand, Proscar caused men's prostates to shrink by 18%, while saw palmetto only caused a 6% decrease in size, a potential advantage for the drug. Although there are many theories about how saw palmetto works, none have been conclusively established. The best evidence suggests that the herb interferes with male hormones.

### Dosages

The standard dosage of saw palmetto is 160 mg twice daily of an extract standardized to contain 85 to 95% fatty acids and sterols. It can also be taken in one daily dose of 320 mg.[9] Taking more than this dose will not give you better results.

**Note:** Make sure to get a full medical checkup to rule out prostate cancer before you self-treat with saw palmetto. Furthermore, all men over the age of 50 should also continue regular prostate checkups with their physicians.

### Safety Issues

Saw palmetto appears to be essentially nontoxic.[10] It's also nearly side-effect free. In a 3-year study involving 435 participants, only 34 complained of side effects, which were mainly the usual mild gastrointestinal distress.[11] No drug interactions are known.

Safety in pregnancy and nursing has not been established. However, because saw palmetto is intended for men only, this is not a terrible drawback. Those with severe liver or kidney disease should not use saw palmetto (or any other herb) except on the advice of a physician.

## Pygeum: Another Well-Documented Natural Choice

The **pygeum** (page 286) tree is a tall evergreen native to central and southern Africa. Its bark has been used since ancient times for urinary problems. In recent years, pygeum has become a popular European treatment for BPH. It's more widely used in France and Italy than in Germany. However, a comparison study with saw palmetto found that pygeum was not as effective.[12] Pygeum is also more expensive and difficult to grow.

Pygeum is also sometimes used for prostatitis, although there is as yet no significant evidence that it works.

### What Is the Scientific Evidence for Pygeum?

At least nine double-blind trials of pygeum have been performed, involving a total of over 600 participants and ranging in length from 45 to 90 days.[13] Overall, the results make a reasonably strong case that pygeum can reduce symptoms such as nighttime urination, urinary frequency, and residual urine volume. We don't know whether pygeum can reduce the need for prostate surgery or whether it affects PSA levels.

### Dosages

The proper dosage of pygeum is 50 to 100 mg twice daily of an extract standardized to contain 14% triterpenes and 0.5% n-docosanol. It is often sold at a slightly lower dose in combination with saw palmetto.

### Safety Issues

Pygeum appears to be essentially nontoxic, both in the short and the long term.[14] The most common side effect is mild gastrointestinal distress. However, safety in those with severe liver or kidney disease has not been established.

## Nettle Root

Anyone who lives in a locale where **nettle** (page 268) grows wild will likely discover the powers of this dark green plant. Depending on the species,

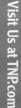

the fine hairs on its leaves and stem cause burning pain that lasts from hours to weeks. Both its leaves and roots can be used as medicine. The root is a popular European treatment for BPH. Over a period of several months, nettle appears to reduce obstruction of urinary flow and decrease the need for nighttime urination.

Nettle leaf (not the root) is sometimes used for **allergies** (page 3).

### What Is the Scientific Evidence for Nettle Root?

Nettle root has not been as well studied as saw palmetto or pygeum.

In a 4- to 6-week double-blind study of 67 men, treatment with nettle root produced a 14% improvement in urine flow and a 53% decrease in residual urine (urine that was not completely expelled from the bladder).[15] Another double-blind study of 40 men showed a significant decrease in frequency of urination after 6 months.[16] A double-blind study of 50 men over 9 weeks showed a significant improvement in urination volume.[17]

### Dosages

According to Germany's Commission E, the proper dosage of nettle root is 4 to 6 g daily of the whole root or a proportional dose of concentrated extract.

### Safety Issues

Nettle root appears to be nearly side-effect free. In one study of 4,087 people who took 600 to 1,200 mg of nettle daily for 6 months, less than 1% reported mild gastrointestinal distress, and only 0.19% experienced allergic reactions (skin rash).[18]

Although detailed safety studies have not been reported, no serious adverse effects have been noted in Germany, where nettle root is widely used. For theoretical reasons, there are some concerns that nettle may interact with conventional medications used for diabetes or high blood pressure, but there are no published reports of such problems occurring.

Safety in those with severe liver or kidney disease has not been established.

### Sitosterol (from *Hypoxis rooperi*)

The South African plant *Hypoxis rooperi* has a long history of native use for bladder and prostate problems. Its tubers contain a family of cholesterol-like compounds called **sitosterols** (page 299), of which the most important is believed to be beta-sitosterolin. In Germany, beta-sitosterol is more widely prescribed for prostate enlargement than saw palmetto.

The scientific evidence for sitosterols is not as strong as that for other BPH treatments widely used in Europe, but there has been at least one solid double-blind study. It followed 200 men with BPH for a period of 6 months.[19] Those treated with sitosterol showed significant improvement in many symptoms of prostate enlargement. Other studies corroborate these results.[20]

The proper dosage of sitosterols should supply 60 to 130 mg daily of beta-sitosterol. Full effects may take 6 months to develop.

Detailed safety studies of sitosterol have not been performed, and safety in those with severe kidney or liver disease has not been established. However, no significant side effects have been observed.[21]

### Grass Pollen

A special extract of grass pollen is widely used in Europe for the treatment of BPH. Although a couple of double-blind and other types of studies have found it to be effective,[22–30] the total evidence is weaker than that for the treatments just described.

Grass pollen extract is just beginning to become widely available in the United States. Look for products that contain rye pollen (*Secale cereale*).

## OTHER NATURAL TREATMENTS

There are a few other treatments often recommended for BPH, but they lack any real scientific evidence. Pumpkin seeds are approved for use in BPH by Germany's Commission E. The mineral **zinc** (page 348) is also commonly recommended in both Europe and the United States as a treatment for prostate disease, as is **flaxseed oil** (page 193). But in the absence of real studies for these treatments I'd suggest sticking with one of the proven herbs above.

# BLADDER INFECTION (URINARY TRACT INFECTION)

*Principal Natural Treatments*
Cranberry, uva ursi

*Other Natural Treatments*
Goldenseal, probiotics, vitamin C, zinc, low-sugar diet, goldenrod, juniper, lapacho, methionine

Bladder infections are a common problem for women, accounting for more than 6 million office visits each year. Men, because of the greater distance between their bladder and urethral opening, only rarely develop bladder infections.

The primary symptoms of a bladder infection are burning during urination, frequency of urination, and urgency to urinate, possibly accompanied by pain in the lower abdomen and cloudy or bloody urine. Occasionally, the infection spreads upward into the kidneys, producing symptoms such as intense back pain, high fever, chills, nausea, and diarrhea.

Conventional treatment for bladder infections consists of appropriate antibiotic treatment guided by urine culture. At press time, a report was released suggesting that it is appropriate for women with frequent bladder infections to have on hand a prescription for antibiotics for the purpose of self-treatment when symptoms arise. Women who have had extremely frequent bladder infections sometimes take antibiotics continuously to prevent the condition.

## PRINCIPAL NATURAL TREATMENTS

Women who do not want to use antibiotics may be able to find some help through the use of herbs. However, if symptoms do not improve or signs of a kidney infection develop, medical attention is essential to prevent serious complications.

### Cranberry: May Help Prevent Infections

**Cranberry** (page 170) juice is commonly used to prevent bladder infections as well as to overcome low-level chronic infections. The cranberry plant is a close relative of the common blueberry. Native Americans used it both as food and as a treatment for bladder and kidney diseases. The Pilgrims learned about cranberry from local tribes and quickly adopted it for their own use. Subsequent physicians used it for bladder infections, for "bladder gravel," and to remove "blood toxins."

In the 1920s, researchers observed that drinking cranberry juice makes the urine more acidic. Because common urine infection bacteria such as *E. coli* dislike acid surroundings, physicians concluded that they had discovered a scientific explanation for the traditional uses of cranberry. This discovery led to widespread medical use of cranberry juice for bladder infections. Cranberry fell out of favor after World War II, only to return in the 1960s as a self-treatment for bladder infections.

More recent research has revised the conclusions reached by scientists in the 1920s. It appears that acidification of the urine is not so important as cranberry's ability to interfere with the bacteria establishing a foothold on the bladder wall.[1–4] If the bacteria can't hold on, they will be washed out with the stream of urine. Furthermore, studies suggest that in women who frequently develop bladder infections, bacteria have an especially easy time holding on to the bladder wall.[5]

When taken regularly, cranberry juice may fix this problem and break the cycle of repeated infection. Cranberry juice also seems to be helpful for chronic bladder infections, those that continue for months with few to no symptoms.

### What Is the Scientific Evidence for Cranberry?

A 6-month study followed 153 women with an average age of 78.5 years.[6] This study looked at chronic bladder infections rather than acute bladder infections. Chronic bladder infections are relatively common in older women and may cause few or no symptoms. The evidence suggests that cranberry can eliminate continuing infections.

Half of the participants were given a standard supermarket cranberry cocktail, and the other

**Bladder Infection**

half were given a placebo drink prepared to look and taste the same. Both treatments contained the same amount of vitamin C, which was important because vitamin C itself may have some antibacterial effects.

Commercial cranberry cocktail is mostly sugar and contains little cranberry juice. It is natural to wonder whether straight cranberry juice would have been more effective. Nonetheless, the results suggest that even cranberry juice cocktail can prevent chronic bladder infections, as well as eliminate ones that have already begun.

There was a 58% lower rate of bacteria in the urine of the women treated with cranberry as compared to those given placebo. Also, if a woman had bacteria in the urine at one point in the study, the chance that she would still have it a month later was 73% lower in the cranberry group.

This study has been criticized for several flaws in its design, especially the method used to analyze the urine. It also doesn't tell us whether regular use of cranberry will prevent ordinary acute bladder infections. Nonetheless, it definitely suggests that cranberry juice does have real potential in the treatment of bladder infections.

## Dosages

The proper dosage of dry cranberry juice extract is 300 to 400 mg twice daily. For those people who prefer juice, 8 to 16 ounces daily should be enough. For best effect, use true cranberry juice, not sugary cranberry juice cocktail.

## Safety Issues

There are no known risks associated with this food for adults, children, and pregnant or nursing women. However, excessive use of cranberry juice may weaken the effect of slightly alkaline drugs, such as many antidepressants and prescription painkillers, by causing them to be excreted more rapidly in the urine.

## Uva Ursi: Appears to Be Effective for Acute Bladder Infections

While cranberry is most often used to prevent bladder infections or to treat simmering chronic infections, **uva ursi** (page 313), also known as bearberry, can be used to treat the classic painful, acute bladder infection. Uva ursi has a long history of use for urinary conditions in both America and Europe. Until the development of sulfa antibiotics, its principal active component, arbutin, was frequently prescribed by physicians as a treatment for bladder and kidney infections.

The uva ursi plant is a low-lying evergreen bush whose berries are a favorite of bears, thus the name bearberry. However, it is the leaves that are used medicinally. We do not know for sure how uva ursi works. It appears that the arbutin contained in uva ursi leaves is broken down in the intestine to another chemical, hydroquinone. This is altered a bit by the liver and then sent to the kidneys for excretion.[7] Hydroquinone then acts as an antiseptic in the bladder.

The European Scientific Cooperative on Phytotherapy (ESCOP) is a scientific organization assigned the task of harmonizing herb policy among European countries. ESCOP recommends uva ursi for "uncomplicated infections of the urinary tract such as cystitis when antibiotic treatment is not considered essential."[8]

**Warning:** This herb is definitely not appropriate for kidney infections. If you develop symptoms such as high fever, chills, nausea, vomiting, diarrhea, or severe back pain, get medical assistance immediately.

Furthermore, hydroquinone can be toxic (see Safety Issues). For this reason it is not a good idea to take uva ursi for a long period of time.

### What Is the Scientific Evidence for Uva Ursi?

Surprisingly little research has been done on uva ursi.[9]

**Treatment**    No double-blind studies have evaluated the clinical effectiveness of uva ursi. Two studies evaluated the antibacterial power of the urine of people who were taking uva ursi and found activity against most major bacteria that infect the urinary tract.[10,11]

**Prevention**    One double-blind study followed 57 women for 1 year.[12] Half were given a standardized dose of uva ursi, and the others received placebo. Over the course of the study, none of the women on uva ursi developed a bladder infection, whereas five of the untreated women did. However, most experts do not believe that continuous treatment with uva ursi is a good idea.

### Dosages

The dosage of uva ursi should be adjusted to provide 400 to 800 mg of arbutin daily.[13,14,15] This dosage should not be exceeded. If the herb is not successful within 1 week, you should definitely seek medical attention. No more than 2 weeks of treatment with uva ursi is recommended even under medical supervision, and it should not be used more than five times a year. Uva ursi should be taken with meals to minimize gastrointestinal upset.

Interestingly, research suggests that arbutin's antibiotic activity depends on the presence of alkaline urine. Many women take vitamin C during bladder infections to acidify the urine and, it is hoped, inhibit the bacteria. However, this may tend to block the effect of uva ursi. For this reason, it may be counterproductive to use both uva ursi and vitamin C. Conversely, supplements thought to alkalinize the urine may improve uva ursi's effectiveness. These include calcium citrate, calcium gluconate, and baking soda.

### Safety Issues

Unfortunately, hydroquinone is a liver toxin, a carcinogen, and an irritant.[16–19] For this reason, uva ursi is not recommended for young children, pregnant or nursing women, and those with severe liver or kidney disease.

However, significant problems are rare among people using uva ursi products in appropriate dosages for a short period of time. Gastrointestinal distress (ranging from mild nausea and diarrhea to vomiting) can occur, especially with prolonged use.[20]

## OTHER NATURAL TREATMENTS

The following treatments are often proposed as treatments for bladder infections, but there is as yet little to no scientific confirmation of their effectiveness.

### Goldenseal

The herb **goldenseal** (page 217) is widely recommended for bladder infections, based on the antibiotic properties of its ingredient berberine. However, we don't know for sure if, when goldenseal is taken by mouth, enough berberine accumulates in the bladder to do anything.

In the past, herbalists would instill goldenseal preparations directly into the bladder, a process that I do not recommend trying yourself. The safety of goldenseal in young children, pregnant or nursing women, and those with severe liver or kidney disease has not been established. For other potential safety issues, see the chapter on goldenseal.

### Probiotics

Probiotics, or "friendly bacteria," particularly those found in live yogurt such as *Lactobacillus* **acidophilus** (page 120), *Bifido bacterium bifidum* (bifidus for short), and *Lactobacillus bulgaricus*, may also be useful in preventing bladder infections. Many bladder infections are caused by the migration of vaginal and rectal bacteria into the urinary tract. When friendly bacteria are present, pathogenic, or disease-causing, bacteria have a difficult time proliferating. Friendly bacteria may be taken orally or introduced in the form of a douche.

Unfortunately, the quality control of acidophilus supplements seems to be very poor. Unless you have a home microbiology lab, it will be difficult for you to tell whether the acidophilus you are buying is really alive. Live culture yogurt may be preferable, unless your store can supply documentation proving that its acidophilus is still alive at time of purchase.

### Other Supplements

Many nutritionally oriented physicians believe that regularly taking **vitamin C** (page 331) and **zinc** (page 348) supplements and decreasing sugar in the diet will help improve immunity against bladder infections. The herbs **goldenrod** (page 216), **juniper** (page 238), cleavers, buchu, and **lapacho** (page 242) and the supplement **methionine** (page 261) may also be helpful.

# CANCER PREVENTION (REDUCING THE RISK)

## Principal Natural Treatments

Vitamin E, selenium, garlic, tomatoes (lycopene), vitamin C, green tea, soy (protein and/or isoflavones)

## Other Natural Treatments

Folic acid, vitamin D, flaxseed oil (lignans), grapes (resveratrol), sulforaphane, turmeric, rosemary, licorice, ginseng, bromelain, melatonin, ellagic acid, quercetin, citrus juices, betulin, papaw tree bark, blue-green algae, probiotics, OPCs, calcium

## Not Recommended Treatments

Beta-carotene

Cancer is the second major cause of death (next to heart disease) in the United States. It claims the lives of more than half a million Americans a year out of the nearly 1.4 million who get the disease. The probability of getting cancer increases with age. Two-thirds of all cases are in people older than 65.[1]

According to the American Cancer Society, one in two men and one in three women will face cancer during their lifetimes. However, it appears that you significantly cut your cancer risk by how you choose to lead your life. That is the bright consensus of an international panel recently convened by the American Institute for Cancer Research and the World Cancer Research Fund.[2]

The panel found four key ways to reduce the odds of getting cancer: Eat the right foods, exercise, watch your weight, and do not smoke. The experts reviewed diet and cancer findings from over 4,500 studies to reach this consensus.

## WHAT CAUSES CANCER?

Cancer is believed to begin with a mutation in a single cell. However, a cell doesn't become cancerous overnight. Several mutations in a row are necessary to create all the characteristic features of cancer. Ordinarily, cells have a self-destruct mechanism that causes them to die when their DNA is damaged. However, in developing cancer cells, something interferes with the self-destruct sequence. It may be that the cancer-causing mutations themselves turn off the countdown.

The DNA alterations that create a cancer cell give it a certain independence from the ordinary rules of cell behavior. Normal cells are highly influenced by nearby cells, with the result that they "get along" well with their neighbors. For example, the growth of a healthy cell is ruled by special growth factors given off by surrounding tissues. However, cancer cells either grow without such growth factors or simply make their own. Many types of cancer cells can also trigger the growth of new blood vessels to feed them.

Cancerous mutations appear to be caused mainly by exposure to carcinogenic substances, of which tobacco is the most common. Many carcinogens exist in the diet as well, such as salt-cured and smoked meats.

Free radicals also appear to play a major role in promoting cancer. These chemically unstable substances are produced by many factors, and are believed to affect heart disease and aging (for more information about free radicals in general, see the chapter on **atherosclerosis** [page 14]). The best documented natural treatments for preventing cancer have antioxidant properties.

Hormones can also help cancer get a start. For example, a newly formed cancer of the prostate or the breast is stimulated by the hormones that ordinarily control tissue in that part of the body. This is why estrogen-replacement therapy can increase the risk of breast cancer and why estrogen suppression is often recommended for women with a history of breast cancer. Substances found in soy may help reduce the incidence of certain cancers by blocking the effects of estrogen and other hormones.

The key to preventing cancer is to minimize your exposure to carcinogens. Quitting smoking is essential, and reducing your intake of smoked, charred, pickled, and salt-cured meats is also believed to be helpful. Eating a diet that is high in fruits, vegetables, and whole grains and low in saturated fat (found primarily in dairy and meat) also lowers your chance of developing cancer.[3] Vegetables in the broccoli family may be particularly helpful.

When it comes to natural cancer prevention, conventional and natural medicine are converging. The dietary suggestions listed previously were originally championed by "alternative" physicians, but they are all presently mainstream. Furthermore, many of the supplements described here are rapidly entering the mainstream as well.

Because the following material is so complex, I have summarized it in the section titled Putting It All Together. You can skip to it now if you want just the conclusions.

For more information, you can also read *The Natural Pharmacist Guide to Reducing Cancer Risk.*

## PRINCIPAL NATURAL TREATMENTS

It is rather difficult to prove that taking a certain supplement will reduce the chance of developing cancer. You really need enormous long-term studies in which some people are given the supplement while others are given placebo. We do have evidence of this type for vitamin E and selenium. These two supplements definitely appear to lower the risk of certain kinds of cancer.

For other supplements, the evidence is more circumstantial. Observational studies have found that people who happen to take in high levels of certain vitamins or herbs in their diets develop a lower incidence of specific cancers. These results are less reliable because such people may also have other healthy lifestyle habits. Researchers attempt to factor out these other influences, however.

Evidence of this type suggests that the herb garlic may reduce the odds of cancer, perhaps because it contains a lot of selenium. Vitamin C supplements do not appear to be very effective, but a substantial intake of vitamin C and beta-

carotene in the form of fruits and vegetables does seem to reduce the incidence of cancer significantly. Beta-carotene taken as a supplement may actually be harmful.

## Vitamin E: Probably Reduces the Odds of Several Types of Cancer

**Vitamin E** (page 337) has the best evidence behind it of any supplement suggested as a preventive treatment for cancer.

In an intervention trial (see the introduction for the definition of an intervention trial) that involved 29,133 smokers, those who were given 50 mg of vitamin E daily for 5 to 8 years showed a 32% reduction in the incidence of prostate cancer and a 41% drop in prostate cancer deaths.[4] Surprisingly, results were seen soon after the beginning of supplementation. This was unexpected because prostate cancer grows very slowly. A cancer that shows up today actually started to develop many years ago. The fact that vitamin E almost immediately lowered the incidence of prostate cancer suggests that it somehow blocks the step at which a hidden prostate cancer makes the leap to being detectable.

The same study also showed that vitamin E supplementation reduced colon cancer by 16%.

The dose of vitamin E used in this study, which corresponds to about 50 to 75 IU of vitamin E, is lower than is usually recommended. It is quite reasonable to assume that a higher dose would be more effective, although this has not been proven.

Observational studies have also shown benefit. Researchers at the Fred Hutchinson Cancer Research Center in Seattle determined that supplemental vitamin E (200 IU or more daily) cut colon cancer risk by 57%.[5,6] Other studies have shown reductions ranging from 29 to 68%, depending on the length of time the participants used vitamin E, as well as other factors.[7,8]

Similarly good results have been seen in stomach cancer; mouth, throat, and laryngeal cancer; and liver cancer.[9–12] However, vitamin E does not appear to be strongly effective against lung cancer.[13]

Vitamin E is typically supplemented at a dose of 400 to 800 IU daily. Realistically, you can't get

this much vitamin E in your diet, so supplements are necessary.

Vitamin E is generally believed to be safe at this dosage level. However vitamin E is known to affect blood clotting and for this reason should not be combined with aspirin or prescription blood thinners except under a physician's supervision.[14] Vitamin E may also present some risk of bleeding on its own. In one study, vitamin E supplementation was associated with an increase in hemorrhagic stroke, the kind of stroke caused by bleeding.[15] For this reason, doses above 800 IU daily should only be used on the advice of a physician.

## Selenium: May Protect Against Lung, Prostate, and Colon Cancer

It has long been known that severe **selenium** (page 297) deficiency increases the risk of cancer.[16] However, by itself, this does not prove that taking selenium supplements will make a difference if you are not deficient in it.

However, a recent double-blind study did find that selenium supplements can dramatically reduce the incidence of cancer. The results were so impressive they caught the researchers by surprise. The study was actually designed to detect selenium's effects on skin cancer.[17] It followed 1,312 individuals, half of whom were given 200 mcg of selenium daily. The participants were treated for an average of 2.8 years and were followed for about 6 years. Although no significant effect on skin cancer was found, the researchers were startled when the results showed that people taking selenium had a 50% reduction in overall cancer deaths and significant decreases in cancer of the lung (40%), colon (50%), and prostate (66%). The findings were so remarkable that the researchers felt obliged to break the blind and allow all the participants to take selenium.

While this evidence is very promising, further research needs to be done to definitively confirm it.

For cancer prevention, the usual recommended therapeutic dosage of selenium is 100 to 200 mcg daily. Of the various sources of selenium, organic forms, such as selenomethionine, selenium-rich yeast, and selenium-enriched garlic, may be preferable to inorganic sodium selen-

ite.[18,19] However, this is a bit controversial.[20,21] When taken at the recommended dosage, selenium is believed to be safe and side-effect free. Long-term use of selenium at a level of 200 mcg daily has been shown to be safe in adults, and doses up to 350 mcg daily are believed to be harmless.[22] Toxic effects begin to be seen at levels above 900 mcg daily and include gastrointestinal distress, central nervous system changes, garlic-like breath odor, and loss of hair and fingernails.

Maximum safe dosages in young children, pregnant or nursing women, and those with severe liver or kidney disease have not been established.

## Garlic: May Reduce the Risk of Colon Cancer

A great deal of evidence from observational studies (see the introduction for the definition of an observational study) suggests that **garlic** (page 197) may help prevent cancer.

In the Iowa Women's Study, a very large and well-conducted observational study, women who ate significant amounts of garlic were found to be about 30% less likely to develop colon cancer.[23] Similar results were seen in other observational studies performed in China, Italy, and the United States.[24,25]

We do not know for sure how garlic might work to prevent cancer. Like vitamin E, whole garlic possesses antioxidant properties.[26,27] Furthermore, various garlic extracts have also been shown to suppress the known DNA-damaging activity of several drugs and toxins.[28] Finally, garlic contains high levels of selenium, which is thought to reduce the risk of cancer (see the previous discussion under the heading Selenium).[29]

It's unclear how much garlic is needed for a cancer-preventive effect, but one or two cloves daily should probably suffice. Side effects (other than bad breath) are rare, and garlic is on the FDA's list of agents that are generally regarded as safe. However, raw garlic in excessive doses can cause stomach upset, heartburn, nausea and vomiting, diarrhea, facial flushing, rapid heartbeat, and insomnia. Garlic appears to interfere with blood clotting, so it should not be combined with blood-thinning drugs such as Coumadin (warfarin), Trental (pentoxifylline), or even aspirin except under medical supervision, nor should it be taken around the time of surgery or labor and delivery. There might also be some risk involved in combining garlic with other blood-thinning herbs or natural supplements, such as **ginkgo** (page 204) and high-dose **vitamin E** (page 337), although no problems have been reported.

## Beta-Carotene: Helpful in the Diet, Harmful As a Supplement?

In the early 1980s, a review of the observational studies clearly showed that people whose diets are high in fruits and vegetables have a significantly decreased risk for cancer.[30,31] Some of the strongest evidence relates to lung cancer, for which a high intake of fruits and vegetables was associated with as much as a 70% reduced risk.

Scientists then set about trying to identify the active principle in fruits and vegetables. One group of substances widely available in these foods are carotenes (named after carrots). A careful examination of the data suggests that the level of carotenes in the diet is strongly connected with protection against lung cancer.[32] Evidence also suggests that carotenes protect against bladder cancer,[33] breast cancer,[34] esophageal cancer,[35] and stomach cancer.[36]

The best-known carotene is **beta-carotene** (page 131), a strong antioxidant that the body can convert to **vitamin A** (page 318). It was a natural step to assume that it was the beta-carotene in these foods that was making the difference. In animal studies, beta-carotene supplements seemed to significantly reduce the incidence of cancer.[37] Unfortunately, studies in which people were actually given beta-carotene supplements (rather than foods containing it) have not shown wonderful results.

The anticancer bubble burst for beta-carotene in 1994 when the results of the Alpha-Tocopherol, Beta-Carotene (ATBC) study came in. Apparently, beta-carotene did not prevent but actually *increased* the risk of getting lung cancer by 18%. This intervention trial had followed 29,133 male smokers in Finland who took supplements of either about 50 IU of vitamin E (alpha-tocopherol) or 20 mg of beta-carotene, or both, or a placebo

daily for 5 to 8 years.[38] This was the same study mentioned previously in which vitamin E reduced the risk of prostate and colon cancer; however, beta-carotene worked in the opposite direction.

In January 1996, researchers monitoring the Beta-Carotene and Retinol Efficacy Trial (CARET) confirmed this bad news with more of their own: The beta-carotene group had 46% more cases of lung cancer deaths.[39] This study involved smokers, former smokers, and workers exposed to asbestos.

Alarmed, the National Cancer Institute (NCI) pushed the brake pedal on the $42 million trial 21 months before it was finished. At about the same time, the 12-year Physicians' Health Study of 22,000 male physicians was finding that 50 mg of beta-carotene taken every other day had no effect at all—good or bad—on the risk of cancer or heart disease.[40] In this study, 11% of the participants were smokers, and 39% were ex-smokers.

Interestingly, in both the ATBC study and the CARET study, higher levels of carotene intake from the diet *were* associated with lower levels of cancer. Apparently, beta-carotene is not effective alone. Other carotenes found in fruits and vegetables appear to be more important for preventing cancer (see, for example, following discussion on lycopene). It is possible that taking beta-carotene depletes the body of other carotenes, thereby producing an overall harmful effect.[41]

These studies also found that beta-carotene supplements may increase the risk of heart disease and stroke as well. Therefore, I recommend getting your beta-carotene from foods, rather than supplements. The best dietary sources of carotenes are yellow-orange vegetables and dark-green vegetables.

## Tomatoes (Lycopene): May Be More Important Than Beta-Carotene

**Lycopene** (page 249), a carotenoid like beta-carotene, is found in high levels in tomatoes and pink grapefruit. Lycopene appears to exhibit about twice the antioxidant activity of beta-carotene and may be more important for preventing cancer than the better known vitamin.

In one study, elderly Americans consuming a diet high in tomatoes reduced their risk for

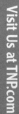

cancers by 50%.[42] Men and women who ate at least seven servings of tomatoes weekly developed less stomach and colorectal cancers compared to those who ate only two servings weekly.

In another study, 47,894 men were followed for 4 years in an observational study looking for influences on prostate cancer.[43] Their diets were evaluated on the basis of how often they ate fruits, vegetables, and foods containing fruits and vegetables. High levels of tomatoes, tomato sauce, and pizza in the diet were strongly connected to the prevention of prostate cancer. After an evaluation of known nutritional factors in these foods as compared to other foods, lycopene appeared to be the common denominator. Additional impetus has been given to this idea by the discovery of lycopene in reasonably high levels in the human prostate.[44] Cooked tomatoes appear to be more bioavailable (more readily used by the body) than raw tomatoes, especially when the tomatoes are cooked in oil. Tomato juice does not seem to be helpful.

## Vitamin C: Helpful in the Diet, Not Helpful As a Supplement?

As with beta-carotene, most of the positive studies of **vitamin C** (page 331) and cancer prevention have looked at the effect of vitamin C in the diet rather than at actual vitamin C supplements. It is possible the other plant substances that come along with vitamin C are equally or more important. Studies involving vitamin C supplements have not produced stellar results.

Several studies have found a strong association between high dietary vitamin C intake and a reduced incidence of stomach cancer.[45,46,47] One way in which vitamin C may work is by preventing the formation of carcinogenic substances known as N-nitroso compounds in the stomach.

Evidence also suggests that vitamin C from food may also provide a protective effect in colon, esophageal, laryngeal, bladder, cervical, rectal, breast, and perhaps lung cancer.[48–52] However, dietary vitamin C intake does not appear to be associated with protection against prostate cancer.[53]

A few studies have used supplemental vitamin C instead of dietary vitamin C. One found that

vitamin C supplementation at 500 mg or more daily was associated with a lower incidence of bladder cancer.[54] However, another study found no connection.[55]

Supplemental vitamin C at 1 g daily failed to prevent new colon cancers after one colon cancer had developed.[56] In another large observational study, 500 mg or more of vitamin C daily over a period of 6 years provided no significant protection against breast cancer.[57] Another study found similar results.[58]

Thus, just as with beta-carotene, it may be that the natural dietary substances that come along with vitamin C are more important for cancer prevention than the vitamin alone. In this case, water-soluble flavonoids may be responsible for the benefit. Eat your fruits and vegetables!

## Green Tea: May Help Prevent Many Types of Cancer

Both **green tea** (page 220) and black tea come from the tea plant called *Camellia sinensis,* which has been cultivated in China for centuries. The key difference between the two is in preparation. For black tea, the leaves are allowed to oxidize, a process believed to lessen the potency of therapeutic compounds known as polyphenols. Green tea is made by lightly steaming the freshly cut leaf, a process that prevents oxidation and possibly preserves more of the therapeutic effects.

Laboratory and animal studies suggest that tea consumption protects against cancers of the stomach, lung, esophagus, duodenum, pancreas, liver, breast, and colon.[59] A 1994 study of skin cancer in mice found that both black and green teas, even decaffeinated versions, inhibited skin cancer in mice exposed to ultraviolet light and other carcinogens.[60,61] After 31 weeks, mice given the teas brewed at the same concentration humans drink had 72 to 93% fewer skin tumors than mice given only water.

However, results from human studies have not been so clear-cut—some have shown a protective effect, and others have not. Nonetheless, the overall weight of the evidence does lean toward the positive side.[62]

One study followed 8,552 Japanese adults for 9 years.[63] Women who drank more than 10 cups daily had a delay in the onset of cancer and also a 43% lower total rate of cancer occurrence. Males had a 32% lower cancer incidence, but this finding was not statistically significant.

A study in Shanghai, China, found that those who drank green tea had significant reductions in the risk of developing cancers of the rectum and pancreas. No significant decrease in colon cancer was found.[64] A total of 3,818 residents aged 30 to 74 were included in the population study. For men, those who drank the most tea had a 28% lower incidence of rectal cancer and a 37% lower incidence of pancreatic cancer compared to those who did not drink tea regularly. For women, the respective reductions in cancer frequency were even greater: 43% and 47%.

Another study in Shanghai found similar results for stomach cancer. Green tea drinkers were 29% less likely to get stomach cancer than nondrinkers, with those drinking the most tea having the least risk.[65] Interestingly, the risk of stomach cancer did not depend on the person's age at which he or she started drinking green tea. Researchers suggested that green tea may disrupt the cancer process at both the intermediate and the late stage.

However, this is a rapidly evolving field, and at press time new information has been released suggesting that there were significant flaws in the green tea studies just described. Other recent evidence indicates that black tea may be more protective than green tea. I suggest talking to your physician about the latest information.

The active ingredients in green tea are believed to be polyphenols, especially one known as epigallocatechin gallate (EGCG). Like vitamin C, polyphenols may block the formation of nitrosamines and other cancer-causing compounds and may trap or detoxify carcinogens.[66] Green tea may also exert an estrogen-blocking effect that is helpful in preventing breast and uterine cancer.[67]

The optimum dosage of green tea is unknown. However, you might want to use the amount correlated with good results in the observational studies. That would mean either drinking 3 cups of green tea daily or taking 100 to 150 mg 3 times daily of a green tea extract standardized for 80% total polyphenols and 55% epigallocatechin content. No significant side effects are associated with green tea, other than those due to its (rather low) caffeine content.

## Soy: May Reduce the Risk of Hormone-Related Cancers

In many animal studies, soybeans, soy protein, or other soy extracts decreased cancer risk, and observational studies show that the same effect may occur in people as well.[68–71] According to the data that we have, soy may help prevent hormone-related cancers such as prostate, breast, and uterine cancer.

Soybeans provide estrogen-like compounds known as **isoflavones** (page 236), especially genistein and daidzein. These substances bind to the same sites in the body as estrogen, occupying these sites and keeping natural estrogen away. Estrogen stimulates certain forms of cancer, but soy estrogens exert a milder estrogen-like effect that may not stimulate cancer as much as natural estrogen. This may partially explain soy's apparent protective effect.[72,73] Soy or soy extracts may also affect cancers in other ways, but more remains to be discovered.

However, in observational studies, it is difficult to tell whether the soy is exerting a directly positive effect on its own or whether some of the benefit is due to the fact that people who eat more soy also eat less meat. For more definitive results, we need studies in which soy or soy extracts are added to the diets of a large group of people while another group is given placebo treatment. Unfortunately, this type of research into soy is still in its infancy.

One or two tofu "burgers" or cups of soy milk daily may be enough to produce a beneficial effect. Soy foods are believed to be safe, although high doses of soy can interfere with mineral absorption. There is also some concern that soy may not be advisable for women who have already had breast cancer.

You can also take concentrated soy protein or soy isoflavones at a dosage of 40 to 60 mg daily.

## OTHER NATURAL TREATMENTS

The substances mentioned in this section have less evidence behind them than the antioxidants

just discussed. However, this is a rapidly growing field. By the time you read this book, new information will undoubtedly be available.

## Folic Acid

**Folic acid** (page 194) deficiency may predispose individuals toward developing cervical cancer,[74] colon cancer,[75,76] lung cancer,[77] and mouth cancer.[78] However, we know very little about whether taking folic acid supplements will help prevent these diseases.

Nonetheless, a deficiency of this essential vitamin is quite common, and if you don't eat a lot of dark-green, leafy vegetables, you will probably find overall benefits from a bit of folic acid supplementation.

A typical dosage is 400 mcg daily. Folic acid is safe, but because it can mask vitamin $B_{12}$ deficiency, it is wise to get your $B_{12}$ level checked before taking high doses (800 mcg or more).

## Vitamin D

Dietary **vitamin D** (page 335) intake was connected to a lower incidence of cancer of the breast, colon, pancreas, and prostate, but the research on this question has yielded mixed results.[79–86] Do not take more than about 800 IU of vitamin D daily except on the advice of a physician.

## Flaxseed Oil (Lignans)

Substances known as *lignans* are found in several foods and may produce anticancer benefits. They are converted in the digestive tract to estrogen-like substances known as enterolactone and enterodiol.[87] Like soy isoflavones (see the previous discussion under the heading Soy), these substances prevent estrogen from attaching to cells and may thereby block its cancer-promoting effects.

Lignans are found most abundantly in flaxseed, a high-fiber grain that has been cultivated since ancient Egyptian times. **Flaxseed oil** (page 193) is also a rich source of an omega-3 fatty acid: alpha-linolenic acid.

Studies in humans and animals suggest that lignans may provide anticancer protection, especially against breast cancer.[88] However, this evidence is not yet strong.

Weak evidence also suggests that the alpha-linolenic acid in flaxseed oil may act against breast cancer. Low levels of alpha-linolenic acid in breast fatty tissues were associated with an increase in cancer and its spread (metastasis) to other areas of the body.[89]

The optimum dose of flaxseed oil is not known. The typical supplemental dosage recommended by some nutritionists is 1 to 2 tablespoons daily. Flaxseed oil is easily damaged by heat and light, so do not cook with it. The most palatable way to take it is by adding it to foods, such as using it as a salad dressing. Flaxseed oil is believed to be safe, although it occasionally causes constipation.

## Grapes (Resveratrol)

**Resveratrol** (page 292) is a phytochemical found in at least 72 different plants, including mulberries and peanuts. Grapes are its richest source. Red wine, which is made from grapes, contains a lot of resveratrol, which may account for some of the beneficial effects attributed to wine in some studies.

Resveratrol is an antioxidant with intriguing anticancer effects as determined in test-tube studies.[90] However, little direct evidence supports the idea that resveratrol is helpful. The proper dosage is not known, and safety studies have not yet been completed.

## Other Treatments on the Horizon

Provocative evidence suggests that a substance called sulforaphane, found in broccoli and related vegetables, may possess anticancer properties. Recently, broccoli sprouts have been touted as a cancer treatment on the basis of their high content of sulforaphane. However, this recommendation is still highly speculative.

Weak or indirect evidence also suggests some cancer-preventive benefits for the spices **turmeric** (page 311) and rosemary as well as for **licorice** (page 244), **ginseng** (page 206), **bromelain** (page 144), **melatonin** (page 258), **OPCs** (page 270), ellagic acid (from grapes, raspberries, strawberries, apples, walnuts, and pecans), **quercetin** (page 288) (a bioflavonoid found in many foods, including apples), citrus juices, betulin (from white birch tree), papaw tree bark, blue-green algae, and probiotics or "friendly" bacteria such as **acidophilus** (page 120).

It has been suggested that **calcium** (page 146) supplementation might reduce the risk of colon cancer, but there is much we still don't know on this subject.[91,92,93]

## PUTTING IT ALL TOGETHER

To prevent cancer, the best thing you can do for yourself is eat a diet high in fruits and vegetables and whole grains and low in smoked, charred, pickled, and salt-cured meats as well as other animal products. Increasing exercise and losing weight also appears to help significantly, and stopping smoking is essential.

The strongest evidence for any supplement in the treatment of cancer concerns vitamin E and prostate cancer. Vitamin E also seems to reduce the incidence of other cancers, especially stomach cancer; mouth, throat, and laryngeal cancer; and liver cancer. A typical dosage is 400 IU daily of alpha-tocopherol.

Selenium supplementation (200 mcg daily) appears to be helpful for preventing lung, colon, and prostate cancers.

Garlic appears to help prevent colon cancer.

Purified beta-carotene has not been shown to prevent cancer (and it may even increase the risk), but carotenes in the diet appear to protect against lung cancer as well as bladder cancer, breast cancer, stomach cancer, and cancer of the upper digestive tract.

Tomatoes seem to reduce the occurrence of prostate cancer as well as stomach and colon cancer, perhaps due to their content of the natural carotene lycopene. Cooked tomatoes appear to be more bioavailable (more readily used by the body) than raw tomatoes, especially when the tomatoes are cooked in oil.

Green tea may help prevent colon cancer, and weaker evidence suggests that it may help prevent cancer of the stomach, small intestine, pancreas, lungs, breast, and uterus.

Soy may help prevent hormone-sensitive cancers, such as those of the breast, prostate, uterus, and colon.

Little direct evidence supports the idea that vitamin C supplements prevent cancer, but foods high in vitamin C seem to lower the incidence of stomach cancer as well as colon, esophageal, laryngeal, bladder, cervical, rectal, and breast cancer.

Folic acid deficiency appears to be associated with cervical, colon, lung, and mouth cancer, but whether taking extra folic acid will help has not been determined.

Please refer to the chapters on these substances to learn about safety issues associated with them.

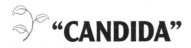 ## "CANDIDA"

### Principal Natural Treatments

There are no well-established natural treatments for "candida."

### Other Natural Treatments

Probiotics, capryllic acid, grapefruit seed extract, betaine hydrochloride, peppermint oil, oregano oil, lavender oil, tea tree oil, barberry, red thyme, lapacho, garlic, low-sugar diet, avoiding foods with high mold content

Candida albicans is a naturally occurring yeast that flourishes in moist areas, such as the digestive tract, the vagina, and skin folds. Ordinarily, its population is kept in check by bacteria that live in the same areas. When normal bacteria are disturbed by antibiotics, however, yeast populations can grow to abnormally high levels.

For women, the most common symptom of excess candida is a vaginal yeast infection, as marked by itchiness, redness, burning on urination, and a yeasty odor. However, candida can also overpopulate in the mouth (thrush), in the warm moist environment under a diaper (diaper rash), and in other areas.

Candida usually confines itself to the surface of mucous membranes and does not penetrate deeply into the body. However, in people whose immune systems are severely depressed, such as those with AIDS or leukemia, candida can become a dangerous, invasive organism. The medical name for this rare and dire condition is *systemic candidiasis.*

Besides this official meaning, systemic candidiasis has another meaning that was coined in the world of alternative medicine. As used there, it is a loose term connoting a whole syndrome of symptoms believed to be related to candida. Equivalent terms are *chronic candida,* the *yeast syndrome,* the *yeast hypersensitivity syndrome* (my favorite), or just plain *candida* for short.

Conventional medicine does not recognize the existence of this alternative syndrome. However, for several years it was practically impossible to walk into an alternative practitioner's office and not walk out with the diagnosis of candida. Fortunately, this excess enthusiasm has cooled in recent years. Among people who believe that they have a candida problem, perhaps 1 in 20 will benefit significantly from treatment for it. Candida is more a fad than a reality. Nonetheless, it has some reality behind it as well.

The story of "the yeast syndrome" begins in 1983, when Orion Truss published *The Missing Diagnosis.* This was followed by William Crook's much more famous *The Yeast Connection.* These books claim that a person who is chronically colonized by too much candida may develop an allergy-like hypersensitivity to it. The symptoms of this allergy are said to be similar to those of other allergies, including sinus congestion, fatigue, intestinal gas, difficulty concentrating, depression, muscle aches, and many other common complaints.

The regimen outlined by Dr. Crook consists of two parts: treatments that tend toward diminishing the total body burden of candida; and less convincing recommendations that attempt to lessen allergic reactions toward yeast in general.

To decrease the amount of yeast in the body, Dr. Crook recommends avoiding certain substances, including antibiotics, corticosteroids, birth control pills, sugar, and most sweet foods (it is his contention that dietary sugar "feeds yeast"). He also recommends the use of various supplements and even strong prescription drugs to directly kill yeast or at least interfere with its growth.

Next, Dr. Crook recommends avoiding foods containing yeast of any type, for he believes that those who are allergic to candida will also be allergic to other members of the fungus family. Thus Dr. Crook forbids fermented foods, such as beer, cheese, breads containing baker's yeast, tomato paste (which has a significant mold content), and even mushrooms.

Some of these recommendations seem farfetched. Although both mushrooms and candida fall into the broad category of fungi, they are not very closely related. Cats and elephants are both mammals, for example, but an allergy to one does not generally imply an allergy to the other. It is difficult to believe that those with sensitivity to candida should also cross-react with food mushrooms, and I have seldom seen it in real life.

Similarly, candida and baker's yeast bear only a distant relationship. Although many people with apparent candida problems do in fact react negatively to bread, it may not be the yeast in the bread that is causing the problem. People with allergies to candida are basically highly allergenic people. They may simply be allergic to the wheat in bread rather than to the yeast. After all, wheat is the second most common food allergen.

There is no conventional medical treatment for yeast hypersensitivity syndrome because conventional medicine does not recognize its existence.

## NATURAL TREATMENTS

There is no scientific evidence that any treatment can reduce the symptoms caused by oversensitivity to candida.

Many treatments can reduce the amount of yeast in the body, and people with a genuine allergy to candida may feel better once this is achieved. Unfortunately, it isn't possible to eliminate *Candida albicans* permanently. No matter how successful a treatment may be, as soon as it is stopped, candida will return. It has to because it is a natural inhabitant of the body. However, we know from other conditions, such as vaginal yeast infections, that sufficient intake of probiotics, or "friendly" bacteria, can help keep yeast regrowth within reasonable bounds. It is probably best to use a mixture of organisms, including **acidophilus** (page 120), bulgaricus, and bifidus. The daily dose should provide 3 to 10 billion viable organisms.

Agents that may reduce the amount of yeast in the body include capryllic acid, grapefruit seed extract, **betaine hydrochloride** (page 134), **peppermint** (page 277) oil, oregano oil, lavender oil, **tea tree** (page 309) oil, barberry, red thyme, pau d'arco (also called **lapacho** [page 242]), and **garlic** (page 197). However, the scientific foundation for the use of these treatments is weak, and the appropriate dosage of each has not been determined. Some of these treatments may be toxic if taken to excess or for prolonged periods.

## Other Treatments

As mentioned earlier, proponents of the candida syndrome further believe that it is important to restrict sugar in the diet, even fruit sugar. This concept is based on the idea that "sugar feeds yeast." However, there is no scientific evidence that dietary sugar increases the growth of candida. They also recommend eliminating all foods with high mold content, such as alcoholic drinks, peanuts, cheeses, bread, and dried fruits. Although these foods cannot increase the amount of candida in your body, they contain yeasts that you could conceivably be allergic to.

 # CANKER SORES

*Principal Natural Treatments*
Deglycyrrhizinated licorice

*Other Natural Treatments*
Acidophilus, calendula, vitamin $B_1$, vitamin $B_2$

Canker sores are small ulcers in the mouth caused by an assortment of viruses. A susceptibility to canker sores tends to run in families. No successful conventional treatment is available.

## PRINCIPAL NATURAL TREATMENTS

A chemically altered form of **licorice** (page 244) known as deglycyrrhizinated licorice (DGL) may be useful in canker sores.

DGL adheres to inflamed mucous membranes, which has made it a useful treatment for **ulcers** (page 112). Although no good scientific evidence supports the use of DGL for canker sores, one preliminary study suggests that it might significantly and rapidly reduce symptoms.[1] Pain levels noticeably decrease within minutes, and remain reduced for hours. According to anecdotal reports, frequent use of DGL throughout the day can almost entirely eliminate the discomfort of canker sores.

This form of licorice is believed to be safe, although safety has not been established in young children, pregnant or nursing women, and those with severe liver or kidney disease. The main problem with DGL is that it must be sucked to coat the canker sores, and some people find its taste objectionable.

## OTHER NATURAL TREATMENTS

Other herbs and supplements sometimes recommended for canker sores include **acidophilus** (page 120), **calendula** (page 150), **vitamin $B_1$** (page 320), and **vitamin $B_2$** (page 321), but there is little evidence as yet that they are effective.

# CARDIOMYOPATHY

*Principal Natural Treatments*
Coenzyme $Q_{10}$, carnitine

Cardiomyopathy is a little understood condition in which the muscle tissue of the heart becomes diseased. There are several distinct forms of cardiomyopathy that may or may not be similar in origin. Medical treatment consists mainly of medications that attempt to compensate for the increasing failure of the heart to function properly. A heart transplant may ultimately be necessary.

## PRINCIPAL NATURAL TREATMENTS

Cardiomyopathy is certainly not a disease that you should treat yourself! For this reason, I deliberately do not discuss dosage or safety issues in this section (although general guidelines can be found for these substances in their chapters in Part Two). However, in consultation with your physician, you may want to consider adding the following two supplements to your treatment regimen.

### Coenzyme $Q_{10}$

There is some evidence that the naturally occurring substance **coenzyme $Q_{10}$ ($CoQ_{10}$)** (page 164) can be beneficial in some forms of cardiomyopathy.[1,2,3]

In a 6-year trial, 143 people with moderately severe cardiomyopathy were given $CoQ_{10}$ daily in addition to standard medical care.[4] The results showed a significant improvement in cardiac function (technically, *ejection fraction*) in 84% of the study participants. Most of them improved by several stages on a scale that measures the severity of heart failure (technically, *NYHA class*). Furthermore, a comparison with individuals on conventional therapy alone appeared to show a reduction in mortality.

This study was an open trial, meaning that participants knew that they were being treated. As explained in the introduction, such studies are not fully reliable due to the power of suggestion. However, these results, including objective measurements of heart function, were so impressive that it is hard to believe the power of suggestion alone could explain them. Nonetheless, double-blind studies are more definitive.

There have been a few such studies of $CoQ_{10}$ in cardiomyopathy. One double-blind controlled trial followed 80 people with various forms of cardiomyopathy over a period of 3 years.[5] Of those treated with $CoQ_{10}$, 89% improved significantly, but when the treatment was stopped, their heart function deteriorated.

No benefit was seen in another double-blind study, but it was a smaller and shorter trial and enrolled only people who had one particular type of cardiomyopathy (idiopathic dilated cardiomyopathy).[6]

### Carnitine

There is a little evidence that the vitamin-like supplement **carnitine** (page 151) may be useful in cardiomyopathy.[7,8] Carnitine is believed to work well with $CoQ_{10}$, and the two treatments are often combined.[9]

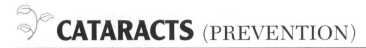

# CATARACTS (PREVENTION)

*Principal Natural Treatments*
   Vitamin C, vitamin E, dietary carotenes (including lutein and lycopene)

*Other Natural Treatments*
   Bilberry, ginkgo, OPCs , turmeric, zinc, riboflavin (vitamin B$_2$), cysteine, lipoic acid, selenium, taurine, niacin (vitamin B$_3$)

Cataracts—an opaque buildup of damaged proteins in the lens of the eye—are the leading cause of visual decline in those over 65. In fact, most people in that age group have at least the beginnings of cataract formation. Many factors contribute to the development of cataracts, but damage by free radicals is believed to play a major role.

Cataracts can be removed surgically. Although this has become a relatively quick, safe, easy, and painless surgery, it does not result in completely normal vision. Clearly, preventing cataracts, if possible, would be preferable.

## PRINCIPAL NATURAL TREATMENTS

Evidence suggests that various antioxidants may help prevent cataracts.

### Vitamin C

In an observational study of 50,800 nurses who were followed for 8 years, a history of taking **vitamin C** (page 331) supplements for more than 10 years was associated with a 45% lower risk of cataracts.[1]

Interestingly, diets high in vitamin C were not found to be protective—only supplemental vitamin C made a difference. This is the opposite of what has been found with vitamin C in the prevention of other diseases. See the discussions of vitamin C in the chapters on **atherosclerosis** (page 14) and **cancer** (page 26) for more details.

Vitamin C is generally believed to be quite safe, at least at dosages up to 500 mg daily. It is often stated that that long-term use of vitamin C can cause kidney stones, but in the large-scale Harvard Prospective Health Professional Follow-Up Study, those taking the most vitamin C

(over 1,500 mg daily) had a lower risk of kidney stones than those taking the least amounts.[2] Nonetheless, individuals with a history of kidney stones and those with kidney failure should probably restrict daily vitamin C intake to about 100 mg daily. Taking more than 1,000 mg daily of vitamin C can deplete the body's **copper** (page 169) stores, so taking 1 to 3 mg of copper daily as a supplement may be advisable.

### Vitamin E

According to observational studies (not as large as the one described under vitamin C), researchers have found that foods high in **vitamin E** (page 337), as well as vitamin E supplements, are associated with a reduced risk of cataracts.[3–8] These results are corroborated by a study in animals,[9] but further work needs to be done to establish vitamin E as a treatment for cataracts.

A typical dosage of vitamin E is 400 IU daily. Vitamin E is generally believed to be safe at this dose. However, in one study, vitamin E supplementation was associated with an increase in hemorrhagic stroke, the kind of stroke caused by bleeding.[10] Considering its ability to reduce blood clotting, vitamin E should not be taken by those with bleeding problems, or combined with aspirin or prescription blood thinners, such as Coumadin (warfarin) and Trental (pentoxifylline), except under a physician's supervision.[11] There also might conceivably be potential risks in combining vitamin E with other natural substances known to thin the blood, such as **garlic** (page 197) and **ginkgo** (page 204), although no problems have been reported.

### Carotenes

Foods high in carotenes (beta-carotene, lutein, lycopene, and others) might protect against cataract

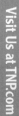

formation.[12,13] In studies, **lutein** (page 248) (found in dark-green vegetables) seemed to be especially helpful for women, whereas the carotenes found in carrots was more helpful in men. **Lycopene** (page 249), a carotene found in tomatoes, was associated with a reduced occurrence of cataracts in both sexes.

However, taking the supplement beta-carotene by itself does not appear to be protective.[14,15] This is one more strike against this antioxidant, which has failed to prove beneficial in other conditions as well (see the discussions of beta-carotene in the chapters on **atherosclerosis** [page 14] and **cancer** [page 26]).

## OTHER NATURAL TREATMENTS

Herbs high in antioxidant flavonoids may also be helpful in protecting against cataracts. The ones most commonly mentioned include **bilberry** (page 135), **ginkgo** (page 204), **OPCs** (page 270), and **turmeric** (page 311). However, of these, only bilberry has any direct evidence in its favor, and that evidence is weak.[16]

Bilberry is a commonly eaten food and as such is believed to be safe, although safety in young children, pregnant or nursing women, and those with severe kidney or liver disease has not been established. The supplements **zinc** (page 348), riboflavin or **vitamin B$_2$** (page 321), cysteine, **lipoic acid** (page 246), **selenium** (page 297), **taurine** (page 308), and niacin or **vitamin B$_3$** (page 323) are sometimes mentioned as helpful for preventing cataracts, but the evidence that they really work is not yet strong.

# CERVICAL DYSPLASIA

*Principal Natural Treatments*
    There are no well-established natural treatments for cervical dysplasia.

*Other Natural Treatments*
    Folic acid (for women on oral contraceptives), multivitamin and mineral supplement, selenium, "emmenagogue herbs" (squaw vine, motherwort, true unicorn, false unicorn, black cohosh, blessed thistle)

Very few cancers can be identified so far ahead of the danger point as cancer of the cervix. The cells lining the surface of the cervix begin to show changes visible under a microscope a decade or more before invasive cancer develops, in plenty of time for definitive treatment. For this reason, a regular, properly performed and interpreted Pap smear is one of medicine's most effective preventive methods.

The stages of progression from a healthy cervix to cancer begin with what is called mild dysplasia: precancerous alterations in structure and activity. Subsequently, altered cells spread from the surface of the cervix down toward the underlying tissue. In the early stages, cancerous changes may disappear on their own, but once these cells fully penetrate the lining, progression to true cancer usually occurs within 5 to 10 years.

Medical treatment consists of watchful waiting for spontaneous regression during the early stages and more aggressive removal of the cervical lining by laser, freezing, or other techniques if no regression occurs. These options are usually successful; however, they are invasive and frequently uncomfortable.

## NATURAL TREATMENTS

It has been claimed that various natural herbs and supplements can improve the odds of early stages of dysplasia changing back to normal cells. If your physician suggests watchful waiting and a

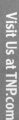
repeat examination, it should be safe to try some of these methods during the waiting period. However, there is no real scientific evidence that these treatments are effective, and in all circumstances close medical supervision is necessary to verify good results or identify failure. Alternative treatment is definitely not advisable for severe cervical dysplasia.

## Folic Acid

**Folic acid** (page 194) deficiency appears to increase the ease with which cervical cancer can develop. Studies suggest that high doses of folic acid, far above nutritional needs, can help reverse cervical dysplasia in women taking oral contraceptives but not in the population at large.[1–4]

The dosage of folic acid used for treatment purposes is often as much as 10 mg daily. Because folic acid can mask **vitamin B$_{12}$** (page 329) deficiency, dosages at this level must be prescribed by a physician. Possible side effects include nausea, flatulence, and loss of appetite as well as an increased rate of seizures in epileptics.

The safety of high doses of folic acid in young children, pregnant or nursing women, and those with severe kidney or liver disease has not been established.

## General Nutritional Support

Studies have found that women with cervical dysplasia tend to show a high frequency of general nutritional deficiencies, as high as 67% in one survey.[5] For this reason, it probably makes sense to take a multivitamin and mineral supplement. Particular vitamins most commonly associated with cervical dysplasia when deficient include **beta-carotene** (page 131), **vitamin C** (page 331), **vitamin B$_6$** (page 326), **selenium** (page 297), and, as previously mentioned, folic acid.[6,7]

## Emmenagogues

Many practitioners of herbal medicine feel that a class of herbs known as emmenagogues can be helpful in cervical dysplasia. These include squaw vine, motherwort, true unicorn, false unicorn, **black cohosh** (page 138), and blessed thistle.

# CHOLESTEROL (ELEVATED)

### Principal Natural Treatments
Garlic, red yeast rice, niacin (vitamin B$_3$), fiber, soy protein or isoflavones

### Other Natural Treatments
Indian mukul myrrh tree (guggulsterone or guggul), pantethine, L-carnitine, aortic glycosaminoglycans, chromium, calcium, flaxseed oil, He shou wu, maitake, chondroitin, copper, gamma oryzanol, lecithin, fenugreek, ashwaganda, multivitamin/mineral, lifestyle changes

One of the most significant discoveries in preventive medicine is that elevated levels of cholesterol in the blood accelerate atherosclerosis, or hardening of the arteries (see the discussion about cholesterol in the chapter on **atherosclerosis** [page 14]). Along with high blood pressure, inactivity, smoking, and diabetes, high cholesterol has proven to be one of the most important promoters of heart disease, strokes, and peripheral vascular disease (blockage of circulation to the extremities, usually the legs).

Cholesterol does not directly clog arteries like grease clogs pipes. The current theory is that elevated levels of cholesterol irritate the walls of blood vessels and cause them to undergo harmful changes. Because most cholesterol is manufactured by the body itself, dietary sources of cholesterol (such as eggs) are not usually the most important problem. The relative proportion of unsaturated fats (from plants) and saturated fats (mainly from animal products) in the diet is more significant. The former lower cholesterol levels, whereas the latter raise them.

There is no question that increasing exercise and improving diet are the most important steps to take when cholesterol is high. These fundamental lifestyle changes are frequently effective and produce many benefits that go beyond simply lowering cholesterol levels.

However, if your cholesterol remains high despite your best efforts, you may need specific cholesterol-lowering treatments. There are a variety of effective drugs to choose from, and some, such as Pravachol (pravastatin), have actually been shown to prevent heart attacks and reduce mortality. While there are known and suspected risks associated with these medications, the benefits of these medications undoubtedly exceed the risks for those with significantly elevated cholesterol levels. In milder cases, however, some of the options described below might be better first choices.

## PRINCIPAL NATURAL TREATMENTS

There are several herbs and supplements that can almost certainly help you lower your cholesterol level. However, before trying them, consult with your physician to find out whether you have time to experiment. If your cholesterol levels are very high and your arteries are already in bad condition, it might be wiser to turn to proven drug treatments. However, if your physician says that you can safely spend some time exploring your options, the treatments described in this section may be worth trying.

## Garlic: Good Evidence It Reduces Total Cholesterol

The most well established herbal treatment for high cholesterol is the kitchen herb **garlic** (page 197). As far back as the first century A.D., Dioscorides wrote of garlic's ability to "clear the arteries." Today, Germany's Commission E authorizes the use of garlic "as an adjunct to dietary measures in patients with elevated blood lipids (cholesterol) and for the prevention of age-related vascular (blood vessel) changes."

The effectiveness of garlic appears to depend heavily on the formulation used. A relatively odorless substance, alliin, is one of the most important compounds in garlic and is believed by many researchers to be a prime active ingredient (or, technically, source of active ingredients). When garlic is crushed or cut, an enzyme called allinase is brought into contact with alliin, turning the latter into allicin. Allicin is most responsible for garlic's strong odor and may also play a major role in lowering cholesterol. The allicin itself then rapidly breaks down into entirely different compounds.

When you powder garlic to put it into a capsule, it acts like cutting the bulb. The chain reaction starts: Alliin contacts allinase, yielding allicin, which then breaks down. Unless something is done to prevent this process, garlic powder will not have any alliin that can be turned into allicin left by the time you buy it.

Some garlic producers declare that alliin and allicin have nothing to do with garlic's effectiveness and simply sell products without either one, such as aged powdered garlic and garlic oil. However, there are serious doubts about the effectiveness of these products. Garlic oil, in particular, seems to be entirely ineffective (see What Is the Scientific Evidence for Garlic?).

Raw garlic is the most reliable source of alliin, but its strong odor keeps many people from using it. To solve this problem, manufacturers have devised ways to produce relatively odor-free garlic that still contains a standardized level of alliin. These are sold as powdered garlic with a guaranteed alliin content and, often, an "allicin potential" or "allicin yield."

### What Is the Scientific Evidence for Garlic?

One of the best studies of garlic standardized to alliin content was conducted in Germany and published in 1990.[1] A total of 261 patients at 30 medical centers were given either 800 mg daily of garlic standardized to alliin content or placebo. Over the course of 16 weeks, patients in the treated group experienced a 12% drop in total cholesterol and a 17% decrease in triglyceride levels. The greatest benefits occurred in patients with initial cholesterol levels of 250 to 300 mg/dL.

All together, at least 28 controlled clinical studies have evaluated the effectiveness of garlic in lowering elevated cholesterol. Although some studies have found no benefit,[2,3] overall the results make a reasonably good case that garlic powder standardized to alliin content can lower total cholesterol by about 9 to 12%.[4,5] We know much less about garlic's effects on LDL ("bad") cholesterol and HDL ("good") cholesterol.

There is also some evidence that aged garlic powder (without alliin) can lower cholesterol levels too, although perhaps to a lesser extent.[6] However, garlic oil appears to be ineffective.[7]

Garlic also appears to modestly reduce blood pressure, making it useful for **hypertension** (page 75). Furthermore, evidence suggests that it may soften artery walls through mechanisms other than lowering cholesterol and blood pressure,[8] perhaps by protecting against free radicals and hindering blood clotting.[9–16] Because of this multifaceted effect, many European physicians regard garlic as one of the best all-around treatments for the prevention of heart disease.

### Dosages

In most of the studies that demonstrated the cholesterol-lowering powers of garlic, the daily dosage supplied at least 10 mg of alliin. This is sometimes stated in terms of how much allicin will be created from that alliin. The number you should look for is 4 to 5 mg of "allicin potential." You must allow at least 1 to 4 months of treatment for full effects.

Aged garlic without alliin may also offer some benefit, but don't bother with garlic oil.

### Safety Issues

As a commonly used food, garlic is on the FDA's GRAS (generally regarded as safe ) list. Rats have been fed gigantic doses of aged garlic (2,000 mg per kilogram body weight) for 6 months without any signs of negative effects.[17] Unfortunately, there is no safety information from animal studies on garlic powder standardized to alliin content, which is by far the most commonly used form of garlic.

The only common side effect of garlic is unpleasant breath odor. Even so-called odorless garlic produces an offensive smell in up to 50% of those who use it.[18]

Other side effects occur only rarely. For example, a study that followed 1,997 people who were given a normal dose of deodorized garlic daily over a 16-week period showed a 6% incidence of nausea, a 1.3% incidence of dizziness on standing (perhaps a sign of low blood pressure), and a 1.1% incidence of allergic reactions.[19] A few reports of bloating, headaches, sweating, and dizziness were also noted.

Raw garlic taken in excessive doses can cause many symptoms, including stomach upset, heartburn, nausea and vomiting, diarrhea, flatulence, facial flushing, rapid pulse, and insomnia.

Because garlic appears to possess blood-thinning effects, it might not be safe to combine garlic with blood thinners, such as Coumadin (warfarin), Trental (pentoxifylline), or aspirin, or with other natural blood-thinning substances like **ginkgo** (page 204) and **vitamin E** (page 337). High doses of garlic should not be taken before surgery or labor and delivery.

Maximum safe doses in young children, pregnant or nursing women, and those with severe kidney or liver disease have not been established.

## Red Yeast Rice:
## May Be Similar to Standard Drugs

Red yeast rice has recently arrived on the market as a treatment for lowering cholesterol. However, because of potential risks, it should only be used under physician supervision.

Red yeast rice is a traditional Chinese substance that is made by fermenting a type of yeast called *Monascus purpureus* over rice. This product (called Hong Qu) has been used in China since at least 800 A.D. as a food and also as a medicinal substance. Recently, it has been discovered that this ancient Chinese preparation contains at least 11 naturally occurring substances similar to prescription drugs in the "statin" family, such as Mevacor and Pravachol.

### What Is the Scientific Evidence for Red Yeast Rice?

A recent major U.S. study on red yeast rice was conducted at the UCLA School of Medicine.[20] This was a 12-week double-blind placebo-controlled trial involving 83 healthy participants (46 men and 37 women, aged 34 to 78 years) with high cholesterol levels. One group was given the recommended dose of red yeast rice, while the other group received a placebo. Both groups were instructed to consume a low-fat diet similar to the American Heart Association Step 1 diet.

The results showed that red yeast rice was significantly more effective than placebo. In the treated group, average total cholesterol (mg/dL) fell by about 18% by 8 weeks. During the same time period, LDL ("bad") cholesterol decreased by 22% and triglycerides by 11%. There was little to no improvement in the placebo group. HDL ("good") cholesterol did not change in either group during the study.

Similar or even better results have been seen in other U.S. and Chinese studies using various forms of red yeast rice.[21,22]

### Dosages

Because red yeast rice products can vary widely in their strength, please refer to the labeling for appropriate dosage.

### Safety Issues

While there have been no serious adverse reactions reported in the studies of red yeast rice, some minor side effects have been reported. In the large study of 446 people, heartburn (1.8%), bloating (0.9%), and dizziness (0.3%) were all mentioned. Formal toxicity studies in rats and mice, giving doses up to 125 times the normal human dose for 3 months, showed no toxic effects, according to unpublished information on file with one of the manufacturers of red yeast rice.[23]

However, because red yeast contains ingredients similar to the statin drugs, there is a theoretical risk of the same side effects and risks that are seen with those drugs. These include elevated liver enzymes, damage to skeletal muscle, and increased risk of cancer. Also, red yeast rice should not be combined with niacin, erythromycin, other statin drugs, or the class of drugs called "fibrates." Serious side effects have occurred when statin drugs were combined with these medications.

This product should not be used by pregnant or nursing mothers or those with severe liver or kidney disease except on a physician's advice.

## Niacin: A Treatment Accepted by Conventional Medicine

The common vitamin niacin, also called **vitamin B₃** (page 323), is an accepted medical treatment for elevated cholesterol with solid science behind

it. According to numerous studies, niacin can lower total cholesterol and LDL cholesterol by 15 to 25%, lower triglycerides by 2 to 50%, and raise HDL cholesterol by 15 to 25%.[24–27] Unfortunately, niacin, if taken in sufficient quantities to lower cholesterol, can cause an annoying flushing reaction and occasionally liver inflammation.[28] It may also worsen blood sugar levels in people with diabetes. Close medical supervision is essential when using niacin to lower cholesterol.

To partially counter some of these problems, a special form of niacin has been developed in Europe: inositol hexaniacinate, or "flushless" niacin.[29] The term *flushless* is not quite accurate—some people do flush with inositol hexaniacinate, but the flush is neither as common nor as severe as with ordinary niacin. It is still necessary to check the liver periodically, so a physician's supervision remains essential.

The proper dosage of inositol hexaniacinate is 500 to 1,000 mg 2 to 3 times daily, taken with food. The usual recommendation is to start with the lower dose and raise it only if the cholesterol doesn't fall sufficiently after about 6 weeks.

Ordinary niacin can be used as well, and there are slow-release forms of niacin available by prescription. However, liver inflammation is a real possibility with all forms of niacin.

## Fiber: Considered "Heart-Healthy" by the FDA

Water-soluble fiber supplements appear to lower cholesterol, and the FDA has permitted products containing this form of fiber to carry a "heart-healthy" label.[30] Many forms are available, ranging from oat bran to expensive fiber products sold through multilevel marketing firms. A good dose of oat bran is 5 to 10 g with each meal and at bedtime, and a good dose of psyllium is 10 g with each meal. However, eating a diet high in fresh fruits and vegetables and whole grains may be even better because of the many healthful nutrients such a diet contains.

## Soy Protein: Soon to Be Labeled "Heart-Healthy"

**Soy protein** (page 301) appears to lower total cholesterol by about 9%, LDL ("bad") cholesterol by 13%, and triglycerides by 10%.[31] At the time of this writing the FDA has proposed allowing foods containing soy protein to make this claim on the label. According to the FDA, it takes about 25 g of soy protein a day to get cholesterol-lowering effects. This amount can be found in ½ pound of tofu or 2½ cups of soy milk.

Soy **isoflavones** (page 236) may be the active ingredient in soy protein.

Soy may not be safe for women with a previous history of breast cancer.

## OTHER NATURAL TREATMENTS

There are also several other promising alternative treatments for high cholesterol. Although the scientific evidence behind them is not yet strong, many alternative practitioners consider them to be highly effective.

A few preliminary double-blind studies suggest that an extract of the Indian mukul myrrh tree, known as gugulipid or **guggul** (page 221), may reduce total cholesterol by about 11% and triglycerides by 17%.[32,33,34] The dosage of standardized guggul should supply 25 mg of guggulsterone 3 times daily. Although side effects appear to be rare, detailed safety studies have not been performed; and safety in young children, pregnant or nursing women, and those with severe kidney or liver disease has not been established.

A special form of the vitamin pantothenic acid, known as **pantethine** (page 275), might significantly lower total blood triglycerides as well as cholesterol, but not all studies agree.[35–38] Further research is necessary to prove the safety and effectiveness of this expensive supplement. **L-carnitine** (page 151) is another expensive supplement that might be able to improve cholesterol levels.[39] A typical dosage is 500 to 1,000 mg 3 times daily.

Carnitine in its three forms (L-carnitine, propionyl-L-carnitine, and acetyl-L-carnitine) appears to be quite safe. However, you should not use forms of the supplement known as "D-carnitine" or "DL-carnitine," as these can cause angina, muscle pain, and loss of muscle function (probably by interfering with carnitine). The maximum safe dosages for young children, pregnant or nursing women, or those with severe liver or kidney disease have not been established.

Preliminary studies suggest that an extract from the lining of the aortas of cows, known as **aortic glycosaminoglycans** (page 125) (GAGs), can improve cholesterol levels.[40,41,42] The typical dosage is 50 mg 2 times daily.

Aortic GAGs are considered safe, as similar substances are widely found in foods. However, if you are taking drugs that powerfully decrease blood clotting, such as Coumadin (warfarin) or heparin, do not use aortic GAGs except under a physician's supervision. Aortic GAGs interfere slightly with blood clotting, and there is at least a chance that the combination could cause bleeding problems.

Supplemental **chromium** (page 161) may improve blood cholesterol in some people but not in others.[43] A typical nutritional dosage is 200 mcg of chromium picolinate daily. **Calcium** (page 146) supplements may also slightly lower cholesterol.[44] A typical nutritional dosage is 500 to 1,200 mg daily.

Other herbs and supplements commonly recommended for high cholesterol include **flaxseed oil** (page 193), **He shou wu** (page 224), **maitake** (page 254), **chondroitin** (page 159), **copper** (page 169), **gamma oryzanol** (page 196), **lecithin** (page 243), **ashwaganda** (page 128), and **fenugreek** (page 185), but there is as yet little solid evidence that they really work.

Finally, because general nutrient deficiencies can alter cholesterol levels, a basic multivitamin and mineral may be useful.

## Lifestyle Approaches

The dietary influence on cholesterol levels is enormous but not entirely understood. Clearly, saturated fats from animal sources raise cholesterol levels, whereas polyunsaturated fats (from plants) lower them.

Much discussion has taken place over precisely which types of nonanimal fats are best. Some studies point toward monounsaturated fats, such as those found in olive oil. Margarine, long thought to be "better than butter," now appears to be generally unhealthful. The hydrogenated or partially hydrogenated oils that make up margarine are found in other foods as well. However, at the time of this writing a special form of margarine from Finland is touted as being heart-healthy.

This is a rapidly evolving field, and anything I write here may be outdated by the time you read this. Consult a qualified health professional for the latest information.

Some observational studies have found an association between coffee intake and elevated cholesterol. However, because coffee use is typically associated with other bad habits, such as smoking and a diet high in animal fat, it is diffi-cult to know for sure whether coffee is really causing the problem.[45]

Finally, other treatments that may help prevent or reverse **atherosclerosis** (page 14) should be considered as well.

For even more information on cholesterol, see *The Natural Pharmacist Guide to Garlic and Cholesterol.*

# COLDS AND FLUS

### *Principal Natural Treatments*
Echinacea, andrographis, zinc, vitamin C, ginseng

### *Other Natural Treatments*
Vitamin E, elderberry, ashwaganda, astragalus, garlic, suma, reishi, maitake, osha, yarrow, kudzu, ginger, mullein, marshmallow, arginine, peppermint

A cold is a respiratory infection caused by one of hundreds of possible viruses. However, because these viruses are so widespread, it is perhaps more accurate to say that colds are caused by a decrease in immunity that allows one of these viruses to take hold.

Colds occur more frequently in winter, but no one knows exactly why. Nearly everyone catches colds occasionally; but some people catch colds quite frequently, and others tend to stay sick an unusually long time.

Conventional medicine can neither cure nor prevent the common cold. Furthermore, none of the over-the-counter treatments have been found to shorten the duration of a cold or even provide significant temporary relief. Some of the natural treatments described in this section may be able to do better.

People often want to take antibiotics for colds, and many physicians will prescribe them—even though antibiotics have no effect on viruses. Many believe that when the mucus turns yellow, it means that a bacterial infection has occurred for which antibiotic treatment is indicated. However, viruses can also produce yellow mucus; and even if bacteria have made a home in the excess mucus, they may be only innocent bystanders and produce no symptoms.

Colds, however, can be complicated by bacterial infections. In such cases antibiotic treatment may be indicated. Decongestants and other symptomatic treatments have not been shown to be dramatically effective.

## PRINCIPAL NATURAL TREATMENTS

Remember the old saying "a cold lasts seven days, but if you treat it properly you will get over it in a week"? Actually, it may be possible to prove folk wisdom wrong by using the right natural supplement. A significant body of research suggests that the herb echinacea can significantly shorten colds and make them less severe. The herb andrographis and the nutritional supplements zinc and vitamin C also seem to help. However, we also don't know whether combining more than one of these treatments together will produce better results.

While these treatments can help you get over a cold faster, there is little evidence that they prevent colds. However, there is one treatment that might have a preventive effect: the herb ginseng.

# Echinacea: Reduces Cold and Flu Symptoms and Helps Recovery

Until the 1930s, **echinacea** (page 179) was the number-one cold and flu remedy in the United States. It lost its popularity with the arrival of sulfa antibiotics. Ironically, sulfa antibiotics are as ineffective against colds as any other antibiotic, while echinacea does seem to be at least somewhat helpful. In Germany, echinacea remains the main remedy for minor respiratory infections.

This herb is thought to be an immune stimulant, a type of treatment not found in conventional medicine. Drugs attack infections, but echinacea appears to activate the body's infection-fighting capacity. However, there is no evidence that echinacea strengthens or "nourishes" the immune system when taken over the long term. There are three main species of echinacea: *Echinacea purpurea, Echinacea angustifolia,* and *Echinacea pallida. E. purpurea* is the most widely used, but the other two are also available. It isn't clear if any one type is better than the others.

## What Is the Scientific Evidence for Echinacea?

An increasingly strong body of evidence suggests that, when taken at the onset of a cold or flu, echinacea can help you get better faster and reduce your symptoms while you are sick. It doesn't seem to have much (if any) effect on preventing colds.

One double-blind study found that in people with flu-like illnesses echinacea can significantly reduce symptoms such as headache, lethargy, cough, and aching limbs.[1] This study followed 100 people who had just become sick. Half received a combination herb product containing *E. angustifolia,* the other half a placebo. The results showed that the echinacea group experienced significantly less intense symptoms than the placebo group.

Another double-blind study of echinacea found similar benefits in 180 people with flu-like illnesses, who were given either placebo or 450 mg or 900 mg of *E. purpurea* daily.[2] By about the third day, those participants receiving the higher dose of echinacea (900 mg) showed noticeable relief in the severity of symptoms. There

was no real benefit in the placebo or low-dose echinacea group.

In another double-blind study, 120 people were given *E. purpurea* or a placebo as soon as they started showing signs of getting a cold.[3] In the treated group, improvement in cold symptoms started much sooner than in the placebo group (4 days instead of 8 days).

Reduction of symptoms was seen in yet another double-blind study of *E. purpurea,* involving about 200 participants.[4]

A double-blind placebo-controlled study using the *E. pallida* species found that treatment reduced the length of colds by about 30%.[5] This study followed 160 adults who had just "caught cold." The results showed that treatment reduced the length of illness from 13 days to about 9.5 days, compared to placebo (these were rather long colds!).

Can regular use of echinacea strengthen your immunity and prevent colds? Probably not. Not only has regular use of echinacea failed to significantly reduce the incidence of colds in most studies,[6–9] a recent study found that it might actually slightly *increase* your risk.[10] The bottom line is that echinacea can be counted on to lessen cold symptoms and help you recover faster, but not to prevent colds altogether.

How does echinacea work? The answer is that we really don't know. Both test-tube and animal studies have shown that the constituents found in echinacea can increase antibody production, raise white blood cell counts, and stimulate the activity of key white blood cells.[11–16] However, it is far from certain that these findings really mean much! Many other substances cause similar changes, including wheat, bamboo, rice, sugarcane, and chamomile, and none of these has ever been considered an immune stimulant.[17]

## Dosages

The three species of echinacea are used interchangeably. The typical daily dosage of echinacea powdered extract is 300 mg 3 times daily. Alcohol tincture (1:5) is usually taken at a dosage of 3 to 4 ml 3 times daily, echinacea juice at 2 to 3 ml 3 times daily, and whole dried root at 1 to 2 g 3 times daily. Echinacea is usually taken at the first sign of a cold and continued for 7 to 14 days. Long-term use is probably not helpful.

There is no broad agreement on which ingredients should be standardized in echinacea tinctures and solid extracts. However, echinacea juice is often standardized to contain 2.4% of beta-1,2-fructofuranoside.

Many herbalists feel that liquid forms of echinacea are more effective than tablets or capsules because they believe that part of echinacea's benefit is due to direct contact with the tonsils and other lymphatic tissues at the back of the throat.[18] These tissues act as an early warning system for infections. By stimulating them, echinacea may encourage the body to fight a cold more promptly.

Finally, **goldenseal** (page 217) is frequently combined with echinacea in cold preparations. However, there is no evidence that oral goldenseal stimulates immunity, nor did traditional herbalists use it for this purpose.[19]

### Safety Issues

Echinacea appears to be very safe. Even when taken in very high doses, it does not appear to cause any toxic effects.[20,21] Side effects are also rare and usually limited to minor gastrointestinal symptoms, increased urination, and allergic reactions.[22]

Germany's Commission E warns against using echinacea if you have an autoimmune disorder such as multiple sclerosis, lupus, or rheumatoid arthritis, as well as tuberculosis or leukocytosis. Rumors say that echinacea should not be used if you have AIDS. These warnings are purely theoretical, being based on fears that echinacea might actually activate immunity in the wrong way. While no evidence shows that echinacea use has actually harmed anyone with these diseases, caution is advisable.

Germany's Commission E also recommends against using echinacea for more than 8 weeks. Since there is no evidence that echinacea is effective when taken long term, this is probably sensible. The safety of echinacea in pregnant or nursing women and those with severe kidney or liver disease has not been established. In German studies from the 1950s and 60s, more than 1,000 children were given injected forms of echinacea, with no apparent harm.[23] Given these

findings, it seems likely that oral echinacea is safe in children, but we don't know this for sure.

## Andrographis: A Promising Treatment for Colds

**Andrographis** (page 123) is a shrub found throughout India and other Asian countries, sometimes called "Indian echinacea" because it is believed to provide much the same benefits. It was widely used during the terrible influenza epidemics that occurred earlier this century. Recently, it has become popular in Scandinavia as a treatment for colds.

### What Is the Scientific Evidence for Andrographis?

According to a few well-designed studies, andrographis can both reduce the symptoms and shorten the duration of colds.

In one double-blind study, 50 people with colds were given either andrographis or placebo.[24] Researchers reported that 55% of the treated participants reported that their colds were less intense than usual, while only 19% of those in the placebo group stated this. The treated group averaged only 0.2 days of sick leave, while the group taking placebo averaged 1 full day of sick leave. Finally, 75% of the treated participants were well after 5 days, compared to less than 40% in the placebo group.

Another double-blind study that enrolled 59 people concluded that andrographis could reduce cold symptoms such as fatigue, sore throat, sore muscles, runny nose, headache, and lymph node swelling.[25] Participants received either 1,200 mg of andrographis (standardized to 4% andrographolides) or a placebo. By the fourth day of the study, the andrographis group showed definite improvement in most of their cold symptoms as compared to the placebo group.

Finally, a double-blind study involving 152 adults compared the effectiveness of andrographis (at either 3 g per day or 6 g per day) versus acetaminophen for sore throat and fever.[26] The higher dose of andrographis (6 g) decreased symptoms of fever and throat pain, as did acetaminophen, while the lower dose of andrographis (3 g) did not. There were no significant side effects in either group.

These studies do not tell us whether andrographis improves immunity or simply relieves symptoms. Still, the results are quite promising and suggest that this herb deserves further study.

### Dosages

A typical dosage of andrographis is 400 mg 3 times daily, taken with lots of liquids at mealtimes. Andrographis is typically standardized to its andrographolide content, usually 4 to 6% in many commercial products.

### Safety Issues

No significant adverse effects have been reported in human studies of andrographis. The 59-person study mentioned earlier asked participants to report side effects, in addition to monitoring lab tests for liver function, complete blood counts, kidney function, and some other laboratory measures of toxicity.[27] All of their tests were within the normal limits for both the placebo and the andrographis groups.

However, full formal safety studies have not been completed. This means that the herb is not recommended for young children, pregnant or nursing women, or those with severe liver or kidney disease.

There are some concerns from animal studies that andrographis may impair fertility. One study showed that male rats became infertile when fed 20 mg of andrographis powder per day.[28] In this case, the rats stopped producing sperm and exhibited physical changes in some of the testicular cells involved in sperm production. Researchers also detected evidence of degeneration of structures in the testicles. However, another study showed no evidence of testicular toxicity in male rats that were given up to 1 g per kilogram of body weight per day for 60 days, so this issue remains unclear.[29]

One group of female mice also did not fare well on andrographis.[30] When fed 2 g per kilogram body weight daily for 6 weeks (thousands of times higher than the usual human dose), all female mice failed to get pregnant when mated with males of proven fertility. Meanwhile, of the control females, 95.2% got pregnant when mated with a similar group of male mice.

While andrographis is probably not a useful form of birth control, these animal studies are somewhat worrisome and warrant further investigation.

## Zinc: Appears Effective, If You Use the Right Form

Another famous alternative treatment for colds is the use of **zinc** (page 348) lozenges. In cases of zinc deficiency, the immune system does not function properly.[31,32] Because zinc is commonly deficient in the diet, especially among senior citizens,[33] nutritional zinc supplementation may certainly be useful for those who get sick easily. Indeed, a recent 2-year, double-blind study suggests that zinc and selenium taken together in nutritional doses can reduce the number of infections in nursing home residents.[34]

However, zinc is most commonly recommended to be used in a different way: sucking on high doses of zinc lozenges at the onset of cold symptoms. This method may work by directly killing viruses in the throat rather than improving the nutritional status of the body.

### What Is the Scientific Evidence for Zinc?

A recent double-blind study concluded that proper use of zinc lozenges can cause many cold symptoms to go away faster than they would otherwise.[35] In this trial, 100 people who were experiencing the early symptoms of a cold were given a lozenge that either contained 13.3 mg of zinc from zinc gluconate or was just a placebo. Participants took the lozenges several times daily until their cold symptoms subsided. The results were impressive. Coughing disappeared within 2.2 days in the treated group versus 4 days in the placebo group. Sore throat disappeared after 1 day versus 3 days in the placebo group, nasal drainage in 4 days (versus 7 days), and headache in 2 days (versus 3 days). Positive results have also been seen in a recent double-blind study of zinc acetate.[36]

Not all studies have shown such positive results.[37] However, the overall results appear to be favorable.[38] It has been suggested that the exact formulation of the zinc lozenge plays a significant role. Flavoring agents, such as citric acid and tartaric acid appear to prevent zinc from killing viruses, and chemical forms of zinc other than zinc gluconate or zinc acetate may not work.[39]

Sweeteners such as sorbitol, sucrose, dextrose, and mannitol are fine, but the information on glycine as a flavoring agent is equivocal.

One recent trial with the right form of zinc lozenge found no benefit, but this may have been due to a cherry flavoring that was added to the lozenges.[40] The bottom line is that certain forms of zinc are probably helpful for colds.

### Dosages

The typical dosage is 13 to 23 mg of zinc as zinc gluconate or zinc acetate, taken every 2 hours at the earliest signs of a cold and continued for no more than a week or two. Lozenges should not contain any other flavorings besides carbohydrate sweeteners such as sorbitol, sucrose, dextrose, and mannitol. Glycine also might be an acceptable flavoring.

For long-term nutritional supplementation of zinc, 10 to 25 mg daily is typically recommended. Zinc can cause **copper** (page 169) deficiency, so it should be combined with 1 to 3 mg of copper daily.

### Safety Issues

The short-term use of zinc every 2 hours is believed to be safe. However, high doses of zinc should not be kept up for more than a week or two because such doses can actually depress the immune system and cause other symptoms if taken for too long. As mentioned previously, zinc can also deplete the body of copper.

## Vitamin C: Not a Cure, but It Helps

**Vitamin C** (page 331) is the most famous of all natural treatments for colds, and it has been subjected to irresponsible hype from both its proponents and opponents. However, if you take a fair look at the research record, it appears that vitamin C can significantly reduce symptoms of colds and help you get over your cold faster.[41,42]

In five studies, in which people took 70 to 200 mg of vitamin C daily, cold symptoms were decreased by about 30%. In 11 other studies that used a higher dosage (1,000 mg or more), symptoms were reduced by 40%.

However, vitamin C does not seem to prevent colds very well, except perhaps those connected with serious endurance exercise such as marathon running.[43,44,45]

A typical dosage is 500 to 1,000 mg 3 to 6 times daily while cold symptoms last. The short-term use of high doses of vitamin C is believed to be safe, although diarrhea may occur.

## Ginseng: May Actually Prevent Colds

Although most people in the West think of **ginseng** (page 206) as a stimulant, in Eastern Europe, ginseng is widely believed to improve overall immunity to illness. As we have seen, echinacea does not seem to prevent colds. But it appears that regular use of ginseng may be able to provide this important benefit.

There are actually three different herbs commonly called ginseng: Asian or Korean ginseng (*Panax ginseng*), American ginseng (*Panax quinquefolius*), and Siberian "ginseng" (*Eleutherococcus senticosus*). The latter herb is actually not ginseng at all, but some herbalists believe that it functions identically.

### What Is the Scientific Evidence for Ginseng?

Unfortunately, most of the scientific studies on ginseng have involved animals who received ginseng injections straight into the abdomen. However, a recent, properly performed, double-blind placebo-controlled study looked at the potential immune-stimulating effects of *Panax ginseng* when taken by mouth.[46] This trial enrolled 227 individuals at three medical offices in Milan, Italy. Half were given ginseng at a dose of 100 mg daily, and the other half took placebo. Four weeks into the study, all participants received influenza vaccine.

The results showed a significant decline in the frequency of colds and flus in the treated group compared to the placebo group (15 versus 42 cases). Also, antibody measurements in response to the vaccination rose higher in the treated group than in the placebo group.

While more research is needed, this study suggests that ginseng may be able to do what echinacea, andrographis, zinc lozenges, and vitamin C cannot: prevent colds.

### Dosages

The typical recommended daily dose of *Panax ginseng* is 1 to 2 g of raw herb, or 200 mg daily of an extract standardized to contain 4 to 7% ginsenosides. *Eleutherococcus* is taken at a dosage of 2 to 3 g whole herb or 300 to 400 mg of extract daily.

Ordinarily, a 2- to 3-week period of using ginseng is recommended, followed by a 1- to 2-week "rest" period. Russian tradition suggests that ginseng should not be used by those under 40 years old.

### Safety Issues

The various forms of ginseng appear to be nontoxic, both in the short and long term, according to the results of studies in mice, rats, chickens, and dwarf pigs. Ginseng also does not seem to be carcinogenic.[47,48,49]

Side effects are rare. Occasionally women report menstrual abnormalities and/or breast tenderness when they take ginseng, and overstimulation and insomnia have also been reported. Unconfirmed reports suggest that highly excessive dosages of ginseng can raise blood pressure, increase heart rate, and possibly cause other significant effects. Whether some of these cases were actually caused by caffeine mixed in with ginseng remains unclear. Ginseng allergy can also occur, as can allergy to any other substance.

In 1979, an article was published in the *Journal of the American Medical Association* claiming that people can become addicted to ginseng and develop blood pressure elevation, nervousness, sleeplessness, diarrhea, and hypersexuality. This report has since been thoroughly discredited and should no longer be taken seriously.[50,51]

However, an unpublished report suggests that ginseng can interfere with drug metabolism, specifically drugs processed by an enzyme called "CYP 3A4." Ask your physician or pharmacist whether you are taking any medications of this type. There have also been specific reports of ginseng interacting with MAO inhibitor drugs and also with a test for digitalis, although again it is not clear whether it was the ginseng or a contaminant that caused the problem.

Safety in young children, pregnant or nursing women, or those with severe liver or kidney disease has not been established. Interestingly, Chinese tradition suggests that ginseng should not be used during pregnancy or lactation.

## OTHER NATURAL TREATMENTS

There is some evidence that **vitamin E** (page 337) may improve immune function, but whether this translates into an effect on colds has not been determined.[52]

A recent study suggests that the herb **elderberry** (page 182) can significantly reduce the length and severity of flu symptoms.[53] Elderberry-flower tea is made by steeping 3 to 5 g of dried flowers in one cup of boiling water for 10 to 15 minutes. A typical dosage is 1 cup 3 times daily. Standardized extracts should be taken according to the directions on the product's label.

Elderberry flower is generally regarded as safe. Side effects are rare and consist primarily of occasional mild gastrointestinal distress or allergic reactions. Nonetheless, safety in young children, pregnant or nursing women, or those with severe liver or kidney disease is not established.

Various herbs are said to work like ginseng and enhance immunity over the long term, including **ashwaganda** (page 128), **astragalus** (page 129), **garlic** (page 197), **suma** (page 307), **reishi** (page 291), and **maitake** (page 254). However, there is as yet no good evidence that they really work. The supplement **arginine** (page 126) might be helpful for preventing colds as well.

Several herbs, including **osha** (page 273), **yarrow** (page 345), **kudzu** (page 241), and **ginger** (page 202), are said to help avert colds when taken at the first sign of infection; but again, there is no scientific evidence that they are effective. Other herbs sometimes recommended to reduce cold symptoms include **mullein** (page 264), **marshmallow** (page 256), and **peppermint** (page 277).

Colds and Flus

Visit Us at TNP.com
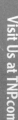

# CONGESTIVE HEART FAILURE

*Principal Natural Treatments*
Coenzyme $Q_{10}$, hawthorn

*Other Natural Treatments*
Taurine, L-carnitine, magnesium, arginine

When the heart sustains injury that weakens its pumping ability, a complicated physiological state called congestive heart failure (CHF) can develop. Fluid builds up in the lungs and lower extremities, the heart enlarges, and many symptoms develop, including severe fatigue, difficulty breathing while lying down, and altered brain function.

Medical treatment for this condition is quite effective and sophisticated and consists of several drugs used in combination.

## PRINCIPAL NATURAL TREATMENTS

CHF is too serious a condition for self-treatment. The supervision of a qualified health-care professional is essential. For this reason, I deliberately do not give detailed dosage information in this section (but you can find them in the chapters on each individual substance). However, given medical supervision, some of the following treatments may be quite useful. In Japan and Europe, coenzyme $Q_{10}$ is frequently added to standard treatment for added benefit. The herb hawthorn alone may be effective for mild CHF.

## Coenzyme $Q_{10}$: Can Be Taken with Standard Medical Treatment

The substance known as **coenzyme $Q_{10}$ ($CoQ_{10}$)** (page 164) appears to be quite helpful when combined with standard treatment for CHF. $CoQ_{10}$ occurs naturally in the energy-producing subunits of all plant and animal cells (the mitochondria). This safe supplement is widely used in Europe, Israel, and Japan as an approved treatment for a variety of cardiovascular conditions.

One double-blind study followed 80 people with CHF and found that adding $CoQ_{10}$ to standard treatment significantly improved heart function.[1]

Another study tracked 641 individuals for 1 full year and found both improved symptoms and a reduced need for hospitalization.[2] $CoQ_{10}$ appears to be essentially nontoxic and side-effect free.[3]

## Hawthorn: Approved in Germany for Mild CHF

The name **hawthorn** (page 222) is derived from "hedgethorn," reflecting this spiny tree's use as a living fence in much of Europe. During the Middle Ages, hawthorn was used to treat dropsy, a condition that we now call CHF. It was also used for other heart ailments and for sore throat.

Hawthorn is widely regarded in modern Europe as a safe and effective treatment for the early stages of CHF. Although not as potent as that other famous heart herb of the Middle Ages, foxglove (digitalis), hawthorn is much safer. The active ingredients in foxglove are the drugs digoxin and digitoxin. However, hawthorn does not appear to have any single active ingredient. This has prevented it from being turned into a drug.

Like digitalis, hawthorn speeds up the heart and increases its force of contraction. However, it may offer one very important advantage. Digitalis and other medications that increase the power of the heart also make it more irritable and liable to dangerous irregularities of rhythm. In contrast, hawthorn appears to have the unique property of both strengthening the heart and stabilizing it against arrythmias.[4,5,6] Also, with digitalis the difference between the proper dose and the toxic dose is very small. Hawthorn has an enormous range of safe dosing.[7]

Between 1981 and 1994, 13 controlled clinical studies of hawthorn were conducted, most of them double-blind.[8] A total of 808 people participated in these trials. The collective results strongly suggest that hawthorn is an effective treatment for early stages of CHF. Comparative studies suggest that hawthorn is about as effective as a low dose of the conventional drug captopril.

**Note:** Although captopril and other standard drugs in the same family have been shown to reduce mortality associated with CHF, there is no similar evidence for hawthorn.

Hawthorn appears to be quite safe. Germany's Commission E lists no known risks, contraindications, or drug interactions with hawthorn, and mice and rats have been given phenomenal doses without showing significant toxicity.[9] However, because hawthorn obviously affects the heart, it should not be combined with other heart drugs without a physician's supervision.

Side effects are also rare and consist mainly of mild stomach upset and occasional allergic reactions (skin rash). Safety in young children, pregnant or nursing women, and those with severe kidney or liver disease has not been established.

## OTHER NATURAL TREATMENTS

Several studies suggest that the amino acid **taurine** (page 308) may be useful in CHF[10–16] and may be more effective than CoQ$_{10}$.[17] Taurine is believed to be safe.

Another treatment for CHF that has some evidence is the expensive supplement **L-carnitine** (page 151), especially when given in the special form called L-propionyl-carnitine.[18–21] Carnitine is frequently combined with CoQ$_{10}$.

There is also some evidence that supplementing with **magnesium** (page 251) or **arginine** (page 126) may be useful.

Finally, it is important to pay attention to all the general considerations that bring health to the heart, such as those described in the chapter on **atherosclerosis** (page 14).

# CONSTIPATION

### *Principal Natural Treatments*

Increased dietary fiber (psyllium husks, debittered fenugreek seeds, and flaxseed) and water intake, cascara sagrada, He shou wu, dandelion

In the nineteenth century, a naturopathic concept came into being whose influence persists today: namely, that regular, frequent, and complete bowel movements are necessary for optimum health. William Harvey Kellogg, of Kellogg's cereal fame, wrote extensively of the dangers of "auto-intoxication" purportedly caused by inadequate elimination. He and others claimed that a concrete-like sludge builds up on the wall of the colon, increasing in thickness over time and destroying the health of the body.

However, in modern times physicians have performed millions of direct examinations of the colon, using the procedure known as colonoscopy, without finding any evidence of such a coating. Caked colons are a myth.

Furthermore, conventional medicine has never observed any connection between elimination and overall health. Many people eliminate only once a week or so, and their health appears to be no worse than that of the population at large. Nonetheless, most people find constipation unpleasant, and for some it becomes a severe chronic problem.

Conventional treatment for constipation involves mainly increasing exercise and intake of dietary fiber and water while reserving laxatives, suppositories, and enemas for emergencies.

## PRINCIPAL NATURAL TREATMENTS

Occasional constipation can be safely self-treated. However, if constipation becomes a chronic problem, it should be evaluated by a physician.

Increasing dietary fiber and water intake is the first treatment to try for chronic constipation. Some of the most useful forms of fiber are psyllium husks, debittered **fenugreek** (page 185) seeds, and flaxseed. A typical dosage is 5 to 10 g 1 to 3 times daily, with at least 16 ounces of liquid. Start with the lower doses and work up gradually, as too much fiber all at once can actually worsen constipation.

The herb cascara sagrada is an approved over-the-counter treatment for constipation. However, when taken by itself, it can occasionally cause dependence. It is often combined in small amounts with other herbs, including barberry, turkey rhubarb, **dandelion** (page 174), **red raspberry** (page 291), **goldenseal** (page 217), and **cayenne**

(page 155), that gently affect the digestive tract. However, the safety and efficacy of these combinations have not been proven. Dandelion used alone and the Chinese herb **He shou wu** (page 224) are also reputed to be effective.

A final point about constipation: Like sleep, elimination is inhibited by thinking too much about it. Part of the key to solving chronic constipation problems is to decrease the sense of worry and anxiety that surrounds the issue. Although constipation is certainly unpleasant, its evils have been greatly exaggerated. Thinking less about it will often go a long way toward solving the problem.

# CYCLIC MASTALGIA
## (CYCLIC MASTITIS, FIBROCYSTIC BREAST DISEASE)

*Principal Natural Treatments*
    Evening primrose oil (GLA), ginkgo, chasteberry, iodine

Some women's breasts are unusually tender and lumpy, with symptoms of pain and dull heaviness that vary with the menstrual cycle. This condition is called cyclic mastalgia or mastitis and is often associated with premenstrual stress syndrome (PMS). When the lumps become significant enough to be called cysts, this condition is sometimes called fibrocystic breast disease.

Besides discomfort, perhaps the worst problem of this condition is that it can mimic the appearance of breast cancer on mammograms, leading to false alarms. To make matters worse, fibrocystic changes can also hide true cancers, and women with fibrocystic breast disease may also have a greater tendency toward breast cancer (although this is controversial).

Conventional treatment of cyclic mastalgia has incorporated many staples of alternative medicine. After screening carefully for breast cancer, physicians typically recommend reducing animal fats, avoiding chocolate and caffeine, and supplementing with vitamin E (400 IU daily) and vitamin $B_6$ (50 mg daily). Some physicians have begun to use evening primrose oil as well. These treatments are more likely to be successful in cases that involve pain but no cysts. Even so, the

response to therapy is slow, often requiring over 6 months for full results.

If these natural methods don't work, physicians may prescribe various hormone or hormone-like medications.

## PRINCIPAL NATURAL TREATMENTS

Cyclic mastalgia often occurs in connection with **PMS** (page 104). (See the chapter on PMS for information on related treatments.)

### Evening Primrose Oil (Source of GLA)

European physicians commonly use evening primrose oil to treat cyclic mastalgia, and the practice has come to be popular among some physicians in the United States as well. Evening primrose oil contains relatively high concentrations of the essential fatty acid gamma-linolenic acid, or **GLA** (page 210). Fatty acid metabolism is known to be disturbed in women with cyclic mastalgia, and abnormalities in essential fatty acid levels have been found in women with PMS and with nonmalignant breast disease.[1] It appears that supplementation with evening primrose oil may be able to correct this imbalance.

## What Is the Scientific Evidence for Evening Primrose Oil?

In uncontrolled studies, evening primrose oil has been found to produce significant benefits in about 44% of women with cyclic mastalgia.[2]

Improvement was also seen in a controlled study of 73 women suffering from cyclic breast pain.[3] Discomfort was significantly reduced in the group taking evening primrose oil, whereas no significant improvement was seen in the placebo group.

However, evening primrose oil does not seem to be helpful when there are breast cysts rather than just pain. In a 1-year double-blind study of 200 women with breast cysts, evening primrose oil did not prove effective.[4,5]

### Dosages

A typical dosage of evening primrose oil for cyclic mastalgia is 3 g daily. It must be taken for at least 4 to 6 weeks for noticeable effect, and maximum benefits may require 4 to 8 months to develop. Borage oil and black currant oil also contain GLA and are sometimes used instead.

### Safety Issues

Animal studies suggest that evening primrose oil is completely nontoxic and noncarcinogenic.[6] Over 4,000 people have taken GLA or evening primrose oil in scientific studies, and no significant adverse effects have ever been noted. However, somewhat less than 2% of the study participants who took evening primrose oil complained of mild headaches and/or gastrointestinal distress, especially at higher dosages.[7,8]

The maximum safe dosage for young children, pregnant or nursing women, or those with severe liver or kidney disease has not been established.

## Ginkgo

Although the herb **ginkgo** (page 204) is primarily used to enhance memory and mental function, it may be helpful for breast tenderness as well. A double-blind study evaluated 143 women with PMS symptoms, 18 to 45 years of age, and followed them for two menstrual cycles.[9] When the study began, each woman received either the ginkgo extract or placebo on day 16 of the first cycle. Treatment was continued until day 5 of the next cycle, and resumed again on day 16 of that cycle.

The results were impressive. As compared to placebo, ginkgo significantly relieved major symptoms of PMS, especially breast pain.

### Dosages

The form of ginkgo used in the study I just described and in all other scientific trials is a highly concentrated extract, in which 50 pounds of the leaf must be used to create 1 pound of product. Such extracts are standardized to contain 24% by weight substances known as ginkgo flavonol glycosides. The proper dosage of ginkgo is 40 to 80 mg 3 times daily. It should be taken from about 2 weeks prior to your menstrual period until bleeding stops.

### Safety Issues

Ginkgo extract appears to be quite safe. A review of nearly 10,000 participants taking ginkgo extract showed that less than 1% experienced side effects, and those that did occur were minor.[10] In another study, overall side effects were no greater in the ginkgo group than in the placebo group.[11] When a medication produces no more side effects than the placebo, we can reasonably regard it as essentially side-effect free. Furthermore, according to animal studies, ginkgo is safe even when taken in massive overdose.[12]

However, taking ginkgo presents one potential concern. The herb possesses a mild blood-thinning effect that could conceivably cause bleeding problems in certain situations. For this reason, people with hemophilia should not take ginkgo except on a physician's advice. Using ginkgo in the weeks prior to or just after major surgery or labor and delivery is also not advisable. Finally, ginkgo should not be combined with blood-thinning drugs such as Coumadin (warfarin), heparin, aspirin, and Trental (pentoxifylline) except under medical supervision. Ginkgo might also conceivably interact with natural products that slightly thin the blood as well, such as **garlic** (page 197) and high-dose **vitamin E** (page 337).

The safety of ginkgo for young children, pregnant or nursing women, and people with kidney or liver disease has not been established.

Depression

## Chasteberry

In Germany, the herb **chasteberry** (page 157) is frequently used to treat cyclic mastalgia and other symptoms of PMS.[13,14,15] (For a detailed discussion of chasteberry use and safety issues, please see the corresponding chapter in Part Two.)

## Other Treatments

The supplement **iodine** (page 233) may also be helpful for cyclic mastalgia in some cases.

 # DEPRESSION (MILD TO MODERATE)

*Principal Natural Treatments*
    St. John's wort

*Other Natural Treatments*
    Phenylalanine, 5-HTP, ginkgo, phosphatidylserine, S-adenosylmethionine, inositol, vitamin $B_6$, vitamin $B_{12}$, folic acid, damiana, beta-carotene, NADH, pregnenolone, tyrosine

*Not Recommended Treatments*
    Yohimbe, DHEA

Depression is a common emotional illness that varies widely in its intensity from person to person. The natural treatments described in this section are useful only for mild to moderate depressive symptoms consisting mainly of depressed mood, fatigue, insomnia, irritability, and difficulty concentrating.

More severe depression includes severely depressed mood complicated by symptoms such as slowed speech, slowed (or agitated) responses, markedly impaired memory and concentration, excessive (or diminished) sleep, significant weight loss (or weight gain), intense feelings of worthlessness and guilt, recurrent thoughts of suicide, and lack of interest in pleasurable activities.

Severe clinical depression is a dangerous and excruciating illness. The emotional structure of the brain has frozen into a pattern of misery that cannot be altered by willpower, a change of scenery, or the most earnest efforts of friends. In a sense, the brain has locked up like a crashed computer. No alternative treatment is especially successful when depression gets this bad.

One of the earliest successful treatments for major depression was shock therapy. This technique is almost the exact equivalent of rebooting a computer, and in cases of major depression its effects were revolutionary. For the first time, a reliable way was available to bring people out of the depths of severe major depression. However, shock treatment was overused at first and became unpopular.

The accidental discovery of antidepressant drugs provided a less interventive route. The original antidepressants, known as MAO inhibitors, could bring people out from the depths of major depression as successfully as shock treatment. However, MAO inhibitors can cause serious and even fatal side effects. No one would ever think of using MAO inhibitors to treat mild to moderate depression.

Subsequently, antidepressants with progressively fewer side effects came on the market, but it was not until the appearance of selective serotonin-reuptake inhibitors (SSRIs), such as Prozac and related drugs, that antidepressants became a viable option for depression that was less than catastrophic. Practically overnight, enormous numbers of people began taking Prozac and similar antidepressants for mild to moderate depression.

The big advantage of the SSRIs is that they don't cause fatigue. Many people find them to be entirely side-effect free. However, side effects are not uncommon and include nausea, insomnia, and sexual disturbances (such as the loss of the ability to experience an orgasm).

# PRINCIPAL NATURAL TREATMENTS

Alternative medicine offers one solidly proven treatment for depression: the herb St. John's wort. The evidence for this herb's effectiveness is nearly as comprehensive as what is required of a drug prior to approval. However, St. John's wort is only useful for mild to moderate depression. For severe depression, conventional antidepressant drugs are necessary and may be lifesaving.

## St. John's Wort:
## A Well-Established Treatment
## for Mild to Moderate Depression

**St. John's wort** (page 303) (*Hypericum perforatum*) is a common perennial herb, with many branches and bright yellow flowers, that grows wild in much of the world. Its name derives from the herb's tendency to flower around the feast of St. John (wort simply means "plant" in Old English). The species name *perforatum* derives from the watermarking of translucent dots that can be seen when a leaf of the plant is held up to the sun.

St. John's wort has a long history of use in emotional disorders. It began to be considered as a treatment for depression early in the twentieth century, and when pharmaceutical antidepressants were invented, German researchers looked for similar properties in St. John's wort.

Today, St. John's wort is one of the best-documented herbal treatments, with a scientific record approaching that of many prescription drugs. Indeed, this herb is a prescription antidepressant in Germany. It is covered by that country's national health-care system and is prescribed more frequently than any synthetic drug. At the time of this writing, St. John's wort has also become the most commonly used antidepressant in the United States.

St. John's wort is used for mild to moderate depression. Typical symptoms include depressed mood, lack of energy, sleep problems, anxiety, appetite disturbance, difficulty concentrating, and poor stress tolerance. Irritability can also be a sign of depression.

St. John's wort appears to be effective in about 55% of cases. As with other antidepressants, the full benefit takes about 4 to 6 weeks to develop. The most common reported effects are brightened mood, increased energy, and improved sleep.

The big advantage of St. John's wort over standard medications is that it rarely, if ever, causes side effects. However, St. John's wort should never be relied on to treat severe depression. If you or a loved one is feeling suicidal, unable to cope with daily life, paralyzed by anxiety, incapable of getting out of bed, unable to sleep, or uninterested in eating, see a physician at once. Drug therapy may save your life.

Like other antidepressants, St. John's wort can also be used to treat chronic insomnia and anxiety when they are related to depression. It may be effective in seasonal affective disorder (SAD) as well.

## What Is the Scientific Evidence for St. John's Wort?

All together, at least 15 double-blind studies comparing St. John's wort to placebo have been reported at the time of this writing.[1,2] A review that evaluated most of these studies found that nine of them were performed according to adequate scientific standards, involving a total of over 600 participants.[3] According to the review author, "on the basis of the published, scientifically compelling evidence, Hypericum represents an effective therapy for the alleviation of the symptoms of depression." This body of research has been criticized by some authorities who point out that none of the studies exceeded 8 weeks in length. However, as it states in the *Physicians' Desk Reference*, Prozac was approved on the basis of studies that lasted no longer than 6 weeks.

## How Does St. John's Wort Work?

We do not really know how St. John's wort acts. Early research suggested that it works like the oldest class of antidepressants, the MAO inhibitors.[4] However, later research essentially discredited this idea.[5,6] More recent research has focused on a connection between St. John's wort and serotonin.[7,8] The substance hyperforin may be a major active ingredient in St. John's wort.[9]

## Dosages

The standard dosage of St. John's wort is 300 mg 3 times daily of an extract standardized to contain 0.3% hypericin. Recently, a new form of the herb has come on the market standardized to

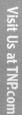

3 to 5% hyperforin instead. However, the dosage amount is the same. Some people take 600 mg of St. John's wort in the morning and 300 mg at night, or 500 mg twice daily. This dosage should not be exceeded, as it is not clear that higher doses produce any better effects, and the chance of side effects might increase.

If the herb bothers your stomach, take it with food. Remember that the full effect takes 4 weeks to develop, so don't give up too soon!

**Warning:** Various systemic diseases, such as hypothyroidism, chronic hepatitis, and anemia, may masquerade as depression. Make sure to find out whether you have an undiagnosed medical illness before treating yourself with St. John's wort.

Also, it can sometimes be difficult to assess the true intensity of your own depression. A physician's evaluation is essential. If you suffer from severe major depression, you should take medications rather than St. John's wort.

### Safety Issues

St. John's wort is essentially side-effect free. Strangely, this good news has an unfortunate consequence: Some people who try St. John's wort decide that it must not be very powerful because it doesn't make them feel ill, so they quit. Be patient!

In a study designed to look for side effects, 3,250 people took St. John's wort for 4 weeks.[10] Overall, about 2.4% experienced side effects. The most common were mild stomach discomfort (0.6%); allergic reactions, mainly rash (0.5%); tiredness (0.4%); and restlessness (0.3%).

In the extensive German experience with St. John's wort as a treatment for depression, no reports of serious adverse consequences have been published.[11] Animal studies involving enormous doses for 26 weeks have not shown any serious toxicity.[12]

Cows and sheep grazing on St. John's wort have sometimes developed severe and even fatal sensitivity to the sun. However, this has never occurred in humans taking St. John's wort at normal doses.[13] In one study, highly sun-sensitive people were given twice the normal dose of the herb.[14] The results showed a mild but measurable increase in reaction to ultraviolet radiation.

The moral of the story is that if you are especially sensitive to the sun, do not exceed the recommended dosage of St. John's wort and continue to take your usual precautions against burning.

A recent report suggests that regular use of St. John's wort might increase the risk of cataracts.[15] While this is preliminary information, it might make sense to wear sunglasses when outdoors if you are taking this herb on a long-term basis.

Older reports suggested that St. John's wort works like the class of drugs known as MAO inhibitors.[16] This led to a number of warnings, including avoiding cheese and decongestants while taking St. John's wort. However, this concern is no longer considered realistic.[17,18]

Safety in young children, pregnant or nursing women, and those with severe liver or kidney disease has not been established.

### Drug Interactions

Herbal experts have warned for some time that combining St. John's wort with drugs in the Prozac family (SSRIs) might raise serotonin too much and cause a number of serious problems. Recently, case reports of such events have begun to trickle in.[19,20] This is a potentially serious risk. Do not combine St. John's wort with prescription antidepressants except on the specific advice of a physician. Since some antidepressants, such as Prozac, linger in the blood for quite some time, you also need to exercise caution when switching from a drug to St. John's wort. If you stop Prozac, you may need to wait 3 weeks or more before starting St. John's wort.

It has been recently reported that St. John's wort lowers blood levels of theophylline, an asthma medication. Unpublished data from the University of Colorado suggest that the hypericin in St. John's wort may increase the activity of an enzyme called cytochrome P-450.[21,22] This substance is responsible for metabolizing many drugs and other chemicals. By increasing P-450 activity, St. John's wort may cause the body to break down these drugs faster, thereby making them less effective. Before taking St. John's wort, it might be a good idea to ask your physician whether any of your medications would be affected by "cytochrome P-450 CYP 1A1 and 1A2 induction."

Another study out of the University of Colorado suggests that St. John's wort may interfere with the action of the antitumor drugs etoposide (VePesid), teniposide (Vumon), mitoxantrone (Novantrone), and doxorubicin (Adriamycin).[23]

## OTHER NATURAL TREATMENTS

There are a number of other herbs and supplements that may be helpful in depression, although the evidence for them is not as strong as that for St. John's wort.

## Phenylalanine: A Promising Treatment for Depression

**Phenylalanine** (page 278) is a naturally occurring amino acid that we all consume in our daily diets. There is some evidence that phenylalanine supplements may help reduce symptoms of depression.

### What Is the Scientific Evidence for Phenylalanine?

Phenylalanine occurs in a right-hand and a left-hand form, known as D- and L-phenylalanine, respectively. Some studies have evaluated the D-form and others the L- form, and still others have evaluated mixtures of both. All seem to be able to provide some measure of relief for symptoms of depression. The mixed form (DLPA) is the type most commonly available in stores.

A 1978 study compared the effectiveness of D-phenylalanine against the antidepressant drug imipramine (taken in daily doses of 100 mg) and found them to be equally effective.[24] A total of 60 individuals were randomly assigned to either one group or the other and followed for 30 days. D-phenylalanine worked more rapidly, producing significant improvement in only 15 days.

Another double-blind study followed 27 people, half of whom received DL-phenylalanine and the other half imipramine in higher doses of 150 to 200 mg daily.[25,26] When the participants were reevaluated in 30 days, the two groups had improved by the same amount.

Unfortunately, there do not seem to have been any properly designed studies that compared phenylalanine to placebo. Until these are performed, phenylalanine cannot be considered a proven treatment for depression, but it is certainly promising.

### Dosages

When used as a treatment for depression, L-phenylalanine is typically started at a dosage of 500 mg daily, and then gradually increased to 3 to 4 g daily.[27] However, side effects may develop at dosages above 1,500 mg daily (see Safety Issues).

D- or DL-phenylalanine may be used for depression as well, but the typical dosage is much lower: 100 to 400 mg daily.[28]

### Safety Issues

Although most people do not report side effects from any type of phenylalanine, daily doses near or above 1,500 mg of L-phenylalanine can reportedly cause anxiety, headache, and even mildly elevated blood pressure.[29]

The long-term safety of phenylalanine in any of its forms is not known.

Both L- and D-phenylalanine must be avoided by those with the rare metabolic disease phenylketonuria (PKU). The safety of high dosages of L-phenylalanine, or any dosage of D-phenylalanine, has not been established for young children, pregnant or nursing women, or those with severe liver or kidney disease.

There are some indications that combining phenylalanine with antipsychotic drugs might increase the risk of developing the long-term side effect known as tardive dyskinesia.[30,31] We also don't know if it is safe to combine phenylalanine with standard antidepressants.

## 5-HTP: May Be Effective, but Use Caution

A new, up-and-coming treatment for depression is **5-HTP (5-hydroxytryptophan)** (page 191). When the body sets about manufacturing serotonin, it first makes 5-HTP. The theory behind taking 5-HTP as a supplement is that providing the one-step-removed raw ingredient might raise serotonin levels. However, this plausible idea has not been proven.

The amino acid tryptophan used to be recommended as a treatment for depression on the

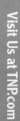

same basis. It is one step back in the chain, being turned by the body into 5-HTP and then to serotonin. However, tryptophan was removed from the market several years ago when a contaminant caused a terrible and often permanent illness in many people who took the supplement. Because 5-HTP is made by a completely different manufacturing process (starting from a plant rather than bacteria), one would not expect the same contaminant to be present. Disturbingly, however, recent reports suggest otherwise (see Safety Issues).

Like St. John's wort, 5-HTP is used mainly in Europe, where many physicians find it an effective treatment for both depression and insomnia.

### What Is the Scientific Evidence for 5-HTP?

There have been several preliminary studies of 5-HTP.[32] The best of these trials was a 6-week study of 63 people given either 5-HTP (100 mg 3 times daily) or an antidepressant in the Prozac family (fluvoxamine, 50 mg 3 times daily).[33] The results showed equal benefit between the supplement and the drug. Actually, 5-HTP worked a little better, but from a mathematical perspective, the difference was not statistically significant.

5-HTP caused fewer and less severe side effects than fluvoxamine. The only real complaint was occasional mild digestive distress.

### Dosages

The typical dosage of 5-HTP is 100 to 200 mg 3 times daily.

### Safety Issues

5-HTP seldom causes noticeable side effects other than occasional digestive distress. However, comprehensive safety studies have not been performed, and there is one significant concern. As I mentioned earlier, the amino acid tryptophan was removed from the stores several years ago when a contaminant caused a terrible and often permanently disabling or fatal illness in many people who took the supplement. Alarmingly, on September 7, 1998, the FDA released a report stating that some commercial 5-HTP preparations had been found to contain a similar contaminant. I suggest you check with your physician for the most recent information.

Like St. John's wort, 5-HTP probably should not be combined with conventional antidepressants. Safety in young children, pregnant or nursing women, and those with severe liver or kidney disease has not been established.

## Ginkgo: Improves Mental Function, but May Help Depression, Too

**Ginkgo** (page 204) is used mainly for age-related mental decline, such as that from **Alzheimer's disease** (page 4). However, during the studies on impaired mental function, researchers frequently observed improvements in mood and relief from symptoms of depression. This incidental discovery led scientists to investigate whether ginkgo might be useful as an antidepressant treatment.

One study, published in 1990, evaluated this effect in 60 people who suffered from depressive symptoms along with other signs of dementia.[34] The results showed significant improvements among participants given ginkgo extract instead of placebo.

Another study followed 40 depressed individuals over the age of 50 who had not responded successfully to antidepressant treatment.[35] Those who were given ginkgo showed an average drop of 50% in scores on the Hamilton Depression scale, whereas the placebo group showed only a 10% improvement.

In 1994 an interesting piece of research was reported that may shed light on the mechanism by which ginkgo could reduce depression.[36] This study examined levels of serotonin receptors in rats of various ages. When older rats were given ginkgo, the level of serotonin-binding sites increased. However, the same effect was not observed in younger rats. The researchers theorized that ginkgo may block an age-related loss of serotonin receptors.

Reduced receptors for serotonin may mean that the body needs more serotonin to produce a normal effect. Instead of raising the level of serotonin, like Prozac does, ginkgo may thus improve the brain's ability to respond to serotonin (at least in older people). However, this is still highly speculative. More experimentation is needed to clarify the mechanism of ginkgo's action and to better quantify its effectiveness in depression.

The proper dose of ginkgo is 40 to 80 mg of a 24% extract taken 3 times daily. As is the case with conventional antidepressants, the full benefit takes up to 6 weeks to develop.

Ginkgo appears to be very safe. Extremely high doses have been given to animals without serious consequences.[37] In all the clinical trials of ginkgo up to 1991, involving a total of almost 10,000 people, only a small number of participants reported side effects produced by ginkgo extract. There were 21 cases of gastrointestinal discomfort and even fewer cases of headaches, dizziness, and allergic skin reactions.[38]

However, because ginkgo slightly thins the blood, it should not be combined with anticoagulant drugs or even aspirin (for more information on this potential risk, see the chapter on ginkgo in Part Two).

Safety in young children, pregnant or nursing women, and those with severe liver or kidney disease has not been established.

## Phosphatidylserine: Good for Mental Function, May Also Help Depression

**Phosphatidylserine** (page 280) is another treatment used mainly for mental decline in the elderly that may also offer antidepressant benefits.[39] (For more information on phosphatidylserine use, see the corresponding chapter in Part Two.)

The proper dosage is 100 mg 3 times daily. Full results take anywhere from 4 weeks to 6 months to manifest. Although no side effects have been reported, this rather expensive supplement usually costs from $50 to $75 per month. Safety in young children, pregnant or nursing women, and those with severe liver or kidney disease has not been established.

## S-Adenosylmethionine: May Be Effective, but Very Expensive

Another European supplement treatment for depression newly arrived in the United States is **SAMe (S-adenosylmethionine)** (page 293). SAMe is a very important biological molecule that occurs throughout the body. Its job is to hand over a chemical fragment called a methyl group to other chemicals that need it.

SAMe is especially popular in Italy, where some physicians report that it is a fast-acting antidepressant. They sometimes use SAMe alongside conventional antidepressants at the very beginning of treatment to provide immediate relief. SAMe is also used as a treatment for osteoarthritis, for which it has a fairly strong research record. Unfortunately, the sum total of evidence for SAMe as an antidepressant remains small and is flawed by the fact that most studies used an intravenous form of the supplement.

In addition to a lack of reliable evidence, SAMe is extremely expensive. The proper dosage is 400 mg 3 to 4 times daily and can cost over $200 per month, although the price is dropping. To minimize stomach distress, most physicians recommend starting at a low dose of perhaps 200 mg twice daily and then gradually working up from there. Once you reach the full dose, stay at it for a month or so. Then, once you are feeling better, you can try reducing the dose again. Some physicians report that a daily dose as low (and as inexpensive!) as 400 mg may be effective for maintaining antidepressant benefits.

SAMe appears to be safe. However, safety in young children, pregnant or nursing women, and those with liver or kidney disease has not been established. It should not be combined with standard antidepressant treatment except under the supervision of a physician.

## Other Herbs and Supplements

Weak evidence suggests that the nutritional substance **inositol** (page 231) might be helpful in depression when taken in extremely high doses (12 g daily).[40] Although this is a nutritional substance, when taken in such enormous doses, its safety cannot be assured.

Diets low in **vitamin B$_6$** (page 326), **vitamin B$_{12}$** (page 329), or **folic acid** (page 194) have been associated with symptoms of depression.[41,42,43] While there is little direct evidence that taking B$_6$ or B$_{12}$ supplements can help depression, an intriguing body of evidence suggests that folic acid supplements really help.[44–51] In any case, since deficiencies of B$_6$ and folic acid are common, and B$_{12}$ deficiencies occur more often with advancing age, there is a lot to be said for taking these vitamins on general principle.

For depression, typical daily doses are 25 to 50 mg of $B_6$, 400 mcg of folic acid, and 10 to 100 mcg of $B_{12}$. These supplements are safe when taken at these doses.

The herbs and supplements **damiana** (page 173), **beta-carotene** (page 131), **NADH** (page 267), **pregnenolone** (page 284), and **tyrosine** (page 312) are also sometimes recommended for depression, but there is little evidence as yet that they really work.

## NOT RECOMMENDED TREATMENTS FOR DEPRESSION

The herb **yohimbe** (page 347) and the hormone **DHEA** (page 176) are sometimes suggested for depression, but because of potential risks I do not suggest using them except under the supervision of a qualified health-care professional (if at all).

 # DIABETES

*Principal Natural Treatments*

*Blood sugar control:*
  Chromium, fenugreek, gymnema, ginseng, garlic, onion, bitter melon, pterocarpus, vanadium, bilberry, *Coccinia indica*, salt bush, vitamin E, biotin, niacinamide

*Treatment of complications:*
  Lipoic acid, evening primrose oil (GLA), bilberry, OPCs, ginkgo, vitamin C, inositol, biotin

*To correct nutritional deficiencies:*
  Magnesium, zinc, vitamin C, vitamin A, taurine, manganese

*Preventing diabetes:*
  Niacinamide

Diabetes has two forms. In the type that develops early in childhood (type 1), the insulin-secreting cells of the pancreas are destroyed (probably by a viral infection), and blood levels of insulin drop nearly to zero. However, in the adult-onset form (type 2), insulin is often plentiful, but the body does not respond normally to it. (This is only an approximate description of the difference between the two types; a full explanation is too technical for this book.) In both forms of diabetes, blood sugar reaches toxic levels, causing injury to many organs and tissues.

Conventional treatment for childhood-onset diabetes includes insulin injections and careful dietary monitoring. The adult-onset form may respond to lifestyle changes alone, such as increasing exercise, losing weight, and improving diet. Various oral medications are also often effective for adult-onset diabetes, although insulin injections may be necessary in some cases.

## PRINCIPAL NATURAL TREATMENTS

Several alternative methods may be helpful when used under medical supervision as an addition to standard treatment. They may help stabilize, reduce, or eliminate medication requirements; reduce the symptoms of diabetic complications; or correct nutritional deficiencies associated with diabetes. However, because diabetes is a dangerous disease with many potential complications, alternative treatment for diabetes should not be attempted as a substitute for conventional medical care.

### Treatments for Improving Blood Sugar Control

The following treatments may be able to improve blood sugar control in type 1 and/or type 2 diabetes. However, keep in mind that if they work, you will need to reduce your medications to avoid hypoglycemia. For this reason, medical supervision is essential.

## Chromium: Helpful in Type 1 and Type 2 Diabetes

**Chromium** (page 161) is an essential trace mineral that plays a significant role in sugar metabolism. Reasonably good evidence suggests that chromium supplementation may help bring blood sugar levels under control in both type 1 and type 2 diabetes.

A 4-month study reported in 1997 followed 180 Chinese men and women with type 2 diabetes, comparing the effects of 1,000 mcg chromium, 200 mcg chromium, and a placebo.[1] The results showed that HbA1c values (a measure of long-term blood sugar control) improved significantly after 2 months in the group receiving 1,000 mcg, and in both chromium groups after 4 months. Fasting glucose was also lower in the group taking the higher dose of chromium.

Another controlled study in 1993 of 243 people with either type 1 or type 2 diabetes found that chromium supplementation at 200 mcg daily decreased insulin or oral medication requirements in 57% of adult-onset and 34% of childhood-onset cases.[2] More women than men responded favorably, and placebo was ineffective. While not all studies have produced positive results,[3] the bulk of the evidence suggests that chromium is indeed effective.

The optimum dosage of chromium is not known. The usual recommended therapeutic dosage is 400 to 600 mcg daily (as chromium picolinate). However, one of the recent studies just described used a higher dose. Since there have been a few worrisome case reports of toxic effects when chromium has been taken at daily doses of 1,200 mcg or higher,[4,5] you should consult with your physician on what might be the appropriate dosage for you.

## Fenugreek: Appears to Be Helpful

The food spice **fenugreek** (page 185) may also help control blood sugar. For millennia, fenugreek has been used both as a medicine and as a spice in Egypt, India, and the Middle East. Numerous animal studies and small-scale trials in humans involving a total of about 100 people have found that fenugreek can reduce blood sugar and serum cholesterol levels in people with diabetes.[6,7,8] It seems to be helpful in both type 1 and type 2 diabetes.

**Dosages**    Because the seeds of fenugreek are somewhat bitter, fenugreek is best taken in capsule form. The typical dosage is 5 to 30 g 3 times a day with meals, taken indefinitely.

**Safety Issues**    As a commonly eaten food, fenugreek is generally regarded as safe. The only common side effect is mild gastrointestinal distress when it is taken in high doses.

Extracts made from fenugreek have been shown to cause uterine contractions in guinea pigs.[9] For this reason, pregnant women should not take fenugreek in doses higher than is commonly used as a spice, perhaps 5 g daily. Safety in young children, nursing women, or those with severe liver or kidney disease has also not been established.

## Gymnema: Preliminary Evidence Suggests It Is Effective

A few preliminary studies suggest that the Ayurvedic (Indian) herb **gymnema** (page 221) may help improve blood sugar control.[10,11,12] In practice, many clinicians report that gymnema is more powerful than the other treatments described in this section. It might be helpful for mild cases of adult-onset diabetes, taken alone or in combination with standard treatment (under a doctor's supervision in either case).

The usual dose of gymnema is 400 to 600 mg daily of an extract standardized to contain 24% gymnemic acids. Because no formal safety studies have been conducted, gymnema should not be taken by young children, pregnant or nursing women, or those with severe kidney or liver disease.

## Ginseng: Promising New Evidence

A double-blind study evaluated the effects of **ginseng** (page 206) in 36 people newly diagnosed with adult-onset diabetes over an 8-week period.[13] The results showed a reduction in glucose levels, improved glycosylated hemoglobin (a measure of long-term blood sugar control), and improved physical capacity. Although ginseng is generally believed to be safe, safety in young children, pregnant or nursing women, and those with severe kidney or liver disease has not been established. (See the chapter on ginseng in Part II for a more detailed discussion of potential safety issues.)

### Other Treatments That May Help Control Blood Sugar

Preliminary evidence suggests that **garlic** (page 197), onion, **bitter melon** (page 137), pterocarpus, **bilberry** (page 135), **vanadium** (page 317), *Coccinia indica,* and salt bush may help some people with diabetes improve blood sugar control.[14-26]

Preliminary studies indicate that **vitamin E** (page 337) may also slightly improve blood sugar control in type 2 diabetes.[27,28] (For a discussion of the safety issues and the proper dosage amounts, see the chapter on vitamin E in Part Two.)

If your child has just developed diabetes, the supplement niacinamide—a form of niacin, also called **vitamin B₃** (page 323)—may prolong what is called the honeymoon period.[29] This is the interval during which the pancreas can still make some insulin, and insulin needs are low. By giving your child niacinamide, you may be able to buy some time to allow him or her to adjust to a life of insulin injections.

When used as therapy for a specific disease, niacinamide is taken in dosages much higher than nutritional needs, about 1 to 4 g daily. Because this dose creates a risk of liver inflammation, medical supervision is essential.

The supplement **biotin** (page 136) is also sometimes said to be helpful in diabetes, for both blood sugar control and reduction of complications, but there is as yet little direct evidence that it works.

## Treating Complications of Diabetes

Several supplements may help prevent or treat some of the common complications of diabetes.

Because atherosclerosis is one of the worst problems with diabetes, all the suggestions discussed in the chapter on **atherosclerosis** (page 14) may be useful.

Other herbs and supplements may be helpful for diabetic neuropathy, diabetic retinopathy, and diabetic cataracts, so the treatments in the chapter on **cataracts** (page 37) may also be of use.

### Lipoic Acid: Standard German Treatment for Diabetic Neuropathy

**Lipoic acid** (page 246) has been widely used in Germany for over 20 years to treat diabetic peripheral neuropathy, a painful nerve condition that often develops after many years of diabetes. This naturally occurring antioxidant may also help prevent and treat cardiac autonomic neuropathy (injury to the nerves controlling the heart) and diabetic cataracts.

Lipoic acid is a vitamin-like substance that plays a role in the body's utilization of energy. Because lipoic acid can be synthesized from other substances, it is not considered an essential nutrient. However, in people with diabetes, levels of lipoic acid are reduced.[30] It is not clear whether lipoic acid supplements correct a deficiency or whether they work in some other way.

Lipoic acid may work especially well when combined with GLA (gamma-linolenic acid).[31,32]

### What Is the Scientific Evidence for Lipoic Acid?

Several double-blind studies support the use of lipoic acid for diabetic neuropathy.[33,34]

In the ALADIN (Alpha-Lipoic Acid in Diabetic Neuropathy) study, 328 people were randomized into four groups and given either a placebo or 100, 600, or 1,200 mg of intravenous lipoic acid daily. Over a course of 3 weeks, the participants were assessed for improvements in sensations such as pain and numbness. The results showed greatest improvement in the 600 mg group, with 82.5% showing adequate response compared to only 57.6% in the placebo group. (As always, the power of placebo is remarkable!) Unfortunately, because in this study the lipoic acid was injected, it is not clear whether the results carry over to oral lipoic acid.

**Warning:** Do not inject lipoic acid products intended for oral use.

Another study used oral lipoic acid. In this 3-month trial, 80 people with diabetes were divided into four groups and treated with oral lipoic acid (660 mg daily), selenium (100 mcg daily), vitamin E (1,200 IU daily), or placebo.[35] Again, lipoic acid significantly improved symptoms compared to the placebo.

However, in this study, **vitamin E** (page 337) and **selenium** (page 297) worked just as well as lipoic acid. This finding gives rise to a suspicion that it may be possible to use cheaper antioxidants instead of lipoic acid. (For more information on the safe use of vitamin E and selenium, see the chapters on these supplements in Part Two.)

The DEKAN (Deutsche Kardiale Autonome Neuropathie) study followed 73 people with diabetes, who had symptoms of cardiac autonomic neuropathy, for 4 months.[36] Treatment with 800 mg of oral lipoic acid daily showed significant improvement compared to placebo and no important side effects.

**Dosages**    The typical dosage of lipoic acid for diabetic peripheral neuropathy is 300 to 600 mg daily, divided into 2 or 3 doses. For cardiac autonomic neuropathy, a higher dosage of 800 mg daily has been used in studies.

Because lipoic acid occasionally improves the body's response to insulin, it may be necessary to start with lower doses and gradually increase while monitoring blood sugar levels under a physician's supervision.

**Safety Issues**    Over the 30 years during which lipoic acid has been used for diabetic peripheral neuropathy in Germany, no serious adverse reactions have been reported. Side effects are rare and generally limited to mild gastrointestinal distress. However, safety in young children, pregnant or nursing women, and those with severe kidney or liver disease has not been established.

### GLA (from Evening Primrose): Probably Helpful, but Slow-Acting

The evening primrose is a native American wildflower, named for the late-afternoon opening of its delicate flowers. Perhaps it should be described as a food supplement rather than an herb, for evening primrose oil has been popularized mainly as a source of **GLA (gamma-linolenic acid)** (page 210), an essential fatty acid also found in black currant and borage oil.

Although many other kinds of fat are unhealthy, essential fatty acids (EFAs) are as necessary as vitamins. The two main kinds of EFAs are called omega-3 and omega-6 fatty acids. The GLA in evening primrose is an omega-6 fatty acid. A growing body of scientific evidence suggests that supplementation with GLA may help relieve symptoms of diabetic neuropathy.

**What Is the Scientific Evidence for GLA?**    Many studies in animals have shown that evening primrose oil can protect nerves from diabetes-induced injury.[37,38] Good results were also seen in a double-blind study that followed 111 people with diabetes from seven medical centers for a period of 1 year.[39] The results showed an improvement in subjective symptoms such as pain and numbness as well as objective signs of nerve injury. Individuals with good blood sugar control improved the most. Earlier double-blind studies also reported positive results.[40]

**Dosages**    A typical dosage of evening primrose oil for diabetic neuropathy is 4 to 6 g daily. It should be taken with food. Keep in mind that full results may take over 6 months to develop.

**Safety Issues**    Animal studies suggest that evening primrose oil is nontoxic and noncarcinogenic.[41] Over 4,000 people have taken GLA or evening primrose oil in scientific studies, and no significant adverse effects have ever been noted.

Somewhat less than 2% of people who take evening primrose oil complain of mild headaches, gastrointestinal distress, or both, especially at higher doses.[42,43]

Early case reports suggested the possibility that GLA might worsen temporal lobe epilepsy or bipolar disorder, but this has not been confirmed.[44,45]

Maximum safe dosages in young children, pregnant or nursing women, and those with severe kidney or liver disease have not been established.

### Other Treatments to Help Treat Complications of Diabetes

The supplement **inositol** (page 231) has also been tried as a treatment for complications of diabetes, but the results have been mixed.[46,47]

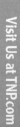

Weak evidence suggests that the herb **bilberry** (page 135) (120 to 240 mg twice daily of an extract standardized to contain 25% anthocyanosides) may help prevent eye damage caused by diabetes.[48,49] For a more complete discussion of bilberry use and safety issues, see the chapter on this herb in Part Two.

**OPCs** (page 270) and **ginkgo** (page 204) are said to provide similar benefits, although the evidence for these is weaker than that of bilberry. See the chapters on these herbs in Part Two for more complete discussions.

**Vitamin C** (page 331) is believed to help prevent cataracts in general.[50,51] It is not known for sure whether vitamin C produces the same benefit in people with diabetes. However, it has been suggested that vitamin C may actually be especially useful because of its relationship to sorbitol, a sugar-like substance that tends to accumulate in the cells of people with diabetes. Sorbitol is believed to play a role in the development of diabetic cataracts, and vitamin C appears to help reduce sorbitol buildup.[52] However, the evidence that vitamin C provides significant benefits through this route is at present indirect and far from conclusive. A daily dose of 500 mg should be safe and sufficient.

## Treating Nutritional Deficiencies in Diabetes

Both diabetes and the medications used to treat it can cause people to fall short of various nutrients. Making up for these deficiencies (either through diet or the use of supplements) may not help your diabetes, but it should make you a healthier person overall.

**Magnesium** (page 251) appears to be the most common mineral deficiency in type 1 diabetes.[53,54] People with either type 1 or type 2 diabetes may also be deficient in the mineral **zinc** (page 348).[55,56,57] **Vitamin C** (page 331) levels have been found to be low in many diabetics on insulin, even though they were consuming seemingly adequate amounts in their diets.[58,59,60] **Vitamin A** (page 318) has been found to be depleted in the bloodstream of diabetics as compared to nondiabetics,[61] partly because of difficulties in getting vitamin A out of the liver, where it is stored.[62,63] Some people with type 1 diabetes appear to be deficient in the amino acid **taurine** (page 308).[64] Finally, **manganese** (page 254) deficiency reportedly can also occur.[65]

### Dosages and Safety Issues

So that you do not take unnecessary supplements, you may want to undergo testing to determine whether you are actually deficient in any of these nutrients. However, such testing is expensive. Because these are safe supplements, you may want to take them simply as insurance.

Typical dosages for nutritional correction in diabetes are as follows: magnesium, 350 to 450 mg daily; zinc 15 to 30 mg daily (combined with 1 to 3 mg daily of **copper** [page 169]); vitamin C, 500 mg daily; and taurine, 2 to 6 g daily. Supplementation with vitamin A is generally recommended at a dose of about 5,000 IU daily; however, women who are or who may become pregnant should not take vitamin A (they should take beta-carotene instead). A general multivitamin and mineral may not be a bad idea, either, for there may be many other marginal deficiencies in diabetes. However, if you suffer from diabetic kidney disease, you should not take any supplements except on the advice of a physician.

People with diabetes should not take high doses of niacin, as it can worsen blood sugar control.

### Preventing Diabetes

Exciting evidence from a huge study conducted in New Zealand suggests that the supplement niacinamide—a form of niacin, also known as **vitamin B$_3$** (page 323)—might be able to reduce the risk of diabetes in children at high risk.[66] In this study, more than 20,000 children were screened for diabetes risk by measuring certain antibodies in the blood (ICA antibodies, believed to indicate risk of developing diabetes). It turned out that 185 of these children had detectable levels. About 170 of these children were then given niacinamide for 7 years (not all parents agreed to give their children niacinamide or stay in the study for that long). About 10,000 other children were not screened, but they were followed to see whether they developed diabetes.

The results were very impressive. In the group in which children were screened and given niacinamide if they were positive for ICA antibodies, the incidence of diabetes was reduced by as much as 60%.

These findings suggest that niacinamide is a very effective treatment for preventing diabetes. (It also shows that tests for ICA antibodies can very accurately identify children at risk for diabetes.)

At present, an enormous-scale, long-term trial called the European Nicotinamide Diabetes Intervention Trial is being conducted to definitively determine whether regular use of niacinamide can prevent diabetes. Results from the German portion of the study have been released at press time, and they were not positive;[67] however, until the entire study is complete, it is not possible to draw conclusions.

For prevention of diabetes in children, the usual dosage of niacinamide is 25 mg per kilogram body weight per day. There are 2.2 pounds in a kilogram, so a 40-pound child would get about 450 mg daily. For safety information, see the chapter on vitamin $B_3$ in Part Two.

**Warning:** Medical supervision is essential before giving your child long-term niacinamide treatment.

For more information on diabetes, see *The Natural Pharmacist Guide to Diabetes.*

# DYSMENORRHEA (PAINFUL MENSTRUATION)

*Principal Natural Treatments*
　Fish oil

*Other Natural Treatments*
　Magnesium, cramp bark, turmeric, white willow, bromelain, black cohosh, *Coleus forskohlii,* manganese, dong quai

We do not know why menstruation is uncomfortable at all, or why it is much more painful for some women than for others and varies so much from month to month.

Occasionally, severe menstrual pain indicates the presence of endometriosis (a condition in which uterine tissue is growing in places other than the uterus) or uterine fibroids (benign tumors in the uterus), but in most cases no such identifiable abnormality can be found. Natural substances known as prostaglandins seem to play a central role in menstrual pain, but the details of the many interactions are scarcely understood, and the available treatments are not specific in their action.

Anti-inflammatory drugs such as ibuprofen usually relieve menstrual pain substantially. However, their blood-thinning effects can increase menstrual flow. Oral contraceptive treatment can also help over the long term, although its success is not guaranteed.

## PRINCIPAL NATURAL TREATMENTS

The best evidence we have for any treatment for dysmenorrhea is in regards to fish oil.

### Fish Oil: Appears to Relieve Cramps

**Fish oil** (page 188) supplements, a good source of omega-3 fatty acids, appear to be quite helpful for the treatment of painful menstruation.

In a 4-month study of 42 adolescents aged 15 to 18, fish oil significantly reduced menstrual pain.[1] Half received 6 g daily of fish oil, providing 1,080 mg of eicosapentaenoic acid (EPA) and 720 mg of docosahexaenoic acid (DHA) daily for 2 months. This was followed by a placebo for 2 months. The other half received the same treatments in the reverse order. The girls in the study reported improvements in their symptoms while they were taking fish oil, but not when they were taking placebo. It is believed that the omega-3 fatty acids in fish oil may help relieve dysmenorrhea by affecting the metabolism of prostaglandins and other factors involved in pain and inflammation.[2]

There are many different types of fish oil products available. A typical daily dose should supply about 1,800 mg of EPA and 900 mg of DHA. Cod liver oil is probably not the best choice due to the potential for excessive intake of **vitamin A** and **vitamin D** (pages 318 and 335). **Flaxseed oil** (page 193) has been proposed as a less smelly alternative to fish oil, but it has not been proven effective.

Because fish oil has a mild "blood-thinning" effect, it should not be combined with powerful blood-thinning medications, such as Coumadin (warfarin) or heparin, except on a physician's advice. However, contrary to some reports, fish oil does not seem to cause bleeding problems when it is taken by itself.[3,4]

Also, fish oil does not appear to raise blood sugar levels in people with diabetes.[5] Nonetheless, if you have diabetes, you should not take any supplement except on the advice of a physician.

Fish oil may temporarily raise the level of LDL ("bad") cholesterol; but this effect seems to be short-lived, and levels return to normal with continued use.[6,7]

If you decide to use cod liver oil as your fish oil supplement, make sure you do not exceed the safe maximum intake of vitamin A and vitamin D. These vitamins are fat-soluble, which means that excess amounts tend to build up in your body, possibly reaching toxic levels. Pregnant women should not take more than 2,500 IU of vitamin A daily because of the risk of birth defects; 5,000 IU

a day is a reasonable upper limit for other individuals. Vitamin D becomes toxic when taken at dosages above 1,000 IU daily for prolonged periods. Look at the bottle label to determine how much of these vitamins you are receiving.

## OTHER NATURAL TREATMENTS

The following natural treatments are widely recommended for painful menstruation, but none have been scientifically proven effective at this time.

### Magnesium

Preliminary studies suggest that **magnesium** (page 251) supplementation may be helpful for dysmenorrhea.[8,9] A typical dosage is 250 to 600 mg daily throughout the cycle, or 500 to 1,000 mg for 3 to 5 days prior to the onset of cramps. Some practitioners believe that magnesium works best when combined with vitamin $B_6$. Magnesium is described in more detail in its own chapter in Part Two.

### Other Herbs and Supplements

The herb cramp bark has traditionally been used to relieve menstrual pain. Unfortunately, it has not received any significant scientific attention.

Herbs with possible anti-inflammatory properties may be helpful as well, including **turmeric** (page 311), **white willow** (page 343), and **bromelain** (page 144). Other potentially helpful treatments include **black cohosh** (page 138), **_Coleus forskohlii_** (page 166), **dong quai** (page 177), and **manganese** (page 254).

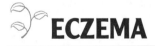

# ECZEMA

*Principal Natural Treatments*
  Evening primrose oil (GLA)

*Other Natural Treatments*
  Topical herbal creams (calendula, chamomile, licorice), burdock, red clover, zinc, *Coleus forskohlii*, quercetin

---

**E**czema is an allergic reaction shown in the skin. It consists mainly of itchy, inflamed patches on the face, elbows, knees, and wrists. Eczema is most commonly found in infants and young children, and many children with eczema also develop hay fever and asthma.

Medical treatment for eczema consists mainly of topical steroid creams.

## PRINCIPAL NATURAL TREATMENTS

Evening primrose oil, a source of the essential fatty acid **GLA (gamma-linolenic acid)** (page 210), is widely used in Europe for eczema, although the evidence that it really works is mixed.

### Evening Primrose Oil: Standard Treatment for Eczema in Europe

A review of all studies reported up to 1989 found that evening primrose oil frequently reduced the symptoms of eczema after several months of use, with the greatest improvement noticeable in the level of itching.[1] However, this review has been criticized because it used unpublished studies as well as studies of poor design.[2] A recent properly designed double-blind study that followed 58 children with eczema for 16 weeks found no difference between the treated and placebo groups.[3] Another double-blind trial followed 39 people with hand dermatitis (inflammation) for 24 weeks. Evening primrose oil at a dosage of 6 g daily produced no significant improvement as compared to the placebo.[4]

A 1985 double-blind study of 123 individuals with moderately severe eczema also found no benefits, but this study appears to have mixed up the treatment and placebo groups![5,6,7]

One recent double-blind trial did find a therapeutic benefit with evening primrose oil, but not for itching![8]

This information is a bit confusing, but putting it all together, it appears likely that evening primrose oil may be mildly effective for treating eczema.

The typical dosage of evening primrose oil is 2 to 4 g daily, taken with food. Full results are said to take over 6 months to develop. Combinations of fish oil and evening primrose oil may be more effective. See the chapter on GLA in Part Two for further details.

## OTHER NATURAL TREATMENTS

The following natural treatments are widely recommended for eczema, but they have not been scientifically proven effective at this time.

### Topical Herbal Creams

Topical creams made from **chamomile** (page 156), **licorice** (page 244), or **calendula** (page 150), alone or in combination, are also widely used in Europe to treat eczema.

### Burdock and Red Clover

The herbs **burdock** (page 145) and **red clover** (page 290) are traditionally drunk as tea to treat eczema. The proper dosage of these herbs varies according to the preparation, so follow the label instructions.

Burdock is a common food in Japan (it is often found in sukiyaki) and as such is believed to be safe.

The safety of red clover is less clear because it contains many blood-thinning and estrogen-like substances. It may not be appropriate for long-term use, especially in girls and adolescents; and it should not be taken by pregnant or nursing women and those on anticoagulant drugs, such as Coumadin (warfarin), Trental (pentoxifylline), or even aspirin.

### Zinc

**Zinc** (page 348) supplementation is said to be effective for eczema in some children. The usual dosage is 10 mg of zinc picolinate daily in children under 10, balanced with 1 mg of **copper** (page 169). For older individuals, the dosage is 15 to 30 mg taken daily, balanced with 1 to 3 mg of copper daily. Too much zinc can be toxic, so dosages should not exceed 30 mg daily.

### Other Treatments

The herb ***Coleus forskohlii*** (page 166) and the supplement **quercetin** (page 288) have also been recommended for eczema, but there is as yet little evidence that they really work.

# GALLSTONES

### Principal Natural Treatments
There are no well-established natural treatments for gallstones.

### Other Natural Treatments
Peppermint, milk thistle, artichoke leaf, boldo, fumitory, greater celandine, turmeric, dandelion, betaine hydrochloride

The job of the gallbladder is to store the bile produced by the liver and to release it on an as-needed basis for digestive purposes. However, it isn't easy to keep this complex mixture of chemicals in liquid form. The various elements of bile have a natural tendency to form sludge, lumps, and hard deposits called gallstones. The body uses several biochemical methods to prevent such condensation from occurring, but this natural chemistry does not always succeed. More than 20% of women and 8% of men develop gallstones at some time in their lives.

You could have gallstones in your body for many years without experiencing any problems. According to current medical guidelines, no treatment is necessary unless pain or other problems begin to develop. However, when a gallstone plugs the duct that leads out of the gallbladder, the organ becomes inflamed and often infected, creating a condition known as cholecystitis.

Generally, gallbladder pain begins with occasional minor attacks that subside rapidly. Perhaps the stones are blocking the duct temporarily and then moving out of the way. However, when full obstruction occurs, the pain often becomes severe and recurrent.

The most reliable symptom of cholecystitis is intense pain beneath the right lower rib cage, often occurring from midnight to 3 A.M. Typically, pain radiates to the right shoulder and is accompanied by a loss of appetite and sometimes nausea. Frequently, fatty meals seem to bring on the pain with particular force.

Techniques for removing the gallbladder have become quite sophisticated. Today, the gallbladder can be removed quickly and usually without complications, bringing full relief of symptoms.

Living without a gallbladder does not seem to bring any long-term consequences. However, many people are opposed on general principle to removing an organ that nature has placed there. The medication Actigall may be able to dissolve gallstones when it is taken for many months.

## NATURAL TREATMENTS

The only time it is appropriate to use alternative treatments for gallstones is before acute cholecystitis develops. Once the gallbladder has become completely blocked, there is a real danger of imminent rupture. Another risk is that a stone may escape the gallbladder and obstruct the common bile duct. When this happens, the liver cannot unload the bile it produces, putting it at risk of permanent injury and creating a true surgical emergency.

However, during the period in which pain is only occasional or intermittent, the risks incurred by postponing surgery are slight. During the same interval when the medication Actigall might be tried, some of the agents described here could be considered as possibilities. Unfortunately, none are well established as effective. Medical supervision is definitely essential.

### Peppermint

Preliminary clinical trials suggest that formulas containing **peppermint** (page 277) and related terpenes (fragrant substances found in plants) can dissolve gallstones.[1] The proper dosage is not clear, but a typical recommendation is 1 or 2 capsules containing 0.2 ml of peppermint oil 3 times daily. The label should say "enteric coated," meaning that it remains intact until it has passed the stomach. Excessive doses of peppermint oil can cause severe gastrointestinal distress and other symptoms, so do not take more than this amount.

## Milk Thistle

**Milk thistle** (page 262), standardized to its silymarin content, has been shown to improve the liquidity of bile,[2] although its actual effects on gallstones in real life are unknown. The standard dosage of milk thistle is 200 mg 2 to 3 times a day of an extract standardized to contain 70% silymarin. For more information on milk thistle use and safety issues, see the corresponding chapter in Part Two.

## Other Herbs and Supplements

Other herbs that are widely prescribed in Germany for gallbladder pain include artichoke leaf, boldo, fumitory, greater celandine, **turmeric** (page 311), and **dandelion** (page 174) root.[3] The supplement **betaine hydrochloride** (page 134) is also sometimes recommended for gallbladder problems, although there is no real evidence as yet that it works.

Consult a qualified physician before using these substances, as they can cause increased pain and may present other risks.

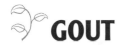

# GOUT

*Principal Natural Treatments*
There are no well-established natural treatments for gout.

*Other Natural Treatments*
Folic acid, devil's claw, fish oil, vitamin E, selenium, bromelain, vitamin A, aspartic acid, cherry juice, celery juice

Gout is an inflammatory condition that is caused by the deposit of uric acid crystals in joints (most famously the big toe) as well as other tissues. Typically, attacks of fierce pain, redness, swelling, and heat punctuate pain-free intervals.

Medical treatment consists of anti-inflammatory drugs for acute attacks and of uric acid–lowering drugs for prevention.

## NATURAL TREATMENTS

The following herbs and supplements are widely recommended for gout, but they have not yet been scientifically proven effective.

## Folic Acid

**Folic acid** (page 194) has been recommended as a preventive treatment for gout for at least 20 years. Some clinicians report that it can be highly effective. However, what little scientific evidence we have on the method is contradictory.[1,2,3] It has been suggested that a contaminant found in folic acid, pterin-6-aldehyde, may actually be responsible for the positive effects observed by some clinicians.

A typical dosage of folic acid for gout is 10 mg daily. However, because folic acid can mask **vitamin B$_{12}$** (page 329) deficiency, it is important to consult with a qualified health-care practitioner before using this method. High doses of folic acid can also cause digestive distress and may worsen seizures in epileptics. The safety of high doses of folic acid in young children, pregnant or nursing women, and those with severe kidney or liver disease has not been established.

## Devil's Claw

The herb **devil's claw** (page 175) is sometimes recommended as a pain-relieving treatment for gout based on evidence for its effectiveness in various forms of arthritis.[4] A typical dosage is 750 mg 3 times daily of a preparation standardized to contain 3% iridoid glycosides.

Devil's claw appears to be quite safe, and there is no evidence of toxicity at dosages many times higher than recommended. However, safety in pregnant or nursing women and those with severe liver or kidney disease has not been established. It is not recommended for use by those with ulcers, as it can sometimes cause stomach irritation.

## Other Supplements

On the basis of interesting reasoning but no concrete evidence of effectiveness, **fish oil** (page 188), **vitamin E** (page 337), **selenium** (page 297), **bromelain** (page 144), **vitamin A** (page 318), and aspartic acid have also been recommended for both prevention and treatment of gout.[5]

## Folk Remedies

A traditional remedy for gout (with negligible scientific evidence) calls for ½ to 1 pound of cherries a day.[6] You can also buy tablets containing concentrated cherry juice.

Celery juice is another folk remedy for gout that is said to be widely used in Australia.

# HEMORRHOIDS

*Principal Natural Treatments*
Hydroxyethylrutosides

*Other Natural Treatments*
Aortic glycosaminoglycans, collinsonia, horse chestnut, OPCs, gotu kola, butcher's broom, bilberry, calendula, slippery elm

Hemorrhoids are swollen, inflamed veins in the rectum that can ache and bleed. They are very common and are usually caused by constipation, a low-fiber diet, a sedentary lifestyle, or pregnancy.

The most important interventions for hemorrhoids aim at reversing their causes. Adopting a high-fiber diet, sitting down less, getting plenty of exercise, and maintaining regular bowel habits can make a significant difference.

Medical treatment consists mainly of stool softeners and moist heat. In more severe cases, surgical procedures may be used.

## PRINCIPAL NATURAL TREATMENTS

Besides the treatments described in this section, the natural treatments used for varicose veins are also often recommended for hemorrhoids because a hemorrhoid is actually a special kind of varicose vein. These include **horse chestnut** (page 228), **OPCs** (page 270), **gotu kola** (page 218), **butcher's broom** (page 146), and **bilberry** (page 135).

### Bioflavonoids

Bioflavonoids are colorful substances that occur widely in the plant kingdom. A certain category of bioflavonoid, called hydroxyethylrutosides (HERs), is extensively used in Europe to relieve hemorrhoid pain. Moderate-size double-blind studies suggest that these safe substances can be beneficial in cases of hemorrhoids, including those that occur during pregnancy.[1,2,3]

These naturally occurring substances are considered very safe, as shown by the fact that researchers felt comfortable giving them to pregnant women. Typical dosages are 500 to 1,000 mg 2 or 3 times daily.

Although it is not known precisely how flavonoids work, it has been suggested that they stabilize the walls of blood vessels, making them less susceptible to injury.

## OTHER NATURAL TREATMENTS

The following natural treatments are widely recommended for hemorrhoids, but they have not been scientifically proven effective at this time.

Preliminary evidence suggests that an extract made from the inner lining of cow aortas called **aortic glycosaminoglycans** (**GAGs**) (page 125) can improve the symptoms of hemorrhoids.[4,5] The recommended dosage is 50 mg twice daily.

See the corresponding chapter in Part Two for detailed safety information.

Collinsonia root (also known as stone root) is a traditional remedy for hemorrhoids. The proper dosage varies according to the preparation and is usually listed on the label. Safety studies have not been performed.

The herb **slippery elm** (page 300) is also sometimes used orally for hemorrhoids; topical **calendula** (page 150) cream is also a popular treatment. However, there is as yet no real evidence that they work.

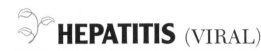

# HEPATITIS (VIRAL)

### Principal Natural Treatments
Milk thistle

### Other Natural Treatments
Licorice, Chinese and Japanese herb combinations, vitamin C, liver extracts, thymus extracts, *Phyllanthus amarus,* astragalus, reishi, lecithin, taurine

Hepatitis is an infection of the liver caused by one of several viruses, the most common of which are named hepatitis A, B, and C. Hepatitis A is spread mainly through contaminated food and water, whereas hepatitis B is transmitted by sexual contact and use of contaminated needles. The route of transmission of hepatitis C is not completely clear but is believed to be similar to that of hepatitis B.

When you first develop hepatitis, it is called acute hepatitis. Hepatitis can also become a long-term disease known as chronic hepatitis. All forms of hepatitis cause jaundice, liver tenderness, and severe fatigue. Hepatitis A is the mildest form and seldom causes symptoms continuing longer than a couple of months. Hepatitis B and C produce more severe symptoms, last two or three times longer, and can go on to become chronic.

Chronic hepatitis consists of persistent liver infection and inflammation that lingers long after the primary symptoms of the disease have disappeared. It can produce subtle symptoms of liver tenderness and continued fatigue and over time can gradually destroy the liver. Chronic hepatitis also appears to increase the risk of liver cancer.

The best treatment for hepatitis is prevention. You can avoid hepatitis A by practicing good hygiene and using the conventional treatment, known as immune globulins, while traveling in areas where the disease is common. Hepatitis B

can be prevented by immunization and the same precautions taken against AIDS. AIDS precautions almost certainly decrease the transmission of hepatitis C as well.

Conventional medicine has little in the way of treatment for the initial hepatitis infection once it has started. Treatment for chronic hepatitis is developing but is still quite imperfect. The most effective methods involve varieties of interferon.

## PRINCIPAL NATURAL TREATMENTS

In Europe, the herb milk thistle is commonly used along with other treatments for hepatitis. Keep in mind, though, that this is a very serious disease. Medical supervision is essential.

### Milk Thistle: May Be Helpful for Chronic Hepatitis

**Milk thistle** (page 262) may be useful as a supportive treatment for chronic hepatitis. Native to Europe and the United States, milk thistle has a long history of use as both a food and a medicine. At the turn of the twentieth century, English gardeners grew milk thistle to use its leaves like lettuce, the stalks like asparagus, the roasted seeds like coffee, and the roots (soaked overnight) like oyster plant. The seeds, fruit, and leaves of milk thistle are also used for medicinal purposes.

German researchers in the 1960s were sufficiently impressed with the history and clinical effectiveness of milk thistle to begin examining it for active constituents. The most important ingredient appears to be silymarin (actually a set of four related substances), which appears to possess a wide variety of liver-protective benefits. It is one of the few herbs that have no real equivalent among standard medications.

In 1986, Germany's Commission E approved an oral extract of milk thistle standardized to 70% silymarin content as a treatment for "toxic liver damage; also the supportive treatment of chronic inflammatory liver diseases and hepatic cirrhosis." The herb is widely used in chronic viral hepatitis as well as alcoholic fatty liver, liver cirrhosis, alcoholic hepatitis, chemical-induced liver toxicity, and abnormal liver enzymes of unknown cause. In addition, milk thistle is often added as a protective agent when drugs that are known to be toxic to the liver are used. An intravenous preparation made from milk thistle is used as an antidote for poisoning by the death-cap mushroom, *Amanita phalloides.*

### What Is the Scientific Evidence for Milk Thistle?

Preliminary double-blind studies of people with chronic hepatitis have shown significant improvement in symptoms such as fatigue, reduced appetite, and abdominal discomfort.[1,2,3] Laboratory signs of liver injury also showed improvement in these trials. However, larger research trials need to be performed before milk thistle can be called a proven treatment for chronic hepatitis. Milk thistle is probably not helpful during the initial acute hepatitis infection.[4]

As for most herbs, the mechanism of action of milk thistle remains in doubt. In mushroom poisoning and other liver-toxic exposure, silymarin is believed to get in the way of toxins trying to bind to liver cell membrane receptors by binding to the receptors itself.[5] This is called *competitive inhibition.* Incidentally, glutathione, a compound that our body normally produces to protect the liver and kidney from reactive chemicals, works in a similar fashion. Many other suggestions of how milk thistle may function have been made, but which one is correct remains unclear.[6–10]

### Dosages

The standard dosage of milk thistle is 200 mg 2 or 3 times daily of an extract standardized to contain 70% silymarin.

Some evidence supports the idea that silymarin bound to phosphatidylcholine is better absorbed.[11,12] This form should be taken at a dosage of 100 to 200 mg twice daily.

### Safety Issues

Milk thistle is believed to possess very little toxicity. Animal studies have not shown any negative effects even when high doses were administered over a long period of time.[13]

A study of 2,637 participants reported in 1992 showed a low incidence of side effects, limited mainly to mild gastrointestinal disturbance.[14]

On the basis of its extensive use as a food, milk thistle is believed to be safe in pregnancy and lactation (milk production), and researchers have enrolled pregnant women in studies.[15] However, safety in young children, pregnant or nursing women, and individuals with severe renal disease has not been formally established. No drug interactions are known.

One report has noted that silibinin (a constituent of silymarin) can inhibit a bacterial enzyme called beta-glucuronidase, which plays a role in the activity of certain drugs, such as oral contraceptives.[16] This could interfere with their action.

## OTHER NATURAL TREATMENTS

The following natural treatments are widely recommended for hepatitis, but they have not been scientifically proven effective at this time.

### Licorice

In Japan, an injectable combination of **licorice** (page 244) (the herb, not the candy) and certain amino acids is used for chronic hepatitis.[17] However, it is not clear whether oral licorice is equally useful, and the high dosages used for treatment of chronic hepatitis may cause an elevation of blood pressure.

**Warning:** Do not inject preparations of licorice designed for oral use.

## Herb Combinations

Chinese and Japanese herbal medicines typically use combinations of herbs rather than just one. A multicenter, randomized, controlled clinical study looked at the effectiveness of a combination containing the herb *Radix bupleuri* in chronic hepatitis and found good results.[18] However, this combination has not been formally tested to verify its safety.

## Other Herbs and Supplements

Other common natural medicine recommendations for hepatitis include high doses of **vitamin C** (page 331); liver extracts; thymus extracts; **taurine** (page 308); **lecithin** (page 243); and the herbs **astragalus** (page 129), **reishi** (page 291), and *Phyllanthus amarus*. However, there is as yet no solid scientific evidence that these approaches really work.

# HERPES (GENITAL HERPES AND COLD SORES)

*Principal Natural Treatments*
  Melissa officinalis, L-lysine

*Other Natural Treatments*
  Vitamin C, astragalus, cat's claw, elderberry, licorice

The common virus known as herpes can cause painful blister-like lesions around the mouth and in the genitalia. Slightly different strains of herpes predominate in each of these two locations, but the infections are essentially identical. In both areas, the herpes virus has the devious habit of hiding out deep in the DNA of nerve ganglia, where it remains inactive for months or years. From time to time the virus reactivates, travels down the nerve, and starts an eruption. Common triggers include stress, dental procedures, infections, and trauma. Flare-ups usually become less severe over time.

Conventional medical treatment consists of antiviral drugs, such as Zovirax. Such medications can shorten the length and intensity of a herpes outbreak or, when taken consistently at lower dosages, reduce the frequency of flare-ups. However, they are not dramatically effective.

## PRINCIPAL NATURAL TREATMENTS

The herb *Melissa officinalis* and the amino acid L-lysine appear to be effective treatments for herpes.

## *Melissa officinalis* (Lemon Balm)

More commonly known in the United States as lemon balm, ***Melissa officinalis*** (page 260) is widely sold in Europe as a topical cream for the treatment of genital and oral herpes. This herb is a native of southern Europe and is widely planted in gardens for the purpose of attracting bees. Its leaves give off a delicate lemon odor when bruised.

Melissa cream appears to be helpful in the treatment of genital and oral herpes. It can be applied only at the first sign of blisters or on a regular basis for the prevention of flare-ups. However, there is no evidence that melissa will stop you from infecting another person.

### What Is the Scientific Evidence for Melissa?

A double-blind placebo-controlled trial involving 116 people found that treatment with melissa cream helped the herpes blisters heal more rapidly.[1] The total number of participants who were completely recovered on the fifth day was 24 of 58 in the melissa group but only 15 of 58 in the placebo group, a statistically significant difference.

The regular use of melissa cream may also decrease the frequency of recurrences.[2]

The most commonly used European melissa product is manufactured using a method that tests the herb's activity against the herpes virus. Here's how it's designed: Human or animal cells are grown in a petri dish and then infected with herpes virus. Left alone, the virus would gradually spread throughout the dish, killing all the cells. However, in this test, standard paper disks containing melissa extract are inserted into the petri dish. The commercial extract is standardized so that a dose of 200 mcg per disk forms a 20 to 30 mm zone of protection from the virus.[3]

We don't really know how melissa works. The leading theory is that the herb makes it more difficult for the herpes virus to attach to cells.

### Dosages

For treatment of an active flare-up of herpes, the proper dosage is four thick daily applications of a standard melissa 70:1 extract cream. This can be reduced to twice daily for preventive purposes.

Pregnant women should not regard melissa as effective prevention against transmission to the newborn. It also will not prevent spread of the disease in sexually active individuals.

### Safety Issues

Topical melissa is not associated with any significant side effects, although allergic reactions are always possible. Safety in young children, pregnant or nursing women, and those with severe liver or kidney disease has not been established.

### L-Lysine

Another famous treatment for herpes involves the amino acid **L-lysine** (page 250). Although study results have been somewhat contradictory, overall the evidence from several double-blind studies suggests that adequate doses of L-lysine can make herpes flare-ups milder and less frequent.[4] Lysine probably works best when it is combined with dietary changes that restrict levels of another amino acid, **arginine** (page 126). (To do this, cut down on gelatin, chocolate, peanuts, almonds and other nuts, seeds, and to a lesser extent wheat.)

A double-blind placebo-controlled trial tested the efficacy of L-lysine in preventing recurring herpes simplex.[5] Twenty-seven individuals were given 1,000 mg of L-lysine 3 times a day for 6 months, while 25 subjects received placebo. Those treated with L-lysine experienced, on average, 2.4 fewer herpes flare-ups than the placebo group, a significant result. The L-lysine group also experienced significantly less severe flare-ups and shorter healing time.

Another placebo-controlled double-blind study on 41 subjects found that 1,250 mg of L-lysine per day also worked, but 624 mg did not.[6] One study found no benefit, but it was very small.[7] Foods high in L-lysine include vegetables, beans, fish, turkey, and chicken. When taken as a supplement, a typical daily dose is 1,000 mg. L-lysine in supplement form has not been associated with any significant side effects. However, high doses of L-lysine in animals have caused gallstones and elevated cholesterol levels.[8,9]

## OTHER NATURAL TREATMENTS

The following natural treatments are widely recommended for herpes, but they have not been scientifically proven effective at this time.

### Other Herbs and Supplements

One study suggests that topical treatment with a **vitamin C** (page 331) solution may speed healing of herpes outbreaks.[10]

Oral vitamin C may also be useful, especially when combined with bioflavonoids.[11] A typical dose is 200 mg of vitamin C combined with 200 mg of mixed bioflavonoids, taken 5 times daily at the very first signs of an impending outbreak. Short-term use of these substances has not been associated with any significant risks.

The herbs **astragalus** (page 129), **cat's claw** (page 154), **elderberry** (page 182), and **licorice** (page 244) are sometimes recommended for herpes as well, but there is little solid evidence as yet that they really work.

# HYPERTENSION (HIGH BLOOD PRESSURE)

### Principal Natural Treatments
Garlic, coenzyme Q$_{10}$

### Other Natural Treatments
Fish oil, calcium, magnesium, potassium, hawthorn, vitamin C, astragalus, maitake, *Coleus forskohlii,* beta-carotene, taurine, flaxseed oil

---

**M**ost people can't tell when their blood pressure is high, which is why hypertension is called the "silent killer." In this case, what you don't know can hurt you. Elevated blood pressure can lead to a greatly increased risk of heart attack, stroke, and many other serious illnesses. Along with high **cholesterol** (page 39) and smoking, hypertension is one of the most important causes of **atherosclerosis** (page 14). In turn, atherosclerosis causes heart attacks, strokes, and other diseases of impaired circulation.

The mechanism by which high blood pressure produces atherosclerosis is similar to a hose fitted with a high-pressure nozzle. All such nozzles come with a warning label that states, "Make sure to discharge pressure in hose after using." Unfortunately, many people (such as myself) frequently fail to pay attention to the warning and leave the hose puffed up with full pressure overnight.

This rather common practice does not produce any immediate consequences. The hose doesn't develop leaks at the seams or burst outright on the first occasion you leave it untended. However, a garden hose that is frequently left under pressure will begin to age more rapidly than it would otherwise. Its lining will begin to crack, its flexibility will diminish, and within a season or two the hose will be sprouting leaks in all directions.

When blood vessels are exposed to constantly high pressure, a similar process is set in motion. Blood pressures as elevated as 220/170 (systolic pressure/diastolic pressure), quite common during activities such as weightlifting, do no harm. Only when excessive pressure is sustained day and night do blood vessel linings begin to be injured and undergo those unhealthy changes known as hardening of the arteries, or atherosclerosis.

Thus, although it is important to lower blood pressure with all deliberate speed, only rarely does it need to be lowered instantly. In most situations, you have plenty of time to work on bringing down your blood pressure. However, that doesn't mean that you should ignore it. Over time, high blood pressure can damage nearly every organ in the body.

The best way to determine your blood pressure is to take several readings at different times of the day and on different days of the week. Blood pressure readings will vary quite a bit from moment to moment; what matters most is the average blood pressure. Thus, if many low readings balance out a few high readings, the net result may be satisfactory.

However, it is essential not to ignore a high value by saying, "I was just stressed then." Stress is part of life, and if it raises your blood pressure once, it will do so again. To come up with an accurate number, you must include every measurement in your calculations.

In most cases, the cause of hypertension is unknown. The kidneys play an important role in controlling blood pressure, and the level of squeezing tension in the blood vessels makes a large contribution as well.

Lifestyle changes can dramatically reduce blood pressure. Increasing exercise, not smoking, and losing weight can all be highly effective. For many years doctors advised patients with hypertension to cut down on salt in the diet. Today, however, the value of this difficult dietary change has undergone significant questioning. Considering how rapidly our knowledge is evolving, I suggest consulting your physician to find the latest recommendations.

If lifestyle changes fail to reduce blood pressure, or if you can't make these alterations, many effective drugs are available. Sometimes you

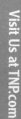

need to experiment with a few to find one that agrees with you.

## PRINCIPAL NATURAL TREATMENTS

Although there are no well-documented natural treatments for hypertension, garlic and coenzyme $Q_{10}$ have some evidence behind them and are reportedly quite effective. Keep in mind that when blood pressure is consistently higher than 160/110, nondrug treatments (other than lifestyle changes) are seldom enough to bring it down.

## Garlic: Appears to Reduce Blood Pressure by 5 to 10%

At least 12 studies have examined the effects of **garlic** (page 197) on blood pressure, although only two of these involved people with hypertension.[1] Overall, it appears that garlic can reduce blood pressure levels by about 5 to 10%.

One of the best of these trials followed 47 subjects with average blood pressures of 171/101.[2] Over a period of 12 weeks, half were given placebo and the other half received 600 mg of garlic powder daily, standardized to 1.3% alliin. This is the most common form of medicinal garlic powder and is used for lowering cholesterol as well.

Compared to the placebo group, garlic reduced systolic blood pressure by 6% and diastolic pressure by 9%. Although this is not a dramatic improvement, it can definitely be useful.

A typical dosage of garlic is 900 mg daily of a garlic powder extract standardized to contain 1.3% alliin, providing about 12,000 mcg of alliin daily. Garlic is generally regarded as safe; however, because it appears to thin the blood it should not be combined with prescription anticoagulants, such as Coumadin (warfarin) or Trental (pentoxifylline). It also might not be a good idea to take garlic in the weeks before or after surgery or labor and delivery, or combine it with blood-thinning natural supplements such as **ginkgo** (page 204) or high-dose **vitamin E** (page 337).

## Coenzyme $Q_{10}$: Appears Effective, but Needs More Study

The supplement **coenzyme $Q_{10}$ ($CoQ_{10}$)** (page 164) is commonly recommended as a treatment for high blood pressure. One small double-blind study found that 100 mg of $CoQ_{10}$ daily can meaningfully reduce blood pressure.[3] Similar results were seen in larger studies, but unfortunately these were not controlled studies.[4,5]

The usual dosage of $CoQ_{10}$ is 30 to 100 mg 3 times daily. This supplement appears to be very safe. For a more complete description of $CoQ_{10}$ see the corresponding chapter in Part Two.

## OTHER NATURAL TREATMENTS

A number of other herbs and supplements may also be somewhat helpful for hypertension.

## Fish Oil

**Fish oil** (page 188), a source of omega-3 fatty acids, is also commonly described as beneficial in the treatment of hypertension. However, the research record is mixed and at best shows a slight benefit.[6] A typical dosage is 3 to 9 g daily. Fish oil frequently causes unpleasant burping. See the chapter on fish oil in Part Two for more information regarding safety issues.

## Minerals: May Be Effective in Case of Deficiency

Adequate intake of **calcium** (page 146), **magnesium** (page 251), and **potassium** (page 282) is necessary for good blood pressure control. When your body lacks adequate amounts of these minerals, supplementation may improve blood pressure.[7–14]

A dosage of 750 to 1,000 mg daily of calcium and 350 mg daily of supplemental magnesium should suffice. Individuals with severe kidney or heart disease, cancer, hyperparathyroidism, sarcoidosis, or a history of kidney stones should not take these supplements except on the advice of a physician. The best source of potassium is fruits and vegetables.

## Hawthorn

The herb **hawthorn** (page 222) is often said to reduce blood pressure, but there is no evidence that this is the case.[15] For more information on hawthorn use and safety issues, see the corresponding chapter in Part Two.

## Vitamin C: Probably Not Effective

Several studies suggest that **vitamin C** (page 331) at a dosage of 1,000 mg or more taken daily may modestly reduce blood pressure.[16,17,18] However, none of these was double-blind. Strange as it may seem, the power of suggestion is quite capable of lowering blood pressure. When a double-blind study performed to evaluate the possible effectiveness of vitamin C found benefits, it found equal benefits in the placebo group as well.[19] One small double-blind study did find a slightly superior effect with vitamin C as compared to placebo.[20]

## Other Treatments

The herbs **astragalus** (page 129), **maitake** (page 254), and *Coleus forskohlii* (page 166) and the supplements **beta-carotene** (page 131), **flaxseed oil** (page 193), and **taurine** (page 308) are sometimes recommended for high blood pressure, but as yet there is no real evidence that they work.

Because **atherosclerosis** (page 14) is the main harm caused by hypertension, treatments listed in that chapter should be considered as well.

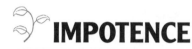

# IMPOTENCE

### *Principal Natural Treatments*
There are no well-established natural treatments for impotence.

### *Other Natural Treatments*
Ginkgo, zinc, L-arginine, pygeum, ginseng, ashwaganda, suma, damiana, muira puama

### *Not Recommended Treatments*
Yohimbe

Impotence, or erectile dysfunction, is the inability to achieve an erection. Impotence may occur for any of at least 15 possible causes, including diabetes, drug side effects, pituitary tumors, hardening of the arteries, hormonal imbalances, and psychological factors. A few of these conditions respond to specific treatment. For example, if a blood pressure drug is causing impotence, the best approach is to change drugs. If a pituitary tumor is secreting the hormone prolactin, treating that tumor may result in immediate improvement. However, in most cases, conventional treatment of impotence is nonspecific.

Generic treatment options include the drug Viagra, mechanical devices that utilize a vacuum to produce an erection, drugs for self-injection, and implantation of penile prostheses. Psychotherapy can also be helpful for treating all varieties of impotence, even when an organic cause can be identified.

## NATURAL TREATMENTS

The following natural treatments are widely recommended for impotence, but they have not been scientifically proven effective at this time.

### Ginkgo

A slight amount of research suggests that **ginkgo** (page 204) may be useful in impotence. One study of 60 men whose impotence was due to poor blood circulation demonstrated a 50% success rate after 6 months.[1] However, because this was not a double-blind study, the improvement noted may have been due to the power of suggestion.

Recent reports suggest that ginkgo may also be useful in reversing the impotence caused by antidepressant drugs in the Prozac family.[2] For more information on ginkgo use and safety issues, see the corresponding chapter in Part Two.

## Zinc

**Zinc** (page 348) deficiency is known to negatively affect sexual function. Because zinc is one of the most commonly deficient minerals in the diet, it is logical to assume that supplementation with zinc may be helpful for some men. A typical dosage for impotence is 15 to 30 mg daily, taken with 1 to 2 mg of **copper** (page 169) as supplemental zinc interferes with copper absorption. Too much zinc can be toxic, so do not exceed this dose.

## L-Arginine

On the basis of minimal evidence, supplementation with **L-arginine** (page 126) has also been recommended as a treatment for impotence. The usual dosage is 2 to 3 g daily, but the safety of L-arginine at this level is not known. However, because arginine restriction is an approach often used to treat **herpes** (page 73), treatment with L-arginine might have the reverse effect.

## Other Treatments

Many other herbs are also reputed to improve sexual function, including **ginseng** (page 206), **ashwaganda** (page 128), **suma** (page 307), **damiana** (page 173), **pygeum** (page 286), and muira puama. However, there is as yet no real evidence that they work.

## Not Recommended Treatments

The herb **yohimbe** (page 347) is the source of the drug yohimbine, which has been shown to be modestly better than placebo for impotence. However, this is a fairly dangerous treatment, and I do not recommend it.

 # INFERTILITY IN MEN

*Principal Natural Treatments*
   There are no well-established natural treatments for infertility in men.

*Other Natural Treatments*
   Vitamin B$_{12}$, zinc, antioxidants (vitamin E, vitamin C), L-carnitine, beta-carotene, coenzyme Q$_{10}$, L-arginine, selenium, ashwaganda, pygeum, PABA

**M**ale infertility, the inability of a man to produce a pregnancy in a woman, can be caused by a great variety of problems, from anatomical defects to hormonal imbalances. In about half of all cases, however, the source of the problem is never discovered.

   The good news is that without any treatment at all, about 25% of supposedly infertile men bring about a pregnancy within a year of the time they first visit a physician for treatment. In other words, infertility is often only low fertility in disguise.

## NATURAL TREATMENTS

The following natural treatments are widely recommended for male infertility, but they have not been scientifically proven effective at this time.

## Vitamin B$_{12}$

Deficiencies in **vitamin B$_{12}$** (page 329) lead to reduced sperm counts and lowered sperm mobility. Thus, vitamin B$_{12}$ supplementation might be expected to improve fertility in men who suffer from a deficiency of this essential vitamin. Mild B$_{12}$ deficiencies are relatively common in people over 60.[1]

   A couple of preliminary studies suggest that B$_{12}$ supplementation (1,000 mcg daily) can sometimes improve sperm counts and sperm activity even when no deficiency exists.[2,3] Unfortunately, improving sperm counts and mobility does not necessarily translate into increased fertility (although it wouldn't hurt). Vitamin $B_{12}$ is believed to be extremely safe.

## Zinc

**Zinc** (page 348) is also an essential nutrient for proper sperm production, and deficiency may result in lowered testosterone levels.[4] One preliminary study found not only an increase in sperm counts, but also an actual increase in pregnancy rate when men with low testosterone were given zinc supplements.[5] However, those whose testosterone levels were normal did not benefit. The usual recommended dosage of zinc is about 15 to 30 mg daily, coupled with 1 mg of **copper** (page 169) for balance. Too much zinc can be toxic, so do not exceed this dose.

## Antioxidants

Free radicals, dangerous chemicals found naturally in the body, may damage sperm. For this reason, a number of studies have evaluated the benefits of antioxidants for male infertility.

In one placebo-controlled study of 52 men whose sperm showed subnormal activity, daily treatment with 100 IU of **vitamin E** (page 337) resulted in improved sperm activity and in-creased rate of pregnancy in their partners.[6] For more information and safety issues, see the chapter on vitamin E in Part Two.

Preliminary studies suggest that **vitamin C** (page 331) may also help.[7] The higher the dose of the vitamin, the quicker the benefit starts; but even low doses produce good results given time. The dosages studied ranged from 200 to 1,000 mg daily. For a discussion of safety issues involving vitamin C, see the corresponding chapter in Part Two.

## Other Herbs and Supplements

Many other substances have been suggested as treatments for infertility, including the herbs **ashwaganda** (page 128) and **pygeum** (page 286), as well as the supplements **PABA** (page 273), **L-carnitine** (page 151), **beta-carotene** (page 131), **coenzyme $Q_{10}$** (**CoQ$_{10}$**) (page 164), **L-arginine** (page 126), and **selenium** (page 297). However, the evidence that they really work is negligible, and studies on the last two supplements have shown more negative than positive results.

All the treatments listed in the chapter on **impotence** (page 77) have also been proposed as treatments for male infertility.

# INFERTILITY IN WOMEN

*Principal Natural Treatments*
   There are no well-established natural treatments for infertility in women.

*Other Natural Treatments*
   Chasteberry, multivitamins, ashwaganda, beta-carotene

There are many possible causes of female infertility. Tubal disease and endometriosis (a condition in which uterine tissue begins to grow where it shouldn't) account for 50% of female infertility; failure of ovulation is the cause of about 30%; and cervical factors cause another 10%.

An immense industry has sprung up around correcting female infertility, using techniques that range from hormone therapy to in vitro (test-tube) babies. Although these methods have their occasional stunning successes, there is con-siderable controversy about the high cost and low rate of effectiveness of fertility treatments in general. The good news is that apparently infertile women often eventually become pregnant with no medical intervention at all.

## NATURAL TREATMENTS

The following natural treatments are widely recommended for female infertility, but they have not been scientifically proven effective at this time.

## Chasteberry

The herb **chasteberry** (page 157) is widely used in Europe as a treatment for infertility.[1] It is believed to work by reducing excessive levels of prolactin, a hormone produced by the pituitary gland.

The typical dose of chasteberry extract is 20 to 40 mg given once a day. Chasteberry is sold often as a liquid extract to be taken at a dosage of 40 drops each morning. However, highly concentrated extracts are also available that require much lower dosing. Chasteberry's safety has not been adequately evaluated. For further discussion of chasteberry use and safety issues, see the corresponding chapter in Part Two.

## Multivitamins

According to one study, general supplementation with multivitamins may improve female fertility.[2]

## Other Treatments

Other treatments sometimes recommended include **ashwaganda** (page 128) and **beta-carotene** (page 131), but there is as yet little real evidence that they work.

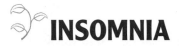# INSOMNIA

### Principal Natural Treatments
Valerian (alone or combined with melissa), melatonin

### Other Natural Treatments
Kava, St. John's wort, 5-HTP, astragalus, hops, passionflower, skullcap, lady's slipper, chamomile, He shou wu, vitamin C, ashwaganda

According to recent reports, many people today have a serious problem getting a good night's sleep. Our lives are simply too busy for us to get the 8 hours we really need. To make matters worse, many of us suffer from insomnia. When we do get to bed, we may stay awake thinking for hours. Sleep itself may be restless instead of refreshing.

Most people who sleep substantially less than 8 hours a night experience a variety of unpleasant symptoms. The most common are headaches, mental confusion, irritability, malaise, immune deficiencies, depression, and fatigue. Complete sleep deprivation can lead to hallucinations and mental collapse.

The best ways to improve sleep are lifestyle changes: eliminating caffeine and sugar from your diet, avoiding stimulating activities before bed, adopting a regular sleeping time, and gradually turning down the lights.

Many drugs can also help with sleep. Such medications as Ambien, Restoril, Ativan, Valium, Xanax, and chloral hydrate are widely used for sleep problems. However, these medications tend to promote tolerance and dependency on the drug, and can even cause addiction.

Recently, physicians have come to regard some forms of insomnia as a variation of depression. This conclusion comes from a kind of reverse reasoning: We know that depression almost always disturbs sleep, and that antidepressants frequently help insomnia. Therefore, maybe some cases of insomnia really are depression in disguise.

Antidepressants can be used in two ways to correct sleep problems. Low doses of certain antidepressants immediately bring on sleep because their side effects include drowsiness. However, this effect tends to wear off with repeated use.

For chronic sleeping problems, full doses of antidepressants may be necessary. Antidepressants are believed to work by actually altering brain chemistry, which produces a beneficial effect on sleep. Trazodone and Serzone are two of the most commonly prescribed antidepressants when improved sleep is desired, but most other antidepressants can be helpful as well.

# PRINCIPAL NATURAL TREATMENTS

Although the scientific evidence isn't yet definitive, the herb valerian and the hormone melatonin are widely accepted as treatments for certain forms of insomnia.

## Valerian: Appears to Improve Sleep Gradually

Over 200 plant species belong to the genus *Valeriana,* but the species used for insomnia is ***Valeriana officinalis*** (page 315). This perennial grows abundantly in moist woodlands in Europe and North America and is under extensive cultivation to meet market demands. The root is used for medicinal purposes.

Valerian has a long traditional use for insomnia. Galen recommended valerian for insomnia in the second century A.D. The herb became popular in Europe from the sixteenth century onward as a sedative and was widely used in the United States as well until the 1950s. Rumors have it that Valium was named to imitate the sound of valerian, although there is no chemical similarity between the two.

Scientific studies of valerian in humans did not begin until the 1970s. The results ultimately led to its approval by Germany's Commission E in 1985. Presently, valerian is an accepted over-the-counter drug for insomnia in Germany, Belgium, France, Switzerland, and Italy.

Valerian is commonly recommended as an aid for occasional insomnia. However, the results of a recent study suggest that it may be more useful for long-term improvement of sleep.[1]

### What Is the Scientific Evidence for Valerian?

Constituents of valerian as well as whole-valerian extracts have been shown to act as sedatives in laboratory animals.[2,3,4] Studies in humans have also found that valerian is an effective sleeping aid.

A recent 28-day, double-blind placebo-controlled study followed 121 people with histories of significant sleep disturbance.[5] This study looked at the effectiveness of 600 mg of an alcohol-based valerian extract taken 1 hour before bedtime.

Valerian didn't work right away. For the first couple of weeks, valerian and placebo were running neck and neck. However, by day 28 valerian had pulled far ahead. Effectiveness was rated as good or very good by participant evaluation in 66% of the valerian group and in 61% by doctor evaluation, whereas in the placebo group, only 29% were so rated by participants and doctors. Only two individuals reported side effects, which were mild.

This study provides good evidence that valerian is effective for insomnia. However, it has one confusing aspect: the 4-week delay before effects were seen. In previous shorter studies, valerian has produced an immediately noticeable effect on sleep,[6–9] and that is what most practitioners believe to be typical. Why valerian took so long to work in this one study has not been explained.

We don't really know how valerian acts to induce sleep. Research suggests that the neurotransmitter GABA may be involved.[10–16] Conventional sleeping pills affect GABA as well.

### Dosages

For insomnia, the standard dosage of valerian is 2 to 3 g of dried root, 270 to 450 mg of a water-based valerian extract (3–6:1), or 600 mg of an alcohol-based extract (4–7:1) taken 30 to 60 minutes before bedtime.[17] If the results of the most recent study are correct, 4 weeks of continuous treatment may be necessary to achieve full results.

Valerian is often combined with the herb **melissa** (page 260); according to one small study, this combination is equally effective as the standard anti-insomnia drug Halcion.[18] However, the study had so few participants, the results aren't reliable. Valerian is not recommended for children under 3 years old.

### Safety Issues

Valerian is listed on the FDA's GRAS (generally regarded as safe) list and is approved for use as a food. Overdoses as high as 20 times the normal dose have not been associated with significant problems.[19] Very high doses have been given to rats without ill effects.[20]

Except for the unpleasant odor, valerian generally produces few to no side effects. In a study of 61 individuals taking normal doses of valerian, only 2 people reported side effects, which consisted of headache and morning grogginess.[21] Mild gastrointestinal distress is also occasionally reported, and, strangely, a few people experience a mild stimulant effect from valerian.

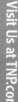

Valerian does not appear to impair driving ability or cause morning grogginess when taken at night.[22,23] However, it can impair alertness for a couple of hours immediately after use. For this reason, driving a car or operating hazardous machinery immediately after taking valerian is not recommended. According to the results of one animal study, valerian should not be combined with other medications that might make you drowsy.[24] However, a study in 1995 found no interaction between alcohol and valerian as measured by concentration, attentiveness, reaction time, and driving performance.[25]

Addiction to valerian has not been observed in studies. However, at the time of this writing there has been a disturbing report of severe withdrawal symptoms in a man who took valerian for many months and then stopped suddenly. This potentially serious problem needs urgent investigation.

The safety of valerian for young children, pregnant or nursing women, and those with liver or kidney disease has not been established.

## Melatonin: Rapid Effect on Sleep

The body uses **melatonin** (page 258) as part of its normal control of the sleep-wake cycle. The pineal gland makes serotonin and then turns it into melatonin when exposure to light decreases. Strong light (such as sunlight) slows melatonin production more than weak light does, and a completely dark room increases the amount of melatonin made more than a partially darkened room does.[26]

Taking melatonin as a supplement seems to stimulate sleep when the natural cycle is disturbed. It is most dramatically effective for jet lag and for those who work the night shift and want to change sleeping time on the weekends.

### What Is the Scientific Evidence for Melatonin?

One double-blind study tracked 320 people who were given 5 mg of standard melatonin, 5 mg of slow-release melatonin, 0.5 mg of standard melatonin, or placebo for 4 nights following plane travel.[27] The results showed improvements only with 5 mg of standard melatonin. Benefits were noted in quality of sleep, the time needed to fall asleep, and daytime drowsiness and fatigue.

Positive results were seen in several other studies,[28,29,30] although at least one negative study has been reported.[31]

According to one review of the literature, treatment is most effective for those who have crossed more than eight time zones.[32] However, melatonin also seems to help bring on sleep for other people, including those with no sleep problems to begin with.

### Dosages

Melatonin is typically taken about 30 minutes before bedtime on the first 4 days after traveling.

The ideal dosage of melatonin is not known. According to some reports, 0.5 mg is the minimum effective dose. However, one study described above found no effect at 0.5 mg but good results at 5 mg.[33] To further complicate matters, this study also found that only quick-release melatonin was effective, while in other studies time-release forms have proved more effective. Clearly, there is much we do not know about melatonin.

### Safety Issues

Melatonin is probably safe for occasional use (as in plane travel), but there is some real concern about using it on a regular basis. Keep in mind that melatonin is not really a food supplement: It is a hormone, just like estrogen, thyroid, or cortisone. Because the body's own production of melatonin is probably the equivalent of a dosage of only *one-tenth* of a milligram per day, when you take melatonin for sleep you are tremendously exceeding natural levels. The consequences of doing so on a regular basis are completely unknown.[34]

Based on theoretical ideas of how melatonin works, some authorities specifically recommend against its use in depression, schizophrenia, autoimmune diseases, and other serious illnesses and for pregnant or nursing women. Do not drive or operate machinery for several hours after taking melatonin.

## OTHER NATURAL TREATMENTS

The following natural treatments are widely recommended for insomnia, but they have not been scientifically proven effective at this time.

## Kava

The antianxiety herb **kava** (page 239) is also said to be helpful for insomnia. A typical dose of standardized extract should provide about 210 mg of kavalactones and should be taken 1 hour before bedtime. For more information on kava use and safety issues, see the corresponding chapter in Part Two.

## St. John's Wort

Because prescription antidepressants can help you sleep, it has been suggested that the herb **St. John's wort** (page 303) may be useful in the same way.

St. John's wort does not cause immediate drowsiness like some pharmaceutical antidepressants. Rather, if it is effective, the results will develop gradually. For more information on St. John's wort use and safety issues, see the corresponding chapter in Part Two.

## Tryptophan and 5-Hydroxytryptophan

For many years, people used tryptophan as a sleeping aid. However, an accidental poisonous contaminant in one batch caused many cases of a terrible illness called eosinophilic myalgia. Tryptophan has since been taken off the shelves.

The substance **5-HTP (5-hydroxytryptophan)** (page 191) has recently become widely available as a substitute. Because it is made by a completely different manufacturing process (starting from a plant rather than bacteria), one would not expect the same contaminant to appear. Surprisingly, however, in September 1998 the FDA released a report stating that there was some evidence that commercial 5-HTP preparations might contain a similar contaminant. Because this is late-breaking news, I suggest you check with your physician for the most recent information.

A typical dosage is 100 to 300 mg at bedtime.

## Other Herbs and Supplements

Many other herbs are reputed to offer sedative or relaxant benefits, including **astragalus** (page 129), **hops** (page 227), **passionflower** (page 276), **skullcap** (page 300), **chamomile** (page 156), **He shou wu** (page 224), **ashwaganda** (page 128), and lady's slipper. **Vitamin C** (page 331) is also sometimes recommended. However, there is as yet little scientific evidence that these treatments really work.

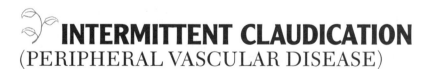

# INTERMITTENT CLAUDICATION
## (PERIPHERAL VASCULAR DISEASE)

*Principal Natural Treatments*
Ginkgo, L-carnitine, inositol hexaniacinate, arginine

The arteries supplying the legs with blood may become seriously blocked in advanced stages of atherosclerosis (hardening of the arteries). This can lead to severe, crampy pain when you walk more than a short distance, because the muscles are starved for oxygen. In fact, the intensity of intermittent claudication is often measured in the distance a person can walk without pain.

Conventional treatment for intermittent claudication consists of measures to combat **atherosclerosis** (page 14), the drug Trental (pentoxifylline), and other medications. In advanced cases, surgery to improve blood flow may be necessary.

## PRINCIPAL NATURAL TREATMENTS

A number of natural treatments may be helpful, but it isn't clear whether it is safe to combine them with the medications that may be prescribed at the same time. Medical supervision is definitely necessary for this serious disease.

Because they work so differently, it has been suggested that the two treatments described in this section, ginkgo and carnitine, might enhance each other's effectiveness when taken together.

## Ginkgo

Germany's Commission E authorizes the use of **ginkgo** (page 204) for the treatment of intermittent claudication. Several preliminary double-blind studies suggest that ginkgo can produce a significant increase in pain-free walking distance, probably by improving circulation.[1,2]

The most recent of these studies enrolled 111 patients and followed them for 24 weeks.[3] Participants were measured for pain-free walking distance by walking up a 12% slope on a treadmill at 2 miles an hour. At the beginning of treatment, both the placebo and ginkgo groups were able to walk about 350 feet without pain.

At the end of the trial, both groups had improved significantly (the power of placebo is amazing!). However, the ginkgo group had improved more, reaching an average of 500 feet compared to 415 feet for the control group.

Bottom line: Ginkgo extract can reduce symptoms and produce measurable if not dramatic improvements in walking distance.

The typical dosage of ginkgo extract is 40 mg 3 times daily. Ginkgo generally does not cause side effects, but fears that it may interact with blood-thinning medications (see the corresponding chapter in Part Two for more details) make its use in intermittent claudication difficult. To safely use ginkgo, you may have to decline conventional treatment, and this could be a very risky decision.

## L-Carnitine

The vitamin-like substance **L-carnitine** (page 151) also appears to be of some benefit in intermittent claudication. Although it does not increase blood flow, carnitine appears to increase walking distance by improving energy utilization in the muscles.

A recent double-blind study followed 245 people, half of whom were treated with a special form of L-carnitine called L-propionyl-carnitine; the other half took placebo.[4] A dosage of 2,000 mg daily produced an average 73% improvement in walking distance, compared to a 46% improvement in the placebo group. Reductions in pain levels were also reported.

The optimum dosage of L-propionyl-carnitine appears to be 1 to 3 g daily. This apparently safe supplement is not associated with any significant side effects, toxicities, or drug interactions. However, individuals on kidney dialysis should not use L-carnitine (or any other supplement) except on medical advice.

## Inositol Hexaniacinate

The supplement inositol hexaniacinate, a special form of **vitamin B$_3$ (niacin)** (page 323), appears to be helpful for intermittent claudication. Double-blind studies involving a total of over 500 individuals have found that it can improve walking distance for people with intermittent claudication.[5–9] For example, in one study, 120 individuals were given either placebo or 2 g of inositol hexaniacinate daily. Over a period of 3 months, walking distance improved significantly in the treated group.[10] The effect was roughly comparable to that of L-carnitine.

The usual dose of inositol hexaniacinate is about 1 to 4 g daily. However, due to the risk of liver inflammation, medical supervision is essential.

## Arginine

The supplement **arginine** (page 126) may be able to improve walking distance for people with intermittent claudication. In one study, after 2 weeks of treatment, participants could walk 66% farther than they could at the beginning of the study.[11]

A typical supplemental dosage of arginine is 2 to 3 g per day.

# IRRITABLE BOWEL SYNDROME (SPASTIC COLON)

*Principal Natural Treatments*
   Peppermint oil

*Other Natural Treatments*
   Acidophilus, *Coleus forskohlii,* glutamine, slippery elm

The symptoms of irritable bowel syndrome (IBS) include one or more of the following: alternating diarrhea and constipation, intestinal gas, bloating and cramping, abdominal pain, painful bowel movements, mucous discharge, and undigested food in the stool. Despite all these distressing symptoms, in IBS the intestines appear to be perfectly healthy when they are examined. Thus the condition belongs to a category of diseases that physicians call *functional*. This term means that while the function of the bowel seems to have gone awry, no injury or disturbance of its structure can be discovered.

The cause of IBS remains unknown. Medical treatment for irritable bowel syndrome consists mainly of increased dietary fiber plus drugs that reduce bowel spasm.

## PRINCIPAL NATURAL TREATMENTS

**Peppermint** (page 277) oil is widely used for IBS. However, the research evidence is a bit contradictory.[1–4] The proper dosage is 1 or 2 capsules (0.2 ml per capsule) 3 times daily between meals. Because dosage amounts of pep-

permint needed to relieve lower bowel cramping can cause heartburn, the best formulations are enteric coated to pass intact through the stomach (this is usually stated on the label).

When taken as directed, peppermint is believed to be reasonably safe in healthy adults.[5] However, peppermint can cause jaundice in newborn babies, so do not try to use it for colic. Excessive intake of peppermint oil can cause nausea, loss of appetite, heart problems, loss of balance, and other nervous system problems.

Safety in pregnant or nursing women or those with severe liver or kidney disease has not been established.

## OTHER NATURAL TREATMENTS

The friendly bacteria **Lactobacillus acidophilus** (page 120) appear to be helpful for IBS.[6]

The herbs **Coleus forskohlii** (page 166) and **slippery elm** (page 300) as well as the supplement **glutamine** (page 215) are also sometimes recommended for IBS, but there is not much evidence as yet that they really work.

 # MACULAR DEGENERATION

*Principal Natural Treatments*
   Antioxidants (vitamin C, vitamin E, selenium, beta-carotene, lutein, zeaxanthin, lycopene, bilberry, ginkgo, grape seed as a source of oligomeric proanthocyanidins, or OPCs), wine

*Other Natural Treatments*
   Zinc

The lens of the eye focuses an image of the world on a portion of the retina called the *macula,* the area of finest visual perception. After

cataracts, damage to the macula is the second most common cause of visual impairment in those over 65. Smoking, high blood pressure, and atherosclerosis are associated with macular degeneration. Bright light also appears to play a role by creating damaging natural substances in the eye, called free radicals. Gradual deterioration of the macula is called macular degeneration.

In the most common form of macular degeneration, a substance known as lipofuscin accumulates in the lining of the retina. No conventional medical treatment is available for this disease, although mainstream researchers are seriously investigating the antioxidants described here.

A much less common form of macular degeneration involves the abnormal growth of blood vessels. This can be treated very successfully, if attended to soon enough, but may lead to irreversible blindness if left untreated. For this reason, medical consultation in all cases of macular degeneration (or any other type of vision loss) is essential.

## PRINCIPAL NATURAL TREATMENTS

Because research suggests that macular degeneration may be related to free radical damage, it's natural to reason that antioxidant nutrients may be able to protect against it. However, more research is necessary for firm conclusions.

An observational study of 2,152 subjects, aged 43 to 86, found that **vitamin C** (page 331) supplementation was associated with a decreased incidence of early age-related macular degeneration.[1] Another observational study enrolling almost 2,000 people found that high intake of vitamin C or **vitamin E** (page 337) was associated with less macular degeneration.[2]

It may be that combinations of many antioxidants, such as those found in foods, are most beneficial. One 18-month, double-blind study found that a daily supplement containing 750 mg of vitamin C, 200 IU of vitamin E, 50 mcg of **selenium** (page 297), and 20,000 IU of **beta-carotene** (page 131) stopped the progression of

macular degeneration.[3] For more information and safety issues for vitamin C, vitamin E, and selenium, see the corresponding chapters in Part Two.

Various dietary carotenes may also be associated with a lower incidence of macular degeneration.[4,5] Carotenes (carotenoids) are a group of substances that are found in many fruits and vegetables, especially yellow-orange and dark-green ones. Beta-carotene is the most famous carotene. However, the less well known carotenes **lutein** (page 248) and zeaxanthin may be more closely correlated with protection from macular degeneration. These are principally found in dark-green leafy vegetables, such as spinach and collard greens. It has been suggested that lutein may protect the macula from light-induced damage by dying it yellow, thereby acting as a kind of natural sunglasses.[6] It also acts in the usual antioxidant fashion by neutralizing free radicals.[7] **Lycopene** (page 249), a carotenoid found in tomatoes, may also be helpful.

Flavonoids are another group of naturally occurring chemicals, found in many plants, that may offer a variety of beneficial effects. Weak but interesting evidence suggests that the flavonoid-rich herbs **bilberry** (page 135), **ginkgo** (page 204), and **OPCs** (page 270) may prevent or treat macular degeneration.[8,9,10]

Moderate wine consumption appears to help prevent macular degeneration.[11] Like these herbs, wine contains high levels of flavonoids.

## OTHER NATURAL TREATMENTS

The mineral **zinc** (page 348) may also help prevent macular degeneration, although the study results are a bit contradictory.[12,13,14] A typical dosage is 15 to 30 mg daily, combined with 1 to 3 mg of **copper** (page 169) to avoid zinc-induced copper deficiency. Too much zinc can be toxic, so do not exceed this dose.

# MENOPAUSAL SYMPTOMS
## (OTHER THAN OSTEOPOROSIS)

*Principal Natural Treatments*
  Black cohosh, soy protein/isoflavones

*Other Natural Treatments*
  Vitamin E, vitamin C, bioflavonoids, essential fatty acids, gamma oryzanol, licorice, chasteberry, dong quai, red clover, suma

The hormonal changes of menopause can produce a wide variety of symptoms, ranging from hot flashes and vaginal dryness to anxiety, depression, and insomnia. Many of these symptoms are undoubtedly caused by the natural decrease in estrogen production that occurs at menopause; however, the human body is so complex that other hormonal factors also play a role.

Menopause is not a disease. It is clearly a natural process, but one that has fallen out of favor in modern society. We no longer consider it as an inevitable transition but instead treat it as a condition requiring treatment. No longer do women accept as merely part of life the decrease in libido, pain during intercourse, years of hot flashes, and other uncomfortable problems that may accompany menopause. This raises an important point: How close to nature do we want to live? One of the most valued ideals of alternative medicine is the desire to trust nature, but sometimes we may want to draw a line. For example, in a state of nature, infant and maternal mortality is high. This process of survival of the fittest helps humanity as a species to be stronger, but it is not something that a compassionate society can tolerate. Thus, no matter what our ideals, we frequently find ourselves tampering with nature. The treatment of menopause is simply one example among many.

Conventional medicine recommends the use of replacement estrogen to provide three benefits: eliminating the symptoms of menopause, protecting against osteoporosis, and maintaining the protection against cardiovascular disease that premenopausal women enjoy.

Estrogen-replacement therapy is quite effective at achieving these goals. However, like most medical treatments, it creates counterbalancing risks. The most frightening issue is the increased risk of breast cancer that appears to be associated with replacement estrogen. The decision whether to use estrogen-replacement therapy should involve a careful examination of the risks and benefits in consultation with a physician. Specially modified estrogens, such as Evista (raloxifene), appear to help osteoporosis and reduce the incidence of breast cancer, but they do not reduce symptoms of menopause.

## PRINCIPAL NATURAL TREATMENTS

Several natural treatments may reduce menopausal symptoms. However, we do not know for sure whether any of these reduce the risk of cardiovascular disease or osteoporosis. See the chapters on **atherosclerosis** (page 14) and **osteoporosis** (page 100) for natural ways to reduce the risk of these conditions.

### Black Cohosh: Widely Used in Europe for Menopausal Symptoms

**Black cohosh** (page 138) is a tall perennial herb that was originally found in the northeastern United States. Native Americans used it mainly for women's health problems but also as a treatment for arthritis, fatigue, and snakebite. European colonists rapidly adopted the herb for similar uses.

In the late nineteenth century, black cohosh was the main ingredient in the wildly popular Lydia E. Pinkham's Vegetable Compound for menstrual cramps. Migrating across the Atlantic, black cohosh became a popular European treatment for women's problems, arthritis, and high blood pressure. In the 1980s, black cohosh was approved by Germany's Commission E for use in menopause.

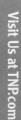

## What Is the Scientific Evidence for Black Cohosh?

Evidence suggests that over a period of 4 to 6 weeks black cohosh can improve all major menopausal symptoms, including hot flashes, sweating, headache, vertigo, heart palpitations, tinnitus, nervousness, irritability, sleep disturbance, anxiety, vaginal dryness, and depression.[1,2,3] Unfortunately, there is no evidence that black cohosh can prevent osteoporosis or heart disease, two of estrogen's most famous benefits.

A double-blind study of 80 participants compared the benefits of black cohosh, estrogen (0.625 mg), and placebo over a period of 12 weeks.[4] Black cohosh proved at least as effective as estrogen in reducing all the major symptoms of menopause. It also helped reverse the menopause-related changes in vaginal cells. Similar results were seen in other studies.[5,6]

Black cohosh is made up of many substances called phytoestrogens, which have shown some estrogen-like activity in test-tube studies. Extracts of the herb reduce levels of the pituitary hormone LH (luteinizing hormone), just like standard estrogen-replacement therapy.[7,8,9] Thus, up until 1998 it was believed that black cohosh worked by imitating some of the effects of estrogen.

However, matters were recently made more complicated when a double-blind study found no evidence of improvement in vaginal cells or other evidence of estrogen-like activity.[10] An animal study has also found no evidence that black cohosh works like estrogen.[11] These surprising findings have upset the apple cart, leaving us quite confused about just how black cohosh really works.

### Dosages

The standard dosage of black cohosh is 1 to 2 tablets twice daily of a standardized extract manufactured to contain 1 mg of 27-deoxyacteine per tablet.

Make sure not to confuse black cohosh with blue cohosh (*Caulophyllum thalictroides*). Blue cohosh is potentially more dangerous because it contains chemicals that are toxic to the heart. A recent case report indicates that it caused severe heart problems in a woman who took blue cohosh during pregnancy.[12]

### Safety Issues

Black cohosh seldom produces any obvious side effects, other than occasional mild gastrointestinal distress. Studies in rats have shown no significant toxicity when black cohosh was given at 90 times the therapeutic dosage for a period of 6 months.[13] Because 6 months in a rat corresponds to decades in a human, this study appears to make a strong statement about the long-term safety of black cohosh.

Unlike estrogen, black cohosh does not stimulate breast cancer cells growing in a test tube, probably because the estrogens it contains are weaker than human estrogen.[14] However, this should not be taken as a guarantee that black cohosh does not increase the risk of breast cancer. Women who have already had breast cancer should not take black cohosh except on the advice of a physician.

Black cohosh has been shown to slightly lower blood pressure and blood sugar in certain animals.[15] For this reason, it's possible that the herb could interact with drugs for high blood pressure or diabetes, although no such problems have been reported.

Black cohosh is generally not recommended for pregnant or nursing mothers, and safety in young children and those with severe liver or kidney disease has not been established.

## Soy Isoflavones: May Reduce Symptoms

Black cohosh isn't the only plant that contains estrogen-like substances. Soy and **soy protein** (page 301) contain phytoestrogens called **isoflavones** (page 236), which appear to produce far-reaching effects in the body. The most famous of these isoflavones are genistein and daidzen. These substances, perhaps along with other constituents of soy protein, appear to be effective in reducing menopausal hot flashes. In one double-blind study of 104 women, daily doses of 60 g of soy protein significantly reduced flushing associated with menopause.[16] However, soy does not appear to reduce vaginal dryness.

It is not known whether soy can prevent osteoporosis.[17] However, a synthetic isoflavone named ipriflavone (chemically similar to what is found in soy) does seem to be effective for this purpose. See the chapters on osteoporosis or isoflavones for more information.

Soy appears to be protective against heart disease and breast and uterine cancer. However, soy possibly may not be safe for those who have already had breast cancer.

The best dosage of soy is unclear. One or two cups of soy milk or slices of tofu daily appear to be helpful.[18]

Various products containing concentrated isoflavones from soy or red clover have recently come on the market. However, although these supplements show promise, more research needs to be done to establish the correct dosage and to verify safety.

## OTHER NATURAL TREATMENTS

**Vitamin E** (page 337), **vitamin C** (page 331); bioflavonoids; essential fatty acids; an extract of rice bran called **gamma oryzanol** (page 196); and the herbs **licorice** (page 244), **red clover** (page 290), **suma** (page 307) and **chasteberry** (page 157) are reportedly helpful for menopause. However, there is as yet little to no scientific evidence to turn to.

The herb **dong quai** (page 177) is also frequently recommended for menopausal symptoms, but a recent double-blind study found it to be entirely ineffective.[19]

For more information on menopause, see *The Natural Pharmacist Guide to Menopause.*

# MIGRAINE HEADACHES

*Principal Natural Treatments*
   Feverfew, magnesium

*Other Natural Treatments*
   5-HTP, fish oil, riboflavin (vitamin B$_2$), chromium, calcium, vitamin C, folic acid, ginger, allergen-free diet, acupuncture

The term *migraine* refers to a class of headaches sharing certain characteristic symptoms. The two main subcategories of migraine are the common and the classic migraine.

In common migraines, headache pain usually occurs in the forehead or temples, often on one side only and typically accompanied by nausea and a preference for a darkened room. Headache attacks last for several hours up to a day or more. They are usually separated by completely pain-free intervals.

In the rarer form of migraine, called classic migraine, headache pain is accompanied by a visual disturbance known as an aura. Otherwise, symptoms are similar to those of the common migraine.

Migraines can be triggered by a variety of causes, including fatigue, stress, hormonal changes, and foods such as alcohol, chocolate, peanuts, and avocados. However, in many people, migraines occur with no obvious triggering factor.

The cause of migraine headaches has been a subject of continuing controversy for over a century. Opinion has swung back and forth between two primary beliefs: that migraines are related to epileptic seizures and originate in the nervous tissue of the brain; or that blood vessels in the skull cause headache pain when they dilate or contract (so-called vascular headaches). Most likely, several factors are involved, and more than one stimulus can light the fuse that leads to a full-blown migraine attack.

Conventional treatment of acute migraines has lately been revolutionized by the drug sumatriptan (Imitrex). This drug can completely abort a migraine headache in many individuals. It works by imitating the action of serotonin on blood vessels, causing them to contract. Drugs made from ergot mold are also effective.

People interested in prevention can choose from a bewildering variety of drugs, including ergot drugs, antidepressants, beta-blockers, calcium channel–blockers, and antiseizure medication. Picking the right one is mostly a matter of trial and error.

## PRINCIPAL NATURAL TREATMENTS

Scientific evidence suggests that the herb feverfew and the mineral magnesium can help prevent migraine headaches.

Keep in mind that serious diseases may occasionally first present themselves as migraine-type headaches. If you suddenly start having migraines without a previous history, or if the pattern of your migraines changes significantly, it is essential to seek medical evaluation.

## Feverfew: Dried Leaf May Reduce Frequency and Severity of Headaches

**Feverfew** (page 186) was widely used in ancient times as a treatment for headaches and other conditions. However, it fell out of favor for several centuries until an unexpected but fortunate event occurred in the late 1970s. At that time, the wife of the chief medical officer of the National Coal Board in England suffered from serious migraine headaches. When this fact became known to workers in the industry, a sympathetic miner suggested that she try a folk treatment he knew about. She followed his advice and chewed feverfew leaves. The results were dramatic: Her migraines almost completely disappeared.

Her husband was impressed, too, and used his high office to gain the ear of a physician who specialized in migraine headaches, Dr. E. Stewart Johnson of the London Migraine Clinic. Johnson subsequently tried feverfew on 10 of his patients. The results were so good that he subsequently gave the herb to 270 of his patients. A whopping 70% reported considerable relief.

Thoroughly excited now, Dr. Johnson enrolled 17 feverfew-using patients in an interesting type of double-blind study.[1] Half were continued on feverfew, and the other half transferred without their knowledge to placebo. Over a period of 6 months, the participants withdrawn from feverfew demonstrated a dramatic increase in headaches, nausea, and vomiting.

Unfortunately, this study had some serious flaws. It was too small, and because the participants were already feverfew users who felt it worked for them, it didn't say anything about the effectiveness of feverfew in the population at large. This type of error in a study is called *self-selection.* Nonetheless, the study brought a flood of response from the public and ultimately led to three preliminary but properly performed double-blind experiments.

Today, feverfew is used mainly for the prevention of chronic, recurrent migraine headaches, especially in the United Kingdom. Those who use it say that their headaches become less frequent and less severe, and may even stop altogether. However, feverfew must be taken religiously every day for best results.

Reportedly, feverfew taken at the onset of a migraine attack can provide some benefit, but no studies have yet been performed to confirm this. It is not at all effective for cluster or tension headaches.

### What Is the Scientific Evidence for Feverfew?

Two double-blind studies suggest that regular use of feverfew leaf can help prevent migraine headaches and reduce their severity when they do come.

The so-called Nottingham trial followed 59 individuals for 8 months.[2] For 4 months, half received a daily capsule of feverfew leaf, and the other half received placebo. The groups were then switched and followed for an additional 4 months. Treatment with feverfew produced a 24% reduction in the number of migraines and a significant decrease in nausea and vomiting during the headaches.

A recent double-blind study of 57 people with migraines, who were given feverfew leaf daily, also showed distinct reductions in headache severity.[3] Unfortunately, the authors did not report whether the frequency of headaches improved.

However, the herb world was surprised when a Dutch study of 50 people showed no difference whatsoever between placebo and a special feverfew extract standardized to its parthenolide content.[4] This unexpected result reversed a widely held view about how feverfew works.

For many years it was assumed that the active ingredient in feverfew was a substance named parthenolide. Many articles were published explaining exactly how parthenolide prevented migraines.[5-8] On the basis of this premature explanation, indignant authors complained that samples of feverfew on the market vary as much as 10 to 1 in their parthenolide content. No less an authority than the herbal expert Varro Tyler said that "standardization of the herbal material on the basis of its parthenolide content is urgently required if this potentially valuable herb is to be used effectively."[9]

However, everyone was jumping the gun. The special feverfew extract used in the negative Dutch study was standardized to a high parthenolide content. Apparently, this extract lacked some essential substance or group of substances that is present in the whole leaf, which was used in the positive studies. Without these unknown constituents, it seems that feverfew does not work. What those substances may have been remains mysterious.

### Dosages

Given the recent confusion surrounding parthenolide, previous dosage recommendations for feverfew based on parthenolide content have been cast in doubt. At the present time, the best recommendation is probably to take 80 to 100 mg of powdered whole feverfew leaf daily.

When taken at the onset of a migraine headache, higher amounts of feverfew are often used. However, the optimum dosage has not been determined.

### Safety Issues

Among the many thousands of people who use feverfew as a folk medicine in England, no reports of serious toxicity have been published.

In the 8-month Nottingham clinical trial of 76 participants (59 completed the study), no significant differences in side effects were found between treated individuals and the placebo group, nor were any changes in measurements on blood tests and urinalysis noted.[10]

In a survey of 300 study participants, 11.3% reported mouth sores after chewing feverfew leaf, occasionally accompanied by general inflammation of tissues in the mouth.[11] A smaller percentage reported mild gastrointestinal dis-

tress.[12] However, mouth sores do not seem to occur in people who use encapsulated feverfew.

Animal studies confirm the safety of feverfew. No adverse effects were seen at doses 100 and 150 times the human daily dose in rats and guinea pigs, respectively.[13]

However, because feverfew was an old folk remedy used to promote abortions, it should probably not be taken during pregnancy. Safety in young children and those with severe liver or kidney disease has also not been established.

## Magnesium: May Help Prevent Migraines

**Magnesium** (page 251) is another natural treatment that appears to be effective for preventing migraine headaches. A recent 12-week double-blind study followed 81 people with recurrent migraines.[14] Half received 600 mg of magnesium daily (in the rather unusual form of trimagnesium dicitrate), and the other half received placebo.

By the last 3 weeks of the study, the frequency of migraine attacks was reduced by 41.6% in the treated group, compared to 15.8% in the placebo group. The only side effects observed were diarrhea (18.6%) and digestive irritation (4.7%).

Similar results have been seen in other double-blind studies.[15,16] There was one study that did not find a benefit,[17] but there were many problems with its design.[18]

Since many people are deficient in magnesium anyway, it's hard to go wrong taking a magnesium supplement. The usual nutritional dose is in the neighborhood of 350 to 450 mg daily, but 600 mg (as used in the study) should be safe, unless you suffer from severe heart or kidney disease.

## OTHER NATURAL TREATMENTS

Several other herbs and supplements are widely recommended for migraine headaches, but as yet there is little scientific proof that they are effective.

## 5-HTP

The supplement **5-HTP (5-hydroxytryptophan)** (page 191) has also been suggested as a treatment for migraine headaches. However, the available scientific evidence is contradictory at best.

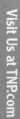

The body manufactures 5-HTP on the way to making serotonin. It is possible, but not yet proven, that supplemental 5-HTP may increase serotonin levels. Serotonin is believed to be involved in the beginning of migraine headaches, and, as described previously, the dramatically effective antimigraine drug Imitrex works by imitating the effects of serotonin on blood vessels. Antidepressants that appear to raise serotonin levels in general, such as Prozac, sometimes seem to help prevent migraines as well. 5-HTP may provide similar benefits.

One study compared the effectiveness of 5-HTP against the standard migraine drug methysergide. In this 6-month trial of 124 participants, 5-HTP proved to be equally effective.[19] Benefits were more dramatic in the strength and duration than in the frequency of attacks. Because methysergide has been proven to be better than placebo, the study results provide meaningful, although not airtight, evidence that 5-HTP is effective as well.

However, in a double-blind study that directly compared 5-HTP to placebo, 5-HTP failed to produce significantly better results than the placebo.[20] And in another study, 5-HTP was not as effective as the drug propranolol.[21] A few studies have found benefits for children and adolescents with various types of headaches, including migraines.[22,23]

Putting all this information together, it appears that 5-HTP is possibly an effective treatment for the prevention of migraines. However, there are some safety concerns regarding 5-HTP.

See the corresponding chapter in Part Two for more information.

## Fish Oil

Preliminary double-blind studies suggest that high doses of **fish oil** (page 188) may be helpful for migraine headaches.[24,25]

## Vitamin B$_2$ (Riboflavin)

According to a recent 3-month double-blind study of 55 people with migraines, 400 mg of **vitamin B$_2$** (page 321) daily can reduce the frequency of migraine headaches by 50%.[26]

## Other Supplements

**Chromium** (page 161), **calcium** (page 146), **vitamin C** (page 331), **folic acid** (page 194), and **ginger** (page 202) have also been reported to be helpful for migraines, but there is as yet not much scientific evidence for any of these treatments.

## Other Treatments

Identifying and eliminating allergenic foods from your diet appears to be helpful in reducing the frequency of migraine attacks.[27]

At least one small double-blind study using real and "sham" treatment suggests that acupuncture can reduce the intensity and number of migraine attacks.[28] Furthermore, the improvements were found to continue for at least a year after the cessation of acupuncture treatment.

For more information on migraine headaches, see *The Natural Pharmacist Guide to Feverfew and Migraines.*

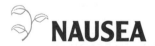 # NAUSEA

*Principal Natural Treatments*
   Ginger, vitamin B$_6$

*Other Natural Treatments*
   Vitamin C, vitamin K, lowfat diet

Nausea can be caused by numerous factors, including stomach flu, viral infections of the inner ear (labyrinthitis), motion sickness, pregnancy, and chemotherapy. If you are continually nauseous, it can be more disabling than chronic pain. Successful treatment can make an enormous difference in your quality of life.

The sensation of nausea can originate in either the nervous system or the digestive tract itself. Most conventional treatments for nausea, such as Dramamine and Compazine, act on the nervous system, but products like Pepto-Bismol soothe the digestive tract directly.

## PRINCIPAL NATURAL TREATMENTS

The herb ginger has become a widely accepted treatment for nausea of various types. Vitamin $B_6$ may be helpful for the nausea of pregnancy.

### Ginger: May Help Several Types of Nausea

Native to southern Asia, **ginger** (page 202) is a 2- to 4-foot perennial that produces grass-like leaves up to a foot long and almost an inch wide. Ginger root, as it is named in the grocery store, actually consists of the underground stem of the plant with its bark-like outer covering scraped off.

Ginger has been used as food and medicine for millennia. Ginger's modern use dates back to the early 1980s, when a scientist named D. Mowrey noticed that ginger-filled capsules reduced his nausea during an episode of flu. Subsequent research ultimately led Germany's Commission E to approve ginger as a treatment for indigestion and motion sickness.

Ginger is typically not as effective as standard drugs for motion sickness, but it has the advantage of not causing drowsiness. Some physicians recommend ginger over other motion sickness drugs for older individuals who are unusually sensitive to drowsiness or loss of balance.

Ginger is also used for the nausea and vomiting of pregnancy, and some conventional medical textbooks mention it. However, physicians are hesitant to recommend any treatment during pregnancy until full safety studies have been performed, and although it is a food, these studies have not yet been completed for ginger (see Safety Issues).

European physicians sometimes give their patients ginger before and just after surgery to prevent the nausea that many people experience when they awaken from anesthesia. However,

this treatment should be attempted only with a physician's approval.

### What Is the Scientific Evidence for Ginger?

Scientific evidence suggests that ginger can be helpful for various forms of nausea.

**Nausea and Vomiting of Pregnancy**    A preliminary double-blind study performed in Denmark concluded that ginger can significantly reduce the nausea and vomiting that often accompany pregnancy.[1] Effects became apparent in 19 of 27 women after 4 days of treatment.

**Motion Sickness**    The first scientific study of ginger for motion sickness followed 36 college students with a known tendency toward motion sickness.[2] They were treated with either ginger or the standard antinausea drug dimenhydrinate and then placed in a rotating chair to see how much motion they could stand. Both treatments seemed about equally effective. Another study also found equivalent benefit between ginger and dimenhydrinate in a group of 60 passengers on a cruise through rough seas.[3] A study of 79 Swedish naval cadets found that ginger could decrease vomiting and cold sweating, but it didn't significantly decrease nausea and vertigo.[4]

However, a 1984 study funded by NASA found that ginger was not any more effective than placebo at reducing the symptoms of nausea caused by a vigorous nausea-provoking method.[5] Negative results were also seen in another study that used a strong nausea stimulus.[6]

Put all together, these studies paint a picture of a treatment that is somewhat effective for motion sickness but cannot overcome severe nausea.

**Post-Surgical Nausea**    A double-blind British study compared the effects of ginger, placebo, and the drug metoclopramide in the treatment of nausea following gynecological surgery.[7] The results in 60 women showed that both treatments produced similar benefits compared to placebo.

A similar British study followed 120 women receiving gynecological surgery.[8] Whereas nausea and vomiting developed in 41% of participants given a placebo, in the groups treated with ginger or metoclopramide (Reglan), these symptoms developed in only 21% and 27%, respectively.

However, a double-blind study of 108 people undergoing similar surgery showed no benefit with ginger as compared to placebo.[9] Negative results were also seen in another study.[10]

**Warning:** Do not use ginger either before or immediately after surgery or labor and delivery without a physician's approval. Not only is it important to have an empty stomach before undergoing anesthesia, there are theoretical concerns that ginger may affect bleeding.

### Dosages

For most purposes, the standard dosage of powdered ginger is 1 to 4 g daily taken in 2 to 4 divided doses.

To prevent motion sickness, it is probably best to begin treatment 1 or 2 days before the trip and continue it throughout the period of travel.

In the nausea and vomiting of pregnancy, the best form of ginger is probably freshly brewed tea made from boiled ginger root or powdered ginger and diluted to taste. If chilled, carbonated, and sweetened, this would become the original form of ginger ale, a famous antinausea beverage.

### Safety Issues

Ginger is on the FDA's GRAS (generally recognized as safe) list and seldom causes any side effects.

Like onions and **garlic** (page 197), extracts of ginger interfere with blood clotting in test tubes.[11,12,13] This has led to a theoretical concern that ginger should not be combined with drugs such as Coumadin (warfarin), Trental (pentoxifylline), or even aspirin. However, European studies with actual oral ginger in normal quantities have not found any effect on clotting. [14,15,16]

Maximum safe dosages for young children, pregnant or nursing women, or those with severe liver or kidney disease have not been established.

### Vitamin B$_6$

A large double-blind study suggests that 30 mg daily of vitamin B$_6$ can reduce the sensation of nausea in morning sickness.[17] At this dose, vitamin B$_6$ should be entirely safe.

## OTHER NATURAL TREATMENTS

Although the following natural treatments are widely recommended to relieve nausea, there is as yet little scientific evidence that they work.

### Vitamin K and Vitamin C

On the basis of studies conducted in the 1950s, a combination of **vitamin K** (page 341) (5 mg) and **vitamin C** (page 331) (25 mg) is sometimes recommended for morning sickness.[18] Please keep in mind that supplemental vitamin K can interfere with prescription blood-thinning drugs such as Coumadin (warfarin) and heparin.

### Other Recommendations

Diets high in saturated fat (animal fat) can increase morning sickness in some people.[19]

# NIGHT VISION (IMPAIRED)

*Principal Natural Treatments*
   Bilberry

*Other Natural Treatments*
   OPCs, vitamin A, zinc

The ability to see in poor light depends on the presence of a substance in the eye called rhodopsin, or visual purple. It is destroyed by bright light but rapidly regenerates in the dark.

However, for some people, the adaptation to darkness or the recovery from glare takes an unusually long time. There is no medical treatment for this condition.

## PRINCIPAL NATURAL TREATMENTS

The herb bilberry is widely used as a treatment for impaired night vision. However, the scientific evidence is not yet as strong as it should be.

### Bilberry: Widely Used in Europe for Impaired Night Vision

The herb **bilberry** (page 135), a close relative of the American blueberry, is the most commonly mentioned natural treatment for impaired night vision. This use dates back to World War II, when pilots in Britain's Royal Air Force reported that a good dose of bilberry jam just before a mission improved their night vision, often dramatically. After the war, medical researchers investigated the constituents of bilberry and found some evidence that it might be effective.

Two preliminary placebo-controlled studies of bilberry found that the herb improved vision in semidarkness, shortened time necessary to adapt to darkness, and speeded recovery from glare.[1,2] Other studies that did not have a placebo group have also found benefits.[3,4,5]

The effects of bilberry are believed to be due to a group of chemicals called anthocyanosides.

These naturally occurring antioxidants have a special attraction to the retina.[6]

The standard dosage of bilberry is 120 to 240 mg twice daily of an extract standardized to contain 25% bilberry anthocyanosides.

As one might expect of a food, bilberry is quite safe. Enormous quantities have been administered to rats without toxic effects.[7,8] One study involving 2,295 participants showed no serious side effects and only a 4% occurrence of mild reactions, such as gastrointestinal distress, skin rashes, and drowsiness.[9] However, safety in young children, pregnant or nursing women, and those with severe liver or kidney disease has not been established.

Bilberry has no known drug interactions.

## OTHER NATURAL TREATMENTS

**OPCs** (page 270) have also been recommended for improving night vision.[10,11]

There is no question that deficiencies of **vitamin A** (page 318) and **zinc** (page 348) can also negatively affect night vision. Since zinc is commonly lacking in many people's diets, taking 15 to 20 mg of zinc daily—along with 1 to 3 mg of **copper** (page 169) for balance—may be advisable.

# OSTEOARTHRITIS

*Principal Natural Treatments*
  Glucosamine, chondroitin sulfate, S-adenosylmethionine, niacinamide

*Other Natural Treatments*
  Devil's claw, healthy diet, boswellia, turmeric, yucca, white willow, boron, copper, D-phenylalanine, selenium, molybdenum, zinc, beta-carotene, cartilage, vitamin C, vitamin E, bromelain, cat's claw, chamomile, dandelion, feverfew

In osteoarthritis, the cartilage in joints has become damaged, disrupting the smooth gliding motion of the joint surfaces. The result is pain, swelling, and deformity.

The pain of osteoarthritis typically increases with joint use and improves at rest. For reasons that aren't clear, although x rays can find evidence of arthritis, the level of pain and stiffness experienced by people does not match the extent of injury noticed on x rays.

Many theories exist about the causes of osteoarthritis, but we don't really know what causes the disease. Osteoarthritis is often described as "wear and tear" arthritis. However, evidence suggests that this simple explanation is not correct. For example, osteoarthritis frequently develops in many joints at the same time, often symmetrically on both sides of the body, even when there is no reason to believe that equal amounts of wear and tear are present. Another intriguing finding is that osteoarthritis of the knee is commonly (and mysteriously) associated with osteoarthritis of the hand. These factors, as well as others, have led to the suggestion that osteoarthritis may actually be a body-wide disease of the cartilage.

During one's lifetime, cartilage is constantly being turned over by a balance of forces that both break down and rebuild it. One prevailing theory suggests that osteoarthritis may represent a situation in which the degrading forces get out of hand. Some of the proposed natural treatments for osteoarthritis described later may inhibit enzymes that damage cartilage.

When the cartilage damage in osteoarthritis begins, the body responds by building new cartilage. For several years, this compensating effort can keep the joint functioning well. Some of the natural treatments described below appear to work by assisting the body in repairing cartilage. Eventually, however, building forces cannot keep up with destructive ones, and what is called end-stage osteoarthritis develops. This is the familiar picture of pain and impaired joint function.

The conventional medical treatment for osteoarthritis consists mainly of analgesic medications, such as Tylenol, and anti-inflammatory drugs, such as Aleve and Orudis. The main problem with anti-inflammatory drugs is that they can cause ulcers. Another possible problem is that they may actually speed the progression of osteoarthritis by interfering with cartilage repair and promoting cartilage destruction.[1–5] In contrast, at least two of the treatments described below may actually slow the course of the disease, although this hasn't been conclusively proven.

Recently, the use of extracts of **cayenne** (page 155) pepper has found its way into conventional medicine. Briefly, it consists of the regular application of cayenne cream to the affected joint, ultimately resulting in a decreased sensation of pain. Unfortunately, this truly natural treatment seldom provides more than modest relief.

## PRINCIPAL NATURAL TREATMENTS

There are several very useful natural treatments for osteoarthritis. Not only do they reduce pain without causing any side effects, some may actually slow the progression of osteoarthritis.

# Glucosamine: Safe Pain Relief That Lasts

One of the best-documented alternative approaches to the treatment of osteoarthritis is the supplement **glucosamine** (page 213). Glucosamine is a small molecule formed of a sugar attached to a chemical structure called an amine. Taking glucosamine supplements provides a natural raw material for rebuilding cartilage. It seems to stimulate the activity of cartilage cells and perhaps also protect cartilage from damage.[6–13]

In Portugal, Spain, and Italy, glucosamine has been a primary treatment for osteoarthritis since the 1980s, and it is also widely used by veterinarians in the United States. Many European physicians believe that it may actually slow the course of the disease, and for this reason they call it a "chondroprotective" drug ("chondro" refers to cartilage). Unfortunately, this wonderful possibility has not been proven. We have more evidence for chondroitin for this purpose.

### What Is the Scientific Evidence for Glucosamine?

Reasonably solid studies have found that supplementation with glucosamine sulfate can relieve the pain of osteoarthritis. For example, one recent double-blind study compared the effectiveness of glucosamine sulfate and placebo in 252 people with osteoarthritis of the knee.[14] The results showed that after 4 weeks the participants treated with glucosamine sulfate were in less pain and could move better than those given a placebo. No more side effects were noted in the participants who took glucosamine than in those who did not.

Another study found glucosamine equally effective to the standard arthritis drug Feldene.[15] A total of 329 participants were given 20 mg of Feldene, glucosamine, a placebo, or glucosamine plus Feldene daily. Improvement was monitored through the Lequesne Index, a rating scale that evaluates the severity of osteoarthritis. Equivalent benefit was seen in all the treated groups. After 90 days, treatment was then stopped, and the participants were followed for an additional 8 weeks.

Interestingly, whereas the benefits of Feldene rapidly disappeared following the end of treatment, glucosamine was still producing a full effect at the end of the post-treatment period.

Other studies, enrolling a total of more than 350 participants, have found equivalent benefit between glucosamine and ibuprofen.[16,17]

### Dosages

Glucosamine is usually taken as glucosamine sulfate, at a dosage of 500 mg 3 times daily. It is not truly a cure because it must be taken forever for good results. It also does not produce complete relief. However, it often appears to help significantly. Pain ordinarily begins to improve in about a week and the benefit continues to increase for a month or more.

### Safety Issues

Glucosamine is believed to be nontoxic and essentially side-effect free.[18,19] This gives it a huge potential advantage over standard drug treatment, which can cause ulcers.

## Chondroitin Sulfate: Relieves Pain and May Slow Progression of Osteoarthritis

Reasonably good evidence supports the use of **chondroitin** (page 159) for the pain of osteoarthritis as well. In addition, provocative evidence suggests that it may help prevent your arthritis from gradually getting worse.

Like glucosamine, chondroitin plays a natural role in the body's manufacture of cartilage. In Europe, chondroitin sulfate is usually injected directly into arthritic joints (under no circumstances should you try this yourself!). However, in the United States, oral chondroitin sulfate is the most popular form of this supplement.

For years it was questioned whether oral chondroitin sulfate could possibly work. Because of its large molecular size it is difficult to see how chondroitin sulfate could find its way through the lining of the digestive tract to be absorbed into the bloodstream. However, in 1995 researchers found evidence that up to 15% of chondroitin is actually absorbed.[20]

Scientists are unsure how chondroitin sulfate works, but one of three theories (or all of them) might explain its mode of action. Some evidence suggests that chondroitin may inhibit the enzymes that break down cartilage in the joints.[21] Another theory holds that chondroitin sulfate increases the amount of hyaluronic acid in the joints. (Hyaluronic acid is a protective fluid that keeps the joints lubricated.) Finally, as a building block of cartilage, available chondroitin might simply help the body rebuild damaged joints.

Perhaps the most exciting development is the recent evidence suggesting that chondroitin sulfate can actually slow the progression of osteoarthritis. This would make it a true chondroprotective drug (see the previous discussion under the heading Glucosamine). However, more research is needed.

Chondroitin sulfate is often sold in combination with glucosamine. Unfortunately, we have no direct evidence that taking both supplements at once is better than taking just one or the other.

### What Is the Scientific Evidence for Chondroitin Sulfate?

Much of the early research on chondroitin sulfate was published in French or Italian journals and has not been translated into English. However, the results of four double-blind placebo-controlled clinical trials were recently published in English. They provide substantial evidence that chondroitin sulfate is an effective treatment for osteoarthritis. Some show evidence that chondroitin sulfate can reduce the symptoms of osteoarthritis, while others suggest that it can actually stop the disease from progressing.

**Reducing Symptoms**    Studies involving a total of more than 250 people and lasting from 3 months to 1 year, have found chondroitin effective for reducing the symptoms of arthritis.

A recent 6-month double-blind placebo-controlled study followed 85 individuals with osteoarthritis of the knee.[22] Participants received either 400 mg of chondroitin sulfate twice a day or placebo. Researchers evaluated improvement in arthritis symptoms by recording the level of pain as judged by the participant, the need for other medications, the time necessary to walk 20 meters on flat ground, and the overall effectiveness of the treatment as rated by physicians and participants.

After 1 month of treatment there was a 23% decrease in joint pain in the chondroitin sulfate group versus only a 12% decrease in the placebo group. By 6 months there was a 43% improvement in the chondroitin sulfate group versus only a 3% improvement in the placebo group (the placebo effect seems to have worn off after a while). While walking speed did not improve in the placebo group, there was a small but significant progressive improvement among individuals taking chondroitin. Physicians judged the improvement as good or very good in 69% of those taking chondroitin sulfate, but only in 32% of those taking placebo.

Another study enrolled more participants (127) and followed them for a period of 3 months.[23] The results were again positive. Finally, a third double-blind study involved only 42 participants, but followed them for a full year. Chondroitin sulfate took months to reach its full effect, but eventually relieved symptoms considerably better than placebo.[24]

**Slowing the Disease**   An exciting feature of this last study was that individuals taking a placebo showed progressive joint damage over the year, but among those taking chondroitin sulfate no worsening of the joints was seen. In other words, chondroitin sulfate seemed to protect the joints of osteoarthritis sufferers from further damage.

No conventional treatment for osteoarthritis protects joints or slows the progression of the disease. If confirmed by larger, properly designed studies, this effect may make chondroitin sulfate a distinctly superior treatment to NSAIDs (nonsteroidal anti-inflammatory drugs) or other conventional medications.

A longer and larger double-blind placebo-controlled trial also found evidence that chondroitin sulfate can slow the progression of osteoarthritis.[25] One hundred and nineteen people were enrolled in this study, which lasted a full 3 years. Thirty-four of the participants received 1,200 mg of chondroitin sulfate per day; the rest received placebo. Over the course of the study researchers took x rays to determine how many joints had progressed to a severe stage.

During the 3 years of the study only 8.8% of those who took chondroitin sulfate developed se-

verely damaged joints, whereas almost 30% of those who took placebo progressed to this extent. Unfortunately, the report did not state whether this difference was statistically significant.

Additional evidence comes from animal studies. Researchers measured the effects of chondroitin sulfate (administered both orally and via injection directly into the muscle) in rabbits, in which cartilage damage had been induced in one knee by the injection of an enzyme.[26] After 84 days of treatment, the damaged knees in the animals who had been given chondroitin sulfate had significantly more cartilage left than the knees of the untreated animals. Receiving chondroitin sulfate by mouth was as effective as taking it through an injection.

### Putting It All Together

Looking at the sum of the evidence, it does appear that chondroitin sulfate may actually protect joints from damage in osteoarthritis. However, better studies are needed to confirm this very important potential benefit. Furthermore, none of this work demonstrates any power to reverse the disease by rebuilding the cartilage. Chondroitin sulfate may simply stop further destruction from occurring, but that in itself is excellent.

### Dosages

The usual dosage of chondroitin sulfate is 400 mg taken 3 times daily. It is frequently combined with glucosamine in commercial products, although there is no direct evidence that such combinations are more effective than either treatment alone.

### Safety Issues

Chondroitin sulfate has not been associated with any serious adverse effects. Participants in clinical trials have found mild digestive system distress to be the only real complaint.

## SAMe: Helpful, but Very Expensive

**SAMe (S-adenosylmethionine)** (page 293) is a substance that occurs naturally in the body, and plays a role in numerous biochemical functions. When used for osteoarthritis, it appears to reduce pain, decrease swelling, and improve mobility about as effectively as standard anti-inflammatory drugs, with significantly fewer side effects and risks. There is also some evidence that SAMe may slow the progression of osteoarthritis. However, this is an extraordinarily expensive supplement.

### What Is the Scientific Evidence for SAMe?

A great deal of good scientific evidence supports the use of SAMe in arthritis.[27] Numerous double-blind studies involving over a thousand participants in total suggest that it is approximately as effective as standard anti-inflammatory drugs.

One of the best double-blind studies enrolled 732 patients and followed them for 4 weeks.[28] Over this period, 235 of the participants received 1,200 mg of SAMe per day, while a similar number took either placebo or 750 mg daily of the standard drug naproxen. The majority of these patients had experienced moderate symptoms of osteoarthritis of either the knee or of the hip for an average of 6 years.

The results indicate that SAMe provided as much pain-relieving effect as naproxen and that both treatments were significantly better than the placebo. However, differences did exist between the two treatments. Naproxen worked more quickly, producing readily apparent benefits at the 2-week follow-up, whereas the full effect of SAMe was not apparent until 4 weeks. By the end of the study, both treatments were producing the same level of benefit. The only problem with this study is that it used a rather low dose of naproxen.

Animal evidence suggests that SAMe may help protect cartilage from damage.[29,30]

### Dosages

SAMe is usually started at an initial dosage of 200 mg twice daily, which is then increased over 1 to 2 weeks up to 1,200 mg per day. The reason for this gradual approach is that if full doses are taken from the beginning many people develop stomach distress.

After symptoms improve, doses as low as 200 mg twice daily may suffice to keep pain under control.

### Safety Issues

SAMe appears to be very safe in general, both in the short and long term.[31–35]

However, people with bipolar disease should not use SAMe except under medical supervision.[36,37] The reason is that SAMe also appears to have antidepressant properties and, like other antidepressants, can cause people with bipolar disease to enter a manic state.

Safety in young children, pregnant or nursing women, or those with severe liver or renal disease has not been fully established.

It has been suggested that SAMe might interact with various drugs (technically, by facilitating their conjugation),[38] but this has not been proven to cause any actual problem. SAMe should definitely not be combined with prescription antidepressants except under the supervision of a physician.[39]

## Niacinamide

There is some evidence that **vitamin B$_3$** (page 323) in the form of niacinamide may provide some benefits for those with osteoarthritis. In a double-blind study, 72 individuals with arthritis were given either 3,000 mg daily of niacinamide (in 5 equal doses) or placebo for 12 weeks.[40] The results showed that treated participants experienced a 29% improvement in symptoms, whereas those given placebo worsened by 10%. However, at this dose, liver inflammation is a concern that must be taken seriously.

## OTHER NATURAL TREATMENTS

The following natural treatments are widely recommended for osteoarthritis, but they have not yet been scientifically proven effective.

## Devil's Claw: Reduces Arthritis Pain

Several preliminary double-blind studies involving a total of over 200 people suggest that the herb **devil's claw** (page 175) can soothe the pain of various types of arthritis.[41]

A typical dosage of devil's claw is 750 mg 3 times daily of a preparation standardized to contain 3% iridoid glycosides. Devil's claw appears to be quite safe, with no evidence of toxicity at doses many times higher than recommended.[42] A 6-month open study of 630 people with arthritis who took devil's claw showed no side effects

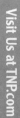

other than occasional mild gastrointestinal distress.[43] For the latter reason, it is recommended that those with ulcers not take devil's claw.

Safety in young children, pregnant or nursing women, or those with severe liver or kidney disease has not been established.

### Healthy Diet: Can Slow the Progression of Arthritis

There is considerable evidence that a diet high in **vitamin C** and **vitamin E** (pages 331 and 337) and beta-carotene can slow the progression of osteoarthritis, by as much as 70%.[44] These nutrients are found in fruits, vegetables, whole grains, nuts, and seeds. However, we don't know whether taking supplements of these vitamins is just as effective. As described in detail in the chapter on **beta-carotene** (page 131), when you get vitamins from foods you also get numerous other healthful substances.

### Miscellaneous Herbs and Supplements

Weak evidence suggests that the herbs **boswellia** (page 143), **turmeric** (page 311), and **yucca** (page 348) may be useful for osteoarthritis.

The herb **white willow** (page 343) contains aspirin-like substances and thus might be helpful. However, whether enough of these natural anti-inflammatories are provided by standard doses of white willow to produce adequate pain relief has not been documented. White willow may irritate the stomach lining like aspirin, and for that reason should not be taken by those with stomach ulcers. Other aspirin warnings apply as well: White willow should not be used by people with aspirin allergies, bleeding disorders, kidney disease, liver disease, or diabetes. It may also interact adversely with alcohol, "blood thinners," other anti-inflammatories, methotrexate, metoclopramide, phenytoin, probenecid, spironolactone, and valproate.

Other substances sometimes recommended for osteoarthritis include **boron** (page 141), **copper** (page 169), **D-phenylalanine** (page 278), **selenium** (page 297), molybdenum, **zinc** (page 348), **beta-carotene** (page 131), **cartilage** (page 153), **vitamin C** (page 331), **vitamin E** (page 337), **bromelain** (page 144), **cat's claw** (page 154), **chamomile** (page 156), **dandelion** (page 174), and **feverfew** (page 186). However, there is little to no evidence as yet that these treatments are effective.

For more information on arthritis, see *The Natural Pharmacist Guide to Arthritis*.

# OSTEOPOROSIS

*Principal Natural Treatments*
   Calcium, vitamin D, ipriflavone, trace minerals, fish oil, GLA

*Other Natural Treatments*
   Vitamin K, copper, magnesium, strontium, vitamin B$_{12}$, folic acid, boron, DHEA, soy isoflavones, manganese, pregnenolone, vanadium, horsetail, progesterone

In centuries past, the fragile bones and stooped stature of the aged were taken for granted. Today, however, prevention of osteoporosis is a real possibility.

Many factors are now known or suspected to accelerate the rate of bone loss. These include smoking, alcohol, low calcium intake, excessive phosphorus intake (such as found in soft drinks), lack of exercise, various medications, and several medical illnesses. Women are much more prone to osteoporosis than men and, for this reason,

the following discussion focuses almost entirely on them.

Conventional medical treatment for osteoporosis in women centers mainly on hormone-replacement therapy. Although supplemental estrogen undoubtedly slows and perhaps even reverses osteoporosis, recent concern about the increased risk of breast cancer has caused many women and their physicians to rethink the use of this therapy. The so-called designer estrogen raloxifene (Evista) may offer benefits without this risk. Other drugs, such as Fosamax (a non-hormonal drug), can also help build bone.

Weight-bearing exercise is strongly recommended.

## PRINCIPAL NATURAL TREATMENTS

There is good evidence that calcium supplements may be able to slow the progression of osteoporosis. A combination of calcium and vitamin D may be able to produce even better effects, and it appears that the semisynthetic substance ipriflavone can actually reverse the disease to some extent. The combination of ipriflavone and calcium has also been tested and found more effective than calcium alone.

## Calcium and Vitamin D

**Calcium** (page 146) is necessary to build and maintain bone. You need **vitamin D** (page 335), too, as the body cannot absorb calcium without it. (Although your body can manufacture vitamin D when exposed to the sun, in this age of sunblock, supplemental vitamin D may be necessary.)

Numerous good studies indicate that calcium supplements can help prevent and slow osteoporosis.[1] Calcium supplementation at the recommended doses appears to be able to reduce bone loss in postmenopausal women in every bone site except the spine.[2,3] Good evidence also tells us that when vitamin D is taken along with calcium the results are even better.[4] Combination treatment may be able to slow osteoporosis in the spine, and in some cases actually reverse osteoporosis to some extent.

While estrogen is more powerful than calcium alone, taking calcium along with estrogen offers additional benefits.[5,6] Calcium supplements also help adolescent girls "put calcium in the bank."[7]

Adding various trace minerals—**zinc** (page 348), 15 mg; **copper** (page 169), 2.5 mg; and **manganese** (page 254), 5 mg—along with calcium and vitamin D seems to produce further improvement.[8,9] Essential fatty acids, such as **fish oil** (page 188) and **GLA** (page 210) from evening primrose oil, may also enhance the effectiveness of calcium.[10,11]

### Dosages

Appropriate dietary intake of calcium is as follows: 210 to 270 mg daily for infants; 500 to 800 mg daily for children up to the age of 8; 1,300 mg daily for children and young adults 9 to 18 years old; 1,000 mg of calcium per day for adults 19 to 50 years old; and 1,200 mg per day for adults 51 years and over. Pregnant or nursing women should take 1,000 mg (unless they are 18 years old or younger, in which case the dosage is 1,300 mg). Because calcium competes with the absorption of other minerals, you should consider taking a multimineral supplement as well.

The usual recommendation for vitamin D ranges from 200 to 400 IU daily depending on age. However, some of the studies cited here used dosages greater than 800 IU daily. Such doses should be taken only under medical supervision.

### Safety Issues

In general, a daily intake of calcium up to 2,000 mg is safe.[12] Greatly excessive intake of calcium can cause numerous side effects, including dangerous or painful deposits of calcium within the body. If you have cancer, hyperparathyroidism, or sarcoidosis, you should only take calcium under the supervision of a physician.

People with kidney stones or a history of kidney stones are often cautioned not to take supplemental calcium. The reason for this warning is that kidney stones are commonly made of calcium oxalate crystals. However, while calcium supplements might increase kidney stone risk, higher intake of calcium from food might actually reduce the risk.[13,14]

Vitamin D is safe when taken at a dosage of 400 IU daily, but can be toxic when taken at doses higher than 1,200 IU daily. Since you may be getting vitamin D from more than one source, I don't recommend exceeding 400 IU except on a physician's advice. Individuals with sarcoidosis or hyperparathyroidism should not take vitamin D at all, except on medical advice.

## Ipriflavone

Various plants contain estrogen-like substances known as phytoestrogens. In 1969, a research project was started to manufacture a type of phytoestrogen that would cause the bone-stimulating effects of phytoestrogens but not the other effects of estrogen. The purpose behind this search was to find a treatment that could prevent osteoporosis without incurring any of estrogen's risks.

The starting point was the research of the phytoestrogens found in soy, called **isoflavones** (page 236). Scientists eventually developed a semisynthetic variation of soy isoflavones named ipriflavone. After 7 successful years of animal experiments with ipriflavone, human research was started in 1981. Today, ipriflavone is available in over 22 countries. Drugstores in the United States can now carry it as a nonprescription dietary supplement.

Ipriflavone appears to help prevent osteoporosis by interfering with the growth of osteoclasts, cells that cause bone breakdown. Estrogen works in much the same way. But, as was intended by its inventors, ipriflavone does not appear to produce estrogenic effects anywhere else in the body. For this reason, it probably doesn't increase the risk of breast or uterine cancer. However, it also doesn't reduce hot flashes, night sweats, mood changes, or vaginal dryness.

### What Is the Scientific Evidence for Ipriflavone?

Numerous double-blind placebo-controlled studies involving a total of over 1,000 participants have examined the effects of ipriflavone on osteoporosis.[15–20] Overall, it appears that ipriflavone can stop the progression of osteoporosis and perhaps reverse it to some extent.

For example, a 2-year double-blind study followed 198 postmenopausal women who had evidence of bone loss.[21] At the end of the study, there was a gain in bone density of 1% in the ipriflavone group compared to a loss of 0.7% in the placebo group.

Taking calcium plus ipriflavone may also be an excellent idea. In one study, 60 women, who had already been diagnosed with osteoporosis and had already suffered one spinal fracture, were given either 1,000 mg of calcium or 1,000 mg of calcium with ipriflavone.[22] After 6 months, the ipriflavone group had an increase of bone density in the spine of 3.5%, compared to a 2.1% net loss in the calcium-only group.

Ipriflavone may also be helpful for preventing osteoporosis in women who are taking Lupron, a medication that accelerates bone loss.[23]

Finally, there is some evidence that combining ipriflavone with estrogen may improve anti-osteoporosis benefits.[24,25] However, we do not know whether such combinations increase or decrease the other benefits and adverse effects of estrogen-replacement therapy.

### Dosages

The proper dosage of ipriflavone has been well established through studies: 200 mg 3 times daily or 300 mg 2 times daily. (A lower dose is necessary for those with kidney failure. Please consult your physician for details.)

### Safety Issues

To date, 2,769 people have been treated with ipriflavone, for an average duration of more than 1 year. The incidence of side effects in those treated with ipriflavone was no more than what was observed in those taking placebo.[26]

However, because ipriflavone is eliminated by the kidneys, concerns have been raised about the use of ipriflavone by patients with kidney problems.

Ipriflavone does not appear to affect the uterus, brain, breast, or vaginal tissue of postmenopausal women or the thyroid gland and uterus of experimental animals.[27] However, given the lack of large long-term cancer-risk studies for ipriflavone, women who have had breast cancer should use ipriflavone only on a physician's advice.

## OTHER NATURAL TREATMENTS

Recent evidence suggests that higher dietary intake of **vitamin K** (page 341) may reduce the risk of hip fracture caused by osteoporosis.[28] Putting this together with other studies, it appears that vitamin K might be helpful,[29–36] although a dose a bit higher than the usual minimum requirement may be required for this benefit: 109 mcg according to one study. See the chapter on vitamin K in Part Two for more information on safety and other issues.

A wide variety of other food supplements have also been suggested as useful for the prevention or reversal of osteoporosis, including **copper** (page 169), **magnesium** (page 251), strontium, **vitamin B**$_{12}$ (page 329), **DHEA** (page 176), natural soy **isoflavones** (page 236), **manganese** (page 254), **pregnenolone** (page 284), **vanadium** (page 317), **horsetail** (page 228), and **folic acid** (page 194). However, there is as yet little direct evidence that they really work.

**Boron** (page 141) is frequently mentioned as a treatment for osteoporosis as well.[37] However, there are some concerns that boron may raise estrogen levels, especially in women on estrogen-replacement therapy, and therefore might present an increased risk of cancer.[38,39]

### The Progesterone Story

Many books promote the idea that natural progesterone prevents or even reduces osteoporosis. In this case, the term *natural* indicates that we are using the same progesterone found in the body. It is still made synthetically, but it is called "natural progesterone" to distinguish it from its chemical cousins known as progestins. Generally, prescription "progesterone" is actually a progestin.

However, although theoretical evidence does suggest that progesterone may help build bone,[40] a recent double-blind study found no actual benefit in women using progesterone cream at the proper doses.[41]

# PERIODONTAL DISEASE (GUM DISEASE)

*Principal Natural Treatments*
Coenzyme $Q_{10}$

*Other Natural Treatments*
Folic acid mouthwash, zinc, vitamin C, calcium, magnesium, bloodroot, tea tree oil, vitamin $B_{12}$

Periodontal disease begins with gum inflammation and progresses to pockets of infection, bone loss, and loosening of the teeth. It is present in 90% of individuals over the age of 65.

Conventional prevention and treatment include regular flossing, using mouthwash that contains extracts of the herb thyme (such as thymol, found in Listerine), and using special toothbrushing appliances. If the condition becomes advanced, special deep-cleaning techniques and even surgery may be necessary.

## PRINCIPAL NATURAL TREATMENTS

The supplement **coenzyme $Q_{10}$ (CoQ$_{10}$)** (page 164), more widely known as a treatment for heart-related conditions, is also used for periodontal disease.

### Coenzyme $Q_{10}$

Several preliminary studies suggest that the supplement CoQ$_{10}$ can help periodontal disease.[1–6]

For example, in one double-blind study, 56 individuals received either 60 mg CoQ$_{10}$ or placebo for 4 weeks. The results showed that CoQ$_{10}$ significantly improved signs of periodontal disease, specifically the depth of gum "pockets."[7] The typical dosage of CoQ$_{10}$ for periodontal disease is 50 to 100 mg daily. CoQ$_{10}$ is essentially side-effect free. For more information on CoQ$_{10}$ use and safety issues, see the corresponding chapter in Part Two.

## OTHER NATURAL TREATMENTS

The following natural treatments are widely recommended for periodontal disease, but they have not been scientifically proven effective at this time.

### Folic Acid

Preliminary studies suggest that **folic acid** (page 194) mouthwash may help in periodontal disease as well. Oral folic acid supplementation does not appear to be especially effective.[8–11]

### Other Herbs and Supplements

Other common recommendations include **zinc** (page 348), **vitamin C** (page 331), **calcium** (page 146), **magnesium** (page 251), **vitamin $B_{12}$** (page 329), **bloodroot** (page 140), and **tea tree** (page 309) oil. However, as yet none of these suggestions can be regarded as proven.

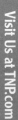

# PMS (PREMENSTRUAL STRESS SYNDROME)

*Principal Natural Treatments*
Calcium, chasteberry

*Other Natural Treatments*
Vitamin E, magnesium, multivitamin and mineral supplements, GLA, ginkgo, progesterone cream

*Probably Ineffective Treatments*
Vitamin $B_6$

Many women experience a variety of unpleasant symptoms in the week or two before menstruating. These include irritability, anger, headaches, anxiety, depression, fatigue, fluid retention, and breast tenderness. These symptoms undoubtedly result from hormonal changes of the menstrual cycle, but we don't know the cause of PMS or exactly how to treat it.

Conventional treatments include antidepressants, antianxiety drugs, beta-blockers, diuretics, oral contraceptives, and other hormonally active formulations. None of these treatments is entirely effective except for those that take the drastic step of inducing artificial menopause.

## PRINCIPAL NATURAL TREATMENTS

There is fairly good evidence that calcium supplements can significantly reduce all the major symptoms of PMS. There is also some evidence that the herbs chasteberry and ginkgo can lessen the symptoms of PMS. Vitamin $B_6$ is widely recommended as well, but its scientific record is mixed at best.

## Calcium: May Improve All Symptoms of PMS

A recent study found surprisingly positive results using **calcium** (page 146) (1,200 mg daily) for the treatment of PMS symptoms. These results have made a big impact because the study was large (about 500 women) and was performed at a prestigious medical center, Columbia University.[1]

Participants took 300 mg of calcium (as calcium carbonate) 4 times daily. Compared to placebo, calcium significantly reduced mood swings, pain, bloating, depression, back pain, and food cravings. Similar findings were also seen in earlier preliminary studies.[2,3]

For healthy women, calcium is safe when taken at this dosage. However, if you have cancer, hyperparathyroidism, or sarcoidosis, you should only take calcium under the supervision of a physician.

## Chasteberry: Especially Effective for Breast Tenderness

The herb **chasteberry** (page 157) is widely used in Europe as a treatment for PMS symptoms. More than most herbs, chasteberry is frequently called by its Latin names: *vitex* or *Vitex agnuscastus*. A shrub in the verbena family, chasteberry is commonly found on riverbanks and nearby foothills in central Asia and around the Mediterranean Sea. After its violet flowers have bloomed, a dark brown, peppercorn-size fruit develops, with a pleasant odor reminiscent of peppermint. It is the fruit that is used medicinally.

The modern use of chasteberry dates back to the 1950s, when the German pharmaceutical firm Madaus Company first produced a standardized extract. It has become a standard European treatment for PMS, cyclical breast tenderness, and menstrual irregularities.

Reportedly, chasteberry can reduce many of the symptoms of PMS, but it is probably most dramatically effective for breast tenderness. This is probably because chasteberry suppresses the release of prolactin, a hormone that affects the breasts. Unlike other herbs used for women's health problems, research has shown that chasteberry does not contain any chemicals that act like estrogen or progesterone. Rather, it acts on the pituitary gland to suppress the release of prolactin.[4–7] Prolactin naturally rises during pregnancy to stimulate milk production and other physiological changes.

### What Is the Scientific Evidence for Chasteberry?

Chasteberry is widely used in Germany as a general treatment for PMS. However, the scientific record for chasteberry lacks properly designed double-blind studies.

German gynecologists clearly believe that chasteberry is effective for PMS. In surveys involving about 3,000 women who had been prescribed chasteberry, physicians rated the overall effect of the treatment as good or very good about 90% of the time.[8,9] Based on the women's own reports, good results were seen in about 60% of participants, but only 30% reported complete relief. Chasteberry may be particularly effective in reducing the cyclic breast pain of PMS.[10]

However, these were not double-blind studies. Since there is a very high level of placebo response in PMS, often reaching 70%,[11] proper double-blind studies are necessary to determine the actual effectiveness of chasteberry.

A recently reported double-blind study followed 175 women with PMS for 3 months. Half of them received a standard chasteberry preparation, and the other half took 200 mg of pyridoxine (vitamin $B_6$) daily.[12] Over the 3-month study period, chasteberry was associated with "a considerably more marked alleviation of typical PMS complaints, such as breast tenderness, edema, inner tension, headache, constipation and depression." Overall, 77% of the participants treated with chasteberry showed improvement.

The main problem with this study is that pyridoxine itself is not a proven treatment for PMS; so the fact that chasteberry proved superior is not necessarily very meaningful (see the following discussion under the heading vitamin $B_6$).

### Dosages

The typical dose of dry chasteberry extract is 20 to 40 mg given once a day. Chasteberry is sold often as a liquid extract to be taken at a dosage of 40 drops each morning. However, highly concentrated extracts are also available that require much lower dosing. I recommend following the label instructions.

### Safety Issues

No detailed studies of the safety of chasteberry have been conducted. However, its widespread use in Germany has not led to any reports of significant adverse effects,[13] with the exception of a single case of excessive ovarian stimulation possibly caused by chasteberry.[14] In a study of over 1,500 women, mild side effects such as nausea, headache, and allergic skin reactions were reported by less than 2.5% of participants.[15]

Because it lowers prolactin levels, chasteberry is not an appropriate treatment for pregnant or nursing mothers. Its safety in adolescents or those with severe liver or kidney disease has not been established.

No known drug interactions are associated with chasteberry. However, it's quite conceivable that the herb could interfere with other hormonal medications, such as birth control pills, or drugs that affect the pituitary, such as bromocriptine.

## Vitamin $B_6$: May Not Be Effective

**Vitamin $B_6$** (page 326) has been used for PMS for many decades, both by European and U.S. physicians. However, the results of scientific studies are mixed at best. A recent properly designed double-blind study found vitamin $B_6$ ineffective.[16] A dozen or more other double-blind studies have investigated the effectiveness of vitamin $B_6$ for PMS, but actually the negative studies cancel out the positive ones.[17] Some books on natural medicine report that the negative studies used too little $B_6$, but in reality there was no clear link between dosage and effectiveness.

The maximum safe dosage of vitamin $B_6$ for self-use is 50 mg twice daily. Higher doses should be used only under a physician's supervision because of the potential risk of nerve injury. Some nutritionally oriented physicians report that the combination of $B_6$ and magnesium is considerably more effective than either treatment alone (see the following discussion under the heading Magnesium).

PMS

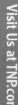

## OTHER NATURAL TREATMENTS

The following treatments are widely recommended for PMS, but they have not yet been scientifically proven effective.

### Vitamin E

Weak evidence suggests that **vitamin E** (page 337) may be helpful for PMS.[18] A typical dosage of vitamin E is 400 IU daily.

### Magnesium

Preliminary studies suggest that **magnesium** (page 251) may also be helpful in PMS.[19,20]

Magnesium is usually supplemented in the range of 200 to 600 mg daily, but for PMS it is sometimes given at a dosage of 500 to 1,000 mg daily starting on day 15 of the menstrual cycle and continuing through the beginning of menstruation. This dosage should be safe in healthy women, but if you suffer from any medical problems, you should check with a physician before trying it. As mentioned earlier, some physicians believe that magnesium should be combined with vitamin $B_6$ for best results.

### Multivitamin and Mineral Supplements

Preliminary evidence suggests that combined treatment with a multivitamin and mineral supplement may be helpful in PMS.[21–24]

## GLA: Primarily for Cyclic Breast Tenderness

Evening primrose oil, a source of **GLA** (page 210), is used for the breast pain that often occurs with premenstrual syndrome called **cyclic mastalgia** (page 52). It may be helpful with other PMS symptoms as well, but the scientific evidence is weak.[25]

A typical dosage of evening primrose oil is 3 g daily. It must be taken for at least 4 to 6 weeks for noticeable effect, and maximum benefits may require 4 to 8 months to develop. Evening primrose oil appears to be safe.

## Ginkgo: For Breast Tenderness and Perhaps Other Symptoms

A recent study suggests that the herb **ginkgo** (page 204) can reduce breast tenderness and other symptoms of PMS. For more information, see the chapter on ginkgo in Part Two.

### Additional Treatments

Progesterone cream is another method widely recommended for PMS, but there is little evidence that it is effective.[26]

For more detailed information on PMS, see *The Natural Pharmacist Guide to PMS*.

---

 **PSORIASIS**

*Principal Natural Treatments*

There are no well-established natural treatments for psoriasis.

*Other Natural Treatments*

Fish oil, *Aloe vera* cream, chromium, selenium, vitamin E, zinc, burdock, red clover, *Coleus forskohlii,* goldenseal, milk thistle, fumaric acid, vitamin D, vitamin A, topical licorice cream, taurine, beta-carotene

---

Up to 2% of Americans suffer from psoriasis, a skin condition that leads to an intensely itchy rash with clearly defined borders and scales that resemble silvery mica. The fingernails are also frequently involved, showing pitting or thickening.

Medical treatment for psoriasis includes applications of topical steroids and peeling agents that expose the underlying skin for the steroid to contact. Ultraviolet light can also be used, sometimes combined with coal tar applications or medications called psoralens. Synthetic versions of vitamin A can also be helpful. For especially problematic psoriasis, low doses of the anti-cancer drug methotrexate have proven quite effective.

## NATURAL TREATMENTS

The following natural treatments are widely recommended for psoriasis, but they have not been scientifically proven effective at this time.

### Fish Oil

There is some evidence that eicosapentaenoic acid (EPA) from **fish oil** (page 188) may be a bit helpful in psoriasis. One 8-week double-blind study followed 28 people with chronic psoriasis.[1] Half received 1.8 mg of EPA daily (supplied by 10 capsules of fish oil), and the other half received placebo. By the end of the study, researchers saw significant improvement in itching, redness, and scaling, but not in the size of the psoriasis patches.

However, another double-blind study followed 145 people with moderate to severe psoriasis for 4 months and found no benefit as compared to placebo.[2]

Fish oil appears to be safe. The most common problem is fishy burps.

However, because fish oil has a mild "blood-thinning" effect, it should not be combined with powerful blood-thinning medications, such as Coumadin (warfarin) or heparin, except on a physician's advice. However, contrary to some reports, fish oil does not seem to cause bleeding problems when it is taken by itself.[3,4]

Also, fish oil does not appear to raise blood sugar levels in people with diabetes.[5] Nonetheless, if you have diabetes, you should not take any supplement except on the advice of a physician.

Fish oil may temporarily raise the level of LDL, or "bad," cholesterol; but this effect seems to be short-lived, and levels return to normal with continued use.[6,7]

If you decide to use cod liver oil as your fish oil supplement, make sure you do not exceed the safe maximum intake of **vitamin A** (page 318) and **vitamin D** (page 335). These vitamins are fat-soluble, which means that excess amounts tend to build up in your body, possibly reaching toxic levels. Pregnant women should not take more than 2,500 IU of vitamin A daily because of the risk of birth defects; 5,000 IU a day is a reasonable upper limit for other individuals. Vitamin D becomes toxic when taken at dosages above 1,000 IU daily for prolonged periods. Look at the bottle label to determine how much of these vitamins you are receiving.

### Aloe

*Aloe vera* (page 122) cream may be helpful for psoriasis, according to a double-blind study that enrolled 60 men and women with mild to moderate symptoms of psoriasis.[8] Participants were treated with either topical *Aloe vera* extract (0.5%) or a placebo cream, applied 3 times daily for 4 weeks. Aloe treatment produced significantly better results than placebo, and these results were said to endure for almost a year after treatment was stopped. The study authors also reported a high level of complete "cure," but what exactly they meant by this was not reported clearly.

### Other Herbs and Supplements

**Chromium** (page 161), **selenium** (page 297), **vitamin E** (page 337), **zinc** (page 348), **burdock** (page 145), **red clover** (page 290), *Coleus forskohlii* (page 166), **goldenseal** (page 217), topical **licorice** (page 244) cream, **taurine** (page 308), **beta-carotene** (page 131), and **milk thistle** (page 262) are sometimes mentioned as possible treatments for psoriasis. However, as yet there is no real evidence that they work.

A somewhat toxic natural substance called fumaric acid is sometimes recommended for psoriasis as well. Vitamin A or special forms of vitamin D taken at high levels may improve symptoms, but these are dangerous treatments that should be used only under the supervision of a physician.

# RAYNAUD'S PHENOMENON

*Principal Natural Treatments*
    There are no well-established natural treatments for Raynaud's phenomenon.

*Other Natural Treatments*
    Inositol hexaniacinate, essential fatty acids (fish oil, GLA), ginkgo

Raynaud's phenomenon is a little understood condition in which the fingers and toes show an exaggerated sensitivity to cold. Classic cases show a characteristic white, blue, and red color sequence as the digits lose blood supply and then rewarm. Some people develop only one or two of these signs.

The cause of Raynaud's phenomenon is unknown.

Conventional treatment consists mainly of reassurance and the recommendation to avoid exposure to cold and the use of tobacco (which can worsen Raynaud's). In severe cases, a variety of drugs can be tried.

## NATURAL TREATMENTS

The following natural treatments are widely recommended for Raynaud's phenomenon, but they have not yet been scientifically proven effective.

### Inositol Hexaniacinate

According to one preliminary double-blind study, the special form of niacin (**vitamin B₃** [page 323]) called inositol hexaniacinate may be helpful for Raynaud's phenomenon.[1] The dosage used in the study was 4 g daily. At this level of supplementation, regular blood tests to rule out liver inflammation are highly recommended. All forms of niacin may cause facial flushing and affect blood sugar levels in people with diabetes.

### Essential Fatty Acids

High doses of **fish oil** (page 188) have also shown good results for Raynaud's phenomenon in preliminary double-blind studies.[2,3] However, a very high dosage must be used, perhaps 12 g daily. See the chapter on fish oil in Part Two for specific safety information.

Another preliminary double-blind study suggests that high doses of **GLA** (page 210) may be useful as well.[4,5] For more information on GLA use and safety issues, see the corresponding chapter in Part Two.

When taking essential fatty acids, it is a good idea to take **vitamin E** (page 337) as well to prevent the fats from being damaged by free radicals. For information on safety issues concerning vitamin E, see the discussion in the corresponding chapter in Part Two.

### Ginkgo

Although no direct evidence shows that **ginkgo** (page 204) is helpful for Raynaud's phenomenon, it has been shown to increase circulation in the fingertips[6] and thus may be useful. For more information on ginkgo use and safety issues, see the corresponding chapter in Part Two.

# RHEUMATOID ARTHRITIS

### Principal Natural Treatments
Fish oil

### Other Natural Treatments
Boswellia, devil's claw, curcumin, bromelain, yucca, GLA, selenium, zinc, boron, magnesium, molybdenum, vitamin C, pantothenic acid, copper, D-phenylalanine, sea cucumber, cartilage extracts, L-histidine, beta-carotene, ginger, burdock, horsetail, Chinese herbs, flaxseed oil, folic acid, manganese, pregnenolone, proteolytic enzymes, cayenne, chamomile, feverfew, white willow, betaine hydrochloride, cat's claw, dietary changes

Rheumatoid arthritis is an autoimmune disease in the general family of lupus. For reasons that are not understood, in rheumatoid arthritis the immune system goes awry and begins attacking innocent tissues, especially cartilage in the joints. Various joints become red, hot, and swollen under the onslaught. The pattern of inflammation is usually symmetrical, occurring on both sides of the body. Other symptoms include inflammation of the eyes, nodules or lumps under the skin, and a general feeling of malaise.

Rheumatoid arthritis is more common in women than in men and typically begins between the ages of 35 and 60. The diagnosis is made by matching the pattern of symptoms with certain characteristic laboratory results.

Medical treatment consists mainly of two categories of drugs: anti-inflammatory drugs in the ibuprofen family (nonsteroidal anti-inflammatory drugs, or NSAIDs) and drugs that may be able to put rheumatoid arthritis into full or partial remission, the so-called disease-modifying antirheumatic drugs (DMARDs).

Anti-inflammatory drugs relieve symptoms of rheumatoid arthritis but do not change the overall progression of the disease, whereas the DMARDs seem to affect the disease itself. A good analogy might be the various options available to "treat" a house "suffering" from a severe termite infestation. You could remove heavy furniture, tiptoe about instead of holding public dances, and put large beams under the joists. However, none of these methods would do anything to stop the gradual destruction of your house. These methods are like NSAIDs and other supportive techniques in that they treat only the symptoms.

A more definitive approach would be to hire an exterminator and kill the termites. In medical terms, this would be described as a disease-modifying treatment. Because medical treatments for chronic diseases are seldom as completely effective as this example, a closer analogy might be spraying a chemical that slows the spread of termites but does not stop them.

In rheumatoid arthritis, the drugs believed to alter the course of the disease (to slow it down or stop it) include gold compounds, D-penicillamine, antimalarials, sulfasalazine, and methotrexate. They are unrelated to one another but work somewhat similarly in practice.

Unfortunately, all the drugs in this category are quite toxic and reliably cause severe side effects. Because of this toxicity, for years a so-called pyramid approach was taken with people with rheumatoid arthritis. Physicians started with NSAIDs to help with the pain and inflammation, and progressed to successively stronger and more toxic medications only when the basic treatments failed. Natural treatments such as those described here might also be useful in early stages.

However, over the last few years, research has found that severe joint damage occurs very early in rheumatoid arthritis. This evidence has caused many authorities to suggest early, aggressive treatment with disease-modifying drugs to prevent joint damage. Nonetheless, this approach has not been universally adopted, and many physicians still prescribe NSAIDs for early stages of rheumatoid arthritis. The treatments described here may be reasonable alternative options.

## PRINCIPAL NATURAL TREATMENTS

Rheumatoid arthritis is a difficult disease, and no alternative approach solves it easily. Even if you choose to use alternative methods, you should maintain regular visits to a rheumatologist to watch for serious complications. Finally, keep in mind that medical treatment may be able to slow the progression of rheumatoid arthritis. It is not likely that any of the alternative options have the same power.

### Fish Oil

**Fish oil** (page 188) is the only natural treatment for rheumatoid arthritis with significant documentation. According to the results of 12 double-blind placebo-controlled studies involving a total of over 500 participants, supplementation with omega-3 fatty acids can significantly reduce the symptoms of rheumatoid arthritis.[1] However, unlike some of the standard treatments, fish oil probably does not slow the progression of rheumatoid arthritis.

The most important omega-3 fatty acids found in fish oil are called EPA (eicosapentaenoic acid) and DHA (docosahexaenoic acid). Many forms of fish oil contain about 18% EPA and 12% DHA, for a total of about 30% by weight of omega-3 oils. In order to match the dosage used in several major studies, you should probably take enough fish oil to supply about 1.8 g of EPA (1,800 mg) and 0.9 g (900 mg) of DHA daily. Results may take 3 to 4 months to develop.

There are many forms of fish oil. If you decide to use cod liver oil as your fish oil supplement, make sure you do not exceed the safe maximum intake of **vitamin A** (page 318) and **vitamin D** (page 335). These vitamins are fat-soluble, which means that excess amounts tend to build up in your body, potentially reaching toxic levels. Otherwise, fish oil appears to be safe. The most common problem is fishy burps. It does have a mild "blood-thinning" effect, so it should not be combined with strong blood-thinning drugs such as Coumadin (warfarin) and heparin unless so instructed by a physician. However, contrary to some reports, fish oil does not seem to cause bleeding problems when it is taken by itself.[2,3] It also does not appear to raise blood sugar levels in people with diabetes. However, if you have diabetes, you should not take any supplement except on the advice of a physician. Fish oil may temporarily raise the level of LDL ("bad") cholesterol, but this effect seems to be short-lived, and levels return to normal with continued use.[4,5]

**Flaxseed oil** (page 193) has been offered as a more palatable substitute for fish oil, but it doesn't seem to work.[6]

Eating a lot of fish may also be helpful.[7]

## OTHER NATURAL TREATMENTS

The following natural treatments are widely recommended for rheumatoid arthritis, but they have not yet been scientifically proven effective.

### Boswellia

**Boswellia serrata** (page 143) is a shrub-like tree that grows in the dry hills of the Indian subcontinent. It is the source of a resin called salai guggal, which has been used for thousands of years in Ayurvedic medicine, the traditional medicine of the region. It is very similar to a resin from a related tree, *Boswellia carteri,* which is also known as frankincense. Both substances have been used historically for arthritis.

Recent research has identified boswellic acids as the likely active ingredients in boswellia. In animal studies, boswellic acids have shown anti-inflammatory effects, but their mechanism of action seems to be quite different from that of standard anti-inflammatory medications.[8,9]

A recent issue of *Phytomedicine* was devoted to boswellia and briefly reviewed previously unpublished studies on the herb.[10] A pair of placebo-controlled trials involving a total of 81 people with rheumatoid arthritis found significant reductions in swelling and pain over the course of 3 months. Furthermore, a comparative study of 60 participants over 6 months found the boswellia extract to relieve symptoms about as well as oral gold therapy.

However, the many details of these studies were not described in this summary review. In particular, while gold shots can induce remission in rheumatoid arthritis, we have no evidence that boswellia can do the same.

Furthermore, another recent double-blind study found no difference between boswellia and placebo.[11] The bottom line is that we need more research to know for sure whether boswellia is an effective treatment for rheumatoid arthritis.

The dosage of boswellia most often recommended is 400 mg 3 times a day of an extract that has been standardized to contain 37.5% boswellic acids. The full effect may take as long as 4 to 8 weeks to develop.

Few side effects have been reported with boswellia, other than an occasional allergic reaction or a mild upset stomach. However, due to the lack of formal safety studies, boswellia is not recommended for young children, pregnant or nursing women, or those with severe liver or kidney disease.

### Devil's Claw

The herb **devil's claw** (page 175) may be beneficial in rheumatoid arthritis. One double-blind study followed 89 people with rheumatoid arthritis for 2 months. The group given devil's claw showed a significant decrease in pain intensity and an improvement in mobility.[12]

Another double-blind study of 50 people with various types of arthritis showed that 10 days of treatment with devil's claw provided significant pain relief.[13]

A typical dosage of devil's claw is 750 mg 3 times daily of a preparation standardized to contain 3% iridoid glycosides.

Devil's claw appears to be quite safe, with no evidence of toxicity at doses many times higher than recommended.[14] A 6-month open study of 630 people with arthritis showed no side effects other than occasional mild gastrointestinal distress.[15] However, devil's claw is not advised for those with ulcers. Safety in young children, pregnant or nursing women, and individuals with severe liver or kidney disease has not been established.

### Curcumin

Curcumin, an extract of the kitchen spice **turmeric** (page 311), is often suggested as a treatment for rheumatoid arthritis. Curcumin appears to possess anti-inflammatory properties,[16] and preliminary studies suggest curcumin may relieve symptoms of rheumatoid arthritis,[17] although much more research is needed.

The typical dosage of curcumin is 400 to 600 mg 3 times daily. Curcumin is sometimes given in combination with an equal dose of an extract of the pineapple plant called **bromelain** (page 144), which appears to possess anti-inflammatory properties of its own.[18]

Curcumin is thought to be quite safe.[19] Side effects are rare and are generally limited to occasional allergic reactions and mild stomach upset. However, safety in very young children, pregnant or nursing women, and those with severe liver or kidney disease has not been established.

### Additional Natural Treatments

One preliminary and rather unimpressive double-blind study suggests that the herb **yucca** (page 348) can help relieve the pain of rheumatoid arthritis.[20]

The essential fatty acid **gamma-linolenic acid (GLA)** (page 210), found in evening primrose oil and borage oil, may help relieve symptoms of rheumatoid arthritis.[21–24] **Zinc** (page 348) has yielded mixed results in studies.[25,26,27]

The following treatments are also sometimes proposed as effective for rheumatoid arthritis, but there is as yet little scientific evidence to turn to: **boron** (page 144), **magnesium** (page 251), molybdenum, **vitamin C** (page 331), **pantothenic acid** (page 275), **copper** (page 169), **D-phenylalanine** (page 278), sea cucumber, **cartilage** (page 153) extracts, **L-histidine** (page 225), **beta-carotene** (page 131), **ginger** (page 202), **burdock** (page 145), **horsetail** (page 229), **folic acid** (page 194), **manganese** (page 254), **pregnenolone** (page 284), **proteolytic enzymes** (page 285), **cayenne** (page 155), **chamomile** (page 156), **feverfew** (page 186), **turmeric** (page 311), **white willow** (page 343), **betaine hydrochloride** (page 134), **cat's claw** (page 154), and Chinese herbal combinations. The antioxidant mineral **selenium** (page 297), while sometimes mentioned as a treatment for rheumatoid arthritis, doesn't seem to work.[28]

Identifying and avoiding food allergens may be helpful in some cases.[29] Adopting a vegetarian diet sometimes brings about improvement in mild rheumatoid arthritis.[30,31]

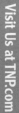

Ulcers

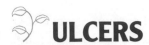 **ULCERS**

*Principal Natural Treatments*
  Deglycyrrhizinated licorice

*Other Natural Treatments*
  Rhubarb, *Aloe vera*, bioflavonoids, vitamin A, zinc, vitamin C, selenium, glutamine, cat's claw, marshmallow, reishi, suma, betaine hydrochloride

The highly concentrated acid produced by the stomach is quite capable of burning a hole through the tissue of the stomach and duodenum (part of the small intestine). That it usually does not do so is a tribute to the effectiveness of the methods that the body uses to protect itself. However, sometimes these protective mechanisms fail, and the ever-present acid begins to produce an ulcer.

Ulcer pain is caused by stomach acid coming into contact with unprotected tissue. Eating generally decreases ulcer pain temporarily because food neutralizes the acid. As soon as the food begins to be digested, the pain returns.

Conventional medical treatment for ulcers has gone through a slow revolution. A few decades ago, the prescribed response to ulcers was a bland diet—one low in spices and high in dairy products, which were believed to coat the stomach. However, eventually it was discovered that spicy foods are innocent and that milk itself is somewhat ulcer forming! The only other option at that time was surgery.

Next came antacids containing magnesium and aluminum (such as Maalox). However, these were seldom strong enough to allow the ulcer to heal fully. Ulcer treatment took a big step forward with the development of Tagamet (cimetidine), followed by Zantac, Pepcid, and others. These drugs dramatically lower the stomach's production of acid. Later, a new class of even more potent acid suppressors appeared, led by Prilosec (omeprazole).

When stomach acid is suppressed, ulcer pain rapidly diminishes, and the ulcer heals. For a time, these drugs were regarded as the definitive answer to ulcers. This early enthusiasm began to fade when it became clear that ulcers frequently returned after the drugs were stopped. In the late 1980s, a new explanation for this problem began to surface. First regarded as a wacky theory, it has now become the accepted explanation.

We now believe that ulcers are caused by the bacteria *Helicobacter pylori*. Apparently, this previously ignored organism has the capacity to infect the stomach and, by so doing, to weaken the stomach lining. Only when antibiotics to kill *Helicobacter pylori* are combined with stomach acid suppressants do ulcers go away and stay away.

## PRINCIPAL NATURAL TREATMENTS

The most famous supplement used for ulcer disease is a special form of **licorice** (page 244) known as deglycyrrhizinated licorice (DGL). This form of licorice eliminates the portion of the herb that can cause serious side effects.

Head-to-head comparison studies involving as many as 100 participants and lasting for up to 2 years suggest that DGL is more effective than the drug Tagamet (cimetidine) at healing ulcers and keeping them from recurring.[1,2,3]

DGL is believed to improve the health of the stomach lining and promote the production of substances that defend against acid. However, DGL has not been shown to kill *Helicobacter pylori*. It probably must be taken continuously to prevent ulcers.

Some natural medicine authorities suggest that DGL may help prevent ulcers caused by medications such as anti-inflammatory drugs and steroids.[4] However, there is no evidence as yet that this is true.

The proper dosage of DGL is two to four 380-mg tablets chewed 20 minutes before meals. For unknown reasons, studies suggest that chewing is essential to achieve full benefit. DGL tastes bad but is believed to be very safe, although extensive safety studies have not been performed. Side effects are rare. Safety in young children, pregnant or nursing women, and those with severe liver or kidney disease has not been established.

**Warning:** Because ulcers can be dangerous, medical supervision of treatment is essential.

## OTHER NATURAL TREATMENTS

The following natural treatments are widely recommended, but they have not been scientifically proven effective at this time.

Rhubarb and **aloe** (page 122) have been suggested as treatments for bleeding ulcers.[5] However, this condition is sufficiently dangerous that conventional medical treatment is far more appropriate.

Highly preliminary studies suggest that various bioflavonoids can inhibit the growth of *Helicobacter pylori*.[6] All fruits and vegetables provide bioflavonoids, but these substances can also be taken as supplements. The dosage depends on the type of bioflavonoid used. A typical dosage for citrus bioflavonoids is 500 mg 3 times daily.

**Vitamin A** (page 318), **zinc** (page 348), **vitamin C** (page 331), **selenium** (page 297), **cat's claw** (page 154), **marshmallow** (page 256), **reishi** (page 291), **suma** (page 307), **betaine hydrochloride** (page 134), and **glutamine** (page 215) have also been suggested as aids to ulcer healing, but there is as yet little to no scientific evidence that they are effective.

 # VARICOSE VEINS

*Principal Natural Treatments*
   Horse chestnut, OPCs, gotu kola, bilberry

*Other Natural Treatments*
   Butcher's broom, aortic glycosaminoglycans, collinsonia, calendula

Walking upright has given our leg veins a difficult task. Although they lack the strong muscular lining of arteries, they must constantly return a large volume of blood to the heart. The movements of the legs act as a pump to push the blood upward while flimsy valves stop gravity from pulling it back down.

However, over time these valves often begin to fail. The blood then begins to pool, stretching the vein wall and injuring its lining. This situation is called *venous insufficiency*. Typically, the legs begin to feel heavy, achy, and tired. When enough injury has occurred, the veins visibly dilate and the cosmetically unpleasant torturous vessels known as varicose veins appear.

For unknown reasons, venous insufficiency affects women about three times as often as men. Occupations involving prolonged standing also increase the incidence of venous insufficiency. Pregnancy and obesity do so as well because of the increase of pressure in the abdomen that makes it more difficult for the blood to flow upward.

Conventional medical treatment of venous insufficiency consists mainly of reducing weight, elevating the legs, and wearing elastic support hose. Unsightly damaged veins can be destroyed by injection therapy or be surgically removed.

## PRINCIPAL NATURAL TREATMENTS

Why are some illnesses luckier than others? Next to prostate enlargement, varicose veins have the most extensive repertoire of scientifically researched herbal treatments: four herbal treatments widely used in Europe for venous insufficiency.

These herbs have much in common. All of them appear to work by strengthening the walls of veins and other vessels. They primarily relieve symptoms of aching and swelling, rather than visible varicose veins. However, it is thought (but not proven) that the regular use of these treatments can prevent visible varicose veins from developing.

**Warning:** Symptoms similar to those caused by varicose veins can actually be due to more dangerous conditions, such as phlebitis. Medical evaluation is necessary prior to self-treating with the natural supplements described here.

## Horse Chestnut: The Best-Documented Treatment for Varicose Veins

The most popular German herbal treatment for venous insufficiency is horse chestnut. Closely related to the Ohio buckeye, its spiny fruits contain a few large seeds known as horse chestnuts. Medical use of this herb dates back to nineteenth-century France, where extracts were used to treat hemorrhoids (which are really a form of varicose veins).

German scientific research into horse chestnut began in the 1960s and ultimately led to Germany's Commission E approving the herb for vein diseases of the legs. In 1995, this herb was the third most common prescription herb in Germany, after **ginkgo** (page 204) and **St. John's wort** (page 303).

### What Is the Scientific Evidence for Horse Chestnut?

The clinical scientific evidence for **horse chestnut** (page 228) as a treatment for venous insufficiency is moderately strong. A total of 558 participants have been involved in double-blind studies.[1] One of the largest followed 212 people over a period of 40 days using a crossover design.[2] Participants initially received either horse chestnut or placebo and then were crossed over to the other treatment (without their knowledge) after 20 days. Horse chestnut treatment significantly reduced leg edema, pain, and sensation of heaviness when compared to placebo.

Another study compared the effectiveness of horse chestnut and compression stockings in 240 people over a course of 12 weeks.[3] Compression stockings worked faster to lessen swelling, but by 12 weeks the results were equivalent between the two treatments.

Unlike many herbs, the active ingredients in horse chestnut have been identified to a reasonable degree of certainty. They appear to be a complex of related chemicals known collectively as aescin. Aescin reduces the rate of fluid leakage from stressed and irritated vessel walls. We don't really know how it does this, but the most prominent theory proposes that aescin plugs leaking capillaries, prevents the release of enzymes that break down collagen and open holes in capillary walls, and forestalls other forms of vein damage.[4,5]

### Dosages

The most common dosage of horse chestnut is 300 mg twice daily, standardized to contain 50 mg aescin per dose, for a total daily dose of 100 mg aescin. After good results have been achieved, the dosage can be reduced by about half for maintenance.

Horse chestnut preparations should certify that a constituent called esculin has been removed. Also, a delayed-release formulation must be used to prevent gastrointestinal upset.

### Safety Issues

After decades of wide usage in Germany, no reports of harmful effects due to properly prepared horse chestnut have been noted, even when it has been taken in large overdose.[6] In animal studies, both horse chestnut and aescin have been found to be very safe. Dogs and rats have been treated for 34 weeks with this herb without harmful effects. However, doses 50 times higher than normal can cause death in animals, and there are two reports out of Italy about kidney damage due to massive overdosage.[7,8] In Japan, where injectable forms are used, occasional serious reactions have been noted.

In clinical studies of horse chestnut, no significant side effects have been reported, other than the usual occasional mild allergic reactions or gastrointestinal distress. However, all these studies involved controlled-release enteric-coated forms of horse chestnut. This allowed it to pass through the stomach without dissolving. Taking horse chestnut in a standard capsule may cause severe stomach upset.

Based on relatively theoretical evidence, horse chestnut is not recommended for those with serious kidney or liver disease, and it should not be combined with blood thinners, such as Coumadin (warfarin), Trental (pentoxifylline), and aspirin. Its safety in pregnancy and nursing has not been established. However, no risks are known in pregnancy, and some studies have enrolled pregnant women.[9]

## OPCs: Reasonably Good Evidence That They Can Help

Grape seed and pine bark contain high levels of special bioflavonoids called **OPCs (oligomeric proanthocyanidin complexes)** (page 270). Similar substances are found in cranberry, bilberry, blueberry, hawthorn, and other plants.

OPCs are interesting antioxidant chemicals that appear to have the ability to improve collagen (a type of strengthening tissue found in many parts of the body), reduce capillary leakage, and control inflammation.[10–13] In Europe, OPCs are widely used to treat venous insufficiency, varicose veins, easy bruising, and **hemorrhoids** (page 70).

### What Is the Scientific Evidence for OPCs?

Controlled studies involving a total of about 400 participants have found that OPCs provide significant benefit for varicose veins.[14,15,16]

For example, a double-blind study comparing OPCs against placebo in 92 individuals showed improvement in 75% of the treated group as compared to 41% in the control group.[17]

### Dosages

OPCs are generally taken at a dosage of 150 to 300 mg daily when used for varicose veins. Lower doses are sometimes recommended as a daily antioxidant supplement.

### Safety Issues

Extensive studies have shown OPCs to be nontoxic.[18] Side effects are rare and are limited to mild gastrointestinal distress. However, safety in young children, pregnant or nursing women, and those with severe liver or kidney disease has not been established. OPCs may have some anticoagulant properties when taken in high doses, and should be used only under medical supervision by individuals on blood-thinner drugs such as Coumadin (warfarin), Trental (pentoxifylline), and heparin.

## Gotu Kola: Also Effective

Another reasonably well documented treatment for venous insufficiency is the tropical creeper **gotu kola** (page 218), which should not be confused with the caffeine-containing kola nut (used in original recipes for Coca-Cola).

In India and Indonesia, gotu kola has a long history of use in promoting wound healing, treating skin diseases, and slowing the progress of leprosy. It was also reputed to prolong life, increase energy, and promote sexual potency.[19] In the 1970s, Italian and other European researchers discovered that gotu kola can significantly improve symptoms of venous insufficiency, and it subsequently became a popular European treatment for this condition.

In practice, 4 weeks of treatment with gotu kola frequently produces welcome benefits in the discomfort of chronic venous insufficiency. The active ingredients in gotu kola are believed to be asiaticoside, asiatic acid madecassic acid, and madecassoside.[20]

### What Is the Scientific Evidence for Gotu Kola?

There is significant scientific evidence for the effectiveness of gotu kola in varicose veins/venous insufficiency.

A vacuum suction chamber has been used in some gotu kola studies to evaluate the rate of fluid leakage in venous insufficiency. It produces swelling when applied to the skin of the ankle. When leg veins are leaking a lot of fluid, this swelling takes longer to disappear.

In one study of people with venous insufficiency, 2 weeks of treatment with gotu kola extracts was shown to reduce the time necessary for the swelling to disappear.[21]

Another study of double-blind design followed 87 people with varicose veins and compared the benefits of gotu kola at 60 mg and 30 mg daily against placebo.[22] The results showed improvements in both treated groups but greater improvement at the higher dose. This kind of dose responsiveness is generally taken as good evidence that a treatment is actually effective.

A double-blind study of 94 individuals with venous insufficiency of the lower limb compared the benefits of gotu kola extract at 120 mg daily and 60 mg daily against a placebo.[23] The results also showed a significant dose-related improvement in the treated groups in symptoms such as subjective heaviness, discomfort, and edema.

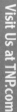

A 1992 review of all the gotu kola studies available concluded that gotu kola extract provides a dose-related improvement in venous insufficiency symptoms, reducing foot swelling, ankle edema, and fluid leakage from the veins.[24]

### Dosages

The usual dosage of gotu kola is 20 to 40 mg 3 times daily of an extract standardized to contain 40% asiaticoside, 29 to 30% asiatic acid, 29 to 30% madecassic acid, and 1 to 2% madecassoside.

### Safety Issues

Studies suggest that oral asiaticoside at a dosage of 1 g per kilogram body weight is safe.[25] This leaves a wide margin of safety, since standard daily doses of gotu kola provide about 2,000 times less asiaticoside for an average adult. Studies have also found that doses of 16 g per kilogram body weight of fresh gotu kola leaves are nontoxic,[26] and studies in rabbits suggest that gotu kola extracts are not harmful to fetal development.[27]

The only reported side effect with gotu kola is rare allergic skin rash. Safety in pregnancy has not been established. However, as with horse chestnut, one gotu kola study did enroll pregnant women.[28] Safety in young children, nursing mothers, and individuals with severe liver or kidney disease has not been established.

## Bilberry: May Be Useful

Although much more famous as a treatment for eye problems such as impaired **night vision** (page 94), there is some evidence that **bilberry** (page 135), a relative of the American blueberry, may be useful in varicose veins as well.

In a placebo-controlled study that followed 60 people with varicose veins for 30 days, bilberry extract significantly decreased pain and swelling.[29] Similar results were seen in another 30-day double-blind trial involving 47 participants.[30] Bilberry contains substances known as anthocyanosides that are closely related to grape seed OPCs. Like OPCs, they appear to strengthen connective tissue, such as the walls of veins.[31,32,33] The standard dosage of bilberry is 120 to 240 mg twice daily of an extract standardized to contain 25% anthocyanosides.

Bilberry is a food and as such is believed to be quite safe. Enormous quantities have been administered to rats without toxic effects.[34] One study of 2,295 people given bilberry extract showed a 4% incidence of side effects, such as mild digestive distress, skin rashes, and drowsiness.[35]

However, safety in young children, pregnant or nursing women, and those with severe liver or kidney disease has not been established.

## OTHER NATURAL TREATMENTS

The following natural treatments are widely recommended for varicose veins, but they have not yet been scientifically proven effective.

## Butcher's Broom

**Butcher's broom** (page 146) is so named because its branches were a traditional source of broom straw used by butchers. This Mediterranean evergreen bush has a long history of traditional use in the treatment of urinary conditions. Recent European interest has focused on the possible value of butcher's broom in the treatment of hemorrhoids and varicose veins, although there is as yet no more than preliminary evidence that it is effective.

Butcher's broom is standardized to its ruscogenin content. A typical oral dose should supply 50 to 100 mg of ruscogenins daily.

Butcher's broom is believed to be safe when used as directed, although detailed studies have not been performed. Noticeable side effects are rare. However, safety in young children, pregnant or nursing women, and those with severe liver or kidney disease has not been established.

## Aortic Glycosaminoglycans

A preparation made from the blood vessels of cows, known as **aortic glycosaminoglycans (GAGs)** (page 125), has been used in Italy as a remedy for varicose veins. Although it is said to be highly effective, the scientific evidence is not yet strong.[36,37,38]

The typical dosage is 100 mg daily. Aortic glycosaminoglycans are believed to be safe because they are widely found in foods. Since aortic GAGs are essentially ground-up blood vessels from cows, they are probably safe to take, even in large quantities. The only concern that has been raised regards their ability to slightly decrease blood clotting. However, safety in young children, pregnant or nursing women, and those with severe liver or kidney disease has not been established.

## Collinsonia

The herb collinsonia, or stone root, has a long traditional history of use as a treatment for varicose veins and hemorrhoids, but it has not been scientifically evaluated to any meaningful extent. The dosage varies with the preparation.

## Calendula

A cream made from the herb **calendula** (page 150) is said to be somewhat cosmetically helpful in varicose veins, although there is little evidence that this is true.

PART

**TWO**

# Herbs and Supplements

# ACIDOPHILUS AND OTHER PROBIOTICS

**Principal Proposed Uses**
Vaginal infections, irritable bowel syndrome, "traveler's diarrhea"

**Other Proposed Uses**
Canker sores, Crohn's disease, ulcerative colitis, colon cancer prevention, yeast hypersensitivity syndrome

**Supplement Forms/Alternative Names**
L. acidophilus, L. bulgaricus, L. thermophilus, L. reuteri, S. bulgaricus, B. bifidus, other "probiotic" bacteria

Acidophilus is a "friendly" strain of bacteria used to make yogurt and cheese. Although we are born without it, acidophilus soon establishes itself in our intestines and helps prevent intestinal infections. Acidophilus also flourishes in the vagina, where it protects women against yeast infections.

Acidophilus is one of several helpful strains of bacteria known collectively as *probiotics* (literally, "pro life," indicating that they are bacteria that help rather than harm). Others include *L. bulgaricus, L. thermophilus, L. reuteri, S. bulgaricus,* and *B. bifidus.* Your digestive tract is like a rain forest ecosystem, with billions of bacteria and yeasts rather than trees, frogs, and leopards. Some of these internal inhabitants are more helpful to your body than others. Acidophilus and related probiotic bacteria not only help the digestive tract function, they also reduce the presence of less healthful organisms by competing with them for the limited space available.

Antibiotics can disturb the balance of your "inner rain forest" by killing friendly bacteria. When this happens, harmful bacteria and yeasts can move in and flourish. This is why women taking antibiotics sometimes develop vaginal infections.

Conversely, it appears that the regular use of probiotics can help prevent vaginal infections and generally improve the health of the gastrointestinal system. Whenever you take antibiotics, you should probably take probiotics as well, and continue them for some time after you are done with the course of treatment. There is also some reason to believe that regular use of probiotics can reduce your risk of developing infectious diarrhea while traveling through foreign countries.

## SOURCES

Although we believe that they are helpful and perhaps even necessary for human health, we don't have a daily requirement for probiotic bacteria. They are living creatures, not chemicals, so they can sustain themselves in your body unless something comes along to damage them, such as antibiotics.

Cultured dairy products such as yogurt and kefir are good sources of acidophilus and other probiotic bacteria. Supplements are widely available in powder, liquid, capsule, or tablet form. Grocery stores and natural food stores both carry milk that contains live acidophilus.

## THERAPEUTIC DOSAGES

Dosages of acidophilus are expressed not in grams or milligrams, but in billions of organisms. A typical daily dose should supply about 3 to 5 billion live organisms. Because this is not a drug but a living organism that you are trying to transplant to your digestive tract, the precise dosage is not so important. But you should take it regularly. Each time you do, you reinforce the beneficial bacterial colonies in your body, which may gradually push out harmful bacteria and yeasts growing there.

The downside of using a living organism is that probiotics may die on the shelf. The container label should guarantee living acidophilus (or bulgaricus, and so on) at the time of purchase, not just at the time of manufacture. Another approach is to eat acidophilus-rich foods such as yogurt, where the bacteria are most likely still alive.

To treat or prevent vaginal infections, mix 2 tablespoons of yogurt or the contents of a couple of capsules of acidophilus with warm water and use as a douche.

Finally, in addition to increasing your intake of probiotics, you can take fructo-oligosaccharides, supplements that can promote thriving colonies of helpful bacteria in the digestive tract. (Fructo-oligosaccharides are carbohydrates found in fruit. *Fructo* means "fruit," and an *oligosaccharide* is a type of carbohydrate.) Taking this supplement is like putting manure in a garden; it is thought to foster a healthy environment for the bacteria you want to have inside you. The typical daily dose of fructo-oligosaccharides is between 2 and 8 g.

## THERAPEUTIC USES

In a few small studies, acidophilus has been found to be effective against vaginal yeast infections as well as those caused by the *Gardnerella* bacteria.[1]

Some evidence also suggests that acidophilus and other probiotics may also be helpful for treating **irritable bowel syndrome** (page 85) and preventing traveler's diarrhea.[2-5]

Probiotic treatment has also been proposed as a treatment for **canker sores** (page 35), Crohn's disease, and ulcerative colitis, and as a preventative measure against colon **cancer** (page 26); but there is no solid evidence that it is effective.

Finally, probiotics may be helpful in a condition known as *yeast hypersensitivity syndrome*, also known as chronic candidiasis, chronic candida, systemic candidiasis, or just **candida** (page 33). Although this syndrome is not recognized by conventional medicine, some practitioners of alternative medicine believe that it is a common problem that leads to numerous symptoms, including fatigue, digestive problems, frequent sinus infections, muscle pain, and mental confusion. Yeast hypersensitivity syndrome is said to consist of a population explosion of the normally benign candida yeast that live in the vagina and elsewhere in the body, coupled with a type of allergic sensitivity to it. Probiotic supplements are widely recommended for this condition because they establish large, healthy populations of friendly bacteria that compete with the candida that is trying to take up residence.

## WHAT IS THE SCIENTIFIC EVIDENCE FOR ACIDOPHILUS?

### Vaginal Yeast Infections

A review of the many studies on the use of oral and topical acidophilus to prevent vaginal yeast infections concluded that the treatment was effective.[6]

### Irritable Bowel Syndrome

People with irritable bowel syndrome (IBS) experience crampy digestive pain as well as alternating diarrhea and constipation and other symptoms. Although the cause of irritable bowel syndrome is not known, one possibility is a disturbance in healthy intestinal bacteria. Based on this theory, acidophilus has been tried as a treatment for IBS.

In a small double-blind study, 18 individuals with irritable bowel syndrome were given either placebo or a capsule containing 5 billion *L. acidophilus* organisms daily for 6 weeks.[7] Greater improvement was seen in the treated group than in the placebo group, but so many people dropped out of the study the results are difficult to evaluate.

### Traveler's Diarrhea

According to several studies conducted on the subject, it appears that regular use of acidophilus can help prevent "traveler's diarrhea" (an illness caused by eating contaminated food, usually in developing countries).[8]

Some evidence suggests that a particular type of probiotic, *L. reuteri*, can help treat diarrhea caused by viral infections in children.[9,10] Keep in mind that diarrhea in young children can be serious. If it persists for more than a day, you should take your child to a physician.

## SAFETY ISSUES

There are no known safety problems with the use of acidophilus or other probiotics. Occasionally, some people notice a temporary increase in digestive gas.

Acidophilus and Other Probiotics

Aloe

## ⚠ INTERACTIONS YOU SHOULD KNOW ABOUT

If you are taking **antibiotics,** it may be beneficial to take probiotic supplements at the same time, and to continue them for a couple of weeks after you have finished the course of drug treatment. This will help restore the balance of natural bacteria in your digestive tract.

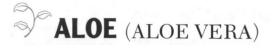

# ALOE (ALOE VERA)

*Principal Proposed Uses*

*Topical uses:*
    Wound and burn healing, psoriasis

*Oral uses:*
    AIDS, diabetes, asthma, ulcers, immune weakness

The succulent aloe plant has been valued since prehistoric times for the treatment of burns, wound infections, and other skin problems. Medicinal aloe is pictured in an ancient cave painting in South Africa, and Alexander the Great is said to have captured an island off Somalia for the sole purpose of possessing the luxurious crop of aloe found there.

Most uses of aloe refer to the gel inside its cactus-like leaves. However, the skin of the leaves themselves can be condensed to form a sticky substance known as "drug aloe" or "aloes." It is a powerful laxative, and an unpleasant one. The uses described below refer only to aloe gel.

## WHAT IS ALOE USED FOR TODAY?

I suspect millions of people (including myself) would swear by their own experience that applying aloe to the skin can drastically reduce the time it takes for a burn to heal. Unfortunately there have never been any properly designed scientific studies that can tell us just how effective aloe really is.[1]

A study in animals suggests that topical aloe gel may improve wound healing.[2] However, one report suggests that aloe can actually impair healing in severe wounds.[3] Aloe is also sometimes used for **psoriasis** (page 106).

Oral *Aloe vera* is also sometimes recommended to treat AIDS, **diabetes** (page 60), **asthma** (page 11), stomach **ulcers** (page 112), and general immune weakness. While the evidence for benefit in these conditions is slight to nonexistent, one of the constituents of aloe, acemannan, does seem to possess numerous interesting effects. Test-tube and animal studies suggest that it may stimulate immunity and inhibit the growth of viruses.[4,5,6] However, it remains to be discovered whether this preliminary research will translate into actual benefits in human beings. *Aloe vera* is definitely not a proven treatment for any of these conditions.

## WHAT IS THE SCIENTIFIC EVIDENCE FOR ALOE?

According to a double-blind study that enrolled 60 men and women with mild to moderate symptoms of psoriasis, *Aloe vera* cream may be helpful for this chronic skin condition.[7] Participants were treated with either topical *Aloe vera* extract (0.5%) or a placebo cream, applied 3 times daily for 4 weeks. Aloe treatment produced significantly better results than placebo, and these results were said to endure for almost a year after treatment was stopped. The study authors also reported a high level of complete "cure," but what exactly they meant by this was not reported clearly.

## DOSAGES

For sunburn and other minor burns, smear aloe gel liberally on the affected area.

For internal use in treating AIDS and other conditions, some authorities recommend a dose of aloe standardized to provide 800 to 1,600 mg of the substance acemannan daily.

## SAFETY ISSUES

Other than occasional allergic reactions, no serious problems have been reported with aloe gel, whether used internally or externally. However, comprehensive safety studies are lacking. Safety in young children, pregnant or nursing women, or those with severe liver or kidney disease has not been established.

## ⚠ INTERACTIONS
## YOU SHOULD KNOW ABOUT

If you are using **hydrocortisone cream,** aloe gel might help it work better.[8]

 # ANDROGRAPHIS (ANDROGRAPHIS PANICULATA)

*Principal Proposed Uses*
Colds (shortening duration and reducing symptoms)

Andrographis is a shrub found throughout India and other Asian countries that is sometimes called "Indian echinacea." It has been used historically in epidemics, including the Indian flu epidemic in 1919, during which andrographis was credited with stopping the spread of the disease.[1]

## WHAT IS ANDROGRAPHIS USED FOR TODAY?

Over the last decade, andrographis has become popular in Scandinavia as a treatment for **colds** (page 44). It is beginning to become available in the United States as well.

## WHAT IS THE SCIENTIFIC EVIDENCE FOR ANDROGRAPHIS?

A few well-designed, double-blind studies that found andrographis to be effective have recently been published in English. The evidence suggests that andrographis reduces the severity of symptoms and shortens the length of colds. One recent, double-blind clinical study of andrographis involved 50 people with colds who received either andrographis or placebo.[2] The results showed that 55% of the treated participants reported that their colds were less intense than usual, while only 19% of those in the placebo group stated this. About 75% of the treated individuals were well after 5 days, compared to less than 40% in the placebo group. These differences are statistically significant and provide meaningful evidence that andrographis is effective.

Another study of 59 people found similar results.[3] Participants received either 1,200 mg of andrographis (standardized to 4% andrographolides) or placebo, and were evaluated for the severity of cold symptoms such as fatigue, sore muscles, runny nose, headache, and lymph node swelling. By the fourth day of the study, the andrographis group showed significant improvement in most of the cold symptoms, including sore throat, muscle aches, and fatigue, as compared to the placebo group.

Finally, a double-blind study involving 152 adults compared the effectiveness of andrographis (in doses of 3 g per day or 6 g per day, for 7 days) to acetaminophen for the treatment of sore throat and fever. The higher dose of andrographis (6 g) decreased symptoms of fever and throat pain, as did acetaminophen, while the lower dose of andrographis (3 g) did not.

There were no significant side effects in either group.[4]

## DOSAGES

A typical dosage of andrographis is 400 mg 3 times a day. Doses as high as 1,000 to 2,000 mg 3 times daily have been used in some studies.

Andrographis

Visit Us at TNP.com

Andrographis is usually standardized to its content of andrographolide, typically 4 to 6%.

## SAFETY ISSUES

Andrographis has not been associated with any side effects in human studies, although animal studies raise concerns about its effects on fertility. In the 59-person study mentioned earlier, participants were monitored for changes in liver function, blood counts, kidney function, and other laboratory measures of toxicity.[5] No problems were found.

However, some studies have raised concerns that andrographis may impair fertility. One study showed that male rats became infertile when fed 20 mg of andrographis powder daily.[6] In this case, the rats stopped producing sperm and showed physical changes in some of the testicular cells involved in sperm production. Researchers also detected evidence of degeneration of other anatomical structures in the testicles. However, another study showed no evidence of testicular toxicity in male rats that were given up to 1 g per kilogram body weight daily for 60 days, so this issue remains unclear.[7]

One group of female mice also did not fare well on high dosages of andrographis.[8] When fed 2 g per kilogram body weight daily for 6 weeks (thousands of times higher than the usual human dose), all female mice failed to get pregnant when mated with males of proven fertility. Meanwhile, of the control females, 95.2% got pregnant when mated with a similar group of male mice.

While andrographis is probably not a useful form of birth control, these results are worrisome and suggest the need for more research. Safety in young children, pregnant or nursing women, or those with severe liver or kidney disease has not been established.

# ANDROSTENEDIONE

*Principal Proposed Uses*
Athletic performance

Androstenedione is a hormone produced naturally in the body by the adrenal glands, the ovaries (in women), and the testicles (in men). The body first manufactures **DHEA** (page 176), then turns DHEA into androstenedione, and finally transforms androstenedione into testosterone, the principal male sex hormone.

Androstenedione is widely used by athletes who believe that it can build muscle and increase strength. However, there is no evidence that it works.

U.S. baseball fans know that the all-time single-season home run champion, Mark McGwire, used androstenedione during his record-setting season. Whether it helped is anyone's guess. Hitting home runs is not only a matter of strength, but of timing and concentration as well. Nonetheless, if McGwire were playing in any other professional sport, or in the Olympics, he would have been suspended for using androstenedione.

## SOURCES

Androstenedione is not an essential nutrient—your body manufactures it from scratch. It is found in meat and in some plants, but to get a therapeutic dosage, you will need to take supplements.

## THERAPEUTIC DOSAGES

Some sports trainers recommend taking 100 mg of androstenedione daily with food.

## THERAPEUTIC USES

Androstenedione is said to enhance athletic performance and strength by increasing muscle.

However, there is no direct evidence that it works.

## WHAT IS THE SCIENTIFIC EVIDENCE FOR ANDROSTENEDIONE?

The German patent for androstenedione claims that 50 mg taken orally by men will raise blood levels of testosterone by about 150%. Blood levels of testosterone start rising 15 minutes after taking androstenedione and stay elevated for 3 hours, then decline to normal. Whether this will improve sports performance, however, is unknown.

## SAFETY ISSUES

In the absence of testosterone deficiency, raising testosterone levels is not known to produce beneficial effects and may be risky. Like other male hormones, androstenedione causes hair loss on the head and growth of body hair.[1] There are also concerns that androstenedione might cause liver cancer and heart disease like other oral strength-building hormones. In addition, the purity of commercial androstenedione is unknown.

Putting all this information together, I think it is fair to say that more research is needed before androstenedione can be recommended.

## ⚠ INTERACTIONS YOU SHOULD KNOW ABOUT

If you are taking any **hormones** or **drugs that affect hormone levels,** it is possible that androstenedione might interfere.

# AORTIC GLYCOSAMINOGLYCANS

*Principal Proposed Uses*
  Atherosclerosis, high cholesterol, varicose veins, hemorrhoids, phlebitis

*Supplement Forms/Alternative Names*
  Aortic GAGs, mesoglycan

Aortic glycosaminoglycans (GAGs) are important substances found in many tissues in the body, including the joints and the lining of blood vessels. Chemically, aortic GAGs are related to the blood-thinning drug heparin and the supplement **chondroitin** (page 159). Unlike chondroitin, aortic GAGs are primarily used to treat diseases of blood vessels. Preliminary evidence suggests that aortic GAGs may be helpful for atherosclerosis, varicose veins, phlebitis, and hemorrhoids.

## SOURCES

Aortic GAGs are not essential nutrients because the body usually manufactures them from scratch. For supplement purposes, aortic GAGs are commercially extracted from the aorta (the largest artery) of cows—hence the name.

## THERAPEUTIC DOSAGES

The usual dosage of aortic GAGs is 100 mg daily.

## THERAPEUTIC USES

Hardening of the arteries due to **atherosclerosis** (page 14) is the major cause of heart disease and strokes. High **cholesterol** (page 39), **hypertension** (page 75), cigarette smoking, and other factors damage the inner lining of blood vessels, causing a series of dangerous changes.

There is some evidence that aortic GAGs may slow the development of atherosclerosis, by lowering cholesterol levels, "thinning" the blood, or through other effects.[1,2]

They may also be useful for various other diseases of blood vessels, including **varicose veins** (page 113), **hemorrhoids** (page 70), and phlebitis.[3–6]

**Warning:** Do not self-treat phlebitis. It is a potentially deadly disease.

## WHAT IS THE SCIENTIFIC EVIDENCE FOR AORTIC GAGS?

### Atherosclerosis

In a recent study, one group of men with early hardening of the coronary (heart) arteries was given 200 mg daily of aortic GAGs, while the other group received no treatment.[7] After 18 months, the layering of the vessel lining was 7.5 times greater in the untreated group than in the aortic GAG group, a significant difference. Additional preliminary evidence that aortic GAGs might help atherosclerosis comes from other studies in animals and people.[8,9] However, in the absence of properly designed double-blind trials, the results can't be taken as truly reliable.

We don't know how aortic GAGs help atherosclerosis. There is some evidence that they can reduce cholesterol levels and also "thin" the blood.[10,11]

### Vein Diseases

Several Italian studies suggest that aortic GAGs may be helpful in varicose veins, phlebitis, and hemorrhoids.[12–15] However, because the full text of these studies is not available in English, it is difficult to evaluate their merits.

## SAFETY ISSUES

Aortic GAGs are essentially ground-up blood vessels from cows, so they are probably safe to take even in large quantities. The only concern that has been raised regards their ability to slightly decrease blood clotting (see Interactions You Should Know About). Maximum safe dosages for young children, pregnant or nursing women, or those with severe liver or kidney disease have not been determined.

## ⚠ INTERACTIONS YOU SHOULD KNOW ABOUT

If you are taking drugs that powerfully decrease blood clotting, such as **Coumadin (warfarin)** or **heparin,** do not use aortic GAGs except under physician supervision. Because aortic GAGs interfere slightly with blood clotting, there is a chance that the combination could cause bleeding problems.

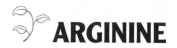

# ARGININE

*Principal Proposed Uses*
  Colds (prevention), intermittent claudication, congestive heart failure, male infertility

*Other Proposed Uses*
  Impotence

*Supplement Forms/Alternative Names*
  Arginine hydrochloride, L-arginine

Arginine is an amino acid found in many foods, including dairy products, meat, poultry, and fish. It plays a role in several important mechanisms in the body, including cell division, the healing of wounds, the removal of ammonia from the body, immune function, and the secretion of important hormones.

The body also uses arginine to make nitric oxide, which relaxes the blood vessels. Based on this, arginine has been proposed as a treatment for various heart conditions, including congestive heart failure, and for impotence, which may be caused by limited blood flow. For reasons that are not at all clear, regular use of arginine may also be able to help reduce the frequency of colds.

## REQUIREMENTS/SOURCES

Normally, the body either gets enough arginine from food, or manufactures all it needs from other widely available nutrients. Certain stresses, such as severe burns, infections, and injuries, can deplete your body's supply of arginine.

Arginine is found in dairy products, meat, poultry, fish, nuts, and chocolate.

## THERAPEUTIC DOSAGES

A typical supplemental dosage of arginine is 2 to 3 g per day. For congestive heart failure, dosages as high as 30 g per day have been tried.

**Warning:** Do not try to self-treat congestive heart failure. If you have this condition, be sure to consult your physician before taking any supplements.

## THERAPEUTIC USES

One preliminary double-blind study suggests that arginine supplementation might help prevent **colds** (page 44).[1]

Other preliminary studies suggest that arginine may relieve some of the symptoms of **intermittent claudication** (page 83)[2] and **congestive heart failure** (page 50).[3,4] The supplement **coenzyme Q$_{10}$ (CoQ$_{10}$)** (page 164), however, has far better evidence as a treatment for the latter condition.

Preliminary evidence suggests that arginine may improve sperm function and thereby help treat **infertility in men** (page 78), but not all studies have found benefit.[5–10]

Arginine has recently become popular as a male aphrodisiac and a cure for **impotence** (page 77), but there is little to no evidence that it works.

## WHAT IS THE SCIENTIFIC EVIDENCE FOR ARGININE?

### Colds

A double-blind study involving 41 children concluded that arginine seemed to provide some protection against respiratory infections.[11] In this study, 20 children were given arginine and 20 received placebo for 60 days of the study. Of the children who received placebo, 15 developed minor respiratory infections (colds) during the 60 days of the study. By contrast, only 5 of the children taking arginine developed colds, a significant difference.

### Intermittent Claudication

People with advanced hardening of the arteries, or **atherosclerosis** (page 14), often have difficulty walking due to lack of blood flow to the legs, a condition known as intermittent claudication. Pain may develop after walking less than half a block. Food bars containing arginine have been found to improve walking distance. After 2 weeks of two food bars daily, study participants could walk 66% farther.[12]

## SAFETY ISSUES

Arginine is an amino acid found naturally in our bodies and our food, and for this reason is believed to be quite safe. However, maximum safe dosages are not known for young children, pregnant or nursing women, or those with severe liver or kidney disease.

Keep in mind that the recommended dosage of arginine is so high that even low percentage levels of a contaminant might cause problems, so be sure to purchase a high-quality product.

## ⚠ INTERACTIONS YOU SHOULD KNOW ABOUT

If you are taking **lysine** (page 250) to treat **herpes** (page 73), arginine might counteract any potential benefit.

Arginine

# ASHWAGANDA (WITHANIA SOMNIFERUM)

## Principal Proposed Uses
Adaptogen (improve ability to withstand stress)

## Other Proposed Uses
Improve exercise ability, immunity, sexual capacity, and fertility; reduce cholesterol; prevent colds and flus; treat insomnia and anxiety

Ashwaganda is sometimes called "Indian ginseng," not because it's related botanically (it's closer to potatoes and tomatoes) but because its uses are similar. Like ginseng, ashwaganda is a "tonic herb" traditionally believed capable of generally strengthening the body. However, it is believed to be milder and less stimulating than ginseng.

## WHAT IS ASHWAGANDA USED FOR TODAY?

Modern herbalists classify ashwaganda as an adaptogen, a substance that increases the body's ability to withstand stress of all types. See the chapter on **ginseng** (page 206) for more information on adaptogens.

Like other adaptogens, ashwaganda is said to improve physical energy, strengthen immunity against **colds and flus** (page 44) and other infections, and increase sexual capacity. It has been suggested as a treatment for **infertility** (pages 78 and 79). Highly preliminary studies suggest that ashwaganda may reduce the negative effects of stress, inhibit inflammation, lower **cholesterol** (page 39), increase sexual performance, produce mild sedation (an effect potentially useful for those troubled by **insomnia** [page 80] or **anxiety** [page 8]), increase hemoglobin levels, and inhibit tumor growth.[1-4] Further studies remain to be performed to evaluate these potential benefits.

## DOSAGES

A typical dosage of ashwaganda is 1 teaspoon of powder twice a day, boiled in milk or water. Herbalists often recommend that those who are young or especially weak should take a lower dosage.

## SAFETY ISSUES

Although formal scientific safety studies have not been completed, ashwaganda appears to be safe when taken in normal doses. However, because some of the constituents of ashwaganda can make you drowsy, it should not be combined with sedative drugs. The herb may also have some steroid-like activity at high dosages. Safety in young children, pregnant or nursing women, or those with severe liver or kidney disease has not been established.

## ⚠ INTERACTIONS YOU SHOULD KNOW ABOUT

If you are taking **sedative drugs,** you should not take ashwaganda at the same time.

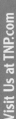

# ASTRAGALUS (ASTRAGALUS MEMBRANACEUS)

### Principal Proposed Uses
Strengthen immunity (against colds, flus, and other illnesses)

### Other Proposed Uses
Atherosclerosis, hypertension (high blood pressure), hyperthyroidism, insomnia, diabetes, chronic active hepatitis, genital herpes, AIDS, chemotherapy side effects

Dried and sliced thin, the root of the astragalus plant is a common component of traditional Chinese herbal formulas. According to Chinese medical theory, astragalus "strengthens the spleen, blood and Qi, raises the yang Qi of the spleen and stomach, and stabilizes the exterior."[1] Don't worry if you didn't understand what you just read, because without many months of training in the unique Chinese approach to illness, there's no way you could have. Suffice it to say that the traditional understanding of the way astragalus works is different from the way it tends to be presented today.

## WHAT IS ASTRAGALUS USED FOR TODAY?

In the United States, astragalus has been presented as an immune stimulant useful for treating **colds and flus** (page 44). Many people have come to believe that they should take astragalus, like **echinacea** (page 179), at the first sign of a cold.

The belief that astragalus can strengthen the immunity has its basis in Chinese tradition. The expression "stabilize the exterior" means helping to create a "defensive shield" against infection.

However, according to Chinese healing tradition, astragalus formulas should not be taken during the early stage of infections. To do so is said to resemble "locking the chicken-coop with the fox inside," causing the infection to be "driven deeper."

Rather, astragalus is supposedly only appropriate for use while you're healthy, for the purpose of preventing future illnesses. Since it was the Chinese who first developed astragalus, perhaps these traditions should be taken seriously.

## WHAT IS THE SCIENTIFIC EVIDENCE FOR ASTRAGALUS?

Although tradition suggests that astragalus should always be used in combination with other herbs, modern Chinese investigators have found various intriguing effects when astragalus is taken by itself. Extracts of astragalus have been shown to stimulate parts of the immune system in mice and humans, and to increase the survival time of mice infected with various diseases.[2,3] Preliminary research also suggests that astragalus might be useful in treating **atherosclerosis** (page 14), hyperthyroidism, **hypertension** (page 75), **insomnia** (page 80), **diabetes** (page 60), chronic active **hepatitis** (page 71), genital **herpes** (page 73), AIDS, and the side effects of cancer chemotherapy.[4–9] However, none of these suggestions can be regarded as proven.

## DOSAGES

A typical daily dosage of astragalus involves boiling 9 to 30 g of dried root to make tea. Newer products use an alcohol-and-water extraction method to produce an extract standardized to astragaloside content, although there is no consensus on the proper percentage.

## SAFETY ISSUES

Astragalus appears to be relatively nontoxic. High one-time doses, as well as long-term administration, have not caused significant harmful effects.[10] Side effects are rare and generally limited to the usual mild gastrointestinal distress or allergic reactions.

As mentioned above, traditional Chinese medicine warns against using astragalus in cases of acute infections. Other traditional contraindications include "deficient yin patterns with heat signs" and "exterior excess heat patterns." Because understanding what these mean would require an extensive education in Chinese medicine, I rec-

ommend using astragalus only under the supervision of a qualified Chinese herbalist.

Safety in young children, pregnant or nursing women, or those with severe liver or kidney disease has not been established.

# BCAAs (BRANCHED-CHAIN AMINO ACIDS)

### Principal Proposed Uses
Loss of appetite (in cancer patients), amyotrophic lateral sclerosis (ALS, Lou Gehrig's disease)

### Other Proposed Uses
Recovery from surgery, improving athletic performance, muscular dystrophy

### Supplement Forms/Alternative Names
Branched-chain amino acids (combined) or leucine, isoleucine, or valine separately

Branched-chain amino acids (BCAAs) are naturally occurring molecules (leucine, isoleucine, and valine) that the body uses to build proteins. The term "branched chain" refers to the molecular structure of these particular amino acids. Muscles have a particularly high content of BCAAs.

For reasons that are not entirely clear, BCAA supplements may improve appetite in cancer patients and slow the progression of amyotrophic lateral sclerosis (ALS, or Lou Gehrig's disease, a terrible condition that leads to degeneration of nerves, atrophy of the muscles, and eventual death).

BCAAs have also been proposed as a supplement to boost athletic performance.

## REQUIREMENTS/SOURCES

Dietary protein usually provides all the BCAAs you need. However, physical stress and injury can increase your need for BCAAs to repair damage, so supplementation may be helpful.

BCAAs are present in all protein-containing foods, but the best sources are red meat and dairy products. Chicken, fish, and eggs are excellent sources as well. Whey protein and egg protein supplements are another way to ensure you're getting enough BCAAs. Supplements may contain all three BCAAs together or simply individual BCAAs.

## THERAPEUTIC DOSAGES

The typical dosage of BCAAs is 1 to 5 g daily.

## THERAPEUTIC USES

Preliminary evidence suggests that BCAAs may improve appetite in cancer patients.[1] There is also some evidence that BCAA supplements may reduce symptoms of amyotrophic lateral sclerosis.[2] Reports, but little real evidence, suggest that BCAAs may reduce muscle loss during recovery from surgery.

BCAAs have also been tried by athletes to build muscle; however, evidence suggests that they do not improve performance or enhance the muscle/fat ratio in the body.[3,4] BCAAs also do not appear to be helpful for muscular dystrophy.[5]

## WHAT IS THE SCIENTIFIC EVIDENCE FOR BCAAS?

### Appetite in Cancer Patients

A double-blind study tested BCAAs on 28 people with cancer who had lost their appetites due to either the disease itself or its treatment.[6] Appetite improved in 55% of those taking BCAAs (4.8 g daily) compared to only 16% of those who took placebo.

## Amyotrophic Lateral Sclerosis (Lou Gehrig's Disease)

A small double-blind study suggested that BCAAs might help protect muscle strength in people with Lou Gehrig's disease.[7] Eighteen individuals were given either BCAAs (taken 4 times daily between meals) or placebo, and followed for 1 year. The results showed that people taking BCAAs declined much more slowly than those receiving placebo. In the placebo group, five of nine participants lost their ability to walk, two died, and another required a respirator. Only one of nine of those receiving BCAAs became unable to walk during the study period. This study is too small to give conclusive evidence, but it does suggest that BCAAs might be helpful for this disease.

## Muscular Dystrophy

One double-blind placebo-controlled study found leucine ineffective at the dose of 0.2 g per kilogram body weight (15 g daily for a 75-kilogram woman) in 96 individuals with muscular dystrophy.[8] Over the course of 1 year, no differences were seen between the effects of leucine and placebo.

## SAFETY ISSUES

BCAAs are believed to be safe; when taken in excess, they are simply converted into other amino acids. However, like other amino acids, BCAAs may interfere with medications for Parkinson's disease.

## ⚠ INTERACTIONS YOU SHOULD KNOW ABOUT

If you are taking **medication for Parkinson's disease,** BCAAs may reduce its effectiveness.

# BETA-CAROTENE

### Principal Proposed Uses
Heart disease prevention, cataract prevention, macular degeneration prevention

### Other Proposed Uses
Osteoarthritis, easy sunburning, abnormal Pap smear, heartburn, Parkinson's disease, rheumatoid arthritis, alcoholism, asthma, depression, epilepsy, psoriasis, infertility, headache, high blood pressure, schizophrenia, AIDS

### Probably Ineffective Uses
Cancer prevention

### Supplement Forms/Alternative Names
Beta-carotene and vitamin A are sometimes described as if they were the same thing. This is because the body converts beta-carotene into vitamin A. However, there are significant differences between the two.
**Note:** All the significant positive evidence for beta-carotene applies to food sources, not supplements.

Beta-carotene belongs to a family of natural chemicals known as carotenes or carotenoids. Scientists have identified nearly 600 different carotenes (other carotenes discussed in this book are **lycopene** [page 249] and **lutein** [page 248]). Widely found in plants, carotenes (along with another group of chemicals, the bioflavonoids) give color to fruits, vegetables, and other plants.

Beta-carotene is a particularly important carotene from a nutritional standpoint, because the body easily transforms it to **vitamin A** (page 318). While vitamin A supplements themselves can be toxic when taken to excess, if you take beta-carotene, your body will make only as much vitamin A as you need. This built-in safety feature makes beta-carotene the best way to get your vitamin A.

Beta-Carotene

Visit Us at TNP.com

Beta-carotene is also often recommended for another reason: It is an antioxidant, like **vitamin E** (page 337) and **vitamin C** (page 331). However, although there is a great deal of evidence that the carotenes found in food can provide a variety of health benefits (from reducing the risk of cancer to preventing heart disease), there is little to no evidence that high doses of purified beta-carotene supplements are good for you.

## REQUIREMENTS/SOURCES

Although beta-carotene is not an essential nutrient, vitamin A is. Three mg (5,000 IU) of beta-carotene supplies about 5,000 IU of vitamin A. (See the chapter on vitamin A for requirements based on age and sex.)

Dark green and orange-yellow vegetables are good sources of beta-carotene. These include carrots, sweet potatoes, squash, spinach, romaine lettuce, broccoli, apricots, and green peppers.

The drugs methotrexate and colchicine can impair beta-carotene absorption.[1]

## THERAPEUTIC DOSAGES

We are not sure at the present time whether it is advisable to take dosages of beta-carotene much higher than the recommended allowance for nutritional purposes. It is probably much better to increase your intake of fresh fruits and vegetables.

## THERAPEUTIC USES

It is difficult to recommend beta-carotene supplements for any use other than to supply nutritional levels of vitamin A.

Evidence suggests that mixed carotenes found in food can protect against **cancer** (page 26) and **heart disease** (page 14).[2–8] However, supplements that contain only purified beta-carotene may actually be harmful.[9–13]

Similarly, although mixed carotenes found in food seem to slow the progression of **cataracts** (page 37) and help prevent **macular degeneration** (page 85), beta-carotene alone does not seem to work.[14–18] Dietary beta-carotene may also slow down the progression of **osteoarthritis**

(page 95), but we don't know whether beta-carotene supplements work for this purpose.[19]

Beta-carotene supplements may be helpful for people with extreme sensitivity to the sun, but the evidence is somewhat contradictory.[20–23] Finally, beta-carotene has been proposed as a treatment for abnormal Pap smears, heartburn, Parkinson's disease, **rheumatoid arthritis** (page 109), alcoholism, **asthma** (page 11), **depression** (page 54), epilepsy, **psoriasis** (page 106), **infertility** (pages 78 and 79), headaches, **hypertension** (page 75), schizophrenia, and AIDS, but there is little to no evidence that it works.

## WHAT IS THE SCIENTIFIC EVIDENCE FOR BETA-CAROTENE?

### Cancer Prevention

The story of beta-carotene and cancer is full of contradictions. It starts in the early 1980s, when the cumulative results of many studies suggested that people who eat a lot of fruits and vegetables are significantly less likely to get cancer.[24,25] A close look at the data pointed to carotenes as the active ingredients in fruits and vegetables. It appeared that a high intake of dietary carotene could dramatically reduce the risk of lung cancer,[26] bladder cancer,[27] breast cancer,[28] esophageal cancer,[29] and stomach cancer.[30]

The next step was to give carotenes to people and see if it made a difference. Researchers used purified beta-carotene instead of mixed carotenes, because it is much more readily available. They studied people in high-risk groups, such as smokers, because it is easier to see results when you look at people who are more likely to develop cancer to begin with. However, the results were surprisingly unfavorable.

The anticancer bubble burst for beta-carotene in 1994 when the results of the Alpha-Tocopherol, Beta-Carotene (ATBC) study came in.[31] These results showed that beta-carotene supplements did not prevent lung cancer, but actually increased the risk of getting it by 18%. This trial had followed 29,133 male smokers in Finland who took supplements of about 50 IU of vitamin E (alpha-tocopherol), 20 mg of beta-carotene, both, or placebo daily for 5 to 8 years. (In contrast, vitamin E was found to reduce the risk of cancer, especially prostate cancer.)

In January 1996, researchers monitoring the Beta-Carotene and Retinol Efficacy Trial (CARET) confirmed the prior bad news with more of their own: The beta-carotene group had 46% more cases of lung cancer deaths.[32] This study involved smokers, former smokers, and workers exposed to asbestos. Alarmed, the National Cancer Institute ended the $42 million CARET trial 21 months before it was planned to end.

At about the same time, the 12-year Physicians' Health Study of 22,000 male physicians was finding that 50 mg of beta-carotene taken every other day had no effect—good or bad—on the risk of cancer or heart disease. In this study, 11% of the participants were smokers and 39% were ex-smokers.[33] Interestingly, higher levels of carotene intake from diet *were* associated with lower levels of cancer.

What is the explanation for this apparent discrepancy? It could be that beta-carotene alone is not effective. The other carotenes found in fruits and vegetables may be more important for preventing cancer than beta-carotene. One researcher has suggested that taking beta-carotene supplements actually depletes the body of other beneficial carotenes.[34]

### Heart Disease Prevention

The situation with beta-carotene and heart disease is rather similar to that of beta-carotene and cancer. Numerous studies suggest that carotenes as a whole can reduce the risk of heart disease.[35] However, isolated beta-carotene may not help prevent heart disease and could actually increase your risk.

The same double-blind intervention trial involving 29,133 Finnish male smokers (mentioned under the discussion of cancer and beta-carotene) found 11% *more* deaths from heart disease and 15 to 20% *more* strokes in those participants taking beta-carotene supplements.[36]

Similar poor results with beta-carotene were seen in another large double-blind study of smokers.[37] Beta-carotene supplementation was also found to increase the incidence of angina in smokers.[38]

The bottom line: As with cancer, the mixed carotenoids found in foods seem to be helpful for heart disease, but beta-carotene supplements do not.

### Osteoarthritis

A high dietary intake of beta-carotene appears to slow the progression of osteoarthritis by as much as 70%, according to a study in which researchers followed 640 individuals over a period of 8 to 10 years.[39] However, again we don't know if purified beta-carotene supplements work the same way as beta-carotene from food sources.[40]

## SAFETY ISSUES

At recommended dosages, beta-carotene is very safe. The only side effects reported from beta-carotene overdose are diarrhea and a yellowish tinge to the hands and feet. These symptoms disappear once you stop taking beta-carotene or move to lower doses.

However, in light of the evidence presented, high-dose beta-carotene may slightly increase the risk of heart disease and cancer. The solution: Eat plenty of fresh fruits and vegetables, and get your beta-carotene that way.

## ⚠ INTERACTIONS YOU SHOULD KNOW ABOUT

If you are taking

- **Colchicine** or **methotrexate:** You may have trouble absorbing beta-carotene.

- The older cholesterol-lowering drugs **colestipol** or **cholestyramine:** You may need extra beta-carotene.

Beta-Carotene

# BETAINE HYDROCHLORIDE

### Principal Proposed Uses

There are no well-documented uses for betaine hydrochloride.

### Other Proposed Uses

Digestive aid, anemia, asthma, atherosclerosis, diarrhea, excess candida (yeast), food allergies, gallstones, hay fever, inner ear infections, rheumatoid arthritis, thyroid conditions, ulcers, heartburn

Betaine hydrochloride is a source of hydrochloric acid, a naturally occurring chemical in the stomach that helps us digest food by breaking up fats and proteins. Stomach acid also aids in the absorption of nutrients through the walls of the intestines into the blood and protects the gastrointestinal tract from harmful bacteria.

A major branch of alternative medicine known as *naturopathy* has long held that low stomach acid is a widespread problem that interferes with digestion and the absorption of nutrients. Betaine hydrochloride is one of the most common recommendations for this condition (along with the more folksy apple cider vinegar).

Betaine is also sold by itself, without the hydrochloride molecule attached. In this form, it is called **TMG (trimethylglycine)** (page 310). TMG is not acidic, but recent evidence suggests that it may provide certain health benefits of its own.

## SOURCES

Betaine hydrochloride is not an essential nutrient, and no food sources exist.

## THERAPEUTIC DOSAGES

Betaine hydrochloride is typically taken in pill form at dosages ranging from 325 to 650 mg with each meal.

## THERAPEUTIC USES

Based on theories about the importance of stomach acid, betaine has been recommended for a wide variety of problems, including anemia, **asthma** (page 11), **atherosclerosis** (page 14), diarrhea, excess **candida** (page 33) yeast, food allergies, **gallstones** (page 68), hay fever and **allergies** (page 3), inner ear infections, **rheumatoid arthritis** (page 109), and thyroid conditions. When one sees such broadly encompassing uses, it is not surprising to find that there is as yet no real scientific research on its effectiveness for any of these conditions.

Many naturopathic physicians also believe that betaine hydrochloride can heal conditions such as **ulcers** (page 112) and esophageal reflux (heartburn). This sounds paradoxical, since conventional treatment for those conditions involves reducing stomach acid, while betaine hydrochloride increases it. However, according to one theory, lack of stomach acid leads to incomplete digestion of proteins, and these proteins cause allergic reactions and other responses that lead to an increase in ulcer pain. Again, scientific evidence is lacking.

## SAFETY ISSUES

Betaine hydrochloride should not be used by those with ulcers or esophageal reflux (heartburn) except on the advice of a physician. This supplement seldom causes any obvious side effects, but it has not been put through rigorous safety studies. In particular, safety for young children, pregnant or nursing women, or those with severe liver or kidney disease has not been established.

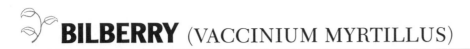

# BILBERRY (VACCINIUM MYRTILLUS)

## Principal Proposed Uses
Eye problems (e.g., poor night vision, diabetic retinopathy, prevention of cataracts, prevention and treatment of macular degeneration)

Strengthen blood vessels (e.g., varicose veins, easy bruising, prevention of post-surgical bleeding)

## Other Proposed Uses
Atherosclerosis, diabetes (blood sugar control)

Often called European blueberry, bilberry is closely related to American blueberry, cranberry, and huckleberry. Its meat is creamy white instead of purple, but it is traditionally used, like blueberries, in the preparation of jams, pies, cobblers, and cakes.

Bilberry fruit also has a long medicinal history. In the twelfth century, Abbess Hildegard of Bingen wrote of bilberry's usefulness for inducing menstruation. Over subsequent centuries, the list of uses for bilberry grew to include a bewildering variety of possible uses, from bladder stones to typhoid fever.

## WHAT IS BILBERRY USED FOR TODAY?

The modern use of bilberry dates back to World War II, when British Royal Air Force pilots reported that a good dose of bilberry jam just prior to a mission improved their **night vision** (page 94), often dramatically. After the war, medical researchers investigated the constituents of bilberry and subsequently recommended it for a variety of eye disorders.

Bilberry is used throughout Europe today for the treatment of poor night vision and day blindness, for which it is believed to be significantly helpful. Regular use of bilberry is also thought to help prevent or treat other eye diseases such as **macular degeneration** (page 85), diabetic retinopathy, and **cataracts** (page 37).

Scientific research also found that bilberry contains biologically powerful substances known as anthocyanosides. Evidence suggests that anthocyanosides strengthen the walls of blood vessels, reduce inflammation, and generally stabilize all tissues containing collagen (such as tendons,

ligaments, and cartilage).[1–5] Grape seed contains related substances with similar properties. However, bilberry's anthocyanosides have a special attraction to the retina, which may explain this herb's apparent usefulness in eye diseases.[6]

There is also some evidence that bilberry can be useful for **varicose veins** (page 113). European physicians additionally believe that bilberry's blood vessel–stabilizing properties also make it useful as a treatment before surgery to reduce bleeding complications, as well as for other blood-vessel problems such as easy bruising, but the evidence as yet is only suggestive.

On the basis of very limited evidence, bilberry has also been suggested as a treatment for improving blood sugar control in people with **diabetes** (page 60) as well as for reducing the risk of **atherosclerosis** (page 14).

## WHAT IS THE SCIENTIFIC EVIDENCE FOR BILBERRY?

Although bilberry is widely used by physicians in Europe based on research performed in the 1960s and earlier, all together the research into bilberry is not yet up to modern standards. However, this is an active area of research, and you can expect new information to be available soon.

### Night Vision

Two early controlled, but not double-blind, studies of bilberry found that the herb temporarily improved night vision.[7,8] However, this effect was not found to persist with continued use. A more recent double-blind placebo-controlled study on 40 healthy subjects found that a single dose of bilberry extract improved visual response for 2 hours.[9]

Visual benefits have also been reported in numerous, more recent trials, but these studies did not use a placebo control group.[10,11,12]

### Diabetic Retinopathy

A double-blind placebo-controlled trial of bilberry extract in 14 people with damage to the retina caused by diabetes and/or hypertension found significant improvements observable by ophthalmoscopic examination (looking in the eye with a machine) and angiography (examining the blood vessels).[13] However, this was a very preliminary study.

Other studies have found similar results, but they were not double-blind.[14,15]

### Cataracts

Although antioxidants in general are believed to help prevent cataracts, direct research into bilberry's effects appears to be limited to one human study that combined the herb with vitamin E.[16] The combination was effective, but whether it was the herb or the vitamin that helped most remains unclear.

### Varicose Veins

In a placebo-controlled study that followed 60 people with varicose veins (technically, venous insufficiency) for 30 days, bilberry extract resulted in a significant decrease in pain and swelling.[17] Similar results were seen in a 30-day double-blind trial involving 47 individuals.[18] Numerous other studies have yielded similarly positive results, although they did not use a placebo group.[19,20] However, there is better evidence for **horse chestnut** (page 228), **OPCs** (page 270), and **gotu kola** (page 218).

## DOSAGES

The standard dosage of bilberry is 120 to 240 mg twice daily of an extract standardized to contain 25% anthocyanosides.

## SAFETY ISSUES

Bilberry is a food and as such is quite safe. Enormous quantities have been administered to rats without toxic effects.[21,22] One study of 2,295 people given bilberry extract found a 4% incidence of side effects such as mild digestive distress, skin rashes, and drowsiness.[23] Although safety in pregnancy has not been proven, studies have enrolled pregnant women.[24] Safety in young children, nursing women, or those with severe liver or kidney disease is not known. There are no known drug interactions. Bilberry does not appear to interfere with blood clotting.[25]

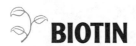

# BIOTIN

*Principal Proposed Uses*
   There are no well-documented uses for biotin.

*Other Proposed Uses*
   Diabetes, "cradle cap" in children, brittle nails

*Supplement Forms/Alternative Names*
   Biocytin (brewer's yeast–biotin complex)

**B**iotin is a water-soluble B vitamin that plays an important role in metabolizing the energy we get from food. Biotin assists four essential enzymes that break down fats, carbohydrates, and proteins.

Very preliminary evidence suggests biotin supplements may be helpful for people with diabetes.

## REQUIREMENTS/SOURCES

Although biotin is a necessary nutrient, we usually get enough from bacteria living in the digestive tract. Actual biotin deficiency is uncommon, unless you frequently eat large quantities of raw egg white. (Raw egg white contains a protein that blocks the absorption of biotin. Fortunately, cooked egg white does not present this problem.)

There is no recommended dietary allowance for biotin, but the Estimated Safe and Adequate Daily Dietary Intake is

- Infants under 6 months, 10 mcg

  6 to 12 months, 15 mcg

- Children 1 to 3 years, 20 mcg

  4 to 6 years, 25 mcg

  7 to 10 years, 30 mcg

- Adults (and children 11 years and older), 30 to 100 mcg

Good dietary sources of biotin include brewer's yeast, nutritional (torula) yeast, whole grains, nuts, egg yolks, sardines, legumes, liver, cauliflower, bananas, and mushrooms.

## THERAPEUTIC DOSAGES

For people with diabetes, the usual recommended dosage of biotin is 7,000 to 15,000 mcg daily.

For treating "cradle cap" (a scaly head rash often found in infants), the usual dosage of biotin is 6,000 mcg daily, *given to the nursing mother* (not the child). A lower dosage of 3,000 mcg daily is used to treat brittle fingernails and toenails.

## THERAPEUTIC USES

There is little hard evidence for any of the proposed uses of biotin. Highly preliminary evidence suggests that supplemental biotin can help reduce blood sugar levels in people with either type 1 (childhood onset) or type 2 (adult onset) **diabetes** (page 60).[1,2] Biotin may also reduce the symptoms of diabetic neuropathy.[3] However, other supplements often recommended for diabetes have much better evidence behind them, such as **chromium** (page 161), **lipoic acid** (page 246), and **GLA** (page 210) from evening primrose oil.

Even weaker evidence suggests that biotin supplements can promote healthy nails[4] and eliminate cradle cap.

## SAFETY ISSUES

Biotin appears to be quite safe. However, maximum safe dosages for young children, pregnant or nursing women, or those with severe liver or kidney disease have not been established.

## ⚠ INTERACTIONS YOU SHOULD KNOW ABOUT

If you are taking

- The antiseizure medications **carbamazepine** or **primidone:** Take biotin supplements at a different time of day.

- **Alcohol:** You may need extra biotin.

 # BITTER MELON (MOMORDICA CHARANTIA)

*Principal Proposed Uses*
Diabetes

Widely sold in Asian groceries as food, bitter melon is also a folk remedy for diabetes, cancer, and various infections.

## WHAT IS BITTER MELON USED FOR TODAY?

Preliminary studies appear to confirm the first of these folk uses, suggesting that bitter melon may improve blood sugar control in people with **diabetes** (page 60).[1,2] If you have diabetes, you might consider adding bitter melon to your diet, but only under a doctor's supervision (see Safety Issues). For more information on bitter melon and diabetes, see *The Natural Pharmacist Guide to Diabetes.*

Bitter melon has also been suggested as a treatment for AIDS, but the evidence thus far is too weak to even mention. There is absolutely no evidence that it can treat cancer.

## DOSAGES

The proper dosage is one small, unripe, raw melon or about 50 ml of fresh juice, each taken in 2 or 3 doses over the course of the day. The only problem is that bitter melon tastes *extremely* bitter. Noted naturopath Michael Murray suggests that you should "simply plug your nose and take a 2-ounce shot."[3]

Tinctures of bitter melon have begun to arrive on the market, which may make the herb a bit easier to swallow. Follow the directions on the label for correct dosage.

## SAFETY ISSUES

As a widely eaten food in Asia, bitter melon is generally regarded as safe. It can cause diarrhea and stomach pain if taken in excessive amounts, but the main risk of bitter melon comes from the fact that it may work! Combining it with standard drugs may reduce blood sugar too well, possibly leading to dangerously low levels. For this reason, if you already take drugs for diabetes, you should add bitter melon to your diet only with a physician's supervision. And definitely don't stop your medication and substitute bitter melon instead! It is not as powerful as insulin or other conventional treatments.

Safety in young children, pregnant or nursing women, or those with severe liver or kidney disease has not been established.

## ⚠ INTERACTIONS YOU SHOULD KNOW ABOUT

If you are taking **insulin** or other **medications to reduce blood sugar,** bitter melon might amplify the effect.[4,5,6]

# BLACK COHOSH (CIMICIFUGA RACEMOSA)

*Principal Proposed Uses*
   Menopausal symptoms

*Other Proposed Uses*
   PMS, dysmenorrhea (painful menstruation)

**B**lack cohosh is a tall perennial herb originally found in the northeastern United States. Native Americans used it primarily for women's health problems, but also as a treatment for arthritis, fatigue, and snakebite. European colonists rapidly adopted the herb for similar uses, and in the late nineteenth century, black cohosh was the principal ingredient in the wildly popular Lydia E. Pinkham's Vegetable Compound for menstrual cramps. Migrating across the Atlantic, black cohosh became a popular European treatment for women's problems, arthritis, and high blood pressure.

## WHAT IS BLACK COHOSH USED FOR TODAY?

Modern German research has found that black cohosh extracts can mimic many of the effects of estrogen. In particular, the herb appears to inhibit the pituitary hormone LH, which rises to sky-high levels in menopause.[1,2,3]

Black cohosh has been approved by Germany's Commission E for use in treating **menopause** (page 87), **dysmenorrhea** (page 65), and **PMS** (page 104). According to the results of studies, menopausal women report distinct improvements in hot flashes, sweating, headache, vertigo, heart palpitations, tinnitus, nervousness, irritability, sleep disturbance, anxiety, vaginal dryness, and depression. Black cohosh takes 4 to 6 weeks to produce its full benefits. Unfortunately, there is no evidence that black cohosh can prevent **osteoporosis** (page 100) or **heart disease** (page 14), two of estrogen's most famous benefits.

Black cohosh appears to be only mildly effective (if at all) for treating **PMS** (page 104) and **dysmenorrhea** (page 65). Some herbalists believe that black cohosh can prevent or treat mild **cervical dysplasia** (page 38), but there is no evidence whatsoever that it really works.

## WHAT IS THE SCIENTIFIC EVIDENCE FOR BLACK COHOSH?

In an open study of 629 menopausal women, standardized black cohosh extract produced significant results in approximately 80% of them.[4] However, these results are made less impressive by the fact that placebo significantly reduces menopausal symptoms in about 50% of cases.[5]

Another open study of black cohosh documented actual improvements in the cells of the vaginal wall.[6] Could the placebo effect produce changes seen by microscope? Perhaps, but it seems unlikely.

The best evidence comes from a double-blind study that followed 80 women for 12 weeks, comparing the benefits of black cohosh, conjugated estrogens (0.625 mg), and placebo.[7] According to the reported results, black cohosh was actually more effective than estrogen both in relieving symptoms and in normalizing the appearance of vaginal cells under microscopic evaluation.

However, a recent double-blind study that evaluated two different dosages of black cohosh did not find any change in vaginal-cell appearance or indeed any other objective measurements that would indicate an estrogen-like effect.[8] An animal study has also found no evidence that black cohosh works like estrogen.[9] These surprising findings have upset the apple cart, leaving us quite confused about just how black cohosh really works.

## DOSAGES

The standard dosage of black cohosh is 1 or 2 tablets twice a day of a standardized extract, manufactured to contain 1 mg of 27-deoxyacteine per tablet.

Make sure not to confuse black cohosh with blue cohosh (*Caulophyllum thalictroides*). Blue cohosh is potentially more dangerous since it contains chemicals that are toxic to the heart; a recent case report indicates that this similarly named herb caused severe heart problems in a pregnant mother.[10]

## SAFETY ISSUES

Black cohosh seldom produces any side effects other than occasional mild gastrointestinal distress. Studies in rats have found no significant toxicity when black cohosh was given at 90 times the therapeutic dosage for a period of 6 months.[11] Since 6 months in a rat corresponds to decades in a human, this study appears to make a strong statement about the long-term safety of black cohosh.

Unlike estrogen, black cohosh does not stimulate breast-cancer cells growing in a test tube.[12] However, black cohosh has not yet been subjected to large-scale studies similar to those conducted for estrogen. For this reason, safety for those with previous breast cancer is not known. Also, because of hormonal activity, black cohosh is not recommended for adolescents or pregnant or nursing women.

Black cohosh has been found to slightly lower blood pressure and blood sugar in certain animals.[13] For this reason, it's possible that the herb could interact with drugs for high blood pressure or diabetes, but there are no reports of any such problems. Safety in young children, or those with severe liver or kidney disease is not known.

## COMBINING BLACK COHOSH WITH ERT

Some women on estrogen-replacement therapy (ERT) choose to take extremely low doses of estrogen (in the 0.312 mg range), hoping to somewhat alleviate the risk of ostcoporosis without increasing the potential for breast cancer. Although there are no studies to tell us whether this will work, it is certainly a logical idea, and some gynecologists endorse it.

However, such a low dose of estrogen may not completely stop symptoms such as hot flashes. Black cohosh has been suggested as an addition to improve symptom control. While this technique has not been studied, it is again a logical idea that is probably safe (but don't ask me to guarantee it!).

## TRANSITIONING FROM ERT TO BLACK COHOSH

Each woman is unique, but in general, many women successfully switch over from 0.625 mg of daily estrogen to the standard dosage of black cohosh without developing symptoms. However, transitioning from higher dosages of estrogen will frequently result in breakthrough hot flashes and other symptoms. Again, remember that black cohosh is not known to offer protection against cardiovascular disease and osteoporosis.

# BLOODROOT (SANGUINARIA CANADENSIS)

### Principal Proposed Uses

*Oral uses:*
   Periodontal disease prevention (used as a toothpaste or mouthwash)

*Topical uses:*
   Warts

*Internal uses:*
   Respiratory illnesses

**B**loodroot is a perennial flowering herb that was widely used by Native Americans both as a reddish-orange dye and as a medicine. Some tribes drank bloodroot tea as a treatment for sore throats, fevers, and joint pain, while others applied the somewhat caustic sap to skin cancers. European herbalists used bloodroot to treat respiratory infections, asthma, joint pain, warts, ringworm, and nasal polyps.

In the mid-1800s, a Dr. Fells of Middlesex Hospital in London developed a cancer treatment consisting of a paste of bloodroot, flour, water, and zinc chloride applied directly to breast tumors and other cancers. Similar formulations were used in various locales up through the turn of the century. Bloodroot was a common constituent of "drawing salves" believed capable of "pulling" tumors out of the body.

## WHAT IS BLOODROOT USED FOR TODAY?

Herbalists frequently recommend bloodroot pastes and salves for the treatment of warts. Bloodroot is an *escharotic,* that is to say a scab-producing substance, and it functions much like commercial wart plasters containing salicylic acid. Although there has not been any real scientific study of the use of bloodroot for warts, based on its immediate effects it is likely to help at least somewhat.

One constituent of bloodroot, sanguinarine, appears to possess topical antibiotic properties.[1] On this basis, the FDA has approved the use of bloodroot in commercially available toothpastes and oral rinses to inhibit the development of dental plaque and **periodontal disease** (page 103) (gingivitis).

Bloodroot is also often combined with other herbs in cough syrups. Some herbalists recommend drinking bloodroot tea for respiratory ailments, but others consider the herb to be too unpredictable in its side effects.

While scientific research has found constituents in bloodroot that possess antitumor properties,[2] there is no evidence that the herb can cure cancer. Undoubtedly bloodroot pastes can nibble away at tumors the same way they dissolve warts. However, such an approach is not likely to cure a malignant tumor, and might actually spread it.

## DOSAGES

For the treatment of warts, bloodroot can be made into a paste and applied directly to the involved area. However, start slowly to see how sensitive you are. Excessive application can lead to severe burns. Once you've discovered your tolerance, apply the herb for a day or so, then remove it and wait for the scab to develop and then

drop off. This process can be repeated until the wart is gone.

Bloodroot tea for treating respiratory illnesses may be made by boiling 1 teaspoon of powdered root in a cup of water and taken 2 or 3 times daily.

## SAFETY ISSUES

Oral bloodroot appears to be relatively safe and nontoxic.[3] However, in large doses, it causes nausea and vomiting, and even at lower dosages it has been known to cause peculiar side effects in some people, such as tunnel vision and pain in the feet. For this reason, many herbalists recommend that it be used only under the supervision of a qualified practitioner.

Topical applications of bloodroot can cause severe burns if used too vigorously and for too long a time. There are also concerns that bloodroot should not be used during pregnancy.[4] Safety in young children, nursing women, or those with severe liver or kidney disease has also not been established.

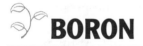 # BORON

Boron

*Principal Proposed Uses*
Osteoarthritis

*Other Proposed Uses*
Osteoporosis, rheumatoid arthritis

*Supplemental Forms/Alternative Names*
Boron chelate, sodium borate

**P**lants need boron for proper health, but it's not known whether humans do. However, boron does seem to assist in the proper absorption of **calcium** (page 146), **magnesium** (page 251), and phosphorus from foods and slows the loss of these minerals through urination. Very preliminary evidence suggests that boron may be helpful for arthritis and osteoporosis.

## SOURCES

No dietary or nutritional requirement for boron has been established, and boron deficiency is not

known to cause any disease. Good sources include leafy vegetables, raisins, prunes, nuts, noncitrus fruits, and grains. A typical American daily diet provides 1.5 to 3 mg of boron.

## THERAPEUTIC DOSAGES

When used as a treatment for arthritis or osteoporosis, boron is often recommended at a dosage of 3 mg per day, an amount similar to the average daily intake from food. However, food sources may be safer (see Safety Issues).

## THERAPEUTIC USES

Although boron is often added to supplements intended for the treatment of **osteoarthritis** (page 95), the evidence that it helps is very weak.[1,2,3] Three other supplements—**glucosamine** (page 213), **chondroitin** (page 159), and **SAMe** (page 293)—are much better-researched treatments for osteoarthritis.

Boron has also been suggested as a treatment for **osteoporosis** (page 100).[4] Other treatments for preventing or even reversing osteoporosis include **isoflavones** (page 236), **calcium** (page 146), and **vitamin D** (page 335).

Finally, boron is sometimes recommended as a treatment for **rheumatoid arthritis** (page 109), but there is no real evidence that it works.

## WHAT IS THE SCIENTIFIC EVIDENCE FOR BORON?

### Osteoarthritis

In areas of the world where people eat relatively high amounts of boron—between 3 and 10 mg per day—the incidence of osteoarthritis is below 10%. However, in regions where there is less boron in the diet—1 mg or less per day—the incidence of arthritis is higher.[5] This observation has given rise to the theory that boron supplements might be helpful for people who already have arthritis symptoms.

However, the only direct evidence we have comes from one preliminary study, which suggests that boron supplements may reduce symptoms of osteoarthritis. Unfortunately, too many participants dropped out of this already very small study for the results to mean much.[6,7]

### Osteoporosis

In one small study, 13 postmenopausal women were first fed a diet that provided 0.25 mg of boron for 119 days; then they were fed the same diet with a boron supplement of 3 mg daily for 48 days.[8] The results revealed that boron supplementation reduced the amount of calcium lost in the urine. This suggests (but certainly doesn't prove) that boron can help prevent osteoporosis. A more recent study failed to support this finding.[9]

## SAFETY ISSUES

Since the therapeutic dosage of boron is about the same as the amount you can get from food, it is probably fairly safe. Unpleasant side effects, including nausea and vomiting, are only reported at about 50 times the highest recommended dose.

One potential concern with boron regards its effect on hormones. In at least two small studies, boron was found to increase levels of estrogen and testosterone, especially in women on estrogen-replacement therapy.[10,11] Because elevated estrogen increases the risk of breast and uterine cancer in women past menopause, this may be a matter of concern for those who wish to take supplemental boron. Further research is necessary to discover whether boron's apparent effects on estrogen is a real problem or not. At the present time, we would recommend getting your boron from fruits and vegetables: We know that they do not increase cancer risk (they reduce it).

## ⚠ INTERACTIONS YOU SHOULD KNOW ABOUT

If you are receiving **hormone-replacement therapy,** use of boron may not be advisable due to the risk of elevating estrogen levels excessively.

# BOSWELLIA (BOSWELLIA SERRATA)

## Principal Proposed Uses
Rheumatoid arthritis, osteoarthritis, bursitis, tendinitis

The gummy resin of the boswellia tree has a long history of use in Indian herbal medicine as a treatment for arthritis, bursitis, respiratory diseases, and diarrhea.

## WHAT IS BOSWELLIA USED FOR TODAY?

Boswellia is often recommended as a treatment for bursitis, tendinitis, **osteoarthritis** (page 95), and **rheumatoid arthritis** (page 109), based on the recent work of Indian scientists. Investigations of boswellia have shown that the herb contains certain substances known as *boswellic acids*, which appear to possess anti-inflammatory properties.[1,2] Other preliminary research suggests that boswellia may improve the biochemical structure of cartilage.[3]

## WHAT IS THE SCIENTIFIC EVIDENCE FOR BOSWELLIA?

According to a recent review of unpublished studies, preliminary double-blind trials have found boswellia effective in relieving the symptoms of rheumatoid arthritis.[4] Two placebo-controlled studies, involving a total of 81 individuals with rheumatoid arthritis, found significant reductions in swelling and pain over the course of 3 months.

Also, a comparative study of 60 people over 6 months found that boswellia extract produced symptomatic benefits comparable to oral gold therapy. However, this review was rather sketchy on details. It did not state whether or not boswellia could induce remission like gold shots, and not enough information was given to evaluate the quality of the research.

However, a recent double-blind placebo-controlled study that enrolled 78 patients found no benefit.[5] About half of the patients dropped out, which diminishes the significance of the results.

There has not been any formal study of boswellia's effectiveness in osteoarthritis.

## DOSAGES

A typical dose of boswellia is 400 mg 3 times a day of an extract standardized to contain 37.5% boswellic acids. The full effect may take 4 to 8 weeks to develop.

## SAFETY ISSUES

Although comprehensive safety testing has not been completed, boswellia appears to be reasonably safe when used as directed. Side effects are rare and consist primarily of occasional allergic reactions or mild gastrointestinal distress. Safety in young children, pregnant or nursing women, or those with severe liver or kidney disease has not been established.

# BROMELAIN (PINEAPPLE STEM)

*Principal Proposed Uses*
   Reducing swelling and inflammation (e.g., recovery after surgery or athletic injuries, vein inflammation, arthritis, dysmenorrhea)
   Digestive problems (e.g., "weak" digestion, food allergies)

*Other Proposed Uses*
   Gout, hemorrhoids

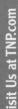
**B**romelain is not actually a single substance, but rather a collection of protein-digesting enzymes found in pineapple juice and in the stem of pineapple plants. It is primarily produced in Japan, Hawaii, and Taiwan, and much of the original research was performed in the first two of those locations. Subsequently, European researchers developed an interest, and by 1995 bromelain had become the thirteenth most common individual herbal product sold in Germany.

## WHAT IS BROMELAIN USED FOR TODAY?

In 1993, Germany's Commission E approved bromelain for "reducing swelling in the nose and sinuses caused by injuries and operations." The reason for this narrow recommendation is that when the commissioners reviewed the available evidence the only reliable studies they could find involved these specific conditions. However, bromelain is actually thought to be useful for other conditions as well, based on its apparent ability to reduce swelling and inflammation. In Europe, bromelain is widely used to aid in recovery from surgery and athletic injuries, as well as to treat **hemorrhoids** (page 70), other diseases of the veins, **osteoarthritis** (page 95), **rheumatoid arthritis** (page 109), **gout** (page 69), and **dysmenorrhea** (page 65) (menstrual pain).

Bromelain is also useful as a digestive enzyme. Unlike most digestive enzymes, bromelain is active both in the acid environment of the stomach and the alkaline environment of the small intestine.[1,2] This may make it particularly effective as an oral digestive aid for those who do not digest proteins properly. Since it is primarily the proteins in foods that cause food allergies, bromelain might reduce food-allergy symptoms as well, although this has not been proven.

## WHAT IS THE SCIENTIFIC EVIDENCE FOR BROMELAIN?

While most large enzymes are broken down in the digestive tract, those found in bromelain appear to be absorbed whole to a certain extent.[3] This finding makes it reasonable to suppose that bromelain can actually produce systemic (whole body) effects. Once in the blood, bromelain appears to produce mild anti-inflammatory and "blood-thinning" effects.[4–7]

In 1993, Germany's Commission E reviewed the evidence for bromelain's effectiveness in reducing the swelling caused by injury or surgery. They found five passable double-blind studies, of which three showed good results and two showed no benefit.[8] In their opinion, the best evidence was for swelling in the nose and sinuses.

Another double-blind study followed 73 people being treated for phlebitis, or inflammation of the veins of the leg.[9] Those who received bromelain in addition to standard treatments showed improved results.

**Warning:** Do not attempt to self-treat phlebitis.

A somewhat informal controlled study of 146 boxers suggested that bromelain helps bruises to heal more quickly.[10]

## DOSAGES

A typical dosage of bromelain is 500 mg 3 times daily between meals, or with meals for use as a digestive aid. The strength of bromelain is measured in MCUs (milk-clotting units). A good preparation should contain 2,000 MCUs per gram.

## SAFETY ISSUES

Bromelain appears to be essentially nontoxic, and it seldom causes side effects other than occasional mild gastrointestinal distress or allergic reactions.[11]

However, because bromelain "thins the blood" to some extent, it shouldn't be combined with drugs such as Coumadin (warfarin) without a doctor's supervision.

Safety in young children, pregnant or nursing women, or those with liver or kidney disease has not been established.

## ⚠ INTERACTIONS YOU SHOULD KNOW ABOUT

If you are taking strong anticoagulants such as **Coumadin (warfarin)** or **heparin,** bromelain might amplify their effect.

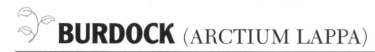

# BURDOCK (ARCTIUM LAPPA)

*Principal Proposed Uses*
Eczema, psoriasis, acne

*Other Proposed Uses*
Cancer?, rheumatoid arthritis

The common burdock, that well-known source of annoying burrs matted in dogs' fur, is also a medicinal herb of considerable reputation. Called *gobo* in Japan, burdock root is said to be a food that provides deep strengthening to the immune system. In ancient China and India, herbalists used it in the treatment of respiratory infections, abscesses, and joint pain. European physicians of the Middle Ages and later used it to treat cancerous tumors, skin conditions, venereal disease, and bladder and kidney problems.

Burdock was a primary ingredient in the famous (or infamous) Hoxsey cancer treatment. Harry Hoxsey was a former coal miner who parlayed a traditional family remedy for cancer into the largest privately owned cancer treatment center in the world, with branches in 17 states. (It was shut down in the 1950s by the FDA. Harry Hoxsey himself subsequently died of cancer.) Other herbs in his formula included **red clover** (page 290), poke, prickly ash, **bloodroot** (page 140), and barberry. Burdock is also found in the famous herbal cancer remedy Essiac.

Despite this historical enthusiasm, there is no significant evidence that burdock is an effective treatment for cancer or any other illness.

## WHAT IS BURDOCK USED FOR TODAY?

Burdock is widely recommended for the relief of dry, scaly skin conditions such as **eczema** (page 66) and **psoriasis** (page 106). It is also used for treating **acne** (page 2). It can be taken internally as well as applied directly to the skin. Burdock is sometimes recommended for **rheumatoid arthritis** (page 109). Unfortunately, there is as yet no real scientific evidence for any of these uses.

## DOSAGES

A typical dosage of burdock is 1 to 2 g of powdered dry root 3 times per day.

## SAFETY ISSUES

As a food commonly eaten in Japan (it is often found in sukiyaki), burdock root is believed to be safe. However, in 1978, the *Journal of the American Medical Association* caused a brief scare by publishing a report of burdock poisoning. Subsequent investigation showed that the herbal product involved was actually contaminated with the poisonous chemical atropine from an unknown source.[1] Safety in young children, pregnant or nursing women, or those with severe liver or kidney disease is not established.

## ⚠ INTERACTIONS YOU SHOULD KNOW ABOUT

If you are taking **insulin,** it is possible that burdock will increase its effect.[2]

# BUTCHER'S BROOM (RUSCUS ACULEATUS)

*Principal Proposed Uses*
  Hemorrhoids, varicose veins

So-named because its branches were a traditional source of broom straw used by butchers, this Mediterranean evergreen bush has a long history of traditional use in the treatment of urinary conditions.

## WHAT IS BUTCHER'S BROOM USED FOR TODAY?

Butcher's broom has been approved by Germany's Commission E as supportive therapy for **hemorrhoids** (page 70) and **varicose veins** (page 113).

Preliminary evidence from animal studies suggests that butcher's broom possesses anti-inflammatory properties and also constricts small veins.[1,2] Double-blind studies in people have not yet been reported.

## DOSAGES

Butcher's broom is standardized to its *ruscogenin* content. A typical oral dose should supply 50 to 100 mg of ruscogenins daily.

For hemorrhoids, butcher's broom can also be applied as an ointment or in the form of a suppository.

## SAFETY ISSUES

Butcher's broom is believed to be safe when used as directed, although detailed studies have not been performed. Noticeable side effects appear to be rare. Safety in young children, pregnant or nursing women, or those with liver or kidney disease has not been established.

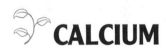

# CALCIUM

*Principal Proposed Uses*
  Osteoporosis, premenstrual syndrome (PMS)

*Other Proposed Uses*
  Colon polyps and cancer prevention, hypertension (high blood pressure), high cholesterol, preeclampsia, attention deficit disorder, migraine headaches, periodontal disease

*Supplement Forms/Alternative Names*
  Calcium carbonate, dolomite, oyster shell calcium, bonemeal, calcium citrate, calcium citrate malate, tricalcium phosphate, calcium lactate, calcium gluconate, calcium aspartate, calcium orotate, calcium chelate

Calcium is the most abundant mineral in the body, making up nearly 2% of total body weight. More than 99% of the calcium in your body is found in your bones, but the other 1% is perhaps just as important for good health. Many enzymes depend on calcium in order to work properly, as do your nerves, heart, and blood-clotting mechanisms.

To build bone, you need to have enough calcium in your diet. But in spite of calcium-fortified orange juice and the best efforts of the dairy industry, most Americans are calcium-deficient.[1] Calcium supplements are a simple way to make sure you're getting enough of this important mineral.

One of the most important uses of calcium is to prevent and treat osteoporosis, the progressive loss of bone mass to which postmenopausal women are especially vulnerable. Calcium works best when combined with vitamin D.

Recent evidence suggests that calcium may have another important use: dramatically reducing PMS symptoms.

## REQUIREMENTS/SOURCES

Although there are some variations between recommendations issued by different groups, a reasonable daily intake for calcium is as follows

- Infants under 6 months, 210 mg
  6 to 12 months, 270 mg

- Children 1 to 3 years, 500 mg
  4 to 8 years, 800 mg

- Males and females 9 to 18 years, 1,300 mg
  19 to 50 years, 1,000 mg
  51 years and older, 1,200 mg

- Pregnant women 18 years and younger,
    1,300 mg
  19 years and older, 1,000 mg

- Nursing women 18 years and younger, 1,300 mg
  19 years and older, 1,000 mg

To absorb calcium, your body also needs an adequate level of vitamin D.

Milk, cheese, and other dairy products are excellent sources of calcium. Other good sources include orange juice or soy milk fortified with calcium, fish canned with its bones (e.g., sardines), dark green vegetables, nuts and seeds, and calcium-processed tofu.

If you wish to use calcium supplements, there are many forms available, each with its pros and cons. The most important ones include naturally derived forms of calcium, refined calcium carbonate, and chelated calcium.

## Naturally Derived Forms of Calcium

These forms of calcium come from bone, shells, or the earth: bonemeal, oyster shell, and dolomite. Animals concentrate calcium in their shells, and calcium is found in minerals in the earth. These forms of calcium are economical, and you can get as much as 500 to 600 mg in one tablet. However, there are concerns that the natural forms of calcium supplements may contain significant amounts of lead.[2] Calcium supplements rarely list the lead content of their source, although they should. The lead concentration should always be less than 2 parts per million.

## Refined Calcium Carbonate

This is the most common commercial calcium supplement, and it is also used as a common antacid. Calcium carbonate is one of the least expensive forms of calcium, but it can cause constipation and bloating, and it may not be well absorbed by people with reduced levels of stomach acid. Taking it with meals improves absorption, because stomach acid is released to digest the food.

## Chelated Calcium

Chelated calcium is calcium bound to an organic acid (citrate, citrate malate, lactate, gluconate, aspartate, or orotate). The chelated forms of calcium offer some significant advantages and disadvantages compared with calcium carbonate.

On the plus side, they are well absorbed regardless of stomach acid and may be more helpful than calcium carbonate for osteoporosis.[3,4,5] On the negative side, chelated calcium is much more expensive and bulkier than calcium carbonate. In other words, you have to take more and larger pills to get enough calcium. It is not at all uncommon to need to take five or six large capsules daily to supply the necessary amount, a quantity some people may find troublesome.

The form of calcium found in beverages is usually the chelated form, calcium citrate malate, or a slightly less well-absorbed form, tricalcium phosphate.

## THERAPEUTIC DOSAGES

Unlike some supplements described in this book, calcium is not taken at extra high doses for

Calcium

Visit Us at TNP.com

special therapeutic benefit. Rather, for all its uses it should be taken in the amounts listed under Requirements/Sources, along with the recommended level of **vitamin D** (page 335) (see the chapter on vitamin D for the proper dosage amounts).

Calcium absorption studies have found that the more calcium you take at one time, the less fully it is absorbed. Therefore, it is most efficient to take your total daily calcium in two or more doses.

It isn't possible to put all the calcium you need in a single multivitamin/mineral tablet, so this is one supplement that should be taken on its own.

Furthermore, calcium may interfere with the absorption of **chromium** (page 161), **manganese** (page 254), **zinc** (page 348), and **magnesium** (page 251).[6–9] This is a potential problem, as magnesium is commonly deficient in the American diet, and we don't need to lower its level further. The answer? Make sure to get enough magnesium in your diet. Also, if you take any of these supplements, it is best to do so at a different time from when you take calcium. This means that it is best to take your multivitamin and mineral pill at a separate time from your calcium supplement.

Calcium may also interfere with **iron** (page 234) absorption.[10,11] However, you shouldn't take extra iron unless you know you are deficient.

## THERAPEUTIC USES

There is little doubt that calcium supplementation is useful in helping prevent and slow down **osteoporosis** (page 100).[12–17] If you are a woman past menopause, this is true whether or not you are taking estrogen. Calcium supplements work best when combined with vitamin D.

A new and rather surprising use of calcium came to light recently when a recent large, well-designed study found that calcium is an effective treatment for **PMS (premenstrual syndrome)** (page 104).[18] Calcium supplementation reduced all major symptoms, including headache, food cravings, moodiness, and fluid retention. The benefits were so impressive that calcium should probably be considered the foremost treatment for PMS.

There may actually be a connection between these two uses of calcium: PMS may be an early sign of future osteoporosis.[19,20]

Recent evidence suggests that getting enough calcium may reduce the risk of developing colon **cancer** (page 26) and colon polyps, a precancerous condition.[21]

Calcium deficiency appears to mildly increase blood pressure levels,[22,23] so if you have **hypertension** (page 75), you should definitely make sure you get enough calcium.

Supplemental calcium appears to reduce total and LDL **cholesterol** (page 39) by about 4% and raise HDL cholesterol by a similar amount.[24]

Calcium is also sometimes recommended for **attention deficit disorder** (page 19), **migraine headaches** (page 89), and **periodontal disease** (page 103), but there is as yet little to no evidence that it is effective.

Finally, calcium has been proposed as a treatment to prevent preeclampsia (a dangerous condition that can develop during pregnancy). However, a recent very large and well-designed study found it to be ineffective.[25]

## WHAT IS THE SCIENTIFIC EVIDENCE FOR CALCIUM?

### Osteoporosis

Numerous studies indicate that calcium supplements are useful in preventing and slowing osteoporosis, the progressive loss of bone mass as we age. Calcium supplementation at the recommended dosages appears to reduce bone loss in postmenopausal women in every part of the body except the spine.[26,27] When vitamin D is taken along with calcium, it may be possible not only to slow down but actually reverse osteoporosis, in the spine as well as in other bones.[28]

If you are taking estrogen to keep your bones strong, additional calcium will provide even more benefit.[29,30] Finally, calcium supplementation is useful for adolescent girls as a way to "put calcium in the bank"—building up a supply for the future.[31]

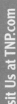

## Premenstrual Syndrome (PMS)

According to a large and well-designed study published in a 1998 issue of *American Journal of Obstetrics and Gynecology,* calcium supplements are a simple and effective treatment for a wide variety of PMS symptoms.[32] In a double-blind placebo-controlled study of 497 women, 1,200 mg daily of calcium as calcium carbonate reduced PMS symptoms by half over a period of three menstrual cycles. These symptoms included mood swings, headaches, food cravings, and bloating. These results corroborate earlier, smaller studies.[33,34]

## Colon Cancer

Recent evidence suggests that the use of calcium carbonate can inhibit the development of precancerous polyps in the colon and rectum. A double-blind placebo-controlled study followed 832 individuals with a history of polyps for 4 years.[35] Participants received either 3 g daily of calcium carbonate or placebo. The calcium group experienced 24% fewer polyps overall than the placebo group.

There is also evidence from observational studies that a high calcium intake is associated with a reduced incidence of colon cancer.[36]

## SAFETY ISSUES

In general, it's safe to take up to 2,000 mg of calcium daily, although this is more than you need.[37] Greatly excessive intake of calcium can cause numerous side effects, including dangerous or painful deposits of calcium within the body.

If you have cancer, hyperparathyroidism, or sarcoidosis, you should take calcium only under a physician's supervision.

People with kidney stones or a history of kidney stones are also often warned not to take supplemental calcium. The reason for this caution is that kidney stones are commonly made of calcium oxalate crystals. However, while calcium supplements might increase kidney stone risk, higher intake of calcium from food might actually reduce the risk.[38,39] If you have a history of kidney stones, consult your physician before taking calcium supplements.

## ⚠ INTERACTIONS YOU SHOULD KNOW ABOUT

If you are taking

- **Corticosteroids, colchicine, heparin, aluminum hydroxide, digoxin, methotrexate** or **phenobarbital:** You may need more calcium.

- **Dilantin (phenytoin):** You may need more calcium; however, you should take it at a different time of day because they interfere with each other's absorption.

- **Antibiotics** in the tetracycline or quinolone **(Cipro, Floxin, Noroxin)** family: Take calcium at a different time of day, because again it interferes with the medications' absorption (and vice versa).

- **Thiazide diuretics, calcium channel-blockers,** or **atenolol:** Do not take extra calcium except on the advice of a physician.

- **Drugs that reduce stomach acid,** such as **Zantac (ranitidine)** or **Prilosec (omeprazole):** You may not be able to absorb calcium carbonate well. You should use a different type of calcium supplement.

- **Calcium:** You may need extra manganese, chromium, zinc, and magnesium. Ideally, take calcium at a different time of day from these minerals, because they interfere with each other's absorption. You may also need extra iron, but don't take iron supplements unless you know that you are iron deficient.

- **Soy:** A constituent of soy called phytic acid can interfere with the absorption of calcium, so take calcium supplements at a different time of day.

Calcium

Visit Us at TNP.com

# CALENDULA A.K.A. MARIGOLD
### (CALENDULA OFFICINALIS)

*Principal Proposed Uses*

*Topical uses:*
    Skin injuries (e.g., cuts, scrapes, burns, nonhealing wounds), skin inflammation (e.g., eczema), hemorrhoids, varicose veins
*Oral uses:*
    Mouth sores

Calendula, well known as one of the ornamental marigolds, blooms month after month from early spring to first frost. Because "calend" means month in Latin, the plant's lengthy flowering season is believed to have given calendula its name. The herb has been used to heal wounds and treat inflamed skin since ancient times.

An active ingredient that might be responsible for calendula's traditional medicinal properties has not been discovered. One theory suggests that volatile oils in the plant act synergistically with other constituents called *xanthophylls*.[1]

## WHAT IS CALENDULA USED FOR TODAY?

Experiments on rats and other animals suggest that calendula cream exerts a wound-healing and anti-inflammatory effect,[2,3] but double-blind studies have not yet been reported.

Creams made with calendula flower are a nearly ubiquitous item in the German medicine chest, used for everything from children's scrapes to **eczema** (page 66), burns, and poorly healing wounds. These same German products are widely available in the United States as well.

Calendula cream is also used to soothe **hemorrhoids** (page 70) and **varicose veins** (page 113), and the tea reportedly reduces the discomfort of mouth sores. However, as yet there is no scientific evidence for these uses.

## DOSAGES

Calendula cream should be applied 2 or 3 times daily to the affected area. For oral use as a mouthwash, pour boiling water over 1 to 2 teaspoons of calendula flowers and allow to steep for 10 to 15 minutes. Rinse your mouth with this liquid several times a day.

## SAFETY ISSUES

Calendula is generally regarded as safe. Neither calendula cream nor calendula taken internally has been associated with any adverse effects other than occasional allergic reactions.

## ⚠ INTERACTIONS YOU SHOULD KNOW ABOUT

If you are taking **sleeping pills** or **antianxiety drugs,** calendula might increase the sedative effect.[4]

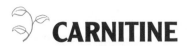 **CARNITINE**

## Principal Proposed Uses

Angina and other heart conditions, intermittent claudication, Alzheimer's disease

## Other Proposed Uses

High cholesterol, performance enhancement, irregular heartbeat, Down's syndrome, muscular dystrophy, impaired sperm motility, chronic obstructive pulmonary disease (emphysema, chronic bronchitis), alcoholic fatty liver disease, toxicity due to AZT (a drug used to treat AIDS)

## Supplement Forms/Alternative Names

L-carnitine, L-acetyl-carnitine (LAC, ALC, acetyl-L-carnitine), L-propionyl-carnitine

Carnitine is an amino acid the body uses to turn fat into energy. It is not normally considered an essential nutrient, because the body can manufacture all it needs. However, supplemental carnitine may improve the ability of certain tissues to produce energy. This effect has led to the use of carnitine in various muscle diseases as well as heart conditions.

## SOURCES

There is no dietary requirement for carnitine. However, a few individuals have a genetic defect that hinders the body's ability to make carnitine. In addition, diseases of the liver, kidneys, or brain may inhibit carnitine production. Certain medications, especially the antiseizure drugs Depakene (valproic acid), and Dilantin (phenytoin), may reduce carnitine levels; however, whether taking extra carnitine would be helpful has not been determined.[1,2,3] Heart muscle tissue, because of its high energy requirements, is particularly vulnerable to carnitine deficiency.

The principal dietary sources of carnitine are meat and dairy products, but to obtain therapeutic dosages a supplement is necessary.

## THERAPEUTIC DOSAGES

Typical dosages for the diseases described here range from 500 to 1,000 mg 3 times daily. Carnitine is taken in three forms: L-carnitine (for heart and other conditions), L-propionyl-carnitine (for heart conditions), and acetyl-L-carnitine

(for Alzheimer's disease). The dosage is the same for all three forms.

## THERAPEUTIC USES

Carnitine is primarily used for heart-related conditions. Fairly good evidence suggests that it can be used along with conventional treatment for **angina** (page 7), or chest pain, to improve symptoms and reduce medication needs.[4–9] When combined with conventional therapy, it may also reduce mortality after a heart attack.[10,11]

Lesser evidence suggests that it may be helpful for pain in the legs after walking due to narrowing of the arteries known as **intermittent claudication** (page 83)[12–20] as well as **congestive heart failure** (page 50).[21–24] Also a few studies suggest that carnitine may be useful for **cardiomyopathy** (page 36).[25,26]

**Warning:** You should not attempt to self-treat any of these serious medical conditions, nor should you use carnitine as a substitute for standard heart drugs.

Evidence also suggests that one particular form of carnitine, L-acetyl-carnitine, may be helpful in **Alzheimer's disease** (page 4),[27–35] although a recent large study found no benefit.[36]

Weak evidence suggests that carnitine may be able to improve **cholesterol** (page 39) and triglyceride levels.[37]

Carnitine is widely touted as a physical performance enhancer, but there is no real evidence that it is effective, and some research indicates that it does not work.[38] Little to no evidence supports other claimed benefits such as treating

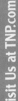

irregular heartbeat, Down's syndrome, muscular dystrophy, impaired sperm motility, chronic obstructive pulmonary disease (emphysema or chronic bronchitis), alcoholic fatty liver disease, and the toxicity of AZT (a drug used to treat AIDS).

## WHAT IS THE SCIENTIFIC EVIDENCE FOR CARNITINE?

### Angina (Chest Pain)

Carnitine might be a good addition to standard therapy for angina. In one double-blind study, 200 individuals with angina (the exercise-induced variety) took either 2 g daily of L-carnitine or placebo. All the study participants continued to take their usual medication for angina. Those taking carnitine showed improvement in several measures of heart function, including a significantly greater ability to exercise without chest pain.[39] They were also able to reduce the dosage of some of their heart medications (under medical supervision) as their symptoms decreased. Similarly positive results were seen in another double-blind trial.[40]

Other studies using L-propionyl-carnitine have shown similar or possibly even greater benefits.[41–44]

### Intermittent Claudication

People with advanced hardening of the arteries, or **atherosclerosis** (page 14), often have difficulty walking due to lack of blood flow to the legs. Pain may develop after walking less than half a block. Although carnitine does not increase blood flow, it appears to improve the muscle's ability to function under difficult circumstances. In a double-blind study of 245 individuals with intermittent claudication, those treated with 2 g daily of L-propionyl-carnitine showed a 73% improvement in walking distance.[45] This result is not quite as good as it sounds, because there was a 46% improvement with placebo (the power of suggestion is always amazing!), but it was nonetheless significant.

Similar results have been seen in most but not all other studies.[46–53] Interestingly, nearly all the studies on carnitine for this condition have been performed by one investigator. L-propionyl-carnitine seems to be more effective for intermittent claudication than plain carnitine.

For another approach, see the discussion of inositol hexaniacinate in the chapter on **vitamin B₃** (page 323) as well as the chapter on **ginkgo** (page 204).

### Congestive Heart Failure

Several small studies have found that carnitine, often in the form of L-propionyl-carnitine, can improve symptoms of congestive heart failure.[54–57] However, there is better evidence for coenzyme $Q_{10}$ for treating this condition.

### After a Heart Attack

Carnitine may help reduce death rate after a heart attack. In a 12-month, placebo-controlled study, 160 individuals who had experienced a heart attack received 4 g of L-carnitine daily or placebo, in addition to other conventional medication. The mortality rate in the treated group was significantly lower than in the placebo group, 1.2% versus 12.5%, respectively. There were also improvements in heart rate, blood pressure, angina (chest pain), and blood lipids.[58] A larger double-blind study of 472 people found that carnitine may improve the chances of survival if given within 24 hours after a heart attack.[59]

**Note:** Carnitine is used along with conventional treatment, not as a substitute for it.

### Alzheimer's Disease

Numerous double- or single-blind clinical studies involving a total of more than 1,400 people have evaluated the potential benefits of acetyl-L-carnitine in the treatment of Alzheimer's disease and other forms of dementia.[60–71] Most have found at least mildly positive results. However, the benefits are slight at best, and one of the best studies found no benefit.

For example, one double-blind trial followed 130 individuals with mild to moderate Alzheimer's disease for 1 full year.[72] All participants worsened over that time, but according to 14 different measurements of mental function and behavior, the treated group deteriorated more slowly. However, the difference was not very large, and it was only statistically significant for a few of the rating scales used.

Some studies, however, have not found any benefit. In particular, a recent double-blind placebo-controlled trial that enrolled 431 participants for 1 year found no significant improvement at all in the group treated with acetyl-L-carnitine.[73]

The most likely explanation for the negative outcome in this well-designed study is that acetyl-L-carnitine produces only a small benefit at most.

## Performance Enhancement

A 1996 review of clinical studies concluded that no scientific basis exists for the belief that carnitine supplements enhance athletic performance.[74] A few studies have found some benefit, but most have not.

## SAFETY ISSUES

L-carnitine in its three forms appears to be safe, even when taken with medications. Individuals should take care, however, not to use forms of the supplement known as "D-carnitine" or "DL-carnitine," as these can cause angina, muscle pain and loss of muscle function (probably by interfering with L-carnitine).

The maximum safe dosages for young children, pregnant or nursing women, or those with severe liver or kidney disease have not been established.

## ⚠ INTERACTIONS YOU SHOULD KNOW ABOUT

If you are taking **antiseizure medications,** particularly **valproic acid (Depakote, Depakene),** but also **phenytoin (Dilantin),** you may need extra carnitine.

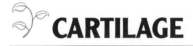

# CARTILAGE

*Principal Proposed Uses*
 There are no well-documented uses for cartilage.

*Other Proposed Uses*
 Cancer treatment, osteoarthritis, rheumatoid arthritis

*Supplement Forms/Alternative Names*
 Shark cartilage, bovine cartilage

---

Cartilage is a tough connective tissue found in many parts of the body. Your ears and nose are made from cartilage, and so is the gliding surface in your joints.

One constituent of cartilage, chondroitin, is widely used in Europe to treat arthritis. Cartilage itself has also been proposed as a treatment for arthritis.

The most commonly used forms of cartilage come from cows (bovine cartilage) and sharks.

Shark cartilage contains chemical compounds that prevent new blood vessel growth in test-tube experiments. Because cancers must create new blood vessels to feed them, shark cartilage has been touted as a cure for cancer. However, there is no direct evidence that it works.

## SOURCES

Unless your uncle works at a slaughterhouse or you're brave enough to prepare your own cartilage from whole sharks, the preferred source of cartilage is your health food store or pharmacy, where you can purchase this supplement in pill or powdered form.

## THERAPEUTIC DOSAGES

Various doses of cartilage have been used in different studies, ranging from 2.5 mg to 60 g daily.

## THERAPEUTIC USES

Cartilage has been proposed as a treatment for the common "wear and tear" type of arthritis known as **osteoarthritis** (page 95). The idea behind this is straightforward: Because osteoarthritis is a disease of the joints, and because cartilage is one of the elements that make up your joints, adding cartilage to the diet might help. This idea sounds a bit too simplistic to be real, but it is the same principle behind the use of **glucosamine** (page 213) and **chondroitin** (page 159) for osteoarthritis, specific substances found in the joints. Since double-blind studies have found those treatments effective, perhaps cartilage itself will ultimately be proven to work. However, studies of cartilage have not yet been performed.

Cartilage has also been proposed for **rheumatoid arthritis** (page 109), again without any particular evidence that it works.

Shark cartilage has been widely hyped as a cure for cancer. However, the evidence that it might work is so preliminary that drawing conclusions from the research available is like calling the results of an election 4 years before it happens based on one small public opinion poll. The science simply hasn't been done yet.

## WHAT IS THE SCIENTIFIC EVIDENCE FOR CARTILAGE?

There is no good clinical evidence yet that cartilage can cure or relieve symptoms of any disease.

A number of test-tube experiments have found that shark cartilage extracts prevent new blood vessels from forming in chick embryos and other test systems.[1,2,3] Developing drugs to prevent blood vessels from forming in tumors is an exciting new approach to treating cancer. Unfortunately, we don't have any research data on human subjects, so we can't say whether shark cartilage really has any effect on tumors in human beings. More study is needed.

## SAFETY ISSUES

Because cartilage is just common, ordinary gristle, it is presumably safe to consume.

#  CAT'S CLAW (UNCARIA TOMENTOSA)

*Principal Proposed Uses*
    Various viral diseases (genital and oral herpes, shingles [herpes zoster], AIDS, feline leukemia virus), allergies, arthritis, ulcers

Cat's claw is a popular herb among the indigenous people of Peru, where it is used to treat cancer, diabetes, ulcers, arthritis, and infections, as well as assist in recovery from childbirth. It is also used as a contraceptive.

Scientific studies of cat's claw conducted in Peru, Italy, Austria, and Germany have yielded numerous intriguing findings, but as yet no conclusive proof of any healing benefit. Nonetheless, with increasing international popularity, cultivation of cat's claw has become a major revenue source for the Ashaninka Indian tribe of Peru.

## WHAT IS CAT'S CLAW USED FOR TODAY?

In Europe and Peru, cat's claw is considered a promising treatment for viral diseases such as **herpes** (page 73), shingles, AIDS, and feline leukemia virus. Its possible use for treating **allergies** (page 3), stomach **ulcers** (page 112), **osteoarthritis** (page 95), and **rheumatoid arthritis** (page 109) is also being studied.[1] However, the best description of the present state of affairs is that we don't yet know whether cat's claw really works. It certainly is not a proven treatment for cancer.

## DOSAGES

The optimum dosage of cat's claw is not clear. Because of the wide variation in the forms and preparations sold, I recommend following the directions on the product's label.

## SAFETY ISSUES

There have not been any reports of serious adverse effects from taking cat's claw. However, European physicians believe that it should not be taken in conjunction with hormone treatments, insulin, or vaccines.[2] Safety in young children, pregnant or nursing women, or those with severe liver or kidney disease has not been established.

 # CAYENNE (CAPSICUM FRUTESCENS, CAPSICUM ANNUUM)

### Principal Proposed Uses

*Topical uses:*
    Post-herpetic neuralgia, arthritis, and other forms of pain

*Oral uses:*
    Heart disease, protecting the stomach from irritation caused by anti-inflammatory drugs

The capsicum family includes red peppers, bell peppers, pimento, and paprika, but the most famous medicinal member of this family is the common cayenne pepper. The substance capsaicin is the common "hot" ingredient in all hot peppers.

Cayenne and related peppers have a long history of use as digestive aids in many parts of the world, but the herb's recent popularity has, surprisingly, come through conventional medicine.

## WHAT IS CAYENNE USED FOR TODAY?

Under the brand name Zostrix, a cream containing concentrated capsaicin has been approved by the FDA for the treatment of the pain that often lingers after an attack of shingles (technically, post-herpetic neuralgia). There is also some evidence that capsaicin creams may be helpful for relieving the pain of various types of **arthritis** (pages 95 and 109) as well as other forms of pain.

Cayenne pepper taken internally has recently been widely touted as a treatment for heart disease by those who have found it useful for themselves or others, but there is no scientific evidence that it is effective. However, a bit of evidence suggests that oral use of cayenne can protect your stomach against damage caused by anti-inflammatory drugs.[1]

## DOSAGES

Capsaicin creams are approved over-the-counter drugs and should be used as directed.

For internal use, cayenne may be taken at a dosage of 1 to 2 standard 00 gelatin capsules 1 to 3 times daily.

## SAFETY ISSUES

As a commonly used food, cayenne is generally regarded as safe. Contrary to some reports, cayenne does not appear to aggravate stomach ulcers.[2]

## ⚠ INTERACTIONS YOU SHOULD KNOW ABOUT

If you are taking

- The asthma drug **theophylline:** Cayenne might increase the amount you absorb, possibly leading to toxic levels.[3]

- **Anti-inflammatory medications:** Cayenne might protect your stomach from damage.

# CHAMOMILE GERMAN (MATRICARIA RECUTITA); ROMAN (CHAMAEMELUM NOBILE)

## Principal Proposed Uses

*Topical uses:*
   Skin inflammation (e.g., dermatitis and eczema), wound healing

*Oral uses:*
   Gastrointestinal discomfort, protection against ulcers, anxiety, insomnia, arthritis, asthma

Two distinct plants are known as chamomile and are used interchangeably: German and Roman chamomile. Although botanically far apart, they both look like miniature daisies and appear to possess similar medicinal benefits.

Over a million cups of chamomile tea are drunk daily, testifying to its good taste and fine reputation. Chamomile was used by early Egyptian physicians for fevers and by ancient Greeks, Romans, and Indians for headaches and disorders of the kidneys, liver, and bladder. Modern-day Germans employ it for digestive upsets and menstrual difficulties, and the British use it for all these purposes.

It has been suggested that chamomile's reported effect is due to the constituents of its bright blue oil, including chamazulene, alpha-bisabolol, and bisaboloxides. However, the water-soluble part of chamomile may play a role, too, especially in soothing stomach upset.

## WHAT IS CHAMOMILE USED FOR TODAY?

The modern use of chamomile dates back to 1921, when a German firm introduced a topical form of chamomile named Kamillosan. This cream became a popular treatment for a wide variety of skin disorders, including **eczema** (page 66), bedsores, post-radiation therapy skin inflammation, and contact dermatitis (e.g., poison ivy).

Chamomile tea is widely used as a folk remedy to soothe colicky pains in the digestive tract and to help **insomnia** (page 80) and **anxiety** (page 8). It might help protect the stomach against irritation caused by alcohol or anti-inflammatory drugs.[1]

Concentrated alcohol extracts of chamomile are also sometimes used to treat the pain caused by various forms of **arthritis** (pages 95 and 109). Finally, it is common practice in Germany for individuals with **asthma** (page 11) or other breathing problems to inhale the steam from boiling chamomile and other herbs.

## WHAT IS THE SCIENTIFIC EVIDENCE FOR CHAMOMILE?

Numerous case reports and controlled (but not blinded) studies have consistently found significant benefits of chamomile cream in inflammatory skin diseases and wound healing.[2]

Animal research suggests that chamomile extracts taken orally can relax the intestines and reduce inflammation.[3] However, properly performed double-blind studies are lacking.

## DOSAGES

Chamomile cream is applied to the affected area 1 to 4 times daily.

Chamomile tea can be made by pouring boiling water over 2 to 3 heaping teaspoons of flowers and steeping for 10 minutes.

Chamomile tinctures and pills should be taken according to the directions on the label. Alcoholic tincture may be the most potent form for internal use.

## SAFETY ISSUES

Chamomile is listed on the FDA's GRAS (generally regarded as safe) list.

Reports that chamomile can cause severe reactions in people allergic to ragweed have received significant media attention. However, when all the evidence is examined, it does not appear that chamomile is actually more allergenic than any other plant.[4] The cause of these reports may be product contaminated with "dog chamomile," a highly allergenic and bad-tasting plant of similar appearance.

Chamomile also contains naturally occurring coumarin compounds that can act as "blood thinners." Excessive use of chamomile is therefore not recommended when taking prescription anticoagulants.

Safety in young children, pregnant or nursing women, or those with liver or kidney disease has not been established, although there have not been any credible reports of toxicity caused by this common beverage tea.

# CHASTEBERRY (VITEX AGNUS-CASTUS)

### Principal Proposed Uses
Cyclic breast discomfort (often associated with PMS), other PMS symptoms, menstrual irregularities, female infertility

### Other Proposed Uses
Menopausal symptoms

Chasteberry is frequently called by its Latin names: *vitex* or, alternatively, *agnus-castus*. A shrub in the verbena family, chasteberry is commonly found on riverbanks and nearby foothills in central Asia and around the Mediterranean Sea. After its violet flowers have bloomed, a dark brown, peppercorn-size fruit with a pleasant odor reminiscent of peppermint develops. This fruit is used medicinally.

As the name implies, for centuries chasteberry was thought to counter sexual desire. A drink prepared from the plant's seeds was used by the Romans to diminish libido, and in ancient Greece, young women celebrating the festival of Demeter wore chasteberry blossoms to show that they were remaining chaste in honor of the goddess. Monks in the Middle Ages used the fruit for similar purposes, yielding the common name "monk's pepper."

## WHAT IS CHASTEBERRY USED FOR TODAY?

The modern use of chasteberry dates back to the 1950s, when the German pharmaceutical firm Madaus Company first produced a standardized extract. This herb has become a standard European treatment for the cyclical breast tenderness that is often associated with PMS, which is sometimes called **cyclic mastalgia** (page 52), cyclic mastitis, mastodynia, or fibrocystic breast disease. Chasteberry is also used for general **PMS** (page 104) symptoms, as well as menstrual irregularities and **infertility in women** (page 79). The herb's full benefits are believed to take several months to develop, so be patient.

Research has shown that, unlike other herbs used for women's health problems, chasteberry does not contain any plant equivalent of estrogen or progesterone. Rather, it acts on the pituitary gland to suppress the release of prolactin.[1–4] Prolactin is a hormone that naturally rises during pregnancy to stimulate milk production. Inappropriately increased production of prolactin may be a factor in cyclic breast tenderness, as well as other symptoms of PMS. Elevated prolactin levels can also cause a woman's period to become irregular and even stop. For this reason, chasteberry is often tried for irregular or absent menstrual flow. However, I recommend that you do not attempt to self-treat significant menstrual irregularities without a full medical evaluation. There could be a serious medical condition causing the problem that you wouldn't want to miss.

High prolactin levels can also cause infertility. For this reason, chasteberry is sometimes tried as a fertility drug.[5]

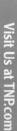

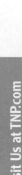
Finally, chasteberry occasionally appears to be dramatically effective at reducing **menopausal symptoms** (page 87). Strangely, it is just as often totally ineffective.

## WHAT IS THE SCIENTIFIC EVIDENCE FOR CHASTEBERRY?

Despite its widespread use in Germany, the scientific record for chasteberry is not as strong as it should be.

### Premenstrual Syndrome (PMS)

German gynecologists clearly believe that chasteberry is effective for PMS. In two rather informal studies enrolling about 3,000 women with PMS, doctors rated chasteberry as effective about 90% of the time.[6,7] Women reported significant or complete improvement in such symptoms as breast pain, fluid retention, headache, and fatigue.

However, this study did not involve a placebo group, and all the patients knew they were being treated. It is impossible to tell from the results what fraction of the benefit was due to the power of suggestion alone. It is a known fact that placebo treatment is highly effective for PMS, often reducing symptoms by as much as 70%.[8] Thus, the results of this study are more a survey of physicians' experiences with chasteberry than actual scientific evidence.

The opinion of experienced physicians is meaningful, but it's definitely not proof. Decades of experience have shown us how easy it is for even seasoned professionals to over- or underestimate the effectiveness of a treatment based on their preconceptions and the power of suggestion. When it comes to medical treatments, well-designed scientific studies are required to produce dependable evidence.

However, a search of medical literature conducted during the writing of this book failed to find any double-blind placebo-controlled studies that directly evaluated the benefits of chasteberry for PMS symptoms. One double-blind study has been performed, but unfortunately it compared chasteberry to **vitamin B$_6$ (pyridoxine)** (page 326) instead of a placebo.[9]

Published in 1997, this study followed 175 women who were given either a standardized chasteberry extract or 200 mg of vitamin B$_6$ daily. Chasteberry proved to be at least as effective as vitamin B$_6$. Both treatments produced significant improvements in all major symptoms of PMS, including breast tenderness, edema, tension, headache, and depression.

Although this study has been widely described as evidence that chasteberry is effective for PMS, it doesn't actually prove anything at all. Vitamin B$_6$ itself has not been proven effective for PMS.[10] Therefore, the fact that chasteberry works just as well as vitamin B$_6$ establishes little! It is quite possible that much of the improvement seen in both groups was due to the placebo effect. We really need a good, large-scale, double-blind placebo-controlled study to discover just how effective chasteberry is, beyond the inevitable effects of suggestion.

### Irregular Menstruation

One double-blind trial followed 52 women with a form of irregular menstruation known as *luteal phase defect*.[11] This condition is believed to be related to excessive prolactin release. After 3 months, the women who took chasteberry showed significant improvements.

## DOSAGES

The typical dose of dry chasteberry extract is 20 to 40 mg given once a day. Chasteberry is sold often as a liquid extract to be taken at a dosage of 40 drops each morning. However, highly concentrated extracts that require much lower dosing are also available. I recommend following the label instructions.

## SAFETY ISSUES

There haven't been any detailed studies of the safety of chasteberry. However, its widespread use in Germany has not led to any reports of significant adverse effects,[12] other than a single case of excessive ovarian stimulation possibly caused by chasteberry.[13]

Because it lowers prolactin levels, chasteberry is not an appropriate treatment for pregnant or nursing women. Safety in young children or those with severe liver or kidney disease has not been established.

There are no known drug interactions associated with chasteberry. However, it is quite conceivable that the herb could interfere with other hormonal medications, such as birth control pills.

## ⚠ INTERACTIONS YOU SHOULD KNOW ABOUT

If you are taking **hormones,** such as **birth control pills,** or **drugs that affect the pituitary,** such as **bromocriptine,** it is possible that chasteberry might interfere with their action.

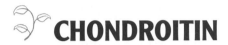

# CHONDROITIN

*Principal Proposed Uses*
  Osteoarthritis

*Other Proposed Uses*
  Atherosclerosis, high cholesterol

*Supplement Forms/Alternative Names*
  Chondroitin sulfate

Chondroitin

Chondroitin sulfate is a naturally occurring substance in the body. It is a major constituent of cartilage—the tough, elastic connective tissue found in the joints.

Based on the evidence of preliminary double-blind studies, chondroitin is widely used in Europe as a treatment for osteoarthritis, the "wear and tear" arthritis that many people suffer as they get older.

Furthermore, chondroitin may go beyond treating symptoms and actually protect joints from damage. Current medical treatments for osteoarthritis, such as NSAIDs (nonsteroidal anti-inflammatory drugs), treat the symptoms but don't actually slow the disease's progression, and they may actually make it get worse faster.[1–5] Chondroitin (along with glucosamine and SAMe) may take the treatment of osteoarthritis to a new level. However, more research needs to be performed to prove definitively that this exciting possibility is real.

## SOURCES

Chondroitin is not an essential nutrient. Animal cartilage is the only dietary source of chondroitin. (When it's on your plate, animal cartilage is called gristle.) Unless you enjoy chewing gristle, you'd do best to obtain chondroitin in pill form from a health food store or pharmacy.

## THERAPEUTIC DOSAGES

The usual dosage of chondroitin is 400 mg taken 3 times daily. Be patient! The results take weeks to develop. In commercial products it is often combined with **glucosamine** (page 213), although there is no direct evidence that such combinations are more effective than either treatment alone.

## THERAPEUTIC USES

Initially, chondroitin was primarily used in an injectable form. But in recent years, double-blind studies using the oral form of chondroitin for **osteoarthritis** (page 95) have been reported.[6,7,8] The best evidence is for a pain-relieving effect, but some studies have found that it can also slow the progression of the disease.[9–12]

Chondroitin has also been proposed as a treatment for other conditions such as **atherosclerosis** (page 14) and high **cholesterol** (page 39), but as yet the evidence that it might help is quite preliminary.[13,14]

## WHAT IS THE SCIENTIFIC EVIDENCE FOR CHONDROITIN?

For years, experts stated that oral chondroitin couldn't possibly work, because its molecules are so big that it seemed doubtful that they could be absorbed through the digestive tract. However, in 1995 researchers laid this objection to rest when they found evidence that up to 15% of chondroitin is absorbed intact.[15]

## Reducing Symptoms of Osteoarthritis

Three recently published double-blind placebo-controlled studies involving a total of about 250 participants suggest that chondroitin can relieve symptoms of osteoarthritis. One enrolled 85 people with osteoarthritis of the knee and followed them for 6 months.[16] Participants received either 400 mg of chondroitin sulfate twice daily or placebo. At the end of the trial, doctors rated the improvement as good or very good in 69% of those taking chondroitin sulfate but in only 32% of those taking placebo.

Another way of comparing the results is to look at maximum walking speed among participants. Whereas individuals in the chondroitin group were able to improve their walking speed gradually over the course of the trial, in the placebo group walking speed did not improve at all. Additionally, there were improvements in other measures of osteoarthritis, such as pain level, with benefits seen as early as 1 month. This suggests that chondroitin was able to stop the arthritis from gradually getting worse (see also Slowing the Progression of Osteoarthritis).

Similar results were found in another study that was shorter (3 months) but followed more individuals (127 people).[17]

A third double-blind study involved only 42 participants; however, it followed them for a full year.[18] Chondroitin took months to reach its full effect but eventually relieved symptoms considerably better than placebo.

Positive results were also seen in earlier studies.[19–22]

## Slowing the Progression of Osteoarthritis

An interesting feature of the full-year study mentioned previously was that, whereas the placebo group showed progressive joint damage over the year, no worsening of the joints was seen in the group taking chondroitin. In other words, chondroitin seemed to protect the joints from damage, thus slowing or perhaps even halting the progression of the disease. Osteoarthritis tends to get worse with time.

As mentioned earlier, no conventional treatment for osteoarthritis protects joints from progressive damage, and some may actually accelerate the process. If further studies confirm that chondroitin prevents progressive damage to the joints, it would make chondroitin distinctly better than any conventional option. Unfortunately, this study was too small to prove anything on its own.

Another, larger study examined the progression of osteoarthritis in 119 people for 3 full years.[23] In this double-blind placebo-controlled trial, those who took 1,200 mg of chondroitin daily showed lower rates of severe joint damage. Only 8.8% of the chondroitin group developed severely damaged joints during the 3 years of the study, compared with almost 30% of the placebo group. This suggests that chondroitin was slowing the progression of osteoarthritis. Unfortunately, the researchers did not report whether this difference was statistically significant.

Additional evidence comes from animal studies. The effect of both oral and injected chondroitin was assessed in rabbits with damaged cartilage in the knee.[24] After 84 days of treatment, the rabbits that were given chondroitin had significantly more healthy cartilage remaining in the damaged knee than the untreated animals. Receiving chondroitin by mouth was as effective as taking it through an injection.

Putting all this information together, it appears quite likely that chondroitin can slow the progression of osteoarthritis. However, more studies are needed to confirm this very exciting possibility. It would also be wonderful if chondroitin could repair damaged cartilage and thus reverse arthritis, but none of the research so far shows such an effect. Chondroitin may simply stop further destruction from occurring.

## How Does Chondroitin Work for Osteoarthritis?

Scientists are unsure how chondroitin sulfate works, but one of several theories (or all of them) might explain its mode of action.

At its most basic level, chondroitin may help cartilage by providing it with the building blocks it needs to repair itself. It is also believed to block enzymes that break down cartilage in the joints.[25,26] Another theory holds that chondroitin increases the amount of hyaluronic acid in the joints.[27] Hyaluronic acid is a protective fluid that keeps the joints lubricated. Finally, chondroitin may have a mild anti-inflammatory effect.[28]

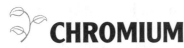

# CHROMIUM

### Principal Proposed Uses
Diabetes, weight loss

### Other Proposed Uses
High cholesterol and triglycerides, Syndrome X, functional hypoglycemia, acne, migraine headaches, psoriasis

### Supplement Forms/Alternative Names
Chromium picolinate, chromium polynicotinate, chromium chloride, high-chromium brewer's yeast

Chromium is a mineral the body needs in very small amounts, but it plays an important role in human nutrition. Most of us are more familiar with chromium's industrial uses—for example, to make chrome-plated steel. Chromium's role in maintaining good health was discovered in 1957, when scientists extracted a substance known as *glucose tolerance factor* (GTF) from pork kidney. GTF, which helps the body maintain normal blood sugar levels, contains chromium.

Chromium's most important function is to help regulate the amount of glucose (sugar) in the blood. Insulin plays a starring role in this fundamental biological process, by regulating the movement of glucose out of the blood and into cells. Scientists believe that insulin uses chromium as an assistant (technically, cofactor) to "unlock the door" to the cell membrane, thus allowing glucose to enter the cell.

Based on chromium's close relationship with insulin, this trace mineral has been studied as a treatment for diabetes. The results have been positive: Chromium supplements appear to improve blood sugar control in people with diabetes.

Recent evidence also suggests that chromium supplements might help dieters lose fat and gain lean muscle tissue.

## SAFETY ISSUES

Chondroitin sulfate has not been associated with any serious side effects, which is not surprising when you consider that taking it by mouth is essentially the same as eating gristle. Subjects in clinical trials have found mild digestive distress to be the only real complaint.

## REQUIREMENTS/SOURCES

No Recommended Dietary Allowance has been established for chromium, but the Estimated Safe and Adequate Daily Dietary Intake is as follows

- Infants under 6 months, 10 to 40 mcg
  6 months to 1 year, 20 to 60 mcg
- Children 1 to 3 years, 20 to 80 mcg
  4 to 6 years, 30 to 120 mcg
- Adults (and children 7 years and older), 50 to 200 mcg

Many Americans may be chromium-deficient.[1] Preliminary research done by the U.S. Department of Agriculture (USDA) in 1985 found low chromium intakes in a small group of people studied. Although large-scale studies are needed to show whether Americans as a whole are chromium-deficient, we do know that many traditional sources of chromium, such as wheat, are depleted of this important mineral during processing.

Some researchers believe that inadequate intake of chromium may be one of the causes for the rising rates of adult-onset diabetes. However, the matter is greatly complicated by the fact that we lack a good test to determine chromium deficiency.[2]

Severe chromium deficiency has only been seen in hospitalized individuals receiving nutrition intravenously. Symptoms include problems with blood sugar control that cannot be corrected by insulin alone.

Chromium is found in drinking water, especially hard water, but concentrations vary so widely throughout the world that drinking water is not a reliable source. The most concentrated sources of chromium are brewer's yeast (not nutritional or torula yeast) and calf liver. Two ounces of brewer's yeast or 4 ounces of calf liver supply between 50 and 60 mcg of chromium. Other good sources of chromium are whole-wheat bread, wheat bran, and rye bread. Potatoes, wheat germ, green peppers, and apples offer modest amounts of chromium.

**Calcium** (page 146) carbonate interferes with the absorption of chromium.[3]

## THERAPEUTIC DOSAGES

The dosage of chromium used in studies ranges from 200 to 1,000 mcg daily. However, there may be potential risks in the higher dosages of chromium (see Safety Issues).

## THERAPEUTIC USES

Chromium has principally been studied for its possible benefits in improving blood sugar control in people with **diabetes** (page 60). Reasonably good evidence suggests that people with adult-onset (type 2) diabetes may show some improvement when given appropriate dosages of chromium.[4] Individuals with childhood-onset (type 1) diabetes may respond as well.[5] Finally, chromium also appears to help treat problems with blood sugar control that are too mild to deserve the name "diabetes."[6,7]

Recent evidence suggests that chromium supplements may also help reduce fat in the body, probably through its effects on insulin.[8]

Weak and sometimes contradictory evidence suggests that chromium may lower **cholesterol** (page 39) and triglyceride levels.[9]

According to some authorities, impaired blood sugar control, high cholesterol, weight gain, and high blood pressure are all part of a bigger picture, given the mysterious-sounding name Syndrome X. Since chromium may be helpful for the first three of these conditions, chromium deficiency has been proposed as the cause of Syndrome X. However, the entire concept of Syndrome X is controversial, and many experts don't believe that it even exists.

Chromium is often suggested as a treatment for the opposite of diabetes, hypoglycemia (low blood sugar). In reality, this condition may not involve lower-than-normal levels of blood sugar at all but rather an abnormal response to normal changes in blood sugar levels. Possible symptoms include anxiety, sweating, and shakiness, which may develop between meals and are relieved by eating. However, there is no direct evidence that chromium is effective for this condition.

Chromium has also been proposed as a treatment for **migraine headaches** (page 89), **psoriasis** (page 106), and **acne** (page 2), but there is as yet no real evidence that it works.

## WHAT IS THE SCIENTIFIC EVIDENCE FOR CHROMIUM?

### Diabetes

Moderately strong evidence supports the use of chromium for diabetes. In a recent double-blind placebo-controlled study, 180 people with type 2 diabetes were given either placebo, 200 mcg of chromium picolinate daily, or a higher dosage of chromium picolinate—1,000 mcg daily. Individuals taking 1,000 mcg showed marked improvements in blood sugar levels. Lesser but still significant benefits were also seen in the 200-mcg group but not in the placebo group.[10]

An earlier controlled study followed 243 people with type 1 or type 2 diabetes, who were given either placebo or 200 mcg daily of chromium. Among those taking chromium, medication requirements decreased in 57% of people with type 2 diabetes and in 34% of those with type 1 diabetes.[11] More women than men responded favorably. The placebo group showed no significant improvement.

Similarly positive results were seen in other small studies.[12,13] However, there have also been negative results.[14]

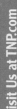

Putting all the results together, it does appear that chromium supplementation can be helpful in treating diabetes, both type 1 and type 2. However, more work needs to be done to determine the optimum dosage.

## Blood Sugar Control in People Without Diabetes

Numerous studies have found that chromium supplementation can improve mild abnormalities in blood sugar control,[15,16,17] although not all studies have shown a positive effect.[18] Because some (but not all) authorities suspect that these relatively slight deviations from the normal indicate a pre-diabetic condition, chromium has been suggested as a treatment to prevent the development of adult-onset diabetes. However, there is no real evidence as yet that it works.

## Weight Loss

Recent evidence suggests that chromium may be an effective aid in weight loss.

A 3-month double-blind study of 122 moderately overweight individuals attempting to lose weight found that 400 mcg of chromium daily resulted in an average loss of 6.2 pounds of body fat, as opposed to 3.4 pounds in the placebo group. There was no loss of lean body mass.[19] These results suggest that chromium can help you lose body fat without losing muscle. It may work by helping the body process its insulin more effectively.

## SAFETY ISSUES

Chromium appears to be safe when taken at a dosage of 50 to 200 mcg daily.[20] No side effects have been noted, except for an interesting one:

Some people who take chromium report that their dreams become more frequent and vivid.

However, chromium is a heavy metal and might conceivably build up and cause problems if taken to excess. Recently, there have been a few reports of kidney damage in people who took a relatively high dosage of chromium: 1,200 mcg or more daily for several months.[21,22]

For this reason, the dosage found most effective for individuals with type 2 diabetes—1,000 mcg daily—might present some health risks. It would be advisable to seek medical supervision if you want to take more than 200 mcg daily.

Also, keep in mind that if you have diabetes and chromium is effective, you may need to cut down your dosage of any medication you take for diabetes. Medical supervision is advised.

Concerns have also been raised over the use of the picolinate form of chromium in individuals suffering from affective or psychotic disorders, because picolinic acids can change levels of neurotransmitters.[23]

The maximum safe dosages of chromium for young children, women who are pregnant or nursing, or those with severe liver or kidney disease have not been established.

## ⚠ INTERACTIONS YOU SHOULD KNOW ABOUT

If you are taking

- **Calcium carbonate supplements:** You should take your chromium supplement at a different time of day, because calcium carbonate may interfere with its absorption.

- **Diabetes medications:** Seek medical supervision before taking chromium.

Chromium

Visit Us at TNP.com

# COENZYME Q$_{10}$

### Principal Proposed Uses

Congestive heart failure, cardiomyopathy, other forms of heart disease, hypertension, periodontal disease, nutrient depletion caused by various medications

### Other Proposed Uses

AIDS, cancer, obesity, muscular dystrophy, enhanced performance for athletes, infertility in men

### Supplement Forms/Alternative Names

CoQ$_{10}$, ubiquinone

---

Coenzyme Q$_{10}$ (CoQ$_{10}$), also known as ubiquinone, is a powerful antioxidant discovered by researchers at the University of Wisconsin in 1957. The name of this supplement comes from the word *ubiquitous*, which means "found everywhere." Indeed, CoQ$_{10}$ is found in every cell in the body. It plays a fundamental role in the mitochondria, the parts of the cell that produce energy from food.

Japanese scientists first discovered the therapeutic properties of CoQ$_{10}$ in the 1960s. Today, it is widely prescribed for heart conditions in Europe and Israel, as well as in Japan. CoQ$_{10}$ appears to assist the heart during times of stress on the heart muscle, perhaps by helping it use energy more efficiently. While CoQ$_{10}$'s best-established use is for congestive heart failure, ongoing research suggests that it may also be useful for other types of heart problems and for a wide variety of additional illnesses.

## SOURCES

Every cell in your body needs CoQ$_{10}$, but no U.S. Recommended Dietary Allowance has been established for this important substance because the body can manufacture CoQ$_{10}$ from scratch.

Because CoQ$_{10}$ is found in all animal and plant cells, we obtain small amounts of this nutrient from our diet. However, it would be hard to get a therapeutic dosage from food.

## THERAPEUTIC DOSAGES

The typical recommended dosage of CoQ$_{10}$ is 30 to 300 mg daily, often divided into 2 or 3 doses.

CoQ$_{10}$ is fat-soluble and is better absorbed when taken in an oil-based soft gel form rather than in a dry form such as tablets and capsules.[1]

## THERAPEUTIC USES

The best-documented use of CoQ$_{10}$ is for treating **congestive heart failure** (page 50).[2–5] Keep in mind that it is taken along with conventional medications, not instead of them.

Weaker evidence suggests that it may be useful for **cardiomyopathy** (page 36) and other forms of **heart disease** (page 14).[6,7,8] CoQ$_{10}$ has been suggested as a treatment for **hypertension** (page 75)[9,10,11] and to prevent the heart damage caused by certain types of cancer chemotherapy. Keep in mind that CoQ$_{10}$ might conceivably interfere with the action of other chemotherapy drugs (although there is no good evidence that it does so). Therefore, if you are a cancer patient, check with your oncologist before using CoQ$_{10}$.

CoQ$_{10}$ may also help **periodontal (gum) disease** (page 103).[12] CoQ$_{10}$ has additionally been proposed as a treatment for a wide variety of other conditions, including **angina** (page 7), **infertility in men** (page 78), AIDS, cancer obesity, and muscular dystrophy. It has also been used as a performance enhancer for athletes. However, as yet the evidence to support these uses remains weak.

CoQ$_{10}$ has become popular as a treatment for possible nutritional depletion caused by various medications. It has been suggested (but not proven) that CoQ$_{10}$ deficiency may play a role in the known side effects of these treatments, and that taking CoQ$_{10}$ supplements might be a good idea.

The best evidence is for the cholesterol-lowering drugs in the statin family, such as lovastatin (Mevacor), simvastatin (Zocor), and pravastatin (Pravachol).[13,14,15]

For several other categories of drugs, the evidence that they cause depletion of $CoQ_{10}$ is fairly indirect. These include oral diabetes drugs (especially glyburide, phenformin, and tolazamide), beta-blockers (specifically propranolol, metoprolol, and alprenolol), antipsychotic drugs in the phenothiazine family, tricyclic antidepressants, methyldopa, hydrochlorothiazide, clonidine, and hydralazine.[16–20]

## WHAT IS THE SCIENTIFIC EVIDENCE FOR COENZYME $Q_{10}$?

### Congestive Heart Failure

Very good evidence tells us that $CoQ_{10}$ can be helpful for people with congestive heart failure (CHF). In this serious condition, the heart muscles become weakened, resulting in poor circulation and shortness of breath.

People with CHF have significantly lower levels of $CoQ_{10}$ in heart muscle cells than healthy people.[21] This fact alone does not prove that $CoQ_{10}$ supplements will help CHF; however, it prompted medical researchers to try using $CoQ_{10}$ as a treatment for heart failure.

The results have been positive. At least nine double-blind studies have found that $CoQ_{10}$ supplements can markedly improve symptoms and objective measurements of heart function when they are taken along with conventional medication.

In the largest of these studies, 641 individuals with moderate to severe congestive heart failure were monitored for 1 year.[22] Half were given 2 mg per kilogram body weight of $CoQ_{10}$ daily; the rest were given placebo. Standard therapy was continued in both groups. The participants treated with $CoQ_{10}$ experienced a significant reduction in the severity of their symptoms. No such improvement was seen in the placebo group. The people who took $CoQ_{10}$ also had significantly fewer hospitalizations for heart failure.

Similarly positive results were also seen in smaller studies involving a total of over 300 participants.[23,24,25]

### Cardiomyopathy

Cardiomyopathy is the general name given to conditions in which the heart muscle gradually becomes diseased. Several small studies suggest that $CoQ_{10}$ supplements are helpful for some forms of cardiomyopathy.[26,27,28]

### Hypertension

Although $CoQ_{10}$ is frequently mentioned as a treatment for hypertension, the scientific evidence for this use is weak. There has only been one double-blind study, and it enrolled only 18 people, too few to prove much.[29]

An uncontrolled study of 109 people with hypertension found significant improvements in systolic and diastolic blood pressure during treatment with an average dosage of 225 mg daily of $CoQ_{10}$ (the dosage was adjusted to achieve a certain blood level). In fact, over 4 months, 51% of treated individuals were able to stop taking one to three blood pressure medications.[30] These marked benefits persisted for the full length of the study (1 year). Similar benefits have been seen in other open studies.[31]

However, although these results are impressive, they can't be taken as fully reliable. When people know that they are being given a treatment, as they did in this study, they may be inspired to make other positive changes in their lives. This factor, along with the power of suggestion, is the reason that properly designed double-blind controlled studies are necessary.

### Periodontal Disease

We're not sure why, but several studies indicate that $CoQ_{10}$ supplementation can help in periodontal (gum) disease. This disease leads to pockets of infection in the gums. According to several small double-blind studies and open trials, $CoQ_{10}$ supplements can significantly reduce the size and improve the health of these pockets.[32]

## SAFETY ISSUES

$CoQ_{10}$ appears to be extremely safe. No significant side effects have been found, even in studies that lasted a year.[33] However, individuals with severe heart disease should not take $CoQ_{10}$ (or any other supplement) except under a doctor's supervision.

The maximum safe dosages of $CoQ_{10}$ for young children, pregnant or nursing women, or those with severe liver or kidney disease have not been determined.

## ⚠ INTERACTIONS YOU SHOULD KNOW ABOUT

If you are taking

- **Cholesterol-lowering drugs** in the "statin" family, **oral diabetes drugs** (especially **glyburide, phenformin,** and **tolazamide**), **beta-blockers** (specifically **propranolol, metoprolol,** and **alprenolol**), **antipsychotic drugs** in the phenothiazine family, **tricyclic antidepressants, methyldopa, hydrochlorothiazide, clonidine,** or **hydralazine:** You may need more coenzyme $Q_{10}$.

# *COLEUS FORSKOHLII*

### *Principal Proposed Uses*
Allergic conditions (e.g., asthma, eczema, allergies)
Muscle contraction (e.g., asthma, high blood pressure, menstrual cramps, irritable bowel [spastic colon], bladder pain, glaucoma)

### *Other Proposed Uses*
Psoriasis

A member of the mint family, *Coleus forskohlii* grows wild on the mountain slopes of Nepal, India, and Thailand. In traditional Asian systems of medicine, it was used for a variety of purposes, including treating skin rashes, asthma, bronchitis, insomnia, epilepsy, and angina. But modern interest is based almost entirely on the work of a drug company, Hoechst Pharmaceuticals.

Like other drug manufacturers, Hoechst regularly screens medicinal plants in hopes of discovering new medications. In 1974, work performed in collaboration with the Indian Central Drug Research Institute found that the rootstock of *Coleus forskohlii* could lower blood pressure and decrease muscle spasms. Intensive study identified a substance named forskolin that appeared to be responsible for much of this effect.

Forskolin is a substance with unique biological activity. It increases the levels of a fundamental natural compound known as *cyclic AMP*.[1,2] Cyclic AMP plays a major role in an immense va-

riety of cellular functions, and, by altering its levels, forskolin has the ability to profoundly alter many aspects of body functioning. Forskolin and synthetic substances patterned after it may eventually form an entirely new class of drugs.

Yet, while all this information about forskolin is interesting, it does not necessarily say anything about the effects of the whole herb itself.

## WHAT IS *COLEUS FORSKOHLII* USED FOR TODAY?

Herb manufacturers have begun to offer extracts of *Coleus forskohlii* that have been specially manufactured to contain high levels of forskolin.

Forskolin has been found to stabilize the cells that release histamine and other inflammatory compounds.[3] This suggests that *Coleus forskohlii* may be a useful treatment for **asthma** (page 11), **eczema** (page 66), and other allergic conditions.

Studies have also found that forskolin relaxes smooth muscle tissue.[4,5] For this reason, *Coleus forskohlii* has been suggested as a treatment for asthma, menstrual cramps or **dysmenorrhea** (page 65), **angina** (page 7), **irritable bowel syndrome** (page 85), crampy bladder pain (as in **bladder infections** [page 23]), and **hypertension** (page 75).

*Coleus forskohlii* has also been proposed as a treatment for **psoriasis** (page 106), because that disease appears to be at least partly related to low levels of cyclic AMP in skin cells.

## WHAT IS THE SCIENTIFIC EVIDENCE FOR *COLEUS FORSKOHLII?*

The scientific evidence for the herb *Coleus forskohlii* as a treatment for any disease is weak. What is known relates to the substance forskolin rather than the whole herb.

Animal studies and open studies in humans suggest that forskolin can reduce blood pressure and dilate bronchial tubes.[6,7,8] A tiny double-blind study indicates that forskolin taken by inhalation may be as effective as standard asthma inhalers,[9] and forskolin eyedrops appear to improve glaucoma.[10]

## DOSAGES

A common dosage recommendation is 50 mg 2 or 3 times a day of an extract standardized to contain 18% forskolin.

However, because such an extract provides significant levels of forskolin, a drug with wide-ranging properties, I recommend that *Coleus forskohlii* extracts should be taken only with a doctor's supervision.

## SAFETY ISSUES

The safety of *Coleus forskohlii* and forskolin has not been fully evaluated, although few significant risks have been noted in studies performed thus far. Caution should be exercised when combining this herb with blood-pressure medications and "blood thinners." Safety in young children, pregnant or nursing women, or those with severe liver or kidney disease has not been established.

## ⚠ INTERACTIONS YOU SHOULD KNOW ABOUT

If you are taking **blood pressure medications** or **anticoagulant drugs,** *Coleus forskohlii* should only be used under the supervision of a physician.

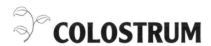

# COLOSTRUM

*Principal Proposed Uses*
Preventing infections

Colostrum is the fluid that new mothers' breasts produce during the first day or two after birth. It gives newborn infants a rich mixture of antibodies and growth factors that help them get a good start.

Although colostrum has been available since the first mammals walked the earth, it is relatively new as a nutritional supplement. The resurgence of breastfeeding in the 1970s sparked a revival of interest in colostrum for both infants and adults. However, most commercial colostrum preparations come from cows, not humans. Whether cow antibodies are good for humans is unclear. Colostrum primarily fights gastrointestinal infections, but a cow's digestive tract is so different from yours and mine that benefits may not cross over.

## REQUIREMENTS/SOURCES

Breastfeeding is the healthiest way to nourish a newborn, and a mother's colostrum is undoubtedly good for a baby. But don't believe claims (by at least one manufacturer) that most babies

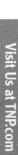

would die without colostrum. Colostrum is good for health, but it's not essential for life.

Colostrum has just become available in capsules that contain its immune proteins in dry form.

## THERAPEUTIC DOSAGES

The usual recommended dosage of colostrum is 10 g daily.

## THERAPEUTIC USES

Colostrum is often sold as an "immune stimulant." However, if it works at all, it should function by directly fighting parasites, bacteria, and viruses.[1-6] There is no particular reason to believe it would strengthen your immune system.

## WHAT IS THE SCIENTIFIC EVIDENCE FOR COLOSTRUM?

### Preventing Infections

There is some evidence that colostrum can help prevent certain infectious diseases, but other studies have found it ineffective.

A specialized form of colostrum was tested for its ability to prevent infection with the common parasite cryptosporidium.[7] One group of healthy volunteers was given colostrum before receiving an infectious dose of cryptosporidium, while the other group was given placebo. Those who took colostrum experienced less diarrhea and appeared to experience a lower-grade infection.

Several other studies indicate that colostrum may relieve diarrhea and other symptoms associated with cryptosporidium in people with AIDS.[8,9]

Another study suggests that colostrum might prevent mild infections with the shigella parasite from becoming severe.[10] However, a different study looking at Bangladeshi children infected with *Helicobacter pylori* (the organism that causes digestive ulcers) found no benefits.[11] Also, no benefit was seen in a study on rotavirus (another parasite that causes diarrhea in children).[12]

## SAFETY ISSUES

Colostrum does not seem to cause any significant side effects. However, comprehensive safety studies have not been performed. Safety in young children or women who are pregnant or nursing has not been established.

# CONJUGATED LINOLEIC ACID

*Principal Proposed Uses*
   There are no well-documented uses for conjugated linoleic acid.

*Other Proposed Uses*
   Reducing body fat

*Supplement Forms/Alternative Names*
   CLA

Conjugated linoleic acid (CLA) is a mixture of different isomers, or chemical forms, of linoleic acid. This is an *essential fatty acid*—a type of fat that your body needs as much as it needs vitamins. Although it has become popular as a "fat-burning" supplement, we don't really know how or even whether CLA really works.

## REQUIREMENTS/SOURCES

Although linoleic acid itself is an important nutritional source of essential fatty acids, there is no evidence that you need to get *conjugated* linoleic acid in your diet. CLA does occur in food, but it would be very difficult to get the recommended dose that way. Supplements are the only practical source.

## THERAPEUTIC DOSAGES

The typical dosage of CLA ranges from 3 to 5 g daily. As with all supplements taken at this high a dosage, it is important to purchase a reputable brand, as even very small amounts of a toxic contaminant could quickly mount up.

## THERAPEUTIC USES

There is some evidence that CLA might help you lose fat while retaining muscle. However, what we know is based primarily on some interesting animal studies and very small human clinical trials.[1,2] Better studies in humans are currently under way, but results are not currently available. At present, there is more evidence that **chromium** (page 161) can provide this benefit.

## SAFETY ISSUES

CLA appears to be a safe nutritional substance. However, maximum safe dosages for young children, pregnant or nursing women, or those with severe liver or kidney disease have not been determined.

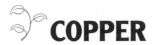

# COPPER

*Principal Proposed Uses*
   There are no well-documented uses for copper.

*Other Proposed Uses*
   High cholesterol, heart disease, osteoporosis, osteoarthritis, rheumatoid arthritis

*Supplement Forms/Alternative Names*
   Copper sulfate, copper picolinate, copper gluconate, copper complexes of various amino acids

The human body contains only 70 to 80 mg of copper, but it's an essential part of many important enzymes. Copper's possible role in treating disease is based on the fact that these enzymes can't do their jobs without it. However, there is little direct evidence that taking extra copper can treat any disease.

## REQUIREMENTS/SOURCES

Although a precise dietary requirement for copper has not been determined, the Estimated Safe and Adequate Daily Dietary Intake is as follows

- Infants under 6 months, 0.4 to 0.6 mg

  6 months to 1 year, 0.6 to 0.7 mg

- Children 1 to 3 years, 0.7 to 1.0 mg

  4 to 6 years, 1.0 to 1.5 mg

  7 to 10 years, 1.0 to 2.0 mg

  11 to 18 years, 1.5 to 2.5 mg

- Adults 19 years and older, 1.5 to 3.0 mg

Marginal copper deficiency appears to be common in Western diets.[1] Excessive **zinc** (page 348) intake reduces copper stores in the body.[2]

Oysters, nuts, legumes, whole grains, sweet potatoes, and dark greens are good sources of copper. Drinking water that passes through copper plumbing is a good source of this mineral, and sometimes it may even provide too much.

## THERAPEUTIC DOSAGES

The typical adult supplemental dosage of copper is 1 to 3 mg daily.

## THERAPEUTIC USES

Copper has been proposed as a treatment for **osteoporosis** (page 100), based primarily on studies that found benefit using mixtures of various trace minerals.[3,4]

One researcher, L. M. Klevay, has claimed in more than a dozen papers that copper deficiencies increase the risk of high **cholesterol** (page

39) and **heart disease** (page 14), but he has failed to supply any real evidence that this idea is true. A double-blind clinical trial of copper supplements for reducing heart disease risk found no benefit.[5]

Similarly, copper has long been mentioned as a possible treatment for **osteoarthritis** (page 95) and **rheumatoid arthritis** (page 109), but there is as yet no real evidence that it works.

## SAFETY ISSUES

Copper is safe when taken at nutritional dosages, but these should not be exceeded. As little as 10 mg of copper daily produces nausea, and 60 mg may cause vomiting. Maximum safe dosages of copper for young children, pregnant or nursing women, or those with severe liver or kidney disease have not been determined.

## ⚠ INTERACTIONS YOU SHOULD KNOW ABOUT

If you are taking

- **Antacids** or other medications that reduce stomach acid, or the drug **ethambutol:** You may need extra copper.
- **Zinc:** You need to make sure to get enough copper.
- **Iron** (page 234) supplements, **manganese** (page 254), high doses of **vitamin C** (page 331), or **antacids:** Your ability to absorb copper may be impaired.[6]
- **Oral contraceptives:** It might not be advisable to take extra copper.
- **Copper:** You may need extra manganese.

 # CRANBERRY (VACCINIUM MACROCARPON)

*Principal Proposed Uses*
   Bladder infections (prevention and possible treatment)

The cranberry plant is a close relative of the common blueberry. Native Americans used it both as food and for the treatment of bladder and kidney diseases. The Pilgrims learned about cranberry from local tribes and quickly adopted it for their own use. Subsequent physicians used it for bladder infections, for "bladder gravel" (small bladder stones), and to remove "blood toxins."

In the 1920s, researchers observed that drinking cranberry juice makes the urine more acidic. Since common urinary tract–infection bacteria such as *E. coli* dislike acidic surroundings, physicians concluded that they had discovered a scientific explanation for the traditional uses of cranberry. This discovery led to widespread medical use of cranberry juice for treating bladder infections. Cranberry fell out of favor with physicians after World War II, but it became popular again during the 1960s—as a self-treatment.

## WHAT IS CRANBERRY USED FOR TODAY?

Cranberry is widely used today to prevent **bladder infections** (page 23). Contrary to the research from the 1920s, it now appears that acidification of the urine is not so important as cranberry's ability to block bacteria from adhering to the bladder wall.[1,2,3] If the bacteria can't hold on they will be washed out with the stream of urine.

Cranberry juice is believed to be most effective as a form of prevention. When taken regularly, it appears to reduce the frequency of recurrent bladder infections in women prone to develop them. Cranberry may also be helpful during a bladder infection but not as reliably.

## WHAT IS THE SCIENTIFIC EVIDENCE FOR CRANBERRY?

Most of the clinical research about cranberry has involved elderly women. The largest study followed 153 women with an average age of 78.5 years for a period of 6 months.[4] Half were given a standard commercial cranberry cocktail drink, the other a placebo drink prepared to look and taste the same. Both treatments contained the same amount of vitamin C to eliminate the possible antibacterial influence of that supplement.

Despite the weak preparation of cranberry used, the results showed a 58% decrease in the incidence of bacteria and white blood cells in the urine.

Interestingly, studies have found that in women who frequently develop bladder infections, bacteria seem to have a particularly easy time holding on to the bladder wall.[5] This suggests that cranberry juice can actually get to the root of their problem, but more research is needed.

## DOSAGES

The proper dosage of dry cranberry juice extract is 300 to 400 mg twice daily. For people who prefer juice, 8 to 16 ounces daily should suffice. Pure cranberry juice and not sugary cranberry juice cocktail with its low percentage of cranberry should be used for best effect.

## SAFETY ISSUES

There are no known risks of this food for adults, children, or pregnant or nursing women. However, cranberry juice may allow the kidneys to excrete certain drugs more rapidly, thereby reducing their effectiveness. All weakly alkaline drugs may be affected, including many antidepressants and prescription painkillers.

## ⚠ INTERACTIONS YOU SHOULD KNOW ABOUT

If you are taking **weakly alkaline drugs,** which include many **antidepressants** and **prescription painkillers,** cranberry might decrease their effectiveness.

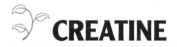

# CREATINE

*Principal Proposed Uses*
   Exercise performance that involves high-intensity, short-term bursts of activity

*Other Proposed Uses*
   Weight loss, improved ratio of body fat to muscle, muscle diseases (e.g., amyotrophic lateral sclerosis or Lou Gehrig's disease, congestive heart failure)

*Supplement Form/Alternative Names*
   Creatine monohydrate

Creatine is a naturally occurring substance that plays an important role in the production of energy in the body. The body converts it to phosphocreatine, a form of stored energy used by muscles.

In recent years, many athletes have tried supplemental creatine as a performance enhancer. If you're a U.S. baseball fan, you probably know that Mark McGwire, the all-time single-season home run champ, takes creatine (along with many other supplements).

Although the evidence for creatine is not definitive, of all sports supplements, it has the most evidence behind it. Numerous small double-blind studies suggest that it can increase athletic performance in sports that involve intense but short bursts of activity.

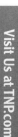

The theory behind its use is that supplemental creatine can build up a reserve of phosphocreatine in the muscles, to help them perform on demand. Supplemental creatine may also help the body make new phosphocreatine faster when it has been used up by intense activity.

## SOURCES

Although some creatine exists in the daily diet, it is not an essential nutrient because your body can make it from the amino acids **L-arginine** (page 126), glycine, and **L-methionine** (page 261). Provided you eat enough protein (the source of these amino acids), your body will make all the creatine you need for good health.

Meat (including chicken and fish) is the most important dietary source of creatine and its amino acid building blocks. For this reason, vegetarian athletes may potentially benefit most from creatine supplementation.

## THERAPEUTIC DOSAGES

For bodybuilding and exercise enhancement, a typical dosage schedule starts with a "loading dose" of 15 to 30 g daily (divided into 2 or 3 separate doses) for 3 to 4 days, followed by 2 to 5 g daily. Some authorities recommend skipping the loading dose. (By comparison, we typically get only about 1 g of creatine in the daily diet.)

Creatine's ability to enter muscle cells can be increased by combining it with glucose, fructose, or other simple carbohydrates. Caffeine appears to block the effects of creatine.[1]

## THERAPEUTIC USES

Creatine is one of the bestselling and best-documented supplements for enhancing athletic performance, but the scientific evidence that it works is far from complete. The best evidence we have points to benefits in forms of exercise that require repeated short-term bursts of high-intensity exercise, such as soccer and basketball.[2,3,4]

Creatine has also been proposed as an aid to promote weight loss and to reduce the proportion of fat to muscle in the body, but there is little evidence that it is effective for this purpose.[5] Better evidence exists for **chromium** (page 161) in this regard.

Preliminary evidence not yet published at press time suggests that creatine may be helpful for certain serious illnesses, including muscle-wasting diseases such as amyotrophic lateral sclerosis (Lou Gehrig's disease) and **congestive heart failure** (page 50). Creatine seems to be able to reduce fatigue and increase strength.

## WHAT IS THE SCIENTIFIC EVIDENCE FOR CREATINE?

### Exercise Performance

Several small double-blind studies suggest that creatine can improve performance in exercises that involve repeated short bursts of high-intensity activity.[6]

For example, in one double-blind study, 16 physical education students exercised 10 times for 6 seconds on a stationary cycle, alternating with a 30-second rest period.[7] The results showed that individuals who took 20 g of creatine for 6 days were better able to maintain cycle speed. Similar results were seen in many other studies.[8,9,10]

Isometric exercise capacity (pushing against a fixed resistance) also seems to improve with creatine.[11]

However, studies of endurance or nonrepeated exercise have *not* shown benefits.[12,13,14] Therefore, creatine probably won't help you for marathon running or single sprints.

## SAFETY ISSUES

Creatine appears to be safe, at least in healthy athletes. No significant side effects have been found with the regimen of several days of a high dosage (15 to 30 g daily) followed by 6 weeks of a lower dosage (2 to 3 g daily). We do not know whether it is safe to use creatine for longer periods.

Two deaths have been reported in individuals taking creatine, but other causes were most likely responsible.[15] Some authorities state that creatine supplements can be harmful for the kidneys, but creatine appears to be safe for those whose kidneys are healthy to begin with.[16] However, individuals with kidney disease, especially those on dialysis, should probably avoid creatine.

As with all supplements taken in very high doses, it is important to purchase a high-quality form of creatine, as contaminants present even in very low concentrations could conceivably build up and cause problems.

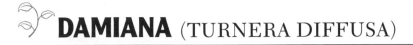

# DAMIANA (TURNERA DIFFUSA)

*Principal Proposed Uses*
Male sexual capacity

*Other Proposed Uses*
Respiratory diseases (e.g., asthma), depression, digestive problems, impotence in men, difficulty achieving orgasm in women, menstrual disorders

---

The herb damiana has been used in Mexico for some time as a male aphrodisiac.[1] Classic herbal literature of the nineteenth century describes it as a "tonic," or general body strengthener.

## WHAT IS DAMIANA USED FOR TODAY?

Damiana continues to be a popular aphrodisiac for males. However, if it works at all, the effect appears to be rather mild. No scientific trials have been reported.

Damiana is also sometimes said to be helpful for treating **asthma** (page 11) and other respiratory diseases, **depression** (page 54), digestive problems, menstrual disorders, and various forms of sexual dysfunction—for example, **impotence** (page 77) in men and inability to achieve orgasm in women.[2,3]

Like the herb **uva ursi** (page 313), damiana contains arbutin, although at a concentration about 10 times lower. Arbutin is a urinary anti-

septic, but the levels present in damiana are probably too small to make this herb a useful treatment for **bladder infections** (page 23).

## DOSAGES

The proper dosage of damiana is 2 to 4 g taken 2 to 3 times daily, or as directed on the label.

## SAFETY ISSUES

Damiana appears to be safe at the recommended dosages. It appears on the FDA's GRAS (generally regarded as safe) list and is widely used as a food flavoring. However, because damiana contains low levels of cyanide-like compounds, excessive doses may be dangerous. Safety in young children, pregnant or nursing women, or those with severe liver or kidney disease is not established. The only common side effect of damiana is occasional mild gastrointestinal distress.

Damiana

Visit Us at TNP.com

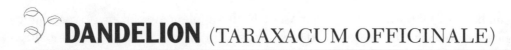

# DANDELION (TARAXACUM OFFICINALE)

## Principal Proposed Uses
Fluid retention (leaves), nutritional supplement (leaves), liver/gallbladder disease (root), constipation (root), various forms of arthritis (root)

The common dandelion, enemy of suburban lawns, is an unusually nutritious food. Its leaves contain substantial levels of vitamins A, C, D, and B complex as well as iron, magnesium, zinc, potassium, manganese, copper, choline, calcium, boron, and silicon.

Worldwide, the root of the dandelion has been used for the treatment of a variety of liver and gallbladder problems. Other historical uses of the root and leaves include the treatment of breast diseases, water retention, digestive problems, joint pain, fever, and skin diseases.

The most active constituents in dandelion appear to be eudesmanolide and germacranolide, substances unique to this herb. Other ingredients include taraxol, taraxerol, and taraxasterol, along with stigmasterol, beta-sitosterol, caffeic acid, and p-hydroxyphenylacetic acid.[1]

## WHAT IS DANDELION USED FOR TODAY?

Dandelion leaves are widely recommended as a food supplement for pregnant and also postmenopausal women because of the many nutrients they contain. They also appear to produce a mild diuretic effect, which may be appreciated by those who suffer from fluid retention.

In the folk medicine of many countries, dandelion root is regarded as a "liver tonic," a substance believed to benefit the liver in an unspecified way. This led to its use for many illnesses traditionally believed to be caused by a "sluggish" or "congested" liver, including constipation, headaches, eye problems, gout, skin problems, fatigue, and boils.

Building on this traditional thinking, some modern naturopathic physicians believe that dandelion can help "detoxify" or clean out the liver and gallbladder.[2] This concept has led to the suggestion that dandelion can reduce the side effects of medications processed by the liver, as well as relieve symptoms of diseases in which impaired liver function plays a role. However, there is as yet no real evidence for any of these uses.

Dandelion root is also used like other bitter herbs to improve appetite and treat minor digestive disorders. When dried and roasted, it is sometimes used as a coffee substitute. Finally, dandelion root has been used for the treatment of "rheumatism" (arthritis) and mild **constipation** (page 51).

The scientific basis for the use of dandelion is scanty. Preliminary studies suggest that dandelion root stimulates the flow of bile.[3,4,5] Dandelion leaves have also been found to produce a mild diuretic effect.[6]

## DOSAGES

A typical dosage of dandelion root is 2 to 8 g 3 times daily of dried root; 250 mg 3 to 4 times daily of a 5:1 extract; or 5 to 10 ml 3 times daily of a 1:5 tincture in 45% alcohol. The leaves may be eaten in salad or cooked.

## SAFETY ISSUES

Dandelion root and leaves are believed to be quite safe, with no side effects or likely risks other than rare allergic reactions.[7–10] It is on the FDA's GRAS (generally regarded as safe) list and approved for use as a food flavoring by the Council of Europe.

However, based on dandelion root's effect on bile secretion, Germany's Commission E has recommended that it not be used at all by individuals with obstruction of the bile ducts or other serious diseases of the gallbladder, and only under physician supervision by those with gallstones.[11]

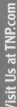

Some references state that dandelion root can cause hyperacidity and thereby increase ulcer pain, but this concern has been disputed.[12]

Because the leaves contain so much **potassium** (page 282), they probably resupply any potassium lost due to dandelion's mild diuretic effect, although this has not been proven.

People with known allergies to related plants, such as **chamomile** (page 156) and **yarrow** (page 345), should use dandelion with caution.

There are no known drug interactions with dandelion. However, based on what we know about dandelion root's effects, there might be some risk when combining it with pharmaceutical diuretics or drugs that reduce blood sugar levels.

Safety in young children, pregnant or nursing women, or those with severe liver or kidney disease has not been established.

## ⚠ INTERACTIONS YOU SHOULD KNOW ABOUT

If you are taking **diuretic drugs** or **medications that reduce blood sugar levels,** use dandelion only under doctor's supervision.

# DEVIL'S CLAW (HARPAGOPHYTUM PROCUMBENS)

*Principal Proposed Uses*
 Pain and inflammation (e.g., various types of arthritis, gout, bursitis, tendinitis)
 Digestive problems (e.g., loss of appetite, mild stomach upset)

**D**evil's claw is a native of South Africa, so named because of its rather peculiar appearance. (An herbalist friend of mine says it looks like "an intelligent alien plant.") Its large tuberous roots are used medicinally, after being chopped up and dried in the sun for 3 days.

Native South Africans used the herb to reduce pain and fever and stimulate digestion. European colonists brought devil's claw back home, where it became a popular treatment for arthritis.

## WHAT IS DEVIL'S CLAW USED FOR TODAY?

In modern Europe, devil's claw is used to treat all types of joint pain, including **osteoarthritis** (page 95), **rheumatoid arthritis** (page 109), and **gout** (page 69). Devil's claw is also used for soft-tissue pain, such as bursitis and tendinitis.

Like other bitter herbs (and this is one of the bitterest!), devil's claw is said to improve appetite and relieve mild stomach upset.

## WHAT IS THE SCIENTIFIC EVIDENCE FOR DEVIL'S CLAW?

One double-blind study followed 89 individuals with rheumatoid arthritis for a 2-month period. The group given devil's claw showed a significant decrease in pain intensity and improved mobility.[1]

Another double-blind study of 50 people with various types of arthritis found that 10 days of treatment with devil's claw provided significant pain relief.[2]

A recent double-blind study of 118 participants suggests that devil's claw may also help relieve soft-tissue pain (muscles, tendons, etc.).[3]

We don't know how devil's claw works. Some studies have found an anti-inflammatory effect but others have not.[4,5] Apparently, the herb doesn't produce the same changes in prostaglandins as standard anti-inflammatory drugs.[6]

## DOSAGES

A typical dosage of devil's claw is 750 mg 3 times daily of a preparation standardized to contain 3% iridoid glycosides.

## SAFETY ISSUES

Devil's claw appears to be quite safe, with no evidence of toxicity at doses many times higher than recommended.[7] A 6-month open study of 630 people with arthritis showed no side effects other than occasional mild gastrointestinal distress. Devil's claw is not recommended for people with ulcers. Safety in young children, pregnant or nursing women, or those with severe liver or kidney disease has not been established.

 # DHEA (DEHYDROEPIANDROSTERONE)

### Principal Proposed Uses
Lupus

### Other Proposed Uses
Osteoporosis, improving general well-being, slowing aging, Alzheimer's disease, depression

### Supplement Forms/Alternative Names
DHEA sulfate

**D**ehydroepiandrosterone (DHEA), a hormone produced by the adrenal glands, is the most abundant hormone in the *steroid* family found in the bloodstream. Your body uses DHEA as the starting material for making the sex hormones testosterone and estrogen.

Numerous popular books have made extravagant claims about DHEA, but in reality we know very little about the effects of DHEA supplements. A growing number of physicians have begun to report that DHEA is helpful for the autoimmune disease lupus, but there are as yet no studies demonstrating its effectiveness for this or any other condition.

Furthermore, keep in mind that DHEA is not a natural supplement. The DHEA you can buy at the store is made by a synthetic chemical process, and it is a hormone, not a nutrient. Although DHEA appears to be safe to use in the short term, its safety when taken for prolonged periods is unknown.

### SOURCES

The body makes its own DHEA; we get very little in our diets. DHEA production peaks early in life and begins to decline as we reach adulthood. By age 60, our bodies produce just 5 to 15% as much as when we were 20. It's not clear whether this decline in DHEA is a bad thing, but some believe that it may contribute to the aging process.

For use as a dietary supplement, DHEA is manufactured synthetically from substances found in soybeans. Contrary to popular belief, there is no DHEA in **wild yam** (page 344).

### THERAPEUTIC DOSAGES

A typical therapeutic dosage of DHEA is 50 to 200 mg daily, although some studies used dosages above and below this range. A cream containing 10% DHEA may also be used; it is typically applied to the skin at a dosage of 3 to 5 g daily.

Physicians sometimes check DHEA levels and adjust the daily dose to achieve blood levels of 20 to 30 nmol/L.

### THERAPEUTIC USES

Preliminary evidence suggests that DHEA may reduce symptoms of lupus.[1] This is an area of active study at present, and may result in a new approach to treating this chronic autoimmune disease.

A very small study (14 participants) suggests that DHEA cream (10%, 3 to 5 g daily) can help fight **osteoporosis** (page 100).[2]

Primarily because DHEA decreases with age, this hormone has been widely hyped as a kind of fountain of youth. However, there is no real evidence that taking DHEA will slow down any of the effects of aging. One study actually found that DHEA does not increase general well-being in healthy people.[3]

DHEA is also sometimes suggested for **depression** (page 54) and for **Alzheimer's disease** (page 4), but there is no evidence as yet that it is either safe or effective for those purposes.

## WHAT IS THE SCIENTIFIC EVIDENCE FOR DHEA?

### Lupus

A preliminary double-blind placebo-controlled study suggests that DHEA may be helpful for treating symptoms of the serious autoimmune disease lupus.[4] However, this study was too small (only 28 participants) to mean a great deal on its own. Larger studies are presently under way.

## SAFETY ISSUES

DHEA appears to be safe when taken in therapeutic doses, at least in the short term. One study found no significant side effects in 50 women who took up to 200 mg daily for up to 1 year.[5] Another study by the same researcher reported an acne-like rash as the only side effect of DHEA treatment.[6]

Concerns have been raised by one study in rats and another in trout that linked DHEA to liver cancer.[7,8] However, at least four other animal studies suggest that DHEA may have some anticancer effects.[9,10]

The long-term safety of DHEA is entirely unknown. This is the case with many supplements, but because there are animal studies suggesting that DHEA might increase the risk of liver cancer, caution is warranted. Estrogen is one example of a hormone that increases the risk for certain forms of cancer, and it took years for researchers to discover that risk. Keep in mind also that the body converts DHEA into other hormones, including estrogen. This effect could be dangerous for women with hormone-influenced diseases such as breast cancer.

The safety of DHEA in young children, pregnant or nursing women, and individuals with severe liver or kidney disease has not been established. We also don't know whether DHEA interacts with other hormone treatments, such as estrogen, although it certainly stands to reason that it might.

## ⚠ INTERACTIONS YOU SHOULD KNOW ABOUT

If you are taking **hormones,** DHEA may interfere with the effects.

DHEA

# DONG QUAI (ANGELICA SINENSIS)

*Principal Proposed Uses*
  Menstrual disorders (dysmenorrhea, PMS, irregular menstruation)

*Probably Ineffective Uses*
  Menopausal symptoms (when taken alone)

One of the major herbs in the Chinese repertoire, *Angelica sinensis* is closely related to European *Angelica archangelica,* a common garden herb and the flavoring in Benedictine and Chartreuse liqueurs. The carrot-like roots of this fragrant plant are harvested in the fall after about 3 years of cultivation and stored in airtight containers prior to processing.

Traditionally, dong quai is said to be one of the most important herbs for strengthening the

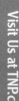

"xue." The Chinese term "xue" is often translated as "blood," but it actually refers to a complex concept of which the blood itself is only a part. In the late 1800s, an extract of dong quai known as Eumenol became popular in Europe as a "female tonic," and this is how most people still understand it in the West.

## WHAT IS DONG QUAI USED FOR TODAY?

Dong quai is often recommended as a treatment for menstrual cramps or **dysmenorrhea** (page 65) and **PMS** (page 104), as well as hot flashes and other **menopausal symptoms** (page 87). The scientific evidence regarding these uses is very weak, consisting primarily of test-tube and animal studies, as well as a few uncontrolled studies of people.[1–5] Furthermore, a recent 24-week study compared the effects of dong quai against a placebo in 71 postmenopausal women.[6] According to the results, dong quai does not reduce menopausal symptoms at all.

Dong quai may be more effective when used in traditional herbal formulas. Two of the most common are Dong Quai and Paeonia, and Bupleurum and Dong Quai. These herbal combinations are frequently used for treating certain types of menopausal symptoms, as well as menstrual pain, fibrocystic breast disease, PMS, abnormal fetal movements, and pelvic inflammatory disease.[7,8,9] However, there is no scientific evidence that they are effective.

Another popular herbal formula is Dong Quai 4, so named because of the total number of herbs involved. This combination, with variations tailored to the individual, is traditionally used to treat certain forms of menstrual irregularity, menstrual pain, anemia, and **insomnia** (page 80).[10,11] A competent Chinese herbalist can tell you which formula would be best for you (according to tradition), as well as adjust the constituents to exactly match your personal needs.

## DOSAGES

I recommend using dong quai under the supervision of a qualified Chinese herbalist, not because the herb is dangerous, but because it is difficult to self-prescribe Chinese herbal formulas.

If you wish to self-treat with dong quai, a typical dosage is 10 to 40 drops of dong quai tincture 1 to 3 times daily, or 1 standard 00 gelatin capsule 3 times daily.

## SAFETY ISSUES

Dong quai is believed to be generally nontoxic. Very large amounts have been given to rats without causing harm.[12] Side effects are rare and primarily consist of mild gastrointestinal distress and occasional allergic reactions (such as rash).

Certain constituents of dong quai can cause increased sensitivity to the sun, but this has not been observed to occur in people using the whole herb.

According to traditional beliefs, inappropriate long-term use of dong quai (such as taking it as a single herb rather than in a combination) can damage the digestive tract and cause other disturbances in overall health. Dong quai is also generally contraindicated during the first 3 months of pregnancy and during acute respiratory infections, and in women with excessively heavy menstruation. However, there is no scientific evidence for these concerns. Safety in young children, pregnant or nursing women, or those with severe liver or kidney disease has not been established.

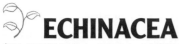 **ECHINACEA**
## (ECHINACEA PURPUREA, E. ANGUSTIFOLIA, E. PALLIDA)

***Principal Proposed Uses***
   Colds and flus (shortening the duration, reducing symptoms)

***Other Proposed Uses***
   Stimulating immunity ("aborting" a cold that has just started, reducing the number of colds during cold season, helping the body fight off other infections)

The decorative plant *Echinacea purpurea,* or purple coneflower, has been one of the most popular herbal medications in both the United States and Europe for over a century.

Native Americans used the related species *Echinacea angustifolia* for a wide variety of problems, including respiratory infections and snakebite. Herbal physicians among the European colonists quickly added the herb to their repertoire. Echinacea became tremendously popular toward the end of the nineteenth century, when a businessman named H. C. F. Meyer promoted an herbal concoction containing *E. angustifolia.* The garish, exaggerated, and poorly written nature of his labeling helped define the characteristics of a "snake oil" remedy.

However, serious manufacturers developed an interest in echinacea as well. By 1920, the respected Lloyd Brothers Pharmaceutical company of Cincinnati, Ohio, counted echinacea as its largest selling product. In Europe, physicians took up the American interest in *E. angustifolia* with enthusiasm. Demand soon outstripped the supply coming from America, and, in an attempt to rapidly plant echinacea locally, the German firm Madeus and Company mistakenly purchased a quantity of *Echinacea purpurea* seeds. This historical accident is the reason why most echinacea today belongs to the *purpurea* species instead of *angustifolia.* Another family member, *Echinacea pallida,* is also used.

Echinacea was the number-one cold and flu remedy in the United States until it was displaced by sulfa antibiotics. Ironically, antibiotics are not effective for colds, while echinacea appears to offer some real help. Echinacea remains the primary remedy for minor respiratory infec-tions in Germany, where over 1.3 million prescriptions are issued each year.

## WHAT IS ECHINACEA USED FOR TODAY?

Germany's Commission E authorizes the use of echinacea juice for "supportive treatment of recurrent infections of the upper respiratory tract and lower urinary tract" and echinacea root extracts for "supportive treatment of flu-like infections." Echinacea has become a wildly popular treatment for **colds and flus** (page 44) in the United States as well, nearing the top of the charts for several years running.

The best scientific evidence about echinacea concerns its ability to help you recover from colds and minor flus more quickly. The old saying goes that a "cold lasts 7 days, but if you treat it, it will be over in a week." However, good evidence tells us that echinacea can actually help you get over colds much faster. It also appears to significantly reduce symptoms while you are sick.

Echinacea may also be able to "abort" a cold, if taken at the first sign of symptoms, but taking echinacea regularly throughout cold season is probably not a great idea. Evidence suggests that it does not work for this purpose, and might actually slightly impair your immunity. For more information on echinacea, see *The Natural Pharmacist Guide to Echinacea and Immunity.*

## WHAT IS THE SCIENTIFIC EVIDENCE FOR ECHINACEA?

Studies of echinacea have used all three species of the herb. We don't know which one is better, or whether they are all equivalent.

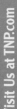

## Reducing the Symptoms and Duration of Colds

Clinical studies with various species of echinacea have found benefits in lessening the symptoms and duration of colds. One double-blind study of 100 individuals with acute flu-like illnesses found that echinacea could significantly reduce cold symptoms.[1] Half of the group received a combination herb product containing *E. angustifolia,* the other half took placebo. The participants rated the severity of symptoms of headache, lethargy, cough, and limb pain. In the treated group, symptoms were significantly less severe.

Another double-blind study of echinacea's effect on flu-like illnesses followed 180 people who were given either 450 mg or 900 mg of *E. purpurea* daily or placebo.[2] By about the third day, those participants receiving the higher dose of echinacea (900 mg) were doing significantly better than those in the placebo or low-dose echinacea groups. Reduction of symptoms was also seen in another double-blind study of *E. purpurea* involving about 200 participants.[3]

Echinacea has also been found to reduce the time needed to get well. A double-blind placebo-controlled study using the *E. pallida* species followed 160 adults with recent onset of cold-like illnesses.[4] The results showed that treatment reduced the average period of illness from 13 days to about 9.5 days, compared to placebo. (These must have been bad colds to last so long!)

Finally, evidence from a double-blind study involving 120 people tells us that *E. purpurea* can cut in half the time it takes for your cold to "turn the corner" and start to get better. This study is described in the next section.

## Preventing Colds

A double-blind study suggests that echinacea can not only make colds shorter and less severe, it can sometimes stop a cold that is just starting.[5] In this study, 120 people were given *E. purpurea* or a placebo as soon as they started showing signs of getting a cold.

Participants took either echinacea or placebo at a dosage of 20 drops every 2 hours for 1 day, then 20 drops 3 times a day for 9 more days. The results over the 10-day study period were prom-

ising. Fewer people in the echinacea group felt that their initial symptoms actually developed into "real" colds (40% of those taking echinacea versus 60% taking the placebo actually became ill). Also, among those who did come down with "real" colds, improvement in the symptoms started sooner in the echinacea group (4 days instead of 8 days). Both of these results were statistically significant. However, echinacea's ability to shorten the duration of colds was more dramatic.

Several studies have attempted to discover whether the daily use of echinacea can prevent colds from even starting, but the results have been less than stellar.

In one double-blind placebo-controlled trial, 302 healthy volunteers were given an alcohol tincture containing either *E. purpurea* root, *E. angustifolia* root, or placebo for 12 weeks.[6] The results showed that *E. purpurea* was associated with perhaps a 20% decrease in the number of people who got sick, and *E. angustifolia* with a 10% decrease. However, the difference was not statistically significant. This means that the benefit, if any, was so small that it could have been due to chance alone.

Actual negative results were seen in a study not yet published at print time.[7] For a period of 6 months, 200 people were given either echinacea or placebo. Use of the herb was actually associated with a 20% higher incidence of sore throat, runny nose, and sinusitis. The authors suggest that long-term use of echinacea might actually slightly impair immune function.

One double-blind placebo-controlled study did find that long-term use of echinacea offered some help, but only for those especially prone to colds.[8] The study involved 609 students at the University of Cologne. Half of the participants were treated with a German product containing *E. angustifolia* for at least 8 weeks; the other half received placebo.

In the group as a whole, echinacea did not significantly decrease the number of colds. However, of the 609 participants, 363 students were rated as particularly prone to infection, based on the number of colds each had developed the winter before. This relatively high-risk group did show a reduction in the number of colds they caught, compared to the control group: The infection-prone students developed on average 20% fewer colds (a statistically significant, although small, improvement).

This study suggests that for those who get sick easily, the regular use of echinacea may slightly decrease the incidence of winter colds. However, considering the other studies in which echinacea had no effect or even a negative one, the bottom line is that echinacea is probably not worth using as a long-term preventive treatment. It is better used directly at the onset of a cold to reduce its severity and duration.

## Immune Stimulation

Both test-tube and animal studies have found that polysaccharides found in echinacea can increase antibody production, raise white blood cell counts, and stimulate the activity of key white blood cells.[9–14] However, the meaningfulness of these studies has been questioned. Many other substances induce similar changes, including wheat, bamboo, rice, sugarcane, and chamomile, and none of these have ever been considered immune stimulants.[15] We don't know whether echinacea produces its effects by stimulating the immune system or in some altogether different way. Its lack of effectiveness in preventing colds when taken over the long term suggests that echinacea does not actually strengthen the immune system overall. See the chapters on **ginseng** (page 206) and **vitamin E** (page 337) for treatments that might offer this benefit.

## DOSAGES

Echinacea is usually taken at the first sign of a cold and continued for 7 to 14 days. The three species of echinacea are used interchangeably. The typical dosage of echinacea powdered extract is 300 mg 3 times a day. Alcohol tincture (1:5) is usually taken at a dosage of 3 to 4 ml 3 times daily, echinacea juice at a dosage of 2 to 3 ml 3 times daily, and whole dried root at 1 to 2 g 3 times daily.

There is no broad agreement on what ingredients should be standardized in echinacea tinctures and solid extracts. However, echinacea juice is often standardized to contain 2.4% of beta-1,2-fructofuranoside.

Many herbalists feel that liquid forms of echinacea are more effective than tablets or capsules, because they feel part of echinacea's benefit is due to activation of the tonsils through direct contact.[16]

Finally, **goldenseal** (page 217) is frequently combined with echinacea in cold preparations. However, there is not a shred of evidence that oral goldenseal stimulates immunity, nor did traditional herbalists use it for this purpose.[17]

## SAFETY ISSUES

Echinacea appears to be safe. Even when taken in very high doses, it has not been found to cause any toxic effects.[18,19] Reported side effects are also uncommon and usually limited to minor gastrointestinal symptoms, increased urination, and mild allergic reactions.[20] Studies dating back to the 1950s suggest that echinacea is safe in children.[21]

Germany's Commission E warns against using echinacea in cases of autoimmune disorders such as multiple sclerosis, lupus, and rheumatoid arthritis, as well as tuberculosis or leukocytosis. There are also rumors that echinacea should not be used by people with AIDS. These warnings are theoretical, based on fears that echinacea might actually activate immunity in the wrong way. But there is no evidence that echinacea use has actually harmed anyone with these diseases.

The Commission E monograph also recommends against using echinacea for more than 8 weeks. The safety of echinacea in young children, pregnant or nursing women, or those with severe liver or kidney disease has not been established. There are no known drug interactions.

Echinacea

Visit Us at TNP.com

# ELDERBERRY (SAMBUCUS NIGRA)

*Principal Proposed Uses*
Flus, colds

*Other Proposed Uses*
HIV, herpes

Native Americans used tea made from elderberry flowers to treat respiratory infections. They also used the leaves and flowers in poultices applied to wounds, and the bark, suitably aged, as a laxative. The berries are frequently made into beverages, pies, and preserves, but they have also been used to treat arthritis.

## WHAT IS ELDERBERRY USED FOR TODAY?

Elderberry flowers are a potential rival for echinacea. Many clinicians feel that elderberry is actually more effective at shortening **colds and flus** (page 44) than the latter, far more famous (and better-studied) herb. According to a preliminary double-blind study performed in Israel, a standardized elderberry extract reduced almost by half the recovery time from a particular strain of epidemic influenza.[1] Elderberry is being studied for potential activity against other viral illnesses as well, including HIV[2] and **herpes** (page 73).[3] Standardized elderberry extracts are seeing increasing use throughout Europe.

## DOSAGES

Elderberry-flower tea is made by steeping 3 to 5 g of dried flowers in 1 cup of boiling water for 10 to 15 minutes. A typical dosage is 1 cup 3 times daily. Standardized extracts should be taken according to the directions on the product's label.

## SAFETY ISSUES

Elderberry flowers are generally regarded as safe. Side effects are rare and consist primarily of occasional mild gastrointestinal distress or allergic reactions. Nonetheless, safety in young children, pregnant or nursing women, or those with severe liver or kidney disease has not been established.

# ELECAMPANE (INULA HELENIUM)

*Principal Proposed Uses*
Chronic respiratory diseases (e.g., asthma), poor digestion

The Latin name of elecampane comes from Helen of Troy, who was supposed to have carried elecampane with her while being abducted from Sparta. Revered by the ancient Greeks and Romans, this herb was recommended for treating such diverse problems as indigestion, melancholy, sciatica, bronchitis, and asthma.

## WHAT IS ELECAMPANE USED FOR TODAY?

Modern herbalists primarily regard elecampane as a long-term treatment for respiratory diseases such as **asthma** (page 11) and bronchitis, especially when excessive mucus is a notable feature. Animal studies suggest that the oil of elecampane

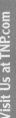

may help suppress coughs.[1] Unfortunately, no human trials of elecampane have been reported.

Elecampane is also sometimes recommended as a daily supplement to improve general digestion.

One of elecampane's constituents, alantolactone, has been used in concentrated form as a treatment for intestinal parasites,[2] but it isn't clear whether the whole herb is particularly effective for this purpose.

## DOSAGES

A typical dosage of elecampane root is 1.5 to 4 g 3 times daily, either in capsule form or boiled in water as tea.

## SAFETY ISSUES

The only reported adverse effects of elecampane are occasional allergic reactions. However, safety in young children, pregnant or nursing women, or those with severe liver or kidney disease has not been established.

# EPHEDRA A.K.A. MA HUANG (EPHEDRA SINICA)

**Principal Proposed Uses**
Effective, but not recommended, for asthma and sinus congestion

**Questionable Proposed Uses**
Weight-loss aid, stimulant

The Chinese herb ma huang is a member of a primitive family of plants that look like thin, branching, connected straws. A related species, *Ephedra nevadensis*, grows wild in the American Southwest and is widely called "Mormon tea." However, only the Asian species of ephedra contains the active compounds ephedrine and pseudoephedrine.

Ma huang was traditionally used by Chinese herbalists during the early stages of respiratory infections and also for the short-term treatment of certain kinds of asthma, eczema, hay fever, narcolepsy, and edema. However, ma huang was not supposed to be taken for an extended period of time, and people with less than robust constitutions were warned to use only low doses or avoid ma huang altogether. If these warnings had been heeded, perhaps some of the current problems with ephedra could have been avoided (see the discussion under What Is Ephedra Used for Today?).

Japanese chemists isolated ephedrine from ma huang at the turn of the century, and it soon became a primary treatment for asthma in the United States and abroad. Ephedra's other major ingredient, pseudoephedrine, became the decongestant Sudafed.

## WHAT IS EPHEDRA USED FOR TODAY?

Although it can still be found in a few over-the-counter drugs for **asthma** (page 11), physicians seldom prescribe ephedrine anymore. The problem is that ephedrine mimics the effects of adrenaline and causes symptoms such as rapid heartbeat, high blood pressure, agitation, insomnia, nausea, and loss of appetite. The newer asthma drugs are much safer and easier to tolerate.

Recently, pills containing ephedrine have been sold as weight-loss aids and "natural" stimulants. Unfortunately, these products have been overused and combined with other stimulants, such as caffeine, resulting in severe overstimulation and even death in some people.[1] In 1997, the FDA proposed stiff limits on dietary supplements containing ephedrine, but they are presently under appeal by manufacturers who say they go too far. The FDA's intervention stemmed from unscrupulous manufacturers, who (mostly via the Internet) promoted ma huang as a natural hallucinogen ("herbal ecstasy") and not as a bronchial decongestant. Dosages of ephedrine required to produce psychoactive effects are exceedingly toxic to the heart; the FDA has documented 38 deaths of otherwise healthy young people who reportedly used ephedrine for psychedelic purposes.

When used properly, ephedra may still be useful as a short-term treatment for sinus congestion and mild asthma, but I would not recommend it as conventional treatments are safer and cause fewer side effects.

## DOSAGES

The dosage of ephedra should be adjusted according to the amount of the ephedrine it provides. A typical adult dosage is 12.5 to 25 mg of ephedrine 3 times daily. It should not be used for more than 1 week. In view of the documented dangers of ephedrine, medical supervision is highly recommended when using ephedra.

## SAFETY ISSUES

Ephedra should *not* be taken by those with enlargement of the prostate, high blood pressure, heart disease, diabetes, hardening of the arteries, glaucoma, or hyperthyroidism.[2] Furthermore, never combine ephedra (or Sudafed) with monoamine-oxidase inhibitors (MAO inhibitors) such as Nardil, or fatal reactions may develop. If symptoms such as a rapid heart rate or a marked increase in blood pressure develop, reduce the dosage or simply stop taking it altogether.

Ephedra is not recommended for young children, pregnant or nursing women, or those with severe liver, heart or kidney disease.

# EYEBRIGHT (EUPHRASIA OFFICINALE L.)

*Principal Proposed Uses*
  Eye infections

The herb eyebright has been used since the Middle Ages as an eyewash for infections and irritations. However, as much as one would like to believe that all traditions are wise, eyebright appears to have been selected for treating eye diseases not because it works particularly well, but because its petals look bloodshot.[1] This follows from the classic medieval philosophic attitude known as the *Doctrine of Signatures*, which states that herbs show their proper use by their appearance.

## WHAT IS EYEBRIGHT USED FOR TODAY?

Like many herbs, eyebright contains astringent substances and volatile oils that are probably at least slightly antibacterial. But there's no evidence that eyebright is particularly effective for treating eye diseases; Germany's Commission E recommends against using it. Warm compresses consisting of nothing but water (or ordinary black tea) are probably equally effective under the same conditions.

Eyebright tea is also sometimes taken internally to treat jaundice, respiratory infections, and memory loss. However, there is no evidence that it is effective for these conditions.

## DOSAGES

Traditionally, eyebright tea is made by boiling 1 tablespoon of the herb in a cup of water. This is then used as an eyewash or taken internally up to 3 times daily.

## SAFETY ISSUES

Eyebright can cause tearing of the eyes, itching, redness, and many other symptoms, probably due to direct irritation.[2] It appears to be safe when taken internally, but not many studies have been performed. Safety in young children, pregnant or nursing women, or those with severe liver or kidney disease has not been established.

# FENUGREEK (TRIGONELLA FOENUMGRAECUM)

**Principal Proposed Uses**
Diabetes (blood sugar control, cholesterol levels), constipation

For millennia, fenugreek has been used both as a medicine and as a food spice in Egypt, India, and the Middle East. It was traditionally recommended for the treatment of wounds, bronchitis, digestive problems, arthritis, kidney problems, and male reproductive conditions.

## WHAT IS FENUGREEK USED FOR TODAY?

Present interest in fenugreek focuses on its benefits for those with **diabetes** (page 60) or high **cholesterol** (page 39). Numerous animal studies and preliminary trials in humans have found that fenugreek can reduce blood sugar and serum cholesterol levels in people with diabetes. Like other high-fiber foods, it may also be helpful for **constipation** (page 51).

## WHAT IS THE SCIENTIFIC EVIDENCE FOR FENUGREEK?

Small double-blind studies suggest that fenugreek can be helpful both for type 1 (childhood onset) and type 2 (adult onset) diabetes.

In one study of 60 people with type 2 diabetes, 25 mg a day of fenugreek led to significant improvements in overall blood sugar control, blood sugar elevations in response to a meal, and cholesterol levels.[1] Another study found benefits with only 15 mg of fenugreek daily.[2]

Finally, in a small double-blind, controlled study, people with type 1 diabetes were randomly prescribed either fenugreek at a dose of 50 gm twice daily as part of their lunch and dinner, or the same meals without the powder, each for 10 days. Those on the fenugreek diet had significant decreases in their fasting blood sugar.[3] (For more information on fenugreek in diabetes, see *The Natural Pharmacist Guide to Diabetes.*)

## DOSAGES

Because the seeds of fenugreek are somewhat bitter, they are best taken in capsule form. The typical dosage is 5 to 30 g of defatted fenugreek taken 3 times a day with meals.

## SAFETY ISSUES

As a commonly eaten food, fenugreek is generally regarded as safe. The only common side effect is mild gastrointestinal distress when it is taken in high doses.

Because fenugreek can lower blood sugar levels, it is advisable to seek medical supervision before combining it with diabetes medications.

Extracts made from fenugreek have been shown to stimulate uterine contractions in guinea pigs.[4] For this reason, pregnant women should not take fenugreek in dosages higher than is commonly used as a spice, perhaps 5 g daily. Besides concerns over pregnant women, safety in young children, nursing women, or those with severe liver or kidney disease has also not been established.

## ⚠ INTERACTIONS YOU SHOULD KNOW ABOUT

If you are taking **diabetes medications,** fenugreek may enhance their effect, possibly causing excessively low blood sugar.

# FEVERFEW (TANACETUM PARTHENIUM)

**Principal Proposed Uses**
Migraine headaches (prevention and treatment)

**Other Proposed Uses**
Arthritis

Originally native to the Balkans, this relative of the common daisy was spread by deliberate planting throughout Europe and the Americas. Feverfew's feathery and aromatic leaves have long been used medicinally to improve childbirth, promote menstruation, induce abortions, relieve rheumatic pain, and treat severe headaches.

Contrary to popular belief, feverfew is not used for lowering fevers. Actually, "feverfew" is a corruption of the name "featherfoil."[1] Featherfoil became featherfew and ultimately feverfew. In a weird historical reversal, this name then led to a widespread belief among herbalists that feverfew could lower fevers. After a while they noticed that it didn't work, and then angrily rejected feverfew as a useless herb! Feverfew remained out of fashion until a serendipitous event occurred in the late 1970s.

At that time, the wife of the chief medical officer of the National Coal Board in England suffered from serious migraine headaches. When workers in the industry learned of this fact, a sympathetic miner suggested she try a folk treatment he had used. She followed his advice and chewed feverfew leaves. The results were dramatic: Her migraines disappeared almost completely.

Her husband was impressed, too. He used his high office to gain the ear of a physician who specialized in migraine headaches, Dr. E. Stewart Johnson of the London Migraine Clinic. Johnson subsequently tried feverfew on 10 of his patients. The results were so good that he subsequently gave the herb to 270 of his patients. A whopping 70% reported considerable relief.

Thoroughly excited now, Dr. Johnson enrolled 17 feverfew-using patients in an interesting type of double-blind study: Half continued to use feverfew, and the other half were transferred, without their knowledge, to a placebo.[2] Over a period of 6 months, the patients withdrawn from feverfew demonstrated a dramatic increase in headaches, nausea, and vomiting.

Unfortunately, this study didn't prove much. It was too small, and because the patients were already feverfew users, it didn't say anything about the effectiveness of feverfew in the population at large. (Presumably, the participants used feverfew because they already knew that the herb worked for them.) Nonetheless, the study brought a flood of response from the public, and ultimately led to the properly performed double-blind experiments described below.

For many years, it was assumed that the active ingredient in feverfew was a substance named parthenolide. Numerous articles were published explaining exactly how parthenolide prevented migraines, stating that it caused platelets to release serotonin and reduce the synthesis of prostaglandins, leukotrienes, and thromboxanes.[3–6] Based on this premature explanation, indignant authors complained that samples of feverfew on the market varied as much as 10 to 1 in their parthenolide content. No less an authority than herbal expert Varro Tyler said, "Standardization of the herbal material on the basis of its parthenolide content is urgently required if this potentially valuable herb is to be used effectively."[7]

However, everyone was jumping the gun. A recent study found that an extract of feverfew standardized to a high-parthenolide content is entirely ineffective.[8] Apparently, this high-parthenolide extract lacked some essential substance or group of substances present in the whole leaf. What those substances may be, however, remains mysterious.

## WHAT IS FEVERFEW USED FOR TODAY?

Feverfew is primarily used for prevention of chronic, recurrent **migraine headaches** (page 89). It must be taken religiously every day for best results.

Feverfew is also sometimes used at the onset of a migraine attack. It is not believed to be effective for cluster or tension headaches.

It is important to remember that serious diseases may occasionally first present themselves as migraine-type headaches. For this reason, proper medical diagnosis is essential if you suddenly start having migraines without a previous history, or if the pattern of your migraines changes significantly.

Feverfew is sometimes recommended as a treatment for various forms of **arthritis** (pages 95 and 109), but there is no evidence that it works.

## WHAT IS THE SCIENTIFIC EVIDENCE FOR FEVERFEW?

Three double-blind studies have been performed to evaluate feverfew's effectiveness as a preventive treatment for migraines. Two returned positive results, the other negative.

The Nottingham trial followed 59 individuals for 8 months.[9] For 4 months, half received a daily capsule of powdered feverfew leaf; the other half took placebo. The groups were then switched and followed for an additional 4 months. Treatment with feverfew produced a 24% reduction in the number of migraines and a significant decrease in nausea and vomiting during the headaches.

A recent Israeli study of 57 people with migraines found a significant decrease in severity of migraine headaches.[10] Unfortunately, it did not report whether there was any change in the frequency of migraines. This study also used powdered feverfew leaf.

However, a Dutch study involving 50 people showed no difference whatsoever between placebo and a special feverfew extract standardized to parthenolide content.[11] As mentioned above, the explanation appears to be that parthenolide is not the active ingredient in feverfew.

## DOSAGES

Given the recent confusion surrounding parthenolide, previous dosage recommendations for feverfew based on parthenolide content have been cast in doubt. At the present time, the best recommendation is probably to take 80 to 100 mg of powdered whole feverfew leaf daily.

When taken at the onset of a migraine headache, higher amounts of feverfew are often used. However, the optimum dosage has not been determined.

## SAFETY ISSUES

Among the many thousands of people who use feverfew as a folk medicine in England, there have been no reports of serious toxicity. Animal studies suggest that feverfew is essentially nontoxic.[12]

In the 8-month Nottingham trial, there were no significant differences in side effects between the treated and control groups.[13] There were also no changes in measurements on blood tests and urinalysis.

In a survey involving 300 people, 11.3% reported mouth sores from chewing feverfew leaf, occasionally accompanied by general inflammation of tissues in the mouth.[14] A smaller percentage reported mild gastrointestinal distress.[15] However, mouth sores do not seem to occur in people who use encapsulated feverfew leaf powder, the usual form.

In view of its use as a folk remedy to promote abortions, feverfew should probably not be taken during pregnancy.

Because feverfew might slightly inhibit the activity of blood-clotting cells known as platelets,[16] it should not be combined with strong anticoagulants, such as Coumadin (warfarin) or heparin, except on medical advice.

Safety in young children, pregnant or nursing women, or those with severe kidney or liver disease has not been established.

## ⚠ INTERACTIONS YOU SHOULD KNOW ABOUT

If you are taking **Coumadin (warfarin)** or **heparin,** do not use feverfew except on medical advice.

Feverfew

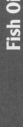

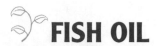 **FISH OIL**

### Principal Proposed Uses

Heart disease prevention, rheumatoid arthritis

### Other Proposed Uses

Dysmenorrhea (menstrual pain), bipolar disease (manic-depressive illness), Raynaud's phenomenon, osteoporosis, lupus, psoriasis, diabetes, ulcerative colitis, Crohn's disease, asthma, allergies, gout, hypertension, migraine headaches

### Supplement Forms/Alternative Names

Eicosapentaenoic acid (EPA), docosahexaenoic acid (DHA), omega-3 oil(s), omega-3 fatty acids

If you're old enough, you may remember your mother giving you cod liver oil. This practice actually began when the smoke-filled skies of nineteenth-century England deprived youngsters of exposure to the sun. Without sun, their bodies couldn't make vitamin D, and they developed rickets. Because cod liver oil contains large amounts of vitamin D, it cured rickets and made a great contribution to public health. Today, however, other constituents of cod liver and other fish oils have become of interest: the omega-3 fatty acids.

Omega-3 fatty acids are one type of *essential fatty acids*, special fats that the body needs as much as it needs vitamins. (The other type is the omega-6 fatty acids. For more information, see the chapter on **GLA** [page 210].) Much of the research into the potential therapeutic benefits of omega-3 fatty acids began when studies of the Inuit (Eskimo) people found that although their diets contain an enormous amount of fat from fish, seals, and whales, they seldom suffer heart attacks or develop rheumatoid arthritis. This is presumably because those sources of fat are very high in omega-3 fatty acids.

Subsequent investigation found that the omega-3 fatty acids found in fish oil can lower blood triglyceride levels, "thin" the blood, and also decrease inflammation in various parts of the body. These effects, as well as others, may explain many of fish oil's apparent benefits.

### REQUIREMENTS/SOURCES

There is no daily requirement for fish oil. However, a healthy diet should provide at least 5 g of essential fatty acids daily.

Many grains, fruits, vegetables, and vegetable oils contain significant amounts of essential omega-6 and/or omega-3 fatty acids. Some authorities believe that it is important to consume several times more omega-3 fatty acids than omega-6 fatty acids. If this theory is true, taking fish oil supplements might help ensure the proper balance.

Cod liver oil is the most common form of fish oil, but it may not be the best for reasons of safety (see Safety Issues). Salmon oil, mackerel oil, halibut oil, and the oils from other coldwater fish might be better choices.

### THERAPEUTIC DOSAGES

Typical dosages of fish oil are 3 to 9 g daily, but this is not the upper limit. In one study, participants ingested 60 g daily.

The most important omega-3 fatty acids found in fish oil are called EPA (eicosapentaenoic acid) and DHA (docosahexaenoic acid). In order to match the dosage used in several major studies, you should probably take enough fish oil to supply about 1.8 g of EPA (1,800 mg) and 0.9 g of DHA daily (900 mg).

Some manufacturers add vitamin E to fish oil capsules to keep the oil from becoming rancid. Another method is to remove all the oxygen from the capsule.

Flaxseed oil also contains omega-3 fatty acids, although of a different kind. It has been suggested as a less smelly substitute for fish oil. However, there is no evidence that it is effective when used for the same therapeutic purposes as fish oil.[1]

## THERAPEUTIC USES

There has been a great deal of excitement about the possibility of using fish oil to help prevent **heart disease** (page 14). Fish oil appears to lower triglyceride levels, raise HDL ("good") cholesterol, "thin" the blood, reduce levels of homocysteine, and perhaps also treat **hypertension** (page 75).[2–11] However, we do not as yet have any direct evidence that it slows down atherosclerosis, reduces the rate of heart attacks, or prevents serious heart disease.

Fish oil has also become recognized as an effective treatment for early stages of **rheumatoid arthritis** (page 109). It appears to significantly reduce symptoms without side effects and may magnify the benefits of standard arthritis drugs.[12] However, we have no evidence that fish oil slows the progress of the disease. Consult your rheumatologist to determine what treatment is best for you.

Various essential fatty acids, including fish oil, **flaxseed oil** (page 193), and **GLA (gamma-linolenic acid)** (page 210), are widely recommended for **dysmenorrhea** (page 65) (menstrual pain), and a study of adolescent women suggests that fish oil may indeed be effective.[13]

A study suggests that fish oil can be very helpful for bipolar disease, more commonly known as manic-depressive disorder.[14] More research is needed, but this appears to be a potential breakthrough for this devastating illness, whose conventional treatment causes a great many side effects.

Small studies also suggest that fish oil may be helpful in **Raynaud's phenomenon** (page 108) (a condition in which a person's hands and feet show abnormal sensitivity to cold temperatures),[15,16] **osteoporosis** (page 100),[17,18] and the autoimmune disease lupus.[19] There is some evidence that eicosapentaenoic acid (EPA) from fish oil may be helpful in **psoriasis** (page 106). One double-blind study followed 28 people with chronic psoriasis for 8 weeks.[20] Half received 1.8 mg of EPA daily (supplied by 10 capsules of fish oil), and the other half received placebo. By the end of the study, researchers saw significant improvement in itching, redness, and scaling, but not in the size of the psoriasis patches. How-

ever, another double-blind study followed 145 people with moderate to severe psoriasis for 4 months and found no benefit as compared to placebo.[21]

Fish oil has also been proposed as a treatment for many other conditions, including **diabetes** (page 60), **allergies** (page 3), **gout** (page 69), **hypertension** (page 75), **migraine headaches** (page 89), ulcerative colitis, and Crohn's disease, but there has been little real scientific investigation of these uses. Fish oil does not appear to be helpful for **asthma** (page 11).[22,23]

## WHAT IS THE SCIENTIFIC EVIDENCE FOR FISH OIL?

### Heart Disease Prevention

Although we have direct evidence that a diet high in fish reduces the incidence of heart disease,[24,25] we don't know for sure if fish oil is as effective.

We do know that fish oil can lower serum triglycerides.[26] Like cholesterol, triglycerides are a type of fat in the blood that tends to damage the arteries, leading to heart disease. Reducing triglyceride levels should help prevent heart disease to some extent.

Fish oil also appears to modestly raise the levels of HDL or "good" cholesterol.[27,28] Additionally, it may help the heart by "thinning" the blood and by reducing blood levels of homocysteine.[29] Blood clots play a major role in heart attacks, and homocysteine is an amino acid that appears to raise the risk of heart disease.

Finally, some studies have found that fish oil can lower blood pressure.[30–34] However, a recent large study involving more than 2,000 subjects found no effect.[35]

### Rheumatoid Arthritis

The omega-3 fatty acids in fish oil can help reduce the symptoms of rheumatoid arthritis, according to 12 double-blind placebo-controlled studies involving a total of over 500 people.[36] This evidence is so strong that it has impressed many conventional physicians. However, unlike some conventional treatments, fish oil probably does not slow the progression of rheumatoid arthritis.

**Fish Oil**

**Visit Us at TNP.com**

## Menstrual Pain

Regular use of fish oil may reduce the pain of menstrual cramps. In a 4-month study of 42 young women aged 15 to 18, half the participants received a daily dose of 6 g of fish oil, providing 1,080 mg of EPA and 720 mg of DHA daily.[37] After 2 months, they were switched to placebo for another 2 months. The other group received the same treatments in reverse order.

The results showed that these young women experienced significantly less menstrual pain while they were taking fish oil.

## Bipolar Disease

A 4-month, double-blind placebo-controlled study of 30 individuals suggests that fish oil can produce striking benefits in bipolar disease, preventing relapse and improving emotional state.[38] Eleven of the 14 individuals who took fish oil improved or remained well during the course of the study, while only 6 out of the 16 participants given placebo responded similarly.

The study will now be repeated by Baylor University and Harvard Medical School/McLean Hospital, enrolling 120 people for a period of 3 years.

## Raynaud's Phenomenon

In small double-blind studies, high dosages of fish oil have been found to reduce the severe finger and toe responses to cold temperatures that occur in Raynaud's phenomenon.[39,40] However, these studies suggest that a very high dosage must be used to get results, perhaps 12 g daily. Gamma-linolenic acid (GLA), an omega-6 fatty acid, may work as well.

## Osteoporosis

Essential fatty acids may also help prevent osteoporosis when taken along with calcium. In one study, 65 postmenopausal women were given calcium along with either placebo or a combination of omega-6 fatty acids (GLA) and omega-3 fatty acids (from fish oil) for 18 months. At the end of the study, the treated groups had denser bones and fewer fractures than the placebo group.[41] Similar results were seen in another study of 40 women.[42]

## Lupus

Lupus is a serious autoimmune disease that can cause numerous problems, including fatigue, joint pain, and kidney disease. One small but well-designed study compared placebo against daily doses (20 g) of EPA from fish oil in 30 individuals with lupus. Fourteen of 17 subjects who took EPA improved significantly, whereas all those on placebo either stayed the same or got worse.[43]

## SAFETY ISSUES

Fish oil appears to be safe. The most common problem is fishy burps.

Because fish oil has a mild "blood-thinning" effect, it should not be combined with powerful blood-thinning medications, such as Coumadin (warfarin) or heparin, except on a physician's advice. However, contrary to some reports, fish oil does not seem to cause bleeding problems when it is taken by itself.[44,45]

Also, fish oil does not appear to raise blood sugar levels in people with diabetes.[46] Nonetheless, if you have diabetes, you should not take any supplement except on the advice of a physician.

Fish oil may temporarily raise the level of LDL, or "bad," cholesterol; but this effect seems to be short-lived, and levels return to normal with continued use.[47,48]

If you decide to use cod liver oil as your fish oil supplement, make sure you do not exceed the safe maximum intake of **vitamin A** (page 318) and **vitamin D** (page 335). These vitamins are fat-soluble, which means that excess amounts tend to build up in your body, possibly reaching toxic levels. Pregnant women should not take more than 2,500 IU of vitamin A daily because of the risk of birth defects; 5,000 IU a day is a reasonable upper limit for other individuals. Vitamin D becomes toxic when taken at dosages above 1,000 IU daily for prolonged periods. Look at the bottle label to determine how much of these vitamins you are receiving.

## ⚠ INTERACTIONS
## YOU SHOULD KNOW ABOUT

If you are taking **Coumadin (warfarin)** or **heparin,** do not take fish oil except on the advice of a physician.

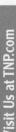

# 5-HTP (5-HYDROXYTRYPTOPHAN)

## Principal Proposed Uses
Depression, migraine headaches

## Other Proposed Uses
Obesity (weight loss), fibromyalgia, insomnia, anxiety

---

Many antidepressant drugs work, at least in part, by raising serotonin levels. The supplement 5-hydroxytryptophan (5-HTP) has been tried in cases of depression for a similar reason: The body uses 5-HTP to make serotonin, so providing the body with 5-HTP might therefore raise serotonin levels.

As a supplement, 5-HTP has also been proposed for all the same uses as other antidepressants, including aiding weight loss, preventing migraine headaches, decreasing the discomfort of fibromyalgia, improving sleep quality, and reducing anxiety.

## SOURCES

5-HTP is not found in foods to any appreciable extent. For use as a supplement, it is manufactured from the seeds of an African plant (*Griffonia simplicifolia*).

## THERAPEUTIC DOSAGES

A typical dosage of 5-HTP is 100 to 200 mg 3 times daily. Once 5-HTP starts to work, it may be possible to reduce the dosage significantly and still maintain good results.

## THERAPEUTIC USES

The primary use of 5-HTP is for **depression** (page 54). Several small, short-term studies have found that it may be as effective as standard antidepressant drugs.[1,2] Since standard antidepressants are also used for **insomnia** (page 80) and **anxiety** (page 8), 5-HTP has also been suggested as a treatment for those conditions, although there is as yet no direct evidence that it works.

Other double-blind studies suggest that 5-HTP may help reduce the frequency and sever-ity of **migraine headaches** (page 89).[3–9] Additionally, preliminary evidence suggests that 5-HTP can reduce symptoms of fibromyalgia[10] and perhaps help you lose weight.[11,12,13]

## WHAT IS THE SCIENTIFIC EVIDENCE FOR 5-HTP?

### Depression

Several small studies have compared 5-HTP to standard antidepressants.[14] The best was a recent 6-week study of 63 people given either 5-HTP (100 mg 3 times daily) or an antidepressant in the Prozac family (fluvoxamine, 50 mg 3 times daily).[15] Researchers found equal benefit between the supplement and the drug. Actually, 5-HTP worked a little better at reducing depressed mood, anxiety, physical symptoms, and insomnia, but the differences were not statistically significant. There was no question that 5-HTP caused fewer and less severe side effects. The only real complaint with 5-HTP was occasional mild digestive distress, which is found with virtually all medications.

### Migraine Headaches

A number of drugs are used to prevent migraine headaches, including antidepressants in the Prozac family. Although we don't know for sure, many of them appear to work by either changing serotonin levels or producing serotonin-like effects in the body. There is some evidence that 5-HTP may be effective as well.

In a 6-month trial of 124 people, 5-HTP proved equally effective as the standard drug methysergide.[16] The most dramatic benefits seen were a reduction in the intensity and duration of migraines. Since methysergide has been proven better than placebo for migraine headaches in earlier studies, the study results provide meaningful, although not airtight, evidence that 5-HTP is also effective.

Similarly good results were seen in another comparative study, using a different medication.[17] However, in one study, 5-HTP was less effective than the drug propranolol.[18]

Other studies sometimes quoted as evidence that 5-HTP is effective for migraines actually enrolled adults or children with many different types of headaches (including migraines).[19–22] Most of them found at least some benefit.

Putting all this evidence together, it appears likely that 5-HTP can help people with frequent migraine headaches, but further research needs to be done. In particular, we need a large double-blind study that compares 5-HTP against placebo over a period of several months.

## Obesity (Weight Loss)

The drug fenfluramine was one member of the now infamous phen-fen treatment for weight loss. Although very successful, fenfluramine was later associated with damage to the valves of the heart, and was removed from the market. Because fenfluramine raises serotonin levels, it seems reasonable to believe that other substances that affect serotonin might also be useful for weight reduction.

Three small placebo-controlled double-blind clinical trials have examined whether 5-HTP can help you lose weight. The first study found that 5-HTP (80 mg daily) could reduce caloric intake despite the fact that the 19 participants made no conscious effort to eat less.[23] The second study, which used a much higher dosage (900 mg daily) in 20 overweight women, found that treatment helped the participants stick to their diets.[24] The result was improved weight loss.

A third study that enrolled 20 obese women confirmed the results of the second, with slightly better results: After 12 weeks the average weight loss in the 5-HTP group was 10.3 pounds versus just 2.28 pounds in the placebo group.[25] These impressive results deserve more study.

For another approach to weight loss, specifically reducing fat, see the chapter on **chromium** (page 161).

## Fibromyalgia

Antidepressants are the primary conventional treatment for fibromyalgia, a little-understood disease characterized by aching, tender muscles, fatigue, and disturbed sleep. One study suggests that 5-HTP may be helpful as well. In this double-blind trial, 50 subjects with fibromyalgia were given either 100 mg of 5-HTP or placebo 3 times daily for a month.[26] Those receiving 5-HTP experienced significant improvements in all symptom categories, including pain, stiffness, sleep patterns, anxiety, and fatigue.

For another approach to fibromyalgia, see the chapter on **SAMe** (page 293).

## SAFETY ISSUES

No significant adverse effects have been reported in clinical trials of 5-HTP. Side effects appear to be limited to occasional mild digestive distress and possible allergic reactions.

However, there is one potentially serious concern. In 1998, the U.S. Food and Drug Administration reported detecting a chemical compound known as "peak X" in some 5-HTP products. Peak X has a frightening history involving a related supplement: tryptophan. Until about 10 years ago, tryptophan was widely used as a sleep aid. However, it was taken off the market when thousands of people using the supplement developed a disabling and sometimes fatal blood disorder. This same contaminant, peak X, was found to be associated with that disaster.

Since the body turns tryptophan into 5-HTP, the latter has been marketed as a safe replacement for the banned amino acid. Until recently, it was assumed that 5-HTP could not possibly present the same risk as tryptophan because it is manufactured completely differently. However, the recent discovery that the same substance exists in batches of 5-HTP is worrisome. As this book goes to press, there is no other information from the FDA regarding specific cautions on using 5-HTP, but you should pay close attention to reports that may follow up on this finding.

Safety in young children, pregnant or nursing women, and those with liver or kidney disease has not been established (although, in some studies children have been given 5-HTP without any apparent harmful effects).

## ⚠ INTERACTIONS
## YOU SHOULD KNOW ABOUT

If you are taking

- **Prescription antidepressants:** Do not take 5-HTP in addition except on a physician's advice. There is a chance you might raise serotonin levels too high.

- The Parkinson's disease medication **carbidopa:** Taking 5-HTP at the same time might increase your chance of developing the disease scleroderma.[27,28,29]

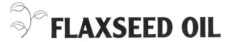

# FLAXSEED OIL

*Principal Proposed Uses*
There are no well-documented uses for flaxseed oil.

*Other Proposed Uses*
Heart disease prevention, rheumatoid arthritis, cancer prevention

*Supplement Forms/Alternative Names*
Linseed oil. Flaxseed oil contains alpha-linolenic acid.

Flaxseed oil is derived from the hard, tiny seeds of the flax plant. It has been proposed as a less smelly alternative to **fish oil** (page 188). Like fish oil, flaxseed oil contains omega-3 fatty acids, a type of fat your body needs as much as it needs vitamins.

However, it's important to realize that the omega-3 fatty acids in flaxseed oil aren't identical to what you get from fish oil. Flaxseed oil contains alpha-linolenic acid (ALA), while fish oil contains eicosapentaenoic acid (EPA) and docosahexaenoic acid (DHA). The effects and potential benefits may not be the same.

Flaxseed oil also contains another important group of chemicals, *lignans.* Lignans are being studied for use in preventing cancer.

## REQUIREMENTS/SOURCES

Flaxseed oil contains both omega-3 and omega-6 fatty acids, which are essential to health. Although the exact daily requirement of these essential fatty acids is not known, deficiencies are believed to be fairly common.[1] Flaxseed oil may be an economical way to ensure that you get enough essential fatty acids in your diet.

The essential fatty acids in flax can be damaged by exposure to heat, light, and oxygen (essentially, they become rancid). For this reason, you shouldn't cook with flaxseed oil. A good product should be sold in an opaque container, and the manufacturing process should keep the temperature under 100 degrees Fahrenheit. Some manufacturers combine the product with vitamin E because it helps prevent rancidity.

## THERAPEUTIC DOSAGES

A typical dosage is 1 to 2 tablespoons of flaxseed oil daily. It can be taken in capsule form or made into salad dressing. Some people find the taste pleasant, although others would politely disagree.

## THERAPEUTIC USES

The best use of flaxseed oil is as a general nutritional supplement to provide essential fatty acids. There is little evidence that it is effective for any specific therapeutic purpose.

Flaxseed oil has been proposed as a less smelly alternative to fish oil for the prevention of **heart disease** (page 14). However, while fish oil lowers blood triglyceride levels as its main effect, flaxseed oil does not affect triglyceride levels.[2] Still, there is some evidence that flaxseed oil or whole flaxseed may reduce LDL ("bad") **cholesterol** (page 39) and perhaps slightly help **hypertension** (page 75).[3,4]

In addition, one study found that a diet high in ALA (from sources other than flaxseed oil) was associated with a reduced risk of heart disease.[5] However, there were so many other factors involved that it is hard to say what caused what.[6]

Although fish oil appears to be effective for reducing symptoms of **rheumatoid arthritis** (page 109), flaxseed oil does not seem to work.[7]

Finally, although flaxseed oil is sometimes recommended as prevention or treatment for **cancer** (page 26), the evidence is still extremely preliminary.[8,9,10]

## SAFETY ISSUES

Flaxseed oil appears to be a safe nutritional supplement when used as recommended.

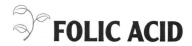

# FOLIC ACID

## Principal Proposed Uses
Preventing birth defects of the brain and spinal cord, preventing heart disease, preventing cancer

## Other Proposed Uses
Gout, depression, osteoporosis, rheumatoid arthritis, vitiligo, migraine headaches, periodontal disease

## Supplement Forms/Alternate Names
Folate, folacin

Folic acid, a B vitamin, plays a critical role in many biological processes. It participates in the crucial biological process known as *methylation,* and plays an important role in cell division: Without sufficient amounts of folic acid, cells cannot divide properly. Adequate folic acid intake can reduce the risk of heart disease and prevent serious birth defects, and it may lessen the risk of developing certain forms of cancer.

Because the chances are good that you don't get enough folic acid in your diet, this is one vitamin really worth paying attention to.

## REQUIREMENTS/SOURCES

Folic acid requirements rise with age. The U.S. Recommended Dietary Allowance is as follows

- Infants under 6 months, 25 mcg
  6 to 12 months, 35 mcg
- Children 1 to 3 years, 150 mcg
  4 to 8 years, 200 mcg

- Males 9 to 13 years, 300 mcg
  14 years and older, 400 mcg
- Females 9 to 13 years, 300 mcg
  14 years and older, 400 mcg
- Pregnant women, 600 mcg
- Nursing women, 500 mcg

Folic acid deficiency is very common, and authorities have suggested adding folic acid to common foods, such as bread, at higher dosages than what is presently required.[1,2]

Various drugs can impair your body's ability to absorb or utilize folic acid, including antacids, alcohol, oral contraceptives, estrogen, sulfasalazine, methotrexate, triamterene, Zantac (ranitidine), corticosteroids (prednisone), cholestyramine, colestipol, and antiseizure medications (valproate, carbamazepine, phenytoin, or phenobarbital).[3,4]

Good sources of folic acid include dark green leafy vegetables (hence the name "folic," for "foliage"), oranges, other fruits, rice, brewer's yeast, beef liver, beans, asparagus, soybeans, and soy flour.

## THERAPEUTIC DOSAGES

For most uses, folic acid should be taken at nutritional doses, about 400 mcg daily for adults. However, higher dosages—up to 10 mg daily—have been used to treat specific diseases. Before taking more than 400 mcg daily, it is important to make sure that you don't have a vitamin $B_{12}$ deficiency (see Safety Issues).

A particular kind of digestive enzyme, pancreatin (see the chapter on **proteolytic enzymes** [page 285]) may interfere with the absorption of folic acid.[5] You can get around this by taking the two supplements at different times of day.

## THERAPEUTIC USES

The use of folic acid supplements by pregnant women dramatically decreases the risk that their children will be born with a serious birth defect called neural tube defect.[6,7] This congenital problem consists of problems with the brain or spinal cord.

Folic acid also lowers blood levels of homocysteine, a suspected risk factor in **heart disease** (page 14).[8–13] According to some experts, increased folate supplementation of foods could reduce heart disease deaths in the United States by as much as 50,000 people annually.[14]

Studies suggest that a deficiency in folic acid might predispose people to develop cancer of the cervix,[15] colon,[16] lung,[17] and mouth.[18] This is yet another reason to make sure you get enough folic acid daily. Although there is no evidence that folic acid supplements can treat cancer, preliminary studies suggest that very high dosages of folic acid (more than 10 mg daily) may be able to reverse precancerous changes found in the cervix among women taking oral contraceptives.[19,20,21]

Very high dosages of folic acid may also be helpful for **gout** (page 69),[22] although some authorities suggest that it was actually a contaminant of folic acid that caused the benefit seen in some studies.[23] Furthermore, other studies have found no benefit at all.[24,25]

Based on intriguing but not yet definitive evidence, folic acid in various dosages has been suggested as a treatment for **depression** (page 54),

bipolar disorder, **osteoporosis** (page 100), **osteoarthritis** (page 95) (in combination with vitamin $B_{12}$), restless legs syndrome, **rheumatoid arthritis** (page 109), and vitiligo (splotchy loss of skin pigmentation).[26–36] Other conditions for which it has been suggested include **migraine headaches** (page 89) and **periodontal disease** (page 103).

## WHAT IS THE SCIENTIFIC EVIDENCE FOR FOLIC ACID?

### Neural Tube Defects

Very strong evidence tells us that regular use of folic acid by pregnant women can reduce the risk of neural tube defect by 50 to 80%.[37,38]

### Heart Disease Prevention

According to a recent study that examined data on 80,000 women, a high intake of folic acid may cut the risk of heart disease in half.[39]

Folic acid is thought to work by reducing blood levels of a substance called homocysteine. Individuals with high homocysteine levels appear to have more than twice the risk of developing heart disease than those with low homocysteine levels,[40] and folic acid supplements, alone or in combination with **vitamin $B_6$** (page 326) and **vitamin $B_{12}$** (page 329), effectively reduce the level of homocysteine in the blood.[41–44]

## SAFETY ISSUES

Folic acid at nutritional doses is extremely safe. The only serious potential problem is that folic acid supplementation can mask the early symptoms of vitamin $B_{12}$ deficiency (a special type of anemia), potentially allowing more irreversible symptoms of nerve damage to develop. For this reason, when taking more than 400 mcg daily, it is important to get your $B_{12}$ level checked. See the chapter on vitamin $B_{12}$ for more information.

Very high dosages of folic acid, greater than 5 mg (5,000 mcg) daily, can cause digestive upset. According to a few reports, folic acid can occasionally cause an increase of seizures in those with epilepsy and may interfere with the anti-seizure drugs phenytoin and phenobarbital.[45,46]

Folic Acid

Visit Us at TNP.com

Gamma Oryzanol

Maximum safe dosages have not been established for young children or pregnant or nursing women.

Contrary to some reports, individuals who are taking the drug methotrexate for rheumatoid arthritis or psoriasis can safely take folic acid supplements at the same time.[47,48]

## ⚠ INTERACTIONS YOU SHOULD KNOW ABOUT

If you are taking

- **Aspirin,** other **anti-inflammatory medications, drugs that reduce stomach acid, sulfa antibiotics, oral contraceptives, estrogen-replacement therapy, triamterene, corticosteroids (prednisone),**

**valproic acid, carbamazepine, nitrous oxide, cholestyramine,** or **colestipol:** You may need to take extra folic acid.

- **Phenytoin, phenobarbital,** or **primidone:** You may need more folic acid. However, too much folic acid can interfere with these medications and cause seizures! Physician supervision is essential.

- **Pancreatin** (a proteolytic enzyme): You should take folic acid at a different time of day to avoid absorption problems.

- **Methotrexate** for rheumatoid arthritis or psoriasis: You can use folic acid without fear of decreasing the medication's effects. However, if you are taking methotrexate for other purposes, do not take folic acid except on the advice of a physician.

# GAMMA ORYZANOL

*Principal Proposed Uses*
Menopausal symptoms ("hot flashes"), high cholesterol

*Other Proposed Uses*
Anxiety, stomach distress, bodybuilding

Gamma oryzanol is a mixture of substances derived from rice bran oil, including sterols and ferulic acid. It has been approved in Japan for several conditions, including menopausal symptoms, mild anxiety, stomach upset, and high cholesterol. Each year Japan manufactures 7,500 tons of gamma oryzanol from 150,000 tons of rice bran. Not surprisingly, most of the research on oryzanol has been performed in Japan and few studies have been translated into English.

Scientists are not certain how gamma oryzanol works. For menopause, it may affect a key hormone, luteinizing hormone (LH). Gamma oryzanol may also interfere with the absorption of cholesterol into the body from food, thus reducing cholesterol levels in the blood.

## SOURCES

There is no daily requirement for gamma oryzanol.

Rice bran oil is the principal source of gamma oryzanol, but it is also found in the bran of wheat and other grains, as well as various fruits, vegetables, and herbs. However, to get enough gamma oryzanol to reach recommended therapeutic dosages, you will need to take supplements.

## THERAPEUTIC DOSAGES

The typical dosage of gamma oryzanol is 300 mg daily.

## THERAPEUTIC USES

Despite the widespread use of gamma oryzanol for **menopausal symptoms** (page 87), the studies available in English provide little evidence that it is effective. The most commonly cited Japanese study was very small and did not have a control group.[1]

Gamma oryzanol may be useful for elevated **cholesterol** (page 39), although the principal evidence appears to be limited to a few animal studies.[2,3] No serious evidence has been presented in English for using gamma oryzanol as a treatment for **anxiety** (page 8) or stomach distress.

Very preliminary evidence suggests that gamma oryzanol may increase testosterone levels and aid muscle development.[4] These findings have created an interest in using gamma oryzanol as a sports supplement.

## WHAT IS THE SCIENTIFIC EVIDENCE FOR GAMMA ORYZANOL?

### Menopausal Symptoms

Gamma oryzanol may be effective in treating hot flashes associated with menopause. An early study examined 21 women, 8 who were experiencing menopause and 13 who had had their ovaries surgically removed. Each woman was given 300 mg daily of gamma oryzanol.[5] After 38 days, more than 67% of the women improved significantly. However, because this study had no control group, there's no way to know whether the benefit was caused by gamma oryzanol or merely the power of suggestion. Keep in mind that at least 50% of menopausal women given placebo experience significant relief from symptoms.[6]

### High Cholesterol

The best evidence that gamma oryzanol can lower cholesterol levels comes from animal studies. In one such study, 32 hamsters with experimentally induced high cholesterol were given a high-saturated–fat diet containing 5% coconut oil and 0.1% cholesterol, with or without 1% oryzanol, for 7 weeks.[7] Despite the unhealthy diet, the hamsters that were given oryzanol absorbed 25% less cholesterol from their food than the control group, and experienced a significant (28%) drop in total cholesterol in the blood. A small, uncontrolled study in people found similar reductions in cholesterol.[8]

### SAFETY ISSUES

No significant side effects have been reported with gamma oryzanol. However, the maximum safe dosages for young children, pregnant or nursing women, or those with severe liver or kidney disease have not been established.

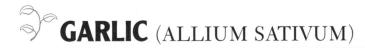

# GARLIC (ALLIUM SATIVUM)

*Principal Proposed Uses*
Atherosclerosis (lowering cholesterol, reducing blood pressure, "thinning" the blood), heart attack prevention

*Other Proposed Uses*
Cancer prevention, topical antibiotic and antifungal, immune stimulant, asthma, candida, colds, diabetes

*Probably Ineffective Uses*
Oral antibiotic, ear infections

The story of garlic's role in human history could fill a book, as indeed it has, many times. Its species name, *sativum*, means cultivated, indicating that garlic does not grow in the wild. So fond have humans been of this herb that garlic can be found almost everywhere in the world, from Polynesia to Siberia. Interestingly, as far back as the first century A.D., Dioscorides wrote of garlic's ability to "clear the arteries."

From Roman antiquity through World War I, garlic poultices were used to prevent wound infections. The famous microbiologist, Louis Pasteur, performed some of the original work showing that garlic could kill bacteria. In 1916, the British government issued a general plea for the public to supply it with garlic in order to meet wartime needs. Garlic was called "Russian penicillin" during World War II because, after running out of antibiotics, the Russian government turned to this ancient treatment for its soldiers.

Conventional doctors in the United States continued to use garlic even when they had abandoned nearly all other herbs. After World War II, Sandoz Pharmaceuticals manufactured a garlic compound for intestinal spasms, and the Van Patten Company produced another for lowering blood pressure.

In the 1950s, garlic finally fell completely out of favor with American physicians. European physicians, continued to investigate garlic.

## WHAT IS GARLIC USED FOR TODAY?

In Europe, garlic has come to be seen as an all-around treatment for preventing **atherosclerosis** (page 14), the cause of heart disease and strokes. As we'll see in the following discussion, moderately good studies have found that certain forms of garlic can lower total **cholesterol** (page 39) levels by about 9 to 12%, as well as possibly improve the ratio of good and bad cholesterol. Garlic also appears to slightly improve **hypertension** (page 75), protect against free radicals, and slow blood coagulation. Putting all these benefits together, garlic may be a broad-spectrum treatment for arterial disease.

Preliminary evidence suggests that regular use of garlic may help prevent **cancer** (page 26). While eating garlic is commonly stated to raise immunity, there is no real evidence that this is the case. Garlic is an effective antibiotic when it contacts the tissue directly, but there is no reason to believe that it will work in this way if you take it by mouth.

Garlic has also been proposed as a treatment for **asthma** (page 11), **candida** (page 33), **colds** (page 44), and **diabetes** (page 60).

Finally, garlic oil products are often recommended for children's ear infections. While these products may reduce pain, it is very unlikely that they have any actual effect on the infection because the eardrum is in the way. For more information on garlic, see *The Natural Pharmacist Guide to Garlic and Cholesterol.*

## WHAT IS THE SCIENTIFIC EVIDENCE FOR GARLIC?

The science behind using garlic to prevent atherosclerosis is moderately strong, although there are some contradictions in the research record.

Garlic preparations have been found to slow hardening of the arteries in animals, reducing the size of plaque deposits by nearly 50%.[1,2] Garlic appears to function somewhat like prescription drugs by interfering with the manufacture of cholesterol.[3,4,5]

Garlic extracts have been found to reduce blood pressure in dogs and rats,[6] and numerous studies in animals and humans suggest that various forms of garlic can reduce blood clotting and neutralize free radicals.[7–13]

### High Cholesterol

At least 28 controlled clinical studies of using garlic to treat elevated cholesterol were published between 1985 and 1995. Together, they suggest that garlic can lower cholesterol by about 9 to 12%.[14,15] Virtually all of these studies used garlic standardized to alliin content (see the discussion under Dosage). Garlic oil does not seem to be effective.

One of the best of these studies was conducted in Germany and published in 1990.[16] A total of 261 patients at 30 medical centers were given either 800 mg of standardized garlic daily or placebo. Over the course of 16 weeks, patients in the treated group experienced a 12% drop in total cholesterol and a 17% decrease in triglyceride levels. The greatest benefits occurred in patients with initial cholesterol levels of 250 to 300 mg/dL.

Another double-blind study, reported in 1996, followed 41 men with cholesterol readings of 220 to 290 mg/dL.[17] The men received either placebo or 7.2 g of aged garlic extract daily for 6 months; then their treatments were switched for 4 months. The results showed a 7% decrease in total serum cholesterol and a 4% decrease in LDL cholesterol in the garlic-treated group. There was also a 5.5% decrease in blood pressure.

One widely quoted study compared garlic to the standard cholesterol-lowering drug bezafibrate.[18] Although the results showed them to be equally effective, the study was not designed properly, so the results mean little. Both groups in the study were asked to improve their diets. The effects of the dietary change could have easily overshadowed real differences between the treatments.

In contrast to these positive results, a couple of other studies have shown no benefit with garlic powder. One study, published in 1996, followed 115 individuals with total cholesterol concentrations of 231 to 328 mg/dL, half of whom received 900 mg daily of a standard garlic extract standardized to contain 1.3% allicin.[19] The results showed no significant difference between the treated and placebo groups. Another negative study was reported in 1995.[20] However, just as in the bezafibrate study, all participants in these two studies were asked to make dietary changes, which may have overwhelmed garlic's anti-hypercholesterolemic effects.

Still, these discrepancies are troubling. However, similar discrepancies occur in the research record of standard drugs as well. Overall, the evidence for garlic powder is strongly favorable.

It can be said with some certainty that garlic oil is not effective for lowering cholesterol.[21]

## Hypertension (High Blood Pressure)

Numerous studies have found that garlic lowers blood pressure slightly, usually in the neighborhood of 5 to 10% more than placebo.[22,23] However, all of these studies suffered from significant flaws, and most were performed on people without high blood pressure.

One of the best studies followed 47 subjects with an average starting blood pressure of 171/101.[24] Over a period of 12 weeks, half were treated with 600 mg of garlic powder daily standardized to 1.3% alliin, the other half were given placebo. The results showed a statistically significant drop of 11% in the systolic blood pressure and 13% in the diastolic pressure. (Blood pressure also fell in the placebo group, by 5% and 4% respectively, so the actual improvement due to garlic is somewhat less than it first appears.) Some garlic studies have been criticized on the basis of the participants being able to tell whether they were being given real garlic or placebo by detecting the garlic odor, but the study authors state that regular questioning of the participants revealed that they could not tell which group they were in.

Another study suggests that garlic's effects increase if it is given a longer time to act. In a 16-week open trial, about 40 subjects with mild hypertension (average blood pressure of 151/96) were given either 600 mg 3 times daily of a garlic preparation standardized to 1.3% alliin (an unusually high dose).[25] The group treated with standardized garlic started with an average blood pressure of 151/96. At 4 weeks, there was a 10% drop in systolic blood pressure, and at 16 weeks the improvement reached 19%. Similar progressive changes occurred in the diastolic blood pressure.

## Direct Effects on Hardening of the Arteries

A recent observational study of 200 individuals suggests that garlic can affect hardening of the arteries by some unidentified means other than lowering cholesterol or blood pressure.[26] The study measured the flexibility of the aorta, the main artery exiting the heart.

## Preventing Heart Attacks

In one study, 432 individuals who had suffered a heart attack were given either garlic juice in milk daily (yum!) or no treatment at all over a period of 3 years.[27] The results showed a significant reduction of second heart attacks and about a 50% reduction in death rate among those taking garlic.

## Cancer Prevention

Several large studies strongly suggest that a diet high in garlic can prevent cancer. In one of the best, the Iowa Women's Study, a group of 41,837 women were questioned as to their lifestyle habits in 1986, and then followed continuously in subsequent years. At the 4-year follow-up, questionnaires showed that women whose diets included significant quantities of garlic were approximately 30% less likely to develop colon cancer.[28]

The interpretations of studies like this one are always a bit controversial. For example, it's possible that the women who ate a lot of garlic also made other healthy lifestyle choices. While

Garlic

Visit Us at TNP.com

researchers looked at this possibility very carefully and concluded that garlic was a common factor, it is not clear that they are right. What is really needed to settle the question is an intervention trial, where some people are given garlic and others are given a placebo. However, none has yet been performed.[29]

## Antimicrobial

There is no question that raw garlic can kill a wide variety of microorganisms by direct contact, including fungi, bacteria, viruses, and protozoa.[30] These findings may explain why garlic was traditionally applied directly to wounds in order to prevent infection (but keep in mind that it can burn the skin). But there is no evidence that taking garlic orally can kill organisms throughout the body.[31–35] Thus, it's not an antibiotic in the usual sense. It's more like Bacitracin ointment.

## DOSAGES

A typical dosage of garlic is 900 mg daily of a garlic powder extract standardized to contain 1.3% alliin, providing about 12,000 mcg of alliin daily. However, a great deal of controversy exists over the proper dosage and form of garlic.

Most everyone agrees that one or two raw garlic cloves a day are adequate for most purposes, but virtual trade wars have taken place over the potency and effectiveness of various dried, aged, or deodorized garlic preparations. The problem has to do with the way garlic is naturally constructed.

A relatively odorless substance, alliin, is one of the most important compounds in garlic. When garlic is crushed or cut, an enzyme called allinase is brought in contact with alliin, turning it into allicin. The allicin itself then rapidly breaks down into entirely different compounds. Allicin is most responsible for garlic's strong odor. It can also blister the skin and kill bacteria, viruses, and fungi. Presumably the garlic plant uses allicin as a form of protection from pests and parasites. It also may provide much of the medicinal benefits of garlic.

When you powder garlic to put it in a capsule, it acts like cutting the bulb. The chain reaction starts: Alliin contacts allinase, yielding allicin, which then breaks down. Unless something is done to prevent this process, garlic powder won't have any alliin or allicin left by the time you buy it.

Some garlic producers declare that alliin and allicin have nothing to do with garlic's effectiveness and simply sell products without it. This is particularly true of aged powdered garlic and garlic oil. But others feel certain that allicin is absolutely essential. However, in order to make garlic relatively odorless, they must prevent the alliin from turning into allicin until the product is consumed. To accomplish this feat, they engage in marvelously complex manufacturing processes, each unique and proprietary. How well each of these methods work is a matter of finger-pointing controversy.

The best that can be said at this point is that in most of the studies that found cholesterol-lowering powers in garlic, the daily dosage supplied at least 10 mg of alliin. This is sometimes stated in terms of how much allicin will be created from that alliin. The number you should look for is 4 to 5 mg of "allicin potential."

Alliin-free aged garlic also appears to be effective when taken at a dose of 1 to 7.2 g daily.

## SAFETY ISSUES

As a commonly used food, garlic is on the FDA's GRAS (generally regarded as safe) list. Rats have been fed gigantic doses of aged garlic (2,000 mg per kilogram body weight) for 6 months without any signs of negative effects.[36] Unfortunately, there do not appear to be any animal toxicity studies on the most commonly used form of garlic—powdered garlic standardized to alliin content.

The only common side effect of garlic is unpleasant breath odor. Even "odorless garlic" produces an offensive smell in up to 50% of those who use it.[37]

Other side effects occur only rarely. For example, a study that followed 1,997 people who were given a normal dose of deodorized garlic daily over a 16-week period showed a 6% incidence of nausea, a 1.3% incidence of dizziness on standing (perhaps a sign of low blood pressure), and a 1.1% incidence of allergic reactions.[38] These are very low percentages in comparison to those usually reported in drug studies. There were also a few reports of bloating, headaches, sweating, and dizziness.

When raw garlic is taken in excessive doses, it can cause numerous symptoms, such as stomach upset, heartburn, nausea, vomiting, diarrhea, flatulence, facial flushing, rapid pulse, and insomnia.

Topical garlic can cause skin irritation, blistering, and even third-degree burns, so be very careful about applying garlic directly to the skin.

Since garlic "thins" the blood, it is not a good idea to take high-potency garlic pills immediately prior to surgery or labor and delivery, due to the risk of excessive bleeding. Similarly, garlic should not be combined with blood-thinning drugs, such as Coumadin (warfarin), heparin, aspirin or Trental (pentoxifylline). Finally, garlic could conceivably interact with natural products with blood-thinning properties, such as **ginkgo** (page 204) or high-dose **vitamin E** (page 337).

Garlic is presumed to be safe for pregnant women (except just before delivery) and nursing mothers, although this has not been proven.

## ⚠ INTERACTIONS YOU SHOULD KNOW ABOUT

If you are taking

- Blood-thinning drugs such as **Coumadin (warfarin), heparin, aspirin,** or **Trental (pentoxifylline):** Do not use garlic except on medical advice.

- **Ginkgo** or **high-dose vitamin E:** Taking garlic at the same time might conceivably cause a risk of bleeding problems.

 # GENTIAN (GENTIANA LUTEA)

### Principal Proposed Uses
Poor appetite, poor digestion

For reasons that aren't entirely clear, bitter plants have the capacity to stimulate appetite, and gentian ranks high on the scale of bitterness. Two of its constituents, gentiopicrin and amarogentin, taste bitter even when diluted by a factor of 50,000![1]

In traditional European herbology, gentian and other bitter herbs are believed to strengthen the digestive system when taken over a period of time. However, in Chinese medicine, gentian is regarded as a rather intense herb that should seldom be taken over the long term. I'm not sure which view is right, although I tend to lean toward the Chinese viewpoint, and only recommend gentian for short-term use.

### WHAT IS GENTIAN USED FOR TODAY?

Gentian extracts are widely sold in liquor stores under the name "bitters," for the purpose of increasing appetite. Tinctures are also sold medicinally for the same purpose.

### DOSAGES

A typical dosage of gentian is 20 drops of tincture 15 minutes before meals. To make the intensely bitter taste more tolerable, you can mix the tincture in juice or water.

### SAFETY ISSUES

Gentian is somewhat mutagenic, meaning that it can cause changes in the DNA of bacteria.[2] For this reason, gentian should not be taken during pregnancy. Safety in young children, nursing women, or those with severe liver or kidney disease is also not established.

In the short term, gentian rarely causes any side effects, except for occasional worsening of ulcer pain and heartburn. (For some people, it relieves stomach problems.)

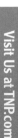

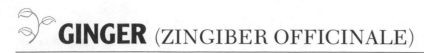

# GINGER (ZINGIBER OFFICINALE)

*Principal Proposed Uses*
Nausea (e.g., motion sickness, morning sickness in pregnancy, post-surgical nausea)

*Other Proposed Uses*
Atherosclerosis, migraine headaches, rheumatoid arthritis

Native to southern Asia, ginger is a 2- to 4-foot perennial that produces grass-like leaves up to a foot long and almost an inch wide. Ginger root, as it is called in the grocery store, actually consists of the underground stem of the plant, with its bark-like outer covering scraped off.

Ginger has been used as food and medicine for millennia. Arabian traders carried ginger root from China and India to be used as a food spice in ancient Greece and Rome, and tax records from the second century A.D. show that ginger was a delightful source of revenue to the Roman treasury. Presently, the annual production of ginger exceeds 2 million pounds.

Chinese medical texts from the fourth century B.C. suggest that ginger is effective in treating nausea, diarrhea, stomachaches, cholera, toothaches, bleeding, and rheumatism. Ginger was later used by Chinese herbalists to treat a variety of respiratory conditions, including coughs and the early stages of colds.

Ginger's modern use dates back to the early 1980s, when a scientist named D. Mowrey noticed that ginger-filled capsules reduced his nausea during an episode of flu. Inspired by this, he performed the first double-blind study of ginger. Germany's Commission E subsequently approved ginger as a treatment for indigestion and motion sickness.

One of the most prevalent ingredients in fresh ginger is the pungent substance gingerol. However, when ginger is dried and stored, its gingerol rapidly converts to the substances shogaol and zingerone. Which, if any, of these substances is most important has not been determined.

## WHAT IS GINGER USED FOR TODAY?

Ginger has become widely accepted as a treatment for **nausea** (page 92). Even some conventional medical texts suggest ginger for the treatment of the nausea and vomiting of pregnancy, although others are more cautious.

Ginger is also used for motion sickness. Medications, such as meclizine, are usually more effective, but they can cause drowsiness. Some conventional physicians recommend ginger over other motion-sickness drugs for older people who are unusually sensitive to drowsiness or loss of balance.

European physicians sometimes give their patients ginger before and just after surgery to prevent the nausea that many people experience on awakening from anesthesia. However, this treatment should only be attempted with a doctor's approval.

Ginger has been suggested as a treatment for numerous other conditions, including **atherosclerosis** (page 14), **migraine headaches** (page 89), **rheumatoid arthritis** (page 109), high **cholesterol** (page 39), burns, **ulcers** (page 112), **depression** (page 54), **impotence** (page 77), and liver toxicity. However, there is negligible evidence for these uses.

In traditional Chinese medicine, hot ginger tea taken at the first sign of a **cold** (page 44) is believed to offer the possibility of averting the infection. However, once more there is no scientific evidence for this use.

## WHAT IS THE SCIENTIFIC EVIDENCE FOR GINGER?

The evidence for ginger's effectiveness is mixed. It has been suggested that, in some negative studies, poor-quality ginger powder might have been used.[1] In general, while most antinausea drugs influence the brain and the inner ear, ginger appears to act only on the stomach.[2]

### Motion Sickness

The first ginger study followed 36 college students with a known tendency toward motion sickness.[3] They were treated with either ginger or the standard nausea drug dimenhydrinate, and then placed in a rotating chair to see how much they could stand. Both treatments seemed about equally effective.

Another study also found equivalent benefit between ginger and dimenhydrinate in a group of 60 passengers on a cruise through rough seas.[4] A later study of 79 Swedish naval cadets found that ginger could decrease vomiting and cold sweating, but didn't significantly decrease nausea and vertigo.[5]

However, a 1984 study funded by NASA found that ginger was not any more effective than placebo.[6] Two other small studies have also failed to find any benefit.[7,8] The reason for the discrepancy may lie in the type of ginger used, or the severity of the stimulant used to bring on motion sickness.

### Nausea and Vomiting of Pregnancy

A preliminary double-blind study performed in Denmark concluded that ginger can significantly reduce the nausea and vomiting often associated with pregnancy. Effects became apparent in 19 of 27 women after 4 days of treatment, although the relief was far from total.[9]

### Post-Surgical Nausea

A double-blind British study compared the effects of ginger, placebo, and metoclopramide in the treatment of nausea following gynecological surgery.[10] The results in 60 women indicated that both treatments produced similar benefits as compared to placebo.

A similar British study followed 120 women receiving elective laparoscopic gynecological surgery.[11] Whereas nausea and vomiting developed in 41% of the participants given placebo, in the groups treated with ginger or metoclopramide (Reglan) these symptoms developed in only 21% and 27% respectively.

However, a double-blind study of 108 people undergoing similar surgery found no benefit with ginger as compared to placebo.[12] Negative re-

sults were also seen in another recent study of 120 women.[13]

## DOSAGES

For most purposes, the standard dosage of powdered ginger is 1 to 4 g daily taken in 2 to 4 divided doses.

To prevent motion sickness, it is probably best to begin treatment 1 or 2 days before the trip and continue it throughout the period of travel.

In the nausea and vomiting of pregnancy, the best form of ginger is probably freshly brewed tea, made from boiled gingerroot and diluted to taste. If chilled, carbonated, and sweetened, this would become the original form of ginger ale, a famous antinausea beverage. Powdered ginger can be used as well.

## SAFETY ISSUES

Ginger is on the FDA's GRAS (generally recognized as safe) list as a food, and the treatment dosages of ginger are comparable to dietary usages.

Like onions and **garlic** (page 197), extracts of ginger inhibit blood coagulation in test-tube experiments.[14,15,16] This has led to a theoretical concern that ginger should not be combined with drugs such as Coumadin (warfarin), heparin, or even aspirin. European studies with actual oral ginger taken alone in normal quantities have not found any significant effect on blood coagulation,[17,18,19] but it is still possible that combination treatment could cause problems.

No side effects have been observed with ginger at recommended dosages.

## ⚠ INTERACTIONS YOU SHOULD KNOW ABOUT

If you are taking strong blood-thinning drugs such as **Coumadin (warfarin)** or **heparin,** ginger might possibly increase the risk of bleeding problems.

**Ginger**

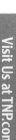

# GINKGO (GINKGO BILOBA)

### Principal Proposed Uses

Memory and mental function (e.g., Alzheimer's disease, non-Alzheimer's dementia, ordinary age-related memory loss)

### Other Proposed Uses

Impaired circulation in the legs (intermittent claudication), fluid retention related to the menstrual cycle, macular degeneration, impotence, tinnitus, depression, complications of diabetes, Raynaud's phenomenon

Traceable back 300 million years, the ginkgo is the oldest surviving species of tree. Although it died out in Europe during the Ice Age, ginkgo survived in China, Japan, and other parts of East Asia. It has been cultivated extensively for both ceremonial and medical purposes, and some particularly revered trees have been lovingly tended for over 1,000 years.

In traditional Chinese herbology, tea made from ginkgo seeds has been used for numerous problems, most particularly asthma and other respiratory illnesses. The leaf was not used. But in the 1950s, German researchers started to investigate the medical possibilities of ginkgo leaf extracts rather than remedies using the seeds. Thus, modern ginkgo preparations are not the same as the traditional Chinese herb, and the comparisons often drawn are incorrect.

## WHAT IS GINKGO USED FOR TODAY?

Presently, ginkgo is the most widely prescribed herb in Germany, reaching a total prescription count of over 6 million in 1995.[1] German physicians consider it to be as effective as any drug treatment for **Alzheimer's disease** (page 4) and other severe forms of memory and mental function decline. We do not know for sure whether ginkgo is helpful in ordinary, age-related memory loss, although there are logical reasons and some preliminary evidence that suggest it might be. See *The Natural Pharmacist Guide to Ginkgo and Memory* for more information.

Germany's Commission E also recommends ginkgo for the treatment of restricted circulation in the legs due to hardening of the arteries known as **intermittent claudication** (page 83).

Recently, ginkgo has attracted interest for possibly reversing the **impotence** (page 77) or difficulty achieving orgasm caused by certain antidepressant drugs.

One study suggests that ginkgo may be helpful in relieving the bloating and fluid retention of **PMS** (page 104).[2]

Additionally, ginkgo is used to treat ringing in the ears (tinnitus), **macular degeneration** (page 85), **depression** (page 54), complications of **diabetes** (page 60), and **Raynaud's phenomenon** (page 108), although as yet there is little evidence that it is effective for these purposes.

## WHAT IS THE SCIENTIFIC EVIDENCE FOR GINKGO?

The scientific record for ginkgo is extensive and impressive.

Numerous studies have found that ginkgo extracts can improve circulation.[3,4] We don't know exactly how ginkgo does this, but unknown constituents in the herb appear to make the blood more fluid, reduce the tendency toward blood clots, extend the life of a natural blood vessel–relaxing substance, and act as an antioxidant.[5,6] However, ginkgo's influence on mental function may have nothing to do with its effects on circulation.

## Impaired Mental Function in the Elderly

In the past, European physicians believed that the cause of mental deterioration with age (senile dementia) was reduced circulation in the brain due to atherosclerosis. Since ginkgo can improve circulation, they assumed that ginkgo was simply getting more blood to brain cells and thereby making them work better.

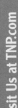

However, the contemporary understanding of age-related memory loss and mental impairment no longer considers chronically restricted circulation the primary issue. Ginkgo (and other drugs used for dementia) may instead function by directly stimulating nerve-cell activity and protecting nerve cells from further injury,[7] although improvement in circulatory capacity may also play a role.

According to a 1992 article published in *Lancet,* over 40 double-blind controlled trials have evaluated the benefits of ginkgo in treating age-related mental decline.[8] Of these, eight were rated of good quality, involving a total of about 1,000 people and producing positive results in all but one study. The authors of the *Lancet* article felt that the evidence was strong enough to conclude that ginkgo extract is an effective treatment for this condition.

Studies since 1992 have verified this conclusion, both in people with Alzheimer's disease and those without the disorder.[9,10] Interestingly, European physicians are so certain that ginkgo is effective that it's become hard for them to perform scientific studies of the herb. To them, it's unethical to give Alzheimer's patients a placebo when they could take ginkgo instead and have additional months of useful life.[11]

This objection doesn't apply in the United States, where physicians generally do not believe that ginkgo is effective. A recent study published in the *Journal of the American Medical Association* reported on the results of a year-long double-blind trial of *Ginkgo biloba* in over 300 individuals with Alzheimer's disease or other forms of severe age-related mental decline.[12] Participants were given either 40 mg of the ginkgo extract or placebo 3 times daily. The results showed significant (but not miraculous) improvements in the treated group.

The results of one double-blind study suggest that ginkgo might be useful for ordinary age-related memory loss as well.[13]

## Impaired Circulation in the Legs (Intermittent Claudication)

In intermittent claudication, impaired circulation can cause a severe, cramp-like pain in one's legs after walking only a short distance. According to Germany's Commission E, at least four reasonably good double-blind studies have found that ginkgo can increase pain-free walking distance by 75 to 500 feet.[14]

One double-blind study enrolled 111 people for 24 weeks.[15] Subjects were measured for pain-free walking distance by walking up a 12% slope on a treadmill at 3 kilometers per hour (about 2 miles per hour). At the beginning of treatment, both the placebo and ginkgo groups were able to walk about 350 feet without pain. By the end of the trial, both groups had improved significantly (the power of placebo is amazing!). However, the ginkgo group improved more: Participants taking ginkgo achieved an average of 500 feet while those in the placebo group reached only 415 feet, an improvement of 85 feet for the ginkgo group. This was not miraculous, but it was still significant.

## Fluid Retention Related to the Menstrual Cycle

One double-blind placebo-controlled study evaluated the benefits of *Ginkgo biloba* extract in women who experience fluid retention related to the menstrual cycle.[16] This trial evaluated 143 women with PMS symptoms, 18 to 45 years of age, and followed them for two menstrual cycles. When the study began, each woman received either the ginkgo extract or placebo on day 16 of the first cycle. Treatment was continued until day 5 of the next cycle, and resumed again on the day 16 of that cycle.

The results were impressive. As compared to placebo, ginkgo significantly relieved major fluid retention symptoms of PMS, especially breast pain.

## Macular Degeneration

One preliminary double-blind study suggests that ginkgo may improve macular degeneration.[17]

## Impotence and Difficulty Achieving Orgasm

Although there is no double-blind evidence at the time of this writing, case reports and open studies suggest that ginkgo can reverse the sexual dysfunction (impotence in men and the inability to

Ginkgo

Visit Us at TNP.com

achieve orgasm in women) caused by drugs in the Prozac family.[18]

## DOSAGES

The standard dosage of ginkgo is 40 to 80 mg 3 times daily of a 50:1 extract standardized to contain 24% ginkgo-flavone glycosides.

## SAFETY ISSUES

Ginkgo appears to be safe. Extremely high doses have been given in animals for long periods of time without serious consequences.[19] Safety in young children, pregnant or nursing women, or those with severe liver or kidney disease, however, has not been established.

In all the clinical trials of ginkgo up through 1991 combined, involving a total of almost 10,000 participants, the incidence of side effects produced by ginkgo extract was extremely small. There were 21 cases of gastrointestinal discomfort, and even fewer cases of headaches, dizziness, and allergic skin reactions.[20]

Contact with live ginkgo plants can cause severe allergic reactions, and ingestion of ginkgo seeds can be dangerous.

German medical authorities do not believe that ginkgo possesses any serious drug interactions.[21] However, because of ginkgo's "blood-thinning" effects, some experts warn that it should not be combined with blood-thinning drugs such as Coumadin (warfarin), heparin, aspirin, and Trental (pentoxifylline), and use of such drugs was prohibited in most of the double-blind trials of ginkgo. It is also possible that ginkgo could cause bleeding problems if combined with natural blood thinners, such as **garlic** (page 197) and high-dose **vitamin E** (page 337). There have been two case reports in highly regarded journals of subdural hematoma (bleeding in the skull) and hyphema (spontaneous bleeding into the iris chamber) in association with ginkgo use.[22,23]

## ⚠ INTERACTIONS YOU SHOULD KNOW ABOUT

If you are taking

- Blood-thinning drugs such as **Coumadin (warfarin), heparin, aspirin,** or **Trental (pentoxifylline):** Simultaneous use of ginkgo might cause bleeding problems.

- Natural substances with blood-thinning properties, such as **garlic, phosphatidylserine,** or high-dose **vitamin E:** It is possible that, again, simultaneous use of ginkgo might cause bleeding problems.

- **Antidepressant drugs** in the SSRI family: Ginkgo might remedy sexual side effects such as impotence or inability to achieve orgasm.

 # GINSENG (PANAX GINSENG, PANAX QUINQUEFOLIUS)

*Principal Proposed Uses*

   Adaptogen (improving resistance to stress), strengthening immunity against colds and flus, enhancing mental function, improving blood sugar control in people with diabetes

*Other Proposed Uses*

   Increasing exercise capacity, preventing cancer, reversing impotence

---

There are actually three different herbs commonly called ginseng: Asian or Korean ginseng *(Panax ginseng)*, American ginseng *(Panax quinquefolius)*, and Siberian "ginseng" *(Eleutherococcus senticosus)*. The latter herb is actually not ginseng at all, but the Russian scientists responsible for promoting it believe that it functions identically.

Asian ginseng is a perennial herb with a taproot resembling the human body. It grows in northern China, Korea, and Russia; its close relative, *Panax quinquefolius,* is cultivated in the United States.

Because ginseng must be grown for 5 years before it is harvested, it commands a high price, with top-quality roots easily selling for more than $10,000. Dried, unprocessed ginseng root is called "white ginseng," and steamed, heat-dried root is "red ginseng." Chinese herbalists believe that each form has its own particular benefits.

Ginseng is widely regarded by the public as a stimulant, but according to everyone who uses it seriously that isn't the right description. In traditional Chinese herbology, *Panax ginseng* was used to strengthen the digestion and the lungs, calm the spirit, and increase overall energy. When the Russian scientist Israel I. Brekhman became interested in the herb prior to World War II, he came up with a new idea about ginseng. He decided that it was an adaptogen.

The term *adaptogen* refers to a hypothetical treatment described as follows: An adaptogen should help the body adapt to stresses of various kinds, whether heat, cold, exertion, trauma, sleep deprivation, toxic exposure, radiation, infection, or psychological stress. Furthermore, an adaptogen should cause no side effects, be effective in treating a wide variety of illnesses, and help return an organism toward balance no matter what may have gone wrong.

Perhaps the only indisputable example of an adaptogen is healthy lifestyle. By eating right, exercising regularly, and generally living a life of balance and moderation, you will increase your physical fitness and ability to resist illnesses of all types. Whether there are any substances that can do as much remains unclear. However, Brekhman felt certain that ginseng produced similarly universal benefits.

Interestingly, traditional Chinese medicine (where ginseng comes from) does not entirely agree. There is no one-size-fits-all in Chinese medical theory. Like any other herb, ginseng is said to be helpful for those people who need its particular effects, and neutral or harmful for others. But in Europe, Brekhman's concept has taken hold, and ginseng is widely believed to be a universal adaptogen.

In the 1940s, Brekhman decided that a much less expensive herb, *Eleutherococcus senticosus,* is just as good as ginseng. A thorny bush that grows much more rapidly than true ginseng, this later received the misleading name of "Siberian" or "Russian ginseng." Contrary to some reports, its chemical makeup is completely unrelated to that of *Panax ginseng.*

## WHAT IS GINSENG USED FOR TODAY?

If Brekhman is right, ginseng (whether *Eleutherococcus* or *Panax*) should be the right treatment for most of us. Modern life is tremendously stressful, and if an herb could help us withstand it, it would be a terrifically useful herb indeed. Ginseng is widely used for this purpose in Russia and Eastern Europe. However, the scientific basis for this use is not strong.

There have been a few good studies of ginseng for certain more specific purposes: strengthening immunity against **colds and flus** (page 44) and other infections, stimulating the mind, helping to control **diabetes** (page 60), and improving physical performance capacity (sports performance).

Ginseng is also said to help prevent **cancer** (page 26), fight chemical dependency, and improve sexual performance, but there is as yet little direct evidence that it really works.[1,2,3]

## WHAT IS THE SCIENTIFIC EVIDENCE FOR GINSENG?

There have been thousands of research papers published on ginseng. Unfortunately, nearly all involved animals that received injections of ginseng extracts directly into the abdomen. There are only a few good double-blind human studies of ginseng taken by mouth.

### Animal Studies

In animals, ginseng injections have been found to increase stamina; improve mental function; protect against radiation, infections, toxins, exhaustion, and stress; and activate white blood cells.[4] If you put these studies together, injected ginseng truly does appear to be an adaptogen, as advertised.

However, having ginseng injected into the abdomen is strikingly different from taking it by mouth. It not only enters the body directly without going through the digestive tract, but for all we know, an injection into the abdomen may itself stimulate numerous bodily changes.

## Open Studies

Although many scientific trials of ginseng involve people, some with enormous numbers of participants, most were not double-blind. This makes the results nearly meaningless.

For example, one widely quoted study followed over 50,000 employees at a Soviet automobile plant who were given *Eleutherococcus* daily during November and December. Plant records showed that the frequency of respiratory infections fell by 40%.[5] However, without a control group, it isn't clear how many infections would have been expected without any treatment. Perhaps it was a milder winter, for example. Furthermore, since the participants knew they were being treated, the placebo effect was given full reign. If they had been given dried shoe leather and it was described as a healing herb, they would have undoubtedly reported fewer illnesses. It doesn't matter how many people were involved: The power of suggestion could be expected to work in all of them. Without a control group and double-blind design, no such study can prove much.

A trial that did use a control group followed 80 women with breast cancer, who were given either *Eleutherococcus* or no treatment.[6] The treated individuals showed a lower incidence of nausea, dizziness, and loss of appetite. Unfortunately, this was not a blinded study. Since treated participants knew they were being treated, and the untreated participants knew they weren't, again it's hard to tell how much of the result was due to the power of suggestion.

## Double-Blind Studies

Out of the thousands of studies performed on *Panax ginseng*, there were only eight double-blind trials published up through 1990.[7] Most (but not all) of them concluded that ginseng does produce a positive effect on such parameters as physical performance, mental ability, cholesterol levels, and blood sugar control. However, most of the studies were too tiny to prove much, and none were conducted according to modern scientific standards.[8] The situation is similar with *Eleuthe-*

*rococcus.* Fortunately, there have been a few better performed studies published subsequently.

### Immune Stimulation

A recent, properly performed, double-blind placebo-controlled study suggests that *Panax ginseng* can improve immunity.[9] This trial enrolled 227 participants at three medical offices in Milan, Italy. Half were given ginseng at a dosage of 100 mg daily, the other half placebo. Four weeks into the study, all participants received influenza vaccine.

The results showed a significant decline in the frequency of colds and flus in the treated group compared to the placebo group (15 versus 42 cases). Also, antibody measurements in response to the vaccination rose higher in the treated group than in the placebo group.

### Diabetes

Another properly performed, double-blind study evaluated the effects of *Panax ginseng* (at dosages of 100 mg or 200 mg daily) on 36 people with adult-onset diabetes.[10] The results showed improvements in blood sugar control. The authors attributed this benefit to a spontaneously increased level of physical activity in the ginseng group.

### Mental Function

A recent study found that *Panax ginseng* can improve some aspects of mental function.[11] Over a period of 2 months, 112 healthy, middle-aged adults were given either ginseng or placebo. The results showed that ginseng improved abstract thinking ability. However, there was no significant change in reaction time, memory, concentration, or overall subjective experience between the two groups.

### Sports Performance

A double-blind study of 20 athletes over an 8-week period found that a standard *Eleutherococcus* formulation produced no improvement in physical performance.[12]

Similarly negative results were seen with *Panax ginseng* in an 8-week double-blind trial that followed 31 healthy men in their twenties.[13] A dose of either 200 or 400 mg per day of standardized *Panax ginseng* root extract standardized to contain 4% ginsenosides produced no change in exercise capacity.

## Observational Study

### Preventing Cancer

A recent observational study (see the introduction for definition) on ginseng and cancer prevention has been widely publicized, but a close look at the data arouses some suspicions. This study was performed in South Korea and followed a total of 4,587 men and women aged 39 years and older from 1987 to 1991.[14] People who regularly consumed *Panax ginseng* were compared with otherwise similar individuals (matched in sex, age, alcohol use, smoking, and education and economic status) who did not.

The results were impressive. Those who used ginseng showed a 60% decrease in risk of death from cancer. Lung cancer and gastric cancer were particularly reduced. The more ginseng consumed, the greater the effect.

However, there is something a bit fishy about this study. Use of ginseng less than three times per year caused a 54% reduction in risk. It seems difficult to believe that so occasional a use of ginseng could reduce cancer mortality by more than half!

## Putting It All Together

Taken together, the scientific record on ginseng is intriguing but not conclusive. If some of the money spent on animal and non-double-blind human studies had been used to fund more double-blind studies in humans, we might know a lot more. At the present state of knowledge, it is hard to know whether ginseng is as effective as its mystique would make it seem.

## DOSAGES

The typical recommended daily dosage of *Panax ginseng* is 1 to 2 g of raw herb, or 200 mg daily of an extract standardized to contain 4 to 7% ginsenosides. *Eleutherococcus* is taken at a dosage of 2 to 3 g whole herb or 300 to 400 mg of extract daily.

Ordinarily, a 2- to 3-week period of using ginseng is recommended, followed by a 1- to 2-week "rest" period. Russian tradition suggests that ginseng should not be used by those under 40.

Finally, because *Panax ginseng* is so expensive, some products actually contain very little. Adulteration with other herbs and even caffeine is not unusual.[15]

## SAFETY ISSUES

The various forms of ginseng appear to be nontoxic, both in the short and long term, according to the results of studies in mice, rats, chickens, and dwarf pigs. Ginseng also does not seem to be carcinogenic.[16,17,18]

Side effects are rare. Occasionally women report menstrual abnormalities and/or breast tenderness when they take ginseng, and overstimulation and insomnia have also been reported. Unconfirmed reports suggest that highly excessive doses of ginseng can raise blood pressure, increase heart rate, and possibly cause other significant effects. Whether some of these cases were actually caused by caffeine mixed in with ginseng remains unclear. Ginseng allergy can also occur, as can allergy to any other substance.

In 1979, an article was published in the *Journal of the American Medical Association* claiming that people can become addicted to ginseng and develop blood pressure elevation, nervousness, sleeplessness, diarrhea, and hypersexuality.[19] This report has since been thoroughly discredited and should no longer be taken seriously.[20,21]

However, there is some evidence that ginseng can interfere with drug metabolism, specifically drugs processed by an enzyme called "CYP 3A4."[22] Ask your physician or pharmacist whether you are taking any medications of this type. There have also been specific reports of ginseng interacting with MAO inhibitor drugs and also with a test for digitalis,[23,24] although again it is not clear whether it was the ginseng or a contaminant that caused the problem. There has also been one report of ginseng reducing the anticoagulant effects of Coumadin.[25]

Safety in young children, pregnant or nursing women, or those with severe liver or kidney disease has not been established. Interestingly,

Chinese tradition suggests that ginseng should not be used by pregnant or nursing mothers.

## ⚠ INTERACTIONS YOU SHOULD KNOW ABOUT

If you are taking

- **Drugs** processed by an enzyme called "CYP 3A4:" Ginseng might interfere. Ask your

physician or pharmacist whether you are taking any medications of this type.

- **MAO inhibitor drugs** or **digitalis:** It is possible that ginseng might cause problems.

- **Insulin:** Ginseng may reduce your dosage need.

- **Coumadin (warfarin):** Ginseng might decrease its effect.

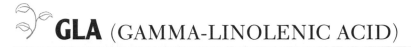

# GLA (GAMMA-LINOLENIC ACID)

*Principal Proposed Uses*
Cyclic mastalgia (also known as fibrocystic breast disease, cyclic mastitis, or mastodynia), general PMS symptoms, diabetic neuropathy, eczema

*Other Proposed Uses*
Rheumatoid arthritis, asthma, Raynaud's phenomenon, osteoporosis, many others

*Supplement Forms/Alternative Names*
GLA found in black currant seed oil, borage oil, evening primrose oil; omega-6 oil(s); omega-6 fatty acids

G LA (gamma-linolenic acid) is one of the two main types of *essential fatty acids*. These are "good" fats that are as necessary for your health as vitamins. Specifically, GLA is an omega-6 fatty acid. For more information on the other major category of essential fatty acids, omega-3, see the chapter on **fish oil** (page 188).

The body uses essential fatty acids to make various prostaglandins and leukotrienes. These substances influence inflammation and pain; some of them increase symptoms, while others decrease them. Taking GLA may swing the balance over to the more favorable prostaglandins and leukotrienes, making it helpful for diseases that involve inflammation.

GLA is widely used in Europe to treat diabetic neuropathy and eczema. Both European and U.S. physicians use GLA to treat cyclic mastalgia, a condition marked by breast pain associated with the menstrual cycle. It may also be useful for other PMS symptoms.

GLA has also been proposed as a treatment for many other conditions.

## REQUIREMENTS/SOURCES

The body ordinarily makes all the GLA it needs from linoleic acid, an omega-6 essential fatty acid found in many foods. In certain circumstances, however, the body may not be able to convert linoleic acid to GLA efficiently. These include advanced age, diabetes, high alcohol intake, eczema, cyclic mastitis, viral infections, excessive saturated fat intake, elevated cholesterol levels, and deficiencies of vitamin $B_6$, zinc, magnesium, biotin, or calcium.[1–6] In such cases, taking GLA supplements may make up for a genuine deficiency.

Very little GLA is found in the diet. Borage oil is the richest supplemental source (17 to 25% GLA), followed by black currant oil (15 to 20%) and evening primrose oil (7 to 10%). Borage and evening primrose are the most common sources.

## THERAPEUTIC DOSAGES

The usual dosage of GLA used to treat cyclic mastitis or eczema is about 200 to 400 mg daily,

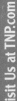

(about 2 to 4 g of evening primrose oil or 1 to 2 g of borage oil). Diabetic neuropathy is typically treated with about 400 to 600 mg daily (about 4 to 6 g of evening primrose or 2 to 3 g of borage oil), and rheumatoid arthritis may require as much as 2,000 to 3,000 mg (best obtained from purified GLA).

GLA should be taken with food. Don't forget that full benefits may take over 6 months to develop, so be patient.

## THERAPEUTIC USES

Most commonly in the form of evening primrose oil, GLA has become a standard treatment for **cyclic mastalgia** (page 52), breast pain that cycles with the menstrual period.[7–10] It is widely used for this purpose by conventional physicians in both Europe and North America, and as a mark of its acceptance it is even mentioned in the AMA's official *Drug Evaluations* textbook.[11]

Evening primrose oil is also said to be useful for other **PMS** (page 104) symptoms, although the evidence is not strong.[12]

Evening primrose oil also appears to be effective for diabetic neuropathy,[13,14] a complication of **diabetes** (page 60). This condition, which develops in many people with diabetes, consists of pain and/or numbness due to progressive nerve damage.

Additionally, evening primrose oil is widely used in Europe as a treatment for **eczema** (page 66). Unfortunately, the scientific evidence that it works is mixed at best, and the most recent studies have not found it to be effective.[15,16,17]

Very high doses of purified GLA may be of some benefit in treating **rheumatoid arthritis** (page 109), especially when combined with conventional treatments.[18–21] GLA may also help in **Raynaud's phenomenon** (page 108) (a condition in which the fingers and toes react to cold in an exaggerated way)[22,23] as well as **osteoporosis** (page 100).[24,25]

Thus far, we've mentioned only a fraction of the conditions for which GLA has been proposed as a treatment. Others include **irritable bowel syndrome** (page 85), **heart disease** (page 14), prostate cancer, bursitis, **allergies** (page 3), Sjögren's disease, endometriosis, **asthma** (page 11), prostate enlargement or **benign prostatic hyperplasia (BPH)** (page 20), chronic fatigue syndrome, and many more. However, none of these potential uses has as yet any strong evidence behind it.

## WHAT IS THE SCIENTIFIC EVIDENCE FOR GLA?

### Cyclic Mastalgia

Cyclic mastalgia, also known as fibrocystic breast disease, cyclic mastitis, and mastodynia, is a condition in which a woman's breasts become painful during the week or two before her menstrual period. The discomfort is accompanied by swelling, inflammation, and sometimes actual cysts that form in the breasts. It is often associated with other symptoms of premenstrual syndrome (PMS).

We do not know the cause of cyclic mastalgia, but researchers have found that it seems to be associated with an imbalance of fatty acids in the body.[26]

Evidence suggests that GLA relieves cyclic mastalgia, perhaps by restoring the balance of essential fatty acids.[27] One report published in 1985 compares the effectiveness of four different therapies in women with severe, painful mastalgia: GLA from evening primrose oil and the pharmaceuticals danazol, bromocriptine, and progestins (often, but not quite accurately, called progesterone).[28]

The results suggest that evening primrose oil was effective in just under 50% of participants. However, this was not actually a study in the usual sense; it was more a collation of records from the Cardiff Clinic, a medical center that specializes in the treatment of breast pain. Contrary to how this study is sometimes reported, it did not have a placebo group.

To really know whether a treatment is effective, you need double-blind placebo-controlled studies to eliminate the power of suggestion. One such study was reported in 1981. This trial followed 73 women suffering from cyclic mastalgia.[29] The results were consistent with the Cardiff Clinic's results, finding that evening primrose oil reduced pain in almost 50% of the women taking it, while only 19% of the women improved in the placebo group.

However, this study was reported only in a very brief form, and many details are missing. We really need better designed and better reported studies to know for sure how effective evening primrose oil really is for cyclic mastalgia.

If you have a severe form of cyclic mastalgia with actual breast cysts, there is some evidence that evening primrose oil will not be completely effective. In a double-blind study of 200 women treated for 1 year, evening primrose oil had no effect on recurrent breast cysts.[30,31] The conclusion appears to be that evening primrose oil relieves breast pain but cannot make breast cysts go away.

## Other PMS Symptoms

Although several small studies suggest that GLA as evening primrose oil is helpful in reducing overall PMS symptoms, all of them suffer from serious flaws.[32]

## Diabetic Neuropathy

Diabetic neuropathy is a gradual degeneration of nerves caused by diabetes. There is some evidence that GLA can be helpful, if you give it long enough to work. In one double-blind placebo-controlled study, 111 people with mild diabetic neuropathy received either 480 mg daily of GLA (about 6 g daily of evening primrose oil) or placebo.[33] After 12 months, the group taking GLA was doing significantly better than the placebo group. Good results were seen in a smaller study as well.[34]

In addition, numerous studies in animals have found that evening primrose oil can protect nerves from diabetes-induced nerve injury.[35,36]

GLA may work especially well for this condition when it is combined with lipoic acid.[37,38]

## Eczema

Despite the fact that GLA (evening primrose oil) is widely used in Europe to treat eczema, the evidence that it works is mixed at best.

A 1989 review of the literature found significant benefit in the nine double-blind controlled studies performed to that date.[39] Evening primrose oil seemed especially effective in relieving itching. However, this review has been criticized because it included the results of unpublished studies that might not have been designed or performed properly.[40] Improvements in symptoms other than itching were seen in a double-blind study of 48 children with eczema.[41]

Other research has failed to find any benefit. For example, a 16-week double-blind study involving 58 children with eczema found no difference between the effects of evening primrose oil and placebo.[42] There have been many other negative studies as well—although some of them too had design and performance problems. (In one, it appears that the placebo group was mixed up with the treatment group.)[43]

## Rheumatoid Arthritis

According to many studies, fish oil, a source of omega-3 essential fatty acids, definitely improves symptoms of rheumatoid arthritis. A few studies suggest that GLA may also work. One double-blind study followed 56 people with rheumatoid arthritis for 6 months.[44] Participants received either 2.8 g daily of GLA or placebo. The group taking GLA experienced significantly fewer symptoms than the placebo group, and the improvements grew over time.

Other small studies have found similar results.[45,46] The overall conclusion appears to be that purified GLA may offer some benefit for rheumatoid arthritis, especially when used along with standard treatment for rheumatoid arthritis.[47]

## Raynaud's Phenomenon

High dosages of evening primrose oil may be useful for Raynaud's phenomenon, a condition in which a person's hands and feet show abnormal sensitivity to cold temperature. A small double-blind study found that GLA produced significantly better results than placebo.[48,49] Similar results have been obtained with the omega-3 fatty acids found in fish oil.

## Osteoporosis

Essential fatty acids, when combined with calcium, may also help prevent osteoporosis. In one study, 65 postmenopausal women were given calcium along with either placebo or a combination of omega-6 fatty acids (from evening primrose oil) and omega-3 fatty acids (from fish oil) for a period of 18 months. At the end of the study period, both treated groups had higher bone density and fewer fractures than the placebo group.[50] Similar results were seen in another study of 40 women.[51]

## SAFETY ISSUES

Most of the safety information we have regarding GLA comes from experience with evening primrose oil.

Animal studies suggest that evening primrose oil is completely nontoxic and noncarcinogenic.[52] Over 4,000 people have taken GLA or evening primrose oil in scientific studies, and no significant adverse effects have ever been noted. However, somewhat less than 2% of the study participants who took evening primrose oil complained of mild headaches and/or gastrointestinal distress, especially at higher dosages.[53,54]

Early case reports suggested the possibility that GLA might worsen temporal lobe epilepsy or bipolar disorder, but there has been no later confirmation.[55,56]

The maximum safe dosage of GLA for young children, pregnant or nursing women, or those with severe liver or kidney disease has not been established.

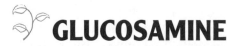

# GLUCOSAMINE

### Principal Proposed Uses
Osteoarthritis

### Other Proposed Uses
Tendinitis, muscle injury prevention

### Supplement Forms/Alternative Names
Glucosamine sulfate, glucosamine hydrochloride, N-acetyl glucosamine

Glucosamine, most commonly used in the form glucosamine sulfate, is a simple molecule derived from glucose, the principal sugar found in blood. In glucosamine, one oxygen atom in glucose is replaced by a nitrogen atom. The chemical term for this modified form of glucose is *amino sugar*.

Glucosamine is produced naturally in the body, where it is a key building block for making cartilage. In Europe, glucosamine is widely used to treat osteoarthritis. Studies show that glucosamine supplements relieve pain and other arthritis symptoms. Interestingly, these improvements seem to last for several weeks after glucosamine supplements are discontinued.

This observation has led to the exciting idea that glucosamine may actually make a deep change in osteoarthritis, rather than simply relieving symptoms. Conventional treatments for arthritis reduce the symptoms but don't slow the actual progress of the disease; in fact, non-steroidal anti-inflammatory drugs, such as indomethacin, may actually speed the progression of osteoarthritis by interfering with cartilage repair and promoting cartilage destruction.[1–5]

In contrast, glucosamine is one of several supplements that may go beyond treating the symptoms to actually slowing the disease itself. (Chondroitin sulfate and SAMe may do the same.) If this is true, it would represent a revolutionary breakthrough in the treatment of arthritis.

However, although the preliminary evidence seems promising, we don't yet have any direct evidence that glucosamine can protect joint cartilage from further damage. See the chapter on **chondroitin** (page 159) for a supplement that has more evidence for this use.

Some athletes use glucosamine, in the (unproved) belief that it can prevent muscle injuries, relieve tendinitis, and repair damaged cartilage.

## SOURCES

There is no U.S. Recommended Dietary Allowance for glucosamine. Your body makes all the glucosamine it needs from building blocks found in foods.

Glucosamine is not usually obtained directly from food. Glucosamine supplements are derived from chitin, a substance found in the shells of shrimp, lobsters, and crabs.

## THERAPEUTIC DOSAGES

For osteoarthritis, a typical dosage of glucosamine is 500 mg 3 times daily. Be patient: Results take weeks to develop. Glucosamine is available in three forms: glucosamine sulfate, glucosamine hydrochloride, and N-acetyl glucosamine. All three forms are sold as tablets or capsules. There is some dispute over which form is best.

Glucosamine is often sold in combination with chondroitin. While the combination does appear to be effective, there is no evidence that combined therapy offers any benefit over either supplement taken alone. (For more information, see the chapter on chondroitin.)

## THERAPEUTIC USES

Glucosamine is used to treat **osteoarthritis** (page 95). The research indicates that it is effective, and about equal in strength to low dosages of nonsteroidal anti-inflammatory drugs such as ibuprofen.[6–10] It reduces pain and swelling and improves mobility with results that continue for weeks after treatment stops.

Glucosamine has also been proposed to treat tendinitis, to prevent muscle injuries, and to repair damaged cartilage, but there is as yet no evidence that it is effective.

## WHAT IS THE SCIENTIFIC EVIDENCE FOR GLUCOSAMINE?

### Osteoarthritis

Solid evidence indicates that glucosamine supplements effectively relieve pain and other symptoms of osteoarthritis. Two types of studies have been performed, those that compared glucosamine against placebo and those that compared it against standard medications.

A recent double-blind study compared glucosamine sulfate against placebo in 252 people with osteoarthritis of the knee.[11] After 4 weeks, the group that was given glucosamine experienced significantly reduced pain and improved movement, to a greater extent than the improvements seen in the placebo group.

Another double-blind study followed 329 people who were divided into four groups. One group was given the standard antiarthritis drug piroxicam (Feldene), a second was given glucosamine, a third received both treatments, and the fourth received placebo only.[12,13] Over 90 days, piroxicam and glucosamine proved equally effective at reducing symptoms. Interestingly, the combination treatment (piroxicam plus glucosamine) didn't produce significantly better results than either treatment taken alone.

After 90 days, treatment was stopped and the participants were followed for an additional 60 days. The benefits of piroxicam rapidly disappeared, but the benefits of glucosamine lasted for the full 60 days.

Similar results have been seen in other studies that compared glucosamine against ibuprofen.[14,15] These studies were well designed and enrolled a total of almost 400 individuals.

We don't know exactly how glucosamine works. However, besides serving as a basic building block for cartilage, glucosamine appears to stimulate cartilage cells in your joints to make proteoglycans and collagen, two proteins essential for the proper function of joints.[16–20]

Glucosamine may also help prevent collagen from breaking down.[21]

## SAFETY ISSUES

Glucosamine appears to be extremely safe for people of all ages. No significant side effects have been reported in any of the studies of glucosamine.

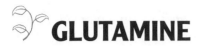 **GLUTAMINE**

### Principal Proposed Uses

There are no well-documented uses for glutamine.

### Other Proposed Uses

Recovery from critical illness, food allergies, digestive disorders (e.g., irritable bowel syndrome, Crohn's disease, ulcerative colitis) "overtraining syndrome," weakened immunity, "brain booster," attention deficit disorder, ulcers

### Supplement Forms/Alternative Names

L-glutamine

Glutamine, or L-glutamine, is an amino acid derived from another amino acid, glutamic acid. Glutamine plays a role in the health of the immune system, digestive tract, and muscle cells, as well as other bodily functions. It appears to serve as a fuel for the cells that line the intestines. Heavy exercise, infection, surgery, and trauma can deplete the body's glutamine reserves, particularly in muscle cells.

The fact that glutamine does so many good things in the body has led people to try glutamine supplements as a treatment for various conditions, including allergies, intestinal problems, and symptoms experienced by athletes who train too hard ("overtraining syndrome").

## SOURCES

There is no daily requirement for glutamine, because the body can make its own supply. As mentioned earlier, various severe stresses may result in a temporary glutamine deficiency.

High-protein foods such as meat, fish, beans, and dairy products are excellent sources of glutamine.

## THERAPEUTIC DOSAGES

Therapeutic dosages of glutamine range from 1.5 to 6 g daily, divided into several separate doses.

## THERAPEUTIC USES

Glutamine might be useful as a nutritional supplement for people undergoing recovery from critical illness.[1]

It has also been suggested as a treatment for food allergies, based on a theory called "leaky gut syndrome." This theory holds that in some people whole proteins leak through the wall of the digestive tract and enter the blood, causing allergic reactions. Preliminary evidence suggests that glutamine supplements might reduce leakage through the intestinal walls.[2,3] On the same principle, glutamine supplements have been suggested for people with other digestive problems, such as **irritable bowel syndrome** (page 85), Crohn's disease, and ulcerative colitis. However, there is little real evidence that it works.

Based on glutamine's role in muscle, it has been suggested that glutamine might be useful for athletes experiencing "overtraining syndrome." As the name suggests, this syndrome is the cumulative effect of a training regimen that allows too little rest and recovery between workouts. Symptoms include depression, fatigue, reduced performance, and physiological signs of stress. Glutamine supplements have additionally been proposed as treatment for immune weakness, **attention deficit disorder** (page 19), **ulcers** (page 112), and as a "brain booster." However, there is little to no scientific evidence for any of these uses.

## WHAT IS THE SCIENTIFIC EVIDENCE FOR GLUTAMINE?

### Recovery from Critical Illness

One small double-blind study found that glutamine supplements might have significant nutritional benefits for seriously ill people.[4] In this study, 84 critically ill hospital patients were divided into two groups. All the patients were being fed through a feeding tube. One group received a normal feeding-tube diet, whereas the other group received this diet plus supplemental glutamine. After 6 months, 14 of the 42 patients receiving glutamine had died, compared with 24 of the control group. The glutamine group also left both the intensive care ward and the hospital significantly sooner than the patients who did not receive glutamine.

## SAFETY ISSUES

As a naturally occurring amino acid, glutamine is thought to be a safe supplement when taken at recommended dosages. However, those who are hypersensitive to monosodium glutamate (MSG) should use glutamine with caution, as the body metabolizes glutamine into glutamate. Also, because many anti-epilepsy drugs work by blocking glutamate stimulation in the brain, high dosages of glutamine may overwhelm these drugs and pose a risk to people with epilepsy.

Maximum safe dosages for young children, pregnant or nursing women, or those with severe liver or kidney disease have not been determined.

## ⚠ INTERACTIONS YOU SHOULD KNOW ABOUT

If you are taking **antiseizure medications,** use glutamine only under medical supervision.

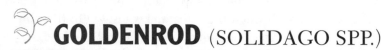

# GOLDENROD (SOLIDAGO SPP.)

### Principal Proposed Uses
Mild bladder infections, bladder/kidney stones

Goldenrod is often falsely accused of being an intensely allergenic plant, because of its unfortunate tendency to bloom brightly at the same time and often in locations quite near to the truly allergenic ragweed. However, actual allergic reactions to this gorgeous plant are unusual.

There are numerous species of goldenrod (27 have been collected in Indiana alone) but all seem to possess similar medicinal properties, and various species are used interchangeably in Europe.[1]

## WHAT IS GOLDENROD USED FOR TODAY?

In Europe, goldenrod is used as a supportive treatment for **bladder infections** (page 23), irritation of the urinary tract, and bladder/kidney stones. Goldenrod increases the flow of urine, helping to wash out bacteria and kidney stones, and may also directly soothe inflamed tissues and calm muscle spasms in the urinary tract.[2] It isn't used as a cure in itself, but rather as a support to other, more definitive treatments such as antibiotics.

We don't really know how well the herb works. Several studies have found that goldenrod increases urine flow,[3] but there is no direct evidence that the herb is effective in resolving bladder infections or bladder/kidney stones. Its active ingredients are not known.

**Warning:** Since urinary conditions are potentially serious, seek a doctor's supervision.

## DOSAGES

A typical dosage is 3 to 4 g of dried herb 2 to 3 times daily. Make sure to drink plenty of water while taking goldenrod, to help it do its job.

## SAFETY ISSUES

The safety of goldenrod hasn't been fully evaluated. However, no significant reactions or side effects have been reported.[4] Safety in young children, pregnant and nursing women, or those with severe liver or kidney disease has not been established.

# GOLDENSEAL (HYDRASTIS CANADENSIS)

*Principal Proposed Uses*

*Topical uses:*
Poorly healing sores, fungal infections, inflamed mucous membranes

*Internal uses:*
Minor digestive problems, sore throat

*Other Proposed Uses*
Urinary tract infections

*Incorrect Proposed Uses*
Masking positive findings on drug screens, "immune stimulant," "antibiotic" for common cold

Although goldenseal root is one of the most popular herbs sold today, it is taken almost entirely for the wrong reasons (see What Is Goldenseal Used for Today?). Originally, it was used by Native Americans both as a dye and as a treatment for skin disorders, digestive problems, liver disease, diarrhea, and eye irritations. European settlers learned of the herb from the Iroquois and other tribes and quickly adopted goldenseal as a part of early colonial medical care.

In the early 1800s, a flamboyant herbalist named Samuel Thompson created a wildly popular system of medicine (some would say personality cult) that swept the country. Thompson spoke of goldenseal in glowing terms, as a nearly magical cure for many conditions. His evangelism led to a dramatic upsurge in demand, followed by overcollection and decimation of the wild plant. Prices skyrocketed and then collapsed when Thompsonianism faded away.

Goldenseal has passed through several more booms and busts. Today, it is again in great demand, but now it is under intentional cultivation.

## WHAT IS GOLDENSEAL USED FOR TODAY?

Contemporary herbalists use goldenseal primarily as a topical antibiotic for wounds that are not healing well. In practice, goldenseal salves, creams, ointments, and powders appear to speed wound healing.

Unfortunately, there are no reliable scientific studies to verify this strong clinical impression.

What we do know is that one of goldenseal's constituents, berberine, possesses strong activity against a wide variety of bacteria and fungi.[1,2] Another factor may be that goldenseal seems to have a soothing effect on inflamed mucous membranes.

Goldenseal is most effective by direct contact. It does not seem to be an effective oral antibiotic, probably because the blood levels of berberine that can be achieved by taking goldenseal orally are far too low to matter.[3] However, goldenseal may also be beneficial in treating sore throats and diseases of the digestive tract because it can contact the affected area directly. Since berberine is concentrated in the bladder, goldenseal may be useful in resolving **bladder infections** (page 23). It may be helpful for treating fungal infections of the skin as well.

Strangely, goldenseal is most commonly used inappropriately. Goldenseal is frequently combined with echinacea to be taken as an "immune booster" and "antibiotic" for the prevention and treatment of **colds** (page 44). However, as the noted herbalist Paul Bergner has pointed out, there are three things wrong with this packaging: (1) there is no credible evidence that goldenseal increases immunity; (2) the herb was never used historically as an early treatment for colds; and (3) antibiotics aren't effective against colds anyway.[4] Nevertheless, the **echinacea** (page 179) in these products may be helpful.

Tradition suggests that goldenseal may help relieve the clogged sinuses and chest congestion that can linger after the acute phase of a cold, although there is no scientific evidence to turn to.

The other myth that has helped drive the sales of goldenseal is the widespread street belief that it can block a positive drug screen. The origin of this false idea dates back to a work of fiction published in 1900 by a pharmacist and author named John Uri Lloyd. In *Stringtown on the Pike,* Lloyd's most successful novel, a dead man is found to have traces of goldenseal in his stomach. In fact, he had taken goldenseal regularly (and correctly) as a digestive aid, but a toxicology expert mistakes the goldenseal for strychnine, and deduces intentional murder.

This work of fiction sufficed to create a folkloric connection between goldenseal and drug testing. Although the goldenseal in the story actually made a drug test come out falsely positive, this has been turned around to become a belief that goldenseal can make urine drug screens come out negative. A word to the wise: It doesn't work.

## DOSAGES

When used as a topical for skin wounds, a sufficient quantity of goldenseal cream, ointment, or powder should be applied to cover the wound. Make sure to clean the wound at least once a day to prevent goldenseal particles from being trapped in the healing tissues.

For mouth sores and sore throats, goldenseal tincture may be swished or gargled. Goldenseal may also be used as strong tea for this purpose, made by boiling 0.5 to 1 g in a cup of water. Goldenseal tea can also be used as a douche for vaginal candidiasis.

For oral use, to aid the digestive tract or loosen clogged sinuses, a typical dosage of goldenseal is 250 to 500 mg 3 times daily. Goldenseal is generally only taken for a couple of weeks at most.

## SAFETY ISSUES

Goldenseal appears to be safe when used as directed. One widespread rumor claims that goldenseal can disrupt the normal bacteria of the intestines. However, there is no scientific evidence that this occurs, and many herbalists believe that such concerns are unwarranted.[5] Another fallacy is that small overdoses of goldenseal are toxic, causing ulcerations of the stomach and other mucous membranes. This idea is based on a misunderstanding of old literature.[6]

However, because berberine has been reported to cause uterine contractions in animals, goldenseal should not be taken by pregnant women.[7] Safety in young children, nursing women, or those with severe liver or kidney disease is also not established.

Side effects of oral goldenseal are uncommon, although there have been reports of gastrointestinal distress and increased nervousness in people who take very high doses.

# GOTU KOLA (CENTELLA ASIATICA)

*Principal Proposed Uses*
   Varicose veins

*Other Proposed Uses*
   Hemorrhoids, keloid scars, scleroderma, burn and wound healing, improving mental performance, anal fissures, bladder ulcers, perineal lesions, liver cirrhosis,

Gotu kola is a creeping plant native to subtropical and tropical climates. In India and Indonesia, gotu kola has a long history of use to promote wound healing and slow the progress of leprosy. It was also reputed to prolong life, increase energy, and enhance sexual potency.[1] Other uses of gotu kola included treating skin diseases, diarrhea, menstrual disorders, vaginal discharge, and venereal disease.

Based on these many traditional indications, gotu kola was accepted as a drug in France in the 1880s. British physicians in Africa used a special extract to treat leprosy.

## WHAT IS GOTU KOLA USED FOR TODAY?

In the 1970s, Italian and other European researchers found evidence that gotu kola could significantly improve symptoms of **varicose veins** (page 113), particularly overall discomfort, tiredness, and swelling. However, the herb is not believed to do much to reduce the unsightliness of veins that are already badly damaged. Some clinicians suggest that regular use of gotu kola can prevent the development of visible varicose veins, but this hasn't been proven. Gotu kola has also been suggested as a treatment for **hemorrhoids** (page 70) because they are a type of varicose vein.

Like other herbs used for the treatment of varicose veins, gotu kola appears to have a generally beneficial effect on connective tissues. Along these lines, it has been used to prevent the development of keloid (bulging, enlarged) scars following surgery, as well as to soften existing keloids. Gotu kola has also been tried as a treatment for improving burn and wound healing and to alleviate the symptoms of the connective tissue disease scleroderma.

Gotu kola has a reputation for improving memory, and the positive results from a study of rats performed in 1992 produced a temporary rush of public interest.[2] However, the benefits in humans, if any, are far from impressive.

Gotu kola should not be confused with the caffeine-containing kola nut, used in original recipes for Coca-Cola.

## WHAT IS THE SCIENTIFIC EVIDENCE FOR GOTU KOLA?

There is significant scientific evidence for the effectiveness of gotu kola in varicose veins/venous insufficiency.

A vacuum suction chamber has been used in some gotu kola studies to evaluate the rate of fluid leakage in venous insufficiency. It produces swelling when applied to the skin of the ankle. When leg veins are leaking a lot of fluid, this swelling takes longer to disappear.

In one study of people with venous insufficiency, 2 weeks of treatment with gotu kola extracts was shown to reduce the time necessary for the swelling to disappear.[3]

Another study of double-blind design followed 87 people with varicose veins and compared the benefits of gotu kola at 60 mg and 30 mg daily against placebo.[4] The results showed improvements in both treated groups but greater improvement at the higher dose. This kind of dose responsiveness is generally taken as good evidence that a treatment is actually effective.

A double-blind study of 94 individuals with venous insufficiency of the lower limb compared the benefits of gotu kola extract at 120 mg daily and 60 mg daily against a placebo.[5] The results also showed a significant dose-related improvement in the treated groups in symptoms such as subjective heaviness, discomfort, and edema.

A 1992 review of all the gotu kola studies available concluded that gotu kola extract provides a dose-related improvement in venous insufficiency symptoms, reducing foot swelling, ankle edema, and fluid leakage from the veins.[6]

Although the subject is far from completely understood, it appears that gotu kola may improve the structure and function of the connective tissue in the body, keeping veins stronger and also possibly reducing the symptoms of other connective-tissue diseases. Along these lines, numerous clinical reports and preliminary studies suggest that gotu kola extracts may be useful in treating keloids, burns, wounds, anal fissures, bladder ulcers, dermatitis, hemorrhoids, perineal lesions, periodontal disease, cellulite, liver cirrhosis, and scleroderma.[7,8] While some of these studies are intriguing and make a good case for further research, none can be regarded as definitive.

## DOSAGES

The usual dosage of gotu kola is 20 to 40 mg 3 times daily of an extract standardized to contain 40% asiaticoside, 29 to 30% asiatic acid, 29 to 30% madecassic acid, and 1 to 2% madecassoside. Be patient, because gotu kola takes at least 4 weeks to work.

For the prevention of keloid scars, the herb is usually taken for 3 months prior to surgery, and for another 3 months afterwards.

Gotu Kola

Visit Us at TNP.com

## SAFETY ISSUES

Orally, gotu kola appears to be nontoxic.[9] It seldom causes any side effects other than the occasional allergic skin rash. However, there are some concerns that gotu kola may be carcinogenic if applied topically to the skin.[10]

Although gotu kola has not been proven safe for pregnant or nursing women, studies in rabbits suggest that it does not harm fetal development,[11] and pregnant women were enrolled in one research trial.[12] Safety in young children and those with severe liver or kidney disease has not been established.

# GREEN TEA (CAMELLIA SINENSIS)

*Principal Proposed Uses*
Cancer prevention

People have been drinking tea for thousands of years, but only in the last couple of decades have we begun to document the potential health benefits of this ancient beverage. Both black and green tea are made from the same plant, but more of the original substances endure in the less-processed green form. Green tea contains high levels of substances called polyphenols, known to possess strong antioxidant, anticarcinogenic, and even antibiotic properties.[1]

A growing body of evidence in both human and animal studies suggests that regular consumption of green tea can reduce the incidence of a variety of cancers, including colon, pancreatic, and stomach cancers.[2] However, the observational studies used to draw these conclusions can be misleading, and not everyone who examines the data concludes that green tea has been proven effective.[3]

## WHAT IS GREEN TEA USED FOR TODAY?

Based on the widely publicized results of the observational studies mentioned earlier, green tea has become popular as a daily drink for **cancer prevention** (page 26).

## DOSAGES

Studies suggest that 3 cups of green tea daily provides protection against cancer. However, because not everyone wants to take the time to drink green tea, manufacturers have offered extracts that can be taken in pill form. A typical dosage is 100 to 150 mg 3 times daily of a green tea extract standardized to contain 80% total polyphenols and 50% epigallocatechin gallate. Whether these extracts work as well as the real thing remains unknown.

## SAFETY ISSUES

As a widely consumed beverage, green tea is generally regarded as safe. It does contain caffeine, although at a lower level than black tea or coffee, and can therefore cause insomnia, nervousness, and the other well-known symptoms of excess caffeine intake. Green tea should not be given to infants and young children.

## ⚠ INTERACTIONS YOU SHOULD KNOW ABOUT

If you are taking **MAO inhibitors,** the caffeine in green tea could cause serious problems.

# GUGGUL (COMMIPHORA MUKUL)

## Principal Proposed Uses
High cholesterol

Guggul, the sticky gum resin from the mukul myrrh tree, plays a major role in the traditional herbal medicine of India. It was traditionally combined with other herbs for the treatment of arthritis, skin diseases, pains in the nervous system, obesity, digestive problems, infections in the mouth, and menstrual problems.

In the early 1960s, Indian researchers discovered an ancient Sanskrit medical text that appears to clearly describe the symptoms and treatment of high cholesterol.[1] One of the main recommendations was guggul. Subsequent tests in animals found that guggul gum both lowered cholesterol levels and also separately protected against the development of hardening of the arteries.

Numerous research trials followed this discovery, culminating in open and double-blind studies examining guggul's effectiveness in humans.[2,3] Although these studies showed positive results, they are small and have real problems in scientific design, making the results less than definitive. Nonetheless, the evidence was strong enough for the Indian government to approve guggul as a treatment for high cholesterol.

## WHAT IS GUGGUL USED FOR TODAY?

It appears that guggul can lower **cholesterol** (page 39) by about 11% and triglycerides by 17%, as well as raise HDL (good) cholesterol levels and lower LDL (bad) cholesterol levels.[4,5] The full benefits take about 4 weeks to develop. See *The Natural Pharmacist Guide to Garlic and Cholesterol* for even more information on guggul and other natural treatments to lower cholesterol.

## DOSAGES

Take a dose of guggul extract standardized to provide 25 mg of gugulsterone 3 times daily. For best results in lowering cholesterol, increase exercise and improve diet as well.

## SAFETY ISSUES

Guggul appears to be reasonably safe, but thorough safety studies have not yet been performed.[6,7] Whole-gum guggul can cause digestive distress. However, extracts standardized to gugulsterone content seldom cause significant immediate problems.

Safety in young children, pregnant or nursing women, or those with severe liver or kidney disease has not been established.

# GYMNEMA (GYMNEMA SYLVESTRE)

## Principal Proposed Uses
Diabetes (blood sugar control)

Native to the forests of India, *Gymnema sylvestre* has a coincidental double relationship to sugar: When placed on the tongue, it blocks the sensation of sweetness, and when taken internally, it appears to help control blood sugar levels in diabetes. There doesn't seem to be any connection between these two effects.

Indian physicians first used gymnema to treat diabetes almost 2,000 years ago. In the 1920s, preliminary scientific studies found that gymnema leaves do indeed reduce blood sugar levels,[1] but nothing much came of this discovery for decades.

## WHAT IS GYMNEMA USED FOR TODAY?

With the recent revival of interest in herbs, gymnema has become increasingly popular in the United States as a supportive treatment for **diabetes** (page 60). A few animal and preliminary human studies suggest that gymnema can increase insulin secretion and also enhance insulin's effectiveness.[2,3,4] Gymnema is most likely to be helpful in mild cases of adult-onset diabetes when insulin injections are not yet required. However, it is also used as a supportive treatment in more serious forms of the disease.

**Warning:** Diabetes is a dangerous illness, thus gymnema should only be used under medical supervision. Under no circumstances should you try to replace insulin with gymnema alone.

## DOSAGES

Gymnema is usually taken at a dosage of 400 to 600 mg daily of an extract standardized to contain 24% gymnemic acid.

## SAFETY ISSUES

When used in appropriate dosages, gymnema appears to be fairly safe, although extensive studies have not been performed. One obvious risk is that if gymnema is successful, it may lower blood sugar levels too far, causing a dangerous hypoglycemic reaction. For this reason, medical supervision is essential.

Safety in young children, pregnant or nursing women, or those with severe kidney or liver disease has not been established.

## ⚠ INTERACTIONS YOU SHOULD KNOW ABOUT

If you are taking **medications to reduce blood sugar levels,** gymnema might cause them to work even better, potentially causing hypoglycemia.

# HAWTHORN (CRATAEGUS OXYACANTHA)

*Principal Proposed Uses*
  Early stages of congestive heart failure, benign heart palpitations, high blood pressure

*Other Proposed Uses*
  Angina, atherosclerosis

---

The name "hawthorn" is derived from "hedgethorn," reflecting this spiny tree's use as a living fence in much of Europe. Besides protecting estates from trespassers, hawthorn has also been used medicinally since ancient times. Roman physicians used hawthorn as a heart drug in the first century A.D., but most of the literature from that period focuses on its symbolic use for religious rites and political ceremonies.

During the Middle Ages, hawthorn was used for the treatment of dropsy, a condition we now call congestive heart failure. It was also used for treating other heart ailments as well as for sore throat.

## WHAT IS HAWTHORN USED FOR TODAY?

Hawthorn is widely regarded in modern Europe as a safe and effective treatment for the early stages of **congestive heart failure** (page 50). Although not as potent as that other famous heart herb of the Middle Ages, foxglove, haw-

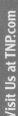

thorn is much safer. The active ingredients in foxglove are the drugs digoxin and digitoxin. However, hawthorn does not appear to have any single active ingredient. This has prevented it from being turned into a drug.

Like foxglove and the drugs made from it, hawthorn appears to improve the heart's pumping ability. But it offers one very important advantage. Digitalis and some other medications that increase the power of the heart also make it more irritable and liable to dangerous irregularities of rhythm. In contrast, hawthorn has the unique property of both strengthening the heart and stabilizing it against arrythmias by lengthening what is called the refractory period.[1,2,3] This term refers to the short period following a heartbeat during which the heart cannot beat again. Many irregularities of heart rhythm begin with an early beat. Digitalis shortens the refractory period, making such a premature beat more likely, while hawthorn protects against such potentially dangerous breaks in the heart's even rhythm. Also, with digitalis the difference between the proper dosage and the toxic dosage is very small. Hawthorn has an enormous range of safe dosing.[4]

Nevertheless, I don't recommend self-treating congestive heart failure! The disease is simply too dangerous. There are also medical treatments (such as ACE inhibitors) that have been proven to save lives in CHF, a benefit that hawthorn may not provide. You need a physician versed in both conventional and alternative medicine to guide you if you wish to use hawthorn for this condition.

There is one condition in which you may be able to safely use hawthorn as a self-treatment: annoying heart palpitations that have been thoroughly evaluated and found to be benign. Common symptoms include occasional thumping as well as episodes of racing heartbeat. These may occur without any identifiable medical cause and may not require any medical treatment, except for purposes of comfort. Although there is little scientific evidence to support it, many people use hawthorn for this condition.

However, because there are many dangerous kinds of heart palpitations, it is absolutely necessary to get a thorough checkup first. You should only self-treat with hawthorn after a doctor tells you that you have no medically significant heart problems. Full benefits may take a month or two to develop.

Finally, hawthorn sometimes lowers blood pressure a little, but seldom enough to make a significant difference.[5,6] It may be helpful for other heart-related conditions, such as **angina** (page 7) and **atherosclerosis** (page 14) in general, but there is as yet little direct evidence.

## WHAT IS THE SCIENTIFIC EVIDENCE FOR HAWTHORN?

There has been a significant amount of solid research regarding the use of hawthorn as a treatment for congestive heart failure. Between 1981 and 1994, 13 controlled clinical studies of hawthorn were performed, most of them double-blind.[7,8] In all, 808 people participated in these trials. The cumulative results strongly suggest that hawthorn is an effective treatment for congestive heart failure. Comparative studies suggest that hawthorn is about as effective as a low dose of the conventional drug captopril, although whether it produces the same long-term benefits as captopril is unknown.[9]

## DOSAGE

The standard dosage of hawthorn is 100 to 300 mg 3 times daily of an extract standardized to contain about 2 to 3% flavonoids or 18 to 20% procyanidins. Full effects appear to take several weeks or months to develop.

## SAFETY ISSUES

Hawthorn appears to be safe. Germany's Commission E lists no known risks, contraindications, or drug interactions with hawthorn, and mice and rats have been given phenomenal doses without showing significant toxicity.[10] However, since hawthorn affects the heart, it shouldn't be combined with other heart drugs without a doctor's supervision. People with especially low blood pressure should also exercise caution.

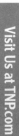

Side effects are rare, mostly consisting of mild stomach upset and occasional allergic reactions (skin rash).

Safety in young children, pregnant or nursing women, or those with severe liver, heart or kidney disease has not been established.

## ⚠ INTERACTIONS YOU SHOULD KNOW ABOUT

If you are taking any **heart medications,** it is possible that taking hawthorn could cause problems.

# HE SHOU WU A.K.A. FO TI
## (POLYGONUM MULTIFLORUM)

### Principal Proposed Uses
High cholesterol, insomnia, constipation

The name of this herb literally means "Black-haired Mr. He," in reference to an ancient story of a Mr. He who restored his vitality, sexual potency, and youthful appearance by taking the herb now named after him. He shou wu is widely used in China for the traditional purpose of restoring black hair and other signs of youth.

More so than with most Chinese herbs, tradition supports taking He shou wu as a single herb, although it also figures as a component in many formulas. He shou wu is also called fo ti; pure unprocessed root is named white fo ti, while herb boiled in black-bean liquid according to a traditional process is called red fo ti. The two forms are believed to have somewhat different properties.

## WHAT IS HE SHOU WU USED FOR TODAY?

Both animal and preliminary human studies performed in China suggest that He shou wu can reduce serum **cholesterol** (page 39) and also improve symptoms of **insomnia** (page 80).[1]

He shou wu is also said to be useful for **constipation** (page 51); although if this is true, the effect is mild.

I tried He shou wu to see if it would turn my graying hair black, but nothing happened. Based on this highly sophisticated scientific research, I suspect that Mr. He's experience is hard to duplicate. (But then again, anecdotal negative data is just as bad as anecdotal positive data!)

## DOSAGES

He shou wu should be taken at a dosage of 9 to 15 g of raw herb per day, or according to the label for processed extracts. For most purposes, the processed or "red" fo ti is said to be superior. However, the raw herb is believed to be more effective for relieving constipation.

## SAFETY ISSUES

Detailed modern safety studies have not been performed on this herb. Immediate side effects are infrequent, primarily limited to mild diarrhea and the rare allergic reaction. Safety for young children, pregnant or nursing women, or those with severe kidney or liver disease has not been established.

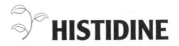

# HISTIDINE

*Principal Proposed Uses*
There are no well-documented uses for histidine.

*Other Proposed Uses*
Rheumatoid arthritis

Histidine is a semiessential amino acid, which means your body normally makes as much as it needs. Like most other amino acids, histidine is used to make proteins and enzymes. The body also uses histidine to make histamine, the culprit behind the swelling and itching you feel in an allergic reaction.

It appears that people with rheumatoid arthritis may have low levels of histidine in their blood. This has led to some speculation that histidine supplements might be a good treatment for this kind of arthritis, but so far no studies have confirmed this.

## SOURCES

Although histidine is not required in the diet, histidine deficiencies can occur during periods of very rapid growth. Dairy products, meat, poultry, fish, and other protein-rich foods are good sources of histidine.

## THERAPEUTIC DOSAGES

A typical therapeutic dosage of histidine is 4 to 5 g daily.

## THERAPEUTIC USES

Individuals with **rheumatoid arthritis** (page 109) appear to have reduced levels of histidine in the blood,[1,2] but this by itself doesn't prove that taking histidine will help. One study designed to evaluate this question directly found no significant benefit.[3]

## SAFETY ISSUES

As a necessary nutrient, histidine is believed to be safe. However, maximum safe dosages of histidine have not been determined for young children, pregnant or nursing women, or those with severe liver or kidney disease. As with other supplements taken in large doses, it is important to purchase a quality product, as contaminants present even in very small percentages could conceivably add up and become toxic.

# HMB (HYDROXYMETHYL BUTYRATE)

*Principal Proposed Uses*
Muscle building for strength athletes and bodybuilders

*Other Proposed Uses*
Weight-loss aid, age-related loss of muscle

*Supplement Forms/Alternative Names*
Beta-hydroxy beta-methylbutyric acid

Technically "beta-hydroxy beta-methylbutyric acid," HMB is a chemical that occurs naturally in the body when the amino acid leucine breaks down.

Leucine is found in particularly high concentrations in muscles. During athletic training, damage to the muscles leads to the breakdown of leucine as well as increased HMB levels. Based on the laws of chemistry, it is possible that taking extra HMB might work in the reverse way, slowing loss of muscle tissue. For this reason, HMB has been proposed as a sports supplement for strength athletes and bodybuilders. It has also been suggested as an aid for preventing normal age-related muscle loss.

## SOURCES

HMB is not an essential nutrient, so there is no established requirement. HMB is found in small amounts in citrus fruit and catfish. To get a therapeutic dosage, however, you need to take a supplement in powder or pill form.

## THERAPEUTIC DOSAGES

A typical therapeutic dosage of HMB is 3 to 5 g daily.

Be careful not to confuse HMB with gamma hydroxybutyrate (GHB), a similar supplement. GHB can cause severe sedation, especially when combined with other sedating substances, such as alcohol or antianxiety drugs.

## THERAPEUTIC USES

Evidence from animal and human studies suggests that HMB may help strength athletes increase muscle mass more rapidly.[1,2] However, due to the absence of proper double-blind studies, we don't know for sure whether it works.

Although it is sometimes proposed as a weight-loss aid, HMB does not appear to help reduce body fat if taken by people who do not exercise while they're taking it.[3]

One author suggests HMB might also help prevent normal age-related muscle loss.[4] Although there is no real evidence for this idea, exercise does prevent muscle loss due to aging and is highly recommended for people of all ages.

## WHAT IS THE SCIENTIFIC EVIDENCE FOR HMB?

### Muscle Building

Studies on chick and rat muscles suggest that HMB reduces the amount of muscle protein that breaks down during exercise.[5]

In a two-part study, 41 male volunteers aged 19 to 29 were given either 0, 1.5, or 3 g of HMB daily for 3 weeks.[6] The participants also lifted weights 3 days a week for 90 minutes.

The results suggest that HMB can enhance strength and muscle mass in direct proportion to how much you take. The improvements increased in relation to dosage: 0.88 pounds of muscle in the group receiving no HMB, 1.76 pounds in the low-HMB group, and 2.64 pounds in the high-HMB group.

In another part of the study, 32 male volunteers took either HMB or no treatment, and then lifted weights for 2 or 3 hours daily, 6 days a week for 7 weeks. The HMB group saw a dramatically greater increase in its bench-press strength—almost *three times* the increase seen in the control group.

Unfortunately, neither part of this study was blinded. Because members of the treated group knew that they were taking HMB, the results could have been largely due to the power of suggestion.

## SAFETY ISSUES

HMB seems to be safe. No side effects were noted in trials of HMB at dosages up to 4 g daily for 4 weeks.[7] However, full safety studies have not been performed, so HMB should not be used by young children, pregnant or nursing women, or those with severe liver or kidney disease, except on the advice of a physician.

As with all supplements taken in very large doses, it is important to purchase a quality product, as an impurity present even in very small percentages could add up to a real problem.

# HOPS (HUMULUS LUPULUS)

## *Principal Proposed Uses*

Anxiety, insomnia, digestive problems

Hops (the fruiting bodies of the hop plant) are most famous as the source of beer's bitter flavor, but they have a long history of use in herbal medicine as well. In Greece and Rome, hops were used as a remedy for poor digestion and intestinal disturbances. The Chinese used the herb for these purposes as well as to treat leprosy and tuberculosis.

As cultivation of hops for beer spread through Europe, it gradually became obvious that workers in hop fields tended to fall asleep on the job, more so than could be explained by the tedium of the work. This observation led to enthusiasm for using hops as a sedative. However, subsequent investigation suggests that much of the sedative effect seen in hop fields is due to an oil that evaporates quickly in storage.

Despite the absence of this oil, dried hop preparations do appear to be somewhat calming. While the exact reason is not clear, it seems that a sedating substance known as methylbutenol develops in the dried herb over a period of time.[1] It may also be manufactured in the body from other constituents of dried hops.

## WHAT ARE HOPS USED FOR TODAY?

Germany's Commission E authorizes the use of hops for "discomfort due to restlessness or anxiety and sleep disturbances." Because its sedative effect is mild at most, the herb is often combined with other treatments for **anxiety** (page 8) and **insomnia** (page 80).

Like other bitter plants, hops are also used to improve appetite and digestion.

Scientists have had difficulty demonstrating that hops cause sedation.[2]

## DOSAGES

The standard dosage of hops is 0.5 g taken 1 to 3 times daily.

## SAFETY ISSUES

Hops are believed to be nontoxic. However, as with all herbs, some people are allergic to it. Interestingly, some species of dogs, greyhounds in particular, appear to be sensitive to hops with reports of deaths occurring.[3] The mechanism of this toxicity is not yet known. Those taken with the popular hobby of brewing beer at home are advised to keep pets away from the relatively large quantity of hops used in this process.

One animal study suggests that hops might increase the effect of sedative drugs,[4] so do not take hops with other medications for insomnia or anxiety except under a physician's supervision.

## ⚠ INTERACTIONS
## YOU SHOULD KNOW ABOUT

If you are taking **sedative drugs,** do not take hops except under a physician's supervision.

Hops

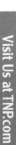

Visit Us at TNP.com

# HORSE CHESTNUT (AESCULUS HIPPOCASTANUM)

*Principal Proposed Uses*
  Vein problems (e.g., varicose veins, phlebitis, hemorrhoids)

*Other Proposed Uses*
  Swelling (sprains and other injuries)

The horse chestnut tree is widely cultivated for its bright white, yellow, or red flower clusters. Closely related to the Ohio buckeye, its spiny fruits contain a few large seeds known as horse chestnuts. A superstition in many parts of Europe suggests that carrying these seeds in your pocket will ward off rheumatism. More serious medical uses date back to nineteenth-century France, where extracts were used to treat hemorrhoids.

## WHAT IS HORSE CHESTNUT USED FOR TODAY?

Serious German research began in the 1960s and ultimately led to the approval of an extract of horse chestnut for vein diseases of the legs. This herb is the third most common single herb product sold in Germany, after ginkgo and St. John's wort. In Japan, an injectable form of horse chestnut is widely used to reduce inflammation after surgery or injury, however it is not available in the United States.

The active ingredients in horse chestnut appear to be a group of chemicals called saponins, of which aescin is considered the most important. Like **OPCs** (page 270) and **bilberry** (page 135), aescin has the capacity to reduce swelling and inflammation, probably by slowing down the rate at which fluid leaks from irritated capillaries.[1] It's not exactly clear how aescin works, but theories include "sealing" leaking capillaries, improving the elastic strength of veins, preventing the release of enzymes (known as glycosaminoglycan hydrolases) that break down collagen and open holes in capillary walls, and blocking other physiological events that lead to vein damage.[2,3]

Horse chestnut is most often used as a treatment for venous insufficiency. This is a condition associated with **varicose veins** (page 113), when the blood pools in the veins of the leg and causes aching, swelling, and a sense of heaviness. While horse chestnut appears to reduce these symptoms, it is not believed to improve visible varicose veins very much.

Because **hemorrhoids** (page 70) are actually a form of varicose veins, horse chestnut is often recommended for them as well.

Based on its known effects on veins, horse chestnut is also sometimes used along with conventional treatment in cases where the veins of the lower legs become seriously inflamed (phlebitis). However, this condition is potentially dangerous and requires a doctor's supervision.

Just like OPCs, extracts of horse chestnut are sometimes recommended to help reduce swelling after sprains and other athletic injuries. Again, this use is based on the known effects of horse chestnut on blood vessels.

## WHAT IS THE SCIENTIFIC EVIDENCE FOR HORSE CHESTNUT?

A total of 558 individuals have been involved in double-blind studies of horse chestnut for treating venous insufficiency.[4] One of the largest trials followed 212 people over a period of 40 days.[5] It was what is called a *crossover study* because the participants initially received horse chestnut or placebo, and then they were crossed over to the other treatment (without their knowledge) after 20 days. The results showed that horse chestnut produced significant improvement in leg edema, pain, and sensation of heaviness.

Another study compared the effectiveness of horse chestnut and compression stockings in 240 people over a course of 12 weeks.[6] Compression stockings worked faster at reducing swelling, but by 12 weeks the results were equivalent.

## DOSAGES

The most common dosage of horse chestnut is 300 mg twice daily, standardized to contain 50 mg aescin per dose, for a total daily dose of 100 mg aescin. After good results have been achieved, the dosage can be reduced by about half for maintenance.

Horse chestnut preparations should certify that a constituent called esculin has been removed. Also, a delayed-release formulation must be used to prevent gastrointestinal upset.

**Warning:** Do not try to inject horse chestnut products designed for oral use!

## SAFETY ISSUES

After decades of wide usage in Germany, there have been no reports of harmful effects due to properly prepared horse chestnut, even when it has been taken in overdose.[7] In animal studies, horse chestnut and its principal ingredient aescin have been found to be very safe, even when taken at dosages eight times higher than normal. Dogs and rats have been treated for 34 weeks with this herb without harmful effects.[8] However, doses 50 times higher than normal can cause death in animals, and there are two reports out of Italy of kidney damage caused by massive overdosage.[9,10] In Japan, where injectable forms are used, dangerous and even fatal reactions have been noted.

For theoretical reasons, horse chestnut is not recommended for people with serious kidney or liver disease. It also should not be combined with anticoagulant or "blood-thinning" drugs, as it may alter their function.[11]

The safety of horse chestnut in young children, and pregnant or nursing women has not been established. However, 13 pregnant women were given horse chestnut in a controlled study without noticeable harm.[12]

In clinical studies of horse chestnut, there have been no significant side effects other than the usual occasional mild allergic reactions or gastrointestinal distress. However, these studies all used controlled-release forms of horse chestnut. Taking this herb in other formulations may cause quite a bit of stomach upset.

## ⚠ INTERACTIONS YOU SHOULD KNOW ABOUT

If you are taking **aspirin** or **anticoagulant drugs,** do not use horse chestnut except under medical supervision.

# HORSETAIL (EQUISETUM ARVENSE)

*Principal Proposed Uses*
Brittle nails, osteoporosis, rheumatoid arthritis

Horsetail is a living fossil, the sole descendent of primitive plants that served as dinosaur snacks 100 million years ago. The herb is unique for its high concentration of silicon, as well as for its ability to dissolve gold and other minerals into itself. Because of its silicon content, horsetail is abrasive enough to be used for polishing.

Medicinally, horsetail has been used for treating urinary disorders, wounds, gonorrhea, nosebleeds, digestive disorders, gout, and many other conditions.[1]

## WHAT IS HORSETAIL USED FOR TODAY?

Silicon plays a role in bone health,[2] and for this reason, horsetail has been recommended to help keep bones and nails strong. The famous German herbalist Rudolf Weiss also suggests that horsetail can relieve symptoms of **rheumatoid arthritis** (page 109).[3] However, there is no real scientific evidence for any of these uses.

## DOSAGES

The standard dosage of horsetail is 1 g in capsule or tea form up to 3 times daily, as needed. Medicinal horsetail should *not* be confused with its highly toxic relative, the marsh horsetail (*Equisetum palustre*).

## SAFETY ISSUES

Noticeable side effects from standard dosages of horsetail tea are rare. However, horsetail contains an enzyme that damages **vitamin B$_1$ (thiamin)** (page 320) and has caused severe illness and even death in livestock that consumed too much of it.[4] In Canada, horsetail products are required to undergo heating or other forms of processing to inactivate this harmful constituent.

Also, perhaps because horsetail contains low levels of nicotine, children have been known to become seriously ill from using the branches as blow guns.[5] This plant can also concentrate toxic metals present in its environment.

For all of the above reasons, horsetail is not recommended for young children, pregnant or nursing women, or those with severe kidney or liver disease.

Horsetail may also cause loss of potassium, which may be dangerous for those taking drugs in the digitalis category.[6]

## ⚠ INTERACTIONS YOU SHOULD KNOW ABOUT

If you are taking **drugs in the digitalis category,** use horsetail only under medical supervision.

# HYDROXYCITRIC ACID

*Principal Proposed Uses*
There are no well-documented uses for hydroxycitric acid.

*Other Proposed Uses*
Weight loss

*Supplement Forms/Alternative Names*
Hydroxycitrate, HCA

Hydroxycitric acid, a derivative of citric acid, is found primarily in certain fruits. Test-tube and animal research suggests that hydroxycitric acid may be helpful in weight loss, because it interferes with the conversion of sugars into fat.

## SOURCES

Hydroxycitric acid is not an essential nutrient. In fact, it is found only in a few plants, primarily the tamarind fruit of Southeast Asia. Supplements are available in many forms, including tablets, capsules, powders, and even snack bars.

## THERAPEUTIC DOSAGES

A typical dosage of HCA is 250 to 1,000 mg 3 times daily.

## THERAPEUTIC USES

According to animal studies, HCA can suppress appetite and thereby encourage weight loss.[1–5] It is thought to work by interfering with the body's ability to produce fat.[6–9] However, no properly designed human studies have yet been reported.

## SAFETY ISSUES

Although no serious side effects have been reported from animal studies or individuals who have used it, hydroxycitric acid has not yet been scientifically tested in humans. Therefore, its safety remains unknown.

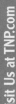

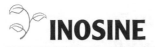

# INOSINE

*Principal Proposed Uses*
   There are no well-documented uses for inosine.

*Other Proposed Uses*
   Athletic performance, heart disease, Tourette's syndrome

Inosine is an important chemical found throughout the body. It plays many roles, one of which is helping to make ATP (adenosine triphosphate), the body's main form of usable energy. Based primarily on this fact, inosine supplements have been proposed as an energy-booster for athletes, as well as a treatment for various heart conditions.

## SOURCES

Inosine is not an essential nutrient. However, brewer's yeast and organ meats, such as liver and kidney, contain considerable amounts. Inosine is also available in purified form.

## THERAPEUTIC DOSAGES

When used as a sports supplement, a typical dosage of inosine is 5 to 6 g daily.

## THERAPEUTIC USES

Inosine has been proposed as a treatment for various forms of heart disease, from inflamma-

tion of the heart lining to irregular heartbeat and heart attacks. However, the evidence that it works is highly preliminary.[1]

Inosine is better known as a performance enhancer for athletes, although most of the available evidence suggests that it *doesn't* work for this purpose.[2–5]

Inosine has also been suggested as a possible treatment for Tourette's syndrome, a neurological disorder.[6]

## SAFETY ISSUES

Although no side effects have been reported with the use of inosine, comprehensive safety studies have not been completed. For this reason, young children, pregnant or nursing women, or those with serious liver or kidney disease should not use inosine.

As with all supplements taken in multigram doses, it is important to purchase a reputable product, because a contaminant present even in small percentages could add up to a real problem.

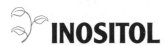

# INOSITOL

*Principal Proposed Uses*
   Depression, panic disorder

*Other Proposed Uses*
   Alzheimer's disease, obsessive-compulsive disorder, attention deficit disorder, diabetic neuropathy

*Supplement Forms/Alternative Names*
   Vitamin $B_8$

Inositol, unofficially referred to as "vitamin $B_8$," is present in all animal tissues, with the highest levels in the heart and brain. It is part of the mem-

branes (outer linings) of all cells, and plays a role in helping the liver process fats as well as contributing to the function of muscles and nerves.

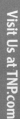

Inositol may also be involved in depression. People who are depressed have much lower-than-normal levels of inositol in their spinal fluid. In addition, inositol participates in the action of serotonin, a neurotransmitter known to be a factor in depression. (Neurotransmitters are chemicals that transmit messages between nerve cells.) For this reason, inositol has been proposed as a treatment for depression, and preliminary evidence suggests that it may be helpful.

Inositol has also been tried for other psychological and nerve-related conditions.

## SOURCES

Inositol is not known to be an essential nutrient. However, nuts, seeds, beans, whole grains, cantaloupe, and citrus fruits supply a substance called phytic acid, which releases inositol when acted on by bacteria in the digestive tract. The typical American diet provides an estimated 1,000 mg daily.

## THERAPEUTIC DOSAGES

Experimentally, inositol dosages of up to 18 g daily have been tried for various conditions.

## THERAPEUTIC USES

Preliminary double-blind studies suggest that high-dose inositol may be useful for **depression** (page 54),[1,2,3] panic disorder,[4] **Alzheimer's disease** (page 4),[5] obsessive-compulsive disorder,[6] and **attention deficit disorder** (page 19).[7]

Inositol is also sometimes proposed as a treatment for complications of **diabetes** (page 60), specifically diabetic neuropathy, but there have been no double-blind placebo-controlled studies, and two uncontrolled studies had mixed results.[8,9]

## WHAT IS THE SCIENTIFIC EVIDENCE FOR INOSITOL?

### Depression

Small double-blind studies have found inositol helpful for depression.[10,11] In one such trial, 28 depressed individuals were given a daily dose of 12 g of inositol for 4 weeks.[12] By the fourth week, the group receiving inositol showed significant improvement compared to the placebo group. However, by itself this study was too small to prove anything.

### Panic Disorder

People with panic disorder frequently develop panic attacks, often with no warning. The racing heartbeat, chest pressure, sweating, and other physical symptoms can be so intense that they are mistaken for a heart attack. A small double-blind study (21 participants) found that people given 12 g of inositol daily had fewer, and less severe, panic attacks as compared to the placebo group.[13] Again, this study was too small to prove anything.

## SAFETY ISSUES

No serious ill effects have been reported for inositol, even with a therapeutic dosage that equals about 18 times the average dietary intake. However, no long-term safety studies have been performed. Safety has not been established in young children, women who are pregnant or nursing, and those with severe liver and kidney disease. As with all supplements used in multigram doses, it is important to purchase a reputable product, because a contaminant present even in small percentages could add up to a real problem.

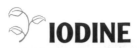

# IODINE

*Principal Proposed Uses*
There are no well-documented uses for iodine other than treating iodine deficiency.

*Other Proposed Uses*
Cyclic mastalgia

*Supplement Forms/Alternative Names*
Iodide, elemental iodine

Your thyroid gland, located just above the middle of your collarbone, needs iodine to make thyroid hormone, which maintains normal metabolism in all cells of the body. Principally found in seawater, dietary iodine can be scarce in many inland areas, and deficiencies were common before iodine was added to table salt. Iodine deficiency causes enlargement of the thyroid, a condition known as goiter. However, if you are not deficient in iodine, taking extra iodine will not help your thyroid work better, and it might even cause problems.

For reasons that are not clear, supplementary iodine might also be helpful for cyclic mastalgia.

## REQUIREMENTS/SOURCES

The U.S. Recommended Dietary Allowance for iodine is

- Infants under 6 months, 40 mcg

  6 to 12 months, 50 mcg

- Children 1 to 3 years, 70 mcg

  4 to 6 years, 90 mcg

  7 to 10 years, 120 mcg

- Adults (and children 11 years and older), 150 mcg

- Pregnant women, 175 mcg

- Nursing women, 200 mcg

Iodine deficiency is rare in developed countries today because of the use of iodized salt.

Seafood and kelp contain very high levels of iodine, as do salty processed foods that use iodized salt.

Most iodine is in the form of iodide, but a few studies suggest that a special form of iodine called *molecular iodine* may be better than iodide (see What Is the Scientific Evidence for Iodine?). However, since the body converts molecular iodine to iodide, it is hard to see why this should be so.

## THERAPEUTIC DOSAGES

A typical therapeutic dosage of iodide or iodine is 200 mcg daily.

## THERAPEUTIC USES

Iodine supplements have been proposed as a treatment for **cyclic mastalgia** (page 52), breast pain and lumpiness that usually cycles in relation to the menstrual period; this condition is also called fibrocystic breast disease or cyclic mastitis.[1]

## WHAT IS THE SCIENTIFIC EVIDENCE FOR IODINE?

### Cyclic Mastalgia

Three clinical studies indicate that iodide supplements may be helpful in treating cyclic mastalgia.[2] These studies, which involved more than 1,000 subjects, suggest that either iodide or iodine (the pure molecular form) might be useful. Researchers found that both iodine and iodide were significantly better than placebo in relieving pain and reducing the size and number of cysts.

One of the studies compared molecular iodine to iodide. Molecular iodine was no more effective than iodide, but was deemed superior because it induced fewer side effects and did not affect the thyroid.

The problem with this study is that the amount of iodine used in either form was very low, much less than the typical daily dose. So it's hard to see how it could really have produced any significant effect.

## SAFETY ISSUES

When taken at the recommended dosage, iodine and iodide appear to be safe nutritional supplements. However, excessive doses of iodide can actually cause thyroid problems! There is also a speculative link between excessive iodide intake and thyroid cancer. For these reasons, iodide intake above about 200 mcg daily is not recommended.

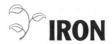

# IRON

## Principal Proposed Uses
Iron deficiency anemia

## Other Proposed Uses
Menorrhagia (heavy menstruation), attention deficit disorder

## Supplement Forms/Alternative Names
Iron sulfate, chelated iron

The element iron is essential to human life. As part of hemoglobin, the oxygen-carrying protein found in red blood cells, iron plays an integral role in nourishing every cell in the body with oxygen. It also functions as a part of myoglobin, which helps muscle cells store oxygen. Without iron, your body could not make ATP (adenosine triphosphate, the body's primary energy source), produce DNA, or carry out many other critical processes.

Iron deficiency can lead to anemia, learning disabilities, impaired immune function, fatigue, and depression. However, you shouldn't take iron supplements unless lab tests show that you are genuinely deficient.

There are two major forms of iron: *heme* iron and *nonheme* iron. Heme iron is bound to the proteins hemoglobin or myoglobin, whereas nonheme iron is an inorganic compound. (In chemistry, "organic" has a very precise meaning that has nothing to do with farming. An organic compound contains carbon atoms. Thus "inorganic iron" is an iron compound containing no carbon.) Heme iron, obtained from red meats and fish, is easily absorbed by the body. Nonheme iron, derived from plants, is less easily absorbed.

## REQUIREMENTS/SOURCES

The U.S. Recommended Dietary Allowance is as follows

- Infants under 6 months, 6 mg
- Children 6 months to 10 years, 10 mg
- Males 11 to 18 years, 12 mg
  19 years and older, 10 mg
- Females 11 to 50 years, 15 mg
  51 years and older, 10 mg
- Menstruating women, 15 mg
- Pregnant women, 30 mg
- Nursing women, 15 mg

Iron deficiency is the most common nutrient deficiency in the world[1] and the number-one cause of anemia. In developed countries, deficiency is much more common in menstruating women than in men. Other groups at high risk are children and pregnant women.[2]

Rich sources of heme iron include oysters, meat, poultry, and fish. The main sources of nonheme iron are dried fruits, molasses, whole grains, legumes, egg yolks, leafy green vegetables, nuts, seeds, and kelp. Acidic foods, such as fruit preserves and tomatoes, are a good source of iron when they've been cooked in iron or stainless steel cookware (some of the iron leaches into the food).

Iron can interfere with the absorption of numerous medications, including captopril, levodopa, carbidopa, penicillamine, cimetidine, thyroid hormone, or antibiotics in the tetracycline or quinolone (Floxin, Cipro) family.[3]

## THERAPEUTIC DOSAGES

The typical short-term therapeutic dosage to correct iron deficiency is 100 to 200 mg daily. Once your body's iron stores reach normal levels, however, this dose should be reduced to the lowest level that can maintain iron balance.

## THERAPEUTIC USES

The most obvious use of iron supplements is to treat iron deficiency anemia. However, don't take iron just because you feel tired. Make sure to get tested to see whether you are indeed deficient. With iron, more is definitely *not* better.

Heavy menstruation (menorrhagia) can certainly cause iron loss. However, for reasons that are not clear, iron supplementation can reportedly lighten up heavy menstrual bleeding, but only if you are iron deficient to begin with.[4] Iron has also been tried as a treatment for **attention deficit disorder** (page 19), but there is as yet no real evidence that it works.

## WHAT IS THE SCIENTIFIC EVIDENCE FOR IRON?

### Menorrhagia

One small double-blind study found good results using iron supplements to treat heavy menstrua-tion. This study, which was performed in 1964, saw an improvement in 75% of the women who took iron (compared to 32.5% of those who took placebo). Women who began with higher iron levels did not respond to treatment.[5] This suggests once more that supplementing with iron is only a good idea if you are deficient in it.

## SAFETY ISSUES

At the recommended dosage, iron is quite safe. Excessive dosages, however, can be toxic—damaging the intestines and liver, and possibly resulting in death. Iron poisoning in children is a surprisingly common problem, so make sure to keep your iron supplements out of their reach.

Mildly excessive levels of iron may be unhealthy for another reason: It acts as an oxidant (the opposite of an antioxidant), perhaps increasing the risk of cancer and heart disease.

## ⚠ INTERACTIONS YOU SHOULD KNOW ABOUT

If you are taking

- **Antibiotics** in the tetracycline or quinolone (**Floxin, Cipro**) family, **ACE inhibitors, levodopa, methyldopa, carbidopa, penicillamine, thyroid hormone, calcium** (page 146), **vitamin E** (page 337), **soy** (page 301),[6] **zinc** (page 348),[7] **copper** (page 169),[8] **or manganese** (page 254)[9,10]: Take iron supplements at a different time of day to avoid absorption problems.

- **Colchicine, cholestyramine, colestipol** or **drugs that reduce stomach acid:** You may need extra iron.

- High doses of **vitamin C** (page 331): You may absorb too much iron.

Iron

Visit Us at TNP.com

**ISOFLAVONES** (SOY ISOFLAVONES AND IPRIFLAVONE)

*Principal Proposed Uses*
  Osteoporosis

*Other Proposed Uses*
  Menopausal symptoms, cancer prevention, bodybuilding

*Supplement Forms/Alternative Names*
  Soy isoflavones

  Note: Soy protein contains a fair amount of isoflavones (see the chapter on soy protein for more information on the relationship between these two supplements).

Isoflavones are water-soluble chemicals found in many plants. In this chapter we will discuss a group of isoflavones known as *phytoestrogens*. They are so named because they cause effects in the body somewhat similar to those of estrogen. The most investigated natural isoflavones, genistein and daidzen, are found in soy products and the herb red clover. Another isoflavone, ipriflavone, is an intentionally modified form of daidzen used as a seminatural drug.

The way soy isoflavones appear to work is interesting. Although they are less powerful than the body's own estrogen, they latch on to the same places (receptor sites) on cells and don't allow actual estrogen to attach. In this way, when there is not enough estrogen in the body, isoflavones can partially make up for it; but when there is plenty of estrogen, they can partially block its influence. The net effect may be to reduce some of the risks of excess estrogen (breast and uterine cancer) while still providing some of estrogen's benefits (preventing osteoporosis).

In 1969, a research project was initiated to manufacture a type of phytoestrogen that would possess the bone-stimulating effects of estrogen without any estrogen-like activity elsewhere in the body. Ipriflavone was the result. After 7 successful years of experiments with animals, human research was started in 1981. Today, ipriflavone is available in over 22 countries and in most drugstores in the United States as a nonprescription dietary supplement. It is an accepted treatment for osteoporosis in Italy, Turkey, and Japan.

Like estrogen, ipriflavone appears to slow bone breakdown. Since it does not appear to have any estrogenic effects anywhere else in the body, it shouldn't increase the risk of breast or uterine cancer. On the other hand, it won't reduce the hot flashes, night sweats, mood changes, or vaginal dryness of menopause, nor prevent heart disease.

Ipriflavone is also touted as a bodybuilding aid, but no real evidence supports this use.

## SOURCES

Although isoflavones are not essential nutrients, they may help reduce the incidence of several diseases. Thus isoflavones may be useful for optimum health, even if they are not necessary for life like a classic vitamin.

Roasted soybeans have the highest isoflavone content, about 167 mg for a 3.5-ounce serving. Tempeh is next, with 60 mg; followed by soy flour, with 44 mg. Processed soy products such as soy protein and soy milk contain about 20 mg per serving. Similar isoflavones are also found in the herb red clover.

The synthetic isoflavone ipriflavone is not found in foods and must be obtained as a supplement.

## THERAPEUTIC DOSAGES

The proper dosage of the synthetic isoflavone ipriflavone has been well established through studies: 200 mg 3 times daily, or 300 mg twice daily.

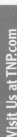

The optimum dosage of natural isoflavones obtained from food is not known. We know that Japanese women eat up to 200 mg of isoflavones daily, but we don't really know what amount of natural isoflavones is ideal. Most experts recommend 25 to 60 mg daily.

## THERAPEUTIC USES

According to the scientific evidence presented in the next section, ipriflavone can definitely help prevent **osteoporosis** (page 100). Much weaker evidence suggests that the natural isoflavones found in soy and **red clover** (page 290) may also be helpful.[1]

Soy isoflavones may also help prevent some forms of **cancer** (page 26) and reduce **menopausal symptoms** (page 87).[2,3,4] However, because most of the studies on this latter subject have used soy protein containing isoflavones rather than pure isoflavones, they are discussed separately in the chapter on **soy protein** (page 301). Studies on the benefits of isoflavones from red clover are pending at the time this book is going to press.

Recently, ipriflavone has been touted as a muscle-building supplement, but there is no evidence that it works.

## WHAT IS THE SCIENTIFIC EVIDENCE FOR ISOFLAVONES?

### Ipriflavone for Osteoporosis

Numerous double-blind placebo-controlled studies involving a total of over 1,000 participants have examined the effects of ipriflavone on osteoporosis.[5–9] Overall, it appears that ipriflavone can stop the progression of osteoporosis, and perhaps reverse it to some extent.

For example, a 2-year double-blind study followed 198 postmenopausal women who showed evidence of bone loss.[10] At the end of the study, there was a gain in bone density of 1% in the ipriflavone group and a loss of 0.7% in the placebo group. These numbers may sound small, but they can add up to a lot of bone over time.

Taking calcium plus ipriflavone may also be an excellent idea. In one study, 60 women who had already been diagnosed with osteoporosis and had already suffered one spinal fracture were given either 1,000 mg of calcium or 1,000 mg of calcium with ipriflavone.[11] After 6 months, the ipriflavone group had an increase of bone density in the spine of 3.5%, compared to a net loss in the calcium-only group.

Ipriflavone may also be helpful for preventing osteoporosis in women who are taking Lupron, a medication that accelerates bone loss.[12]

Finally, combining ipriflavone with estrogen may enhance anti-osteoporosis benefits.[13,14] However, we do not know whether such combinations increase or decrease the other benefits and adverse effects of estrogen-replacement therapy.

### Soy Isoflavones for Osteoporosis

One study evaluated the benefits of natural soy isoflavones in osteoporosis. A total of 66 postmenopausal women took either placebo (soy protein with isoflavones removed) or 56 or 90 mg of isoflavones daily for 6 months.[15] The group that took the higher dosage of isoflavones showed significant gains in spinal bone density. There was little change in the placebo or low-dose isoflavone groups. This study suggests that natural isoflavones may be effective.

Similar benefits have been seen in many animal studies involving either soy isoflavones or soy proteins.[16–22]

## SAFETY ISSUES

Natural soy isoflavones have not been subjected to rigorous safety studies. However, because they are consumed in very high quantities among those who eat traditional Asian diets, they are thought to be safe when used at the recommended dosages. However, because isoflavones work somewhat like estrogen, there are at least theoretical concerns that they may not be safe for women who have already had breast cancer.

Nearly 3,000 people have used the seminatural isoflavone ipriflavone in clinical studies, with no more side effects than those taking placebo. However, because ipriflavone is metabolized by the kidneys, individuals with severe kidney disease should have their ipriflavone dosage monitored by a physician.[23]

# JUNIPER BERRY (JUNIPERUS COMMUNIS)

## Principal Proposed Uses

Bladder infections

In Dutch, juniper is called "geniver," from which came the name "gin." But juniper is not only good for making martinis. Its berries (actually not berries at all, but a portion of the cone) were used by the Zuni Indians to assist in childbirth, by British herbalists to treat congestive heart failure and stimulate menstruation, and by American nineteenth-century herbalists to treat congestive heart failure, gonorrhea, and urinary tract infections.

The explanation for some of these uses may be found in juniper's diuretic properties. Its volatile oils have been shown to increase the rate of kidney filtration,[1] thereby perhaps helping to remove the accumulated fluid in congestive heart failure, and "wash out" the offending bacteria in urinary tract infections. However, there is no direct scientific evidence that juniper is effective for these purposes.

## WHAT IS JUNIPER BERRY USED FOR TODAY?

Contemporary herbalists primarily use juniper as a component of herbal formulas designed to treat **bladder infections** (page 23). A typical combination might include **uva ursi** (page 313), parsley, cleavers, and buchu. Such formulas are said to be most effective when taken at the first sign of symptoms and may not work well once the infection has really taken hold. Unfortunately, double-blind studies of juniper have not been performed.

Recently, gin-soaked raisins have been touted as an arthritis treatment. This is probably just a fad, but some weak evidence suggests that juniper may possess anti-inflammatory properties.[2] In the test tube, juniper has also been shown to inhibit herpes virus.[3]

## DOSAGES

You can make juniper tea by adding 1 cup of boiling water to 1 tablespoon of juniper berries, covering, and allowing the berries to steep for 20 minutes. The usual dosage is 1 cup twice a day. However, juniper is said to work better as a treatment for bladder infections when combined with other herbs. Combination products should be taken according to label instructions.

**Warning:** Bladder infections can go on to become kidney infections. For this reason, seek medical supervision if your symptoms don't resolve in a few days, or if you develop intense low back pain, fever, chills, or other signs of serious infection.

## SAFETY ISSUES

Although juniper is regarded as safe and is widely used in foods, I don't recommend taking it during pregnancy. (I also recommend not drinking gin.) Remember, juniper was used historically to stimulate menstruation and childbirth. It has also been shown to cause miscarriages in rats.[4]

Juniper seldom causes any noticeable side effects. Prolonged use of juniper could possibly deplete the body of potassium, the way other diuretics do, but this hasn't been proven. Combining juniper with conventional diuretics, however, may cause excessive fluid loss.

Some texts warn that juniper oil may be a kidney irritant, but there is no real evidence that this is the case.[5] Nonetheless, people with serious kidney disease probably shouldn't take juniper. Safety for young children, nursing women, or those with severe liver disease has also not been established.

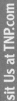

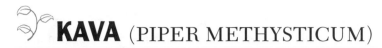

# KAVA (PIPER METHYSTICUM)

*Principal Proposed Uses*
   Anxiety, insomnia

*Other Proposed Uses*
   Alcohol withdrawal, tension headaches

Kava is a member of the pepper family that has long been cultivated by Pacific Islanders for use as a social and ceremonial drink. The first description of kava came to the West from Captain James Cook on his celebrated voyages through the South Seas. Cook reported that on occasions when village elders and chieftains gathered together for significant meetings, they would hold an elaborate kava ceremony at the beginning to break the ice (if there's any ice in the South Seas). Typically, each participant would drink two or three bowls of chewed-up kava mixed with coconut milk. Kava was also drunk in less formal social settings as a mild intoxicant.

When they learned about kava's effects, European scientists set to work trying to isolate its active ingredients. However, it wasn't until 1966 that substances named kavalactones were isolated and found to be effective sedatives. One of the most active of these is dihydrokavain, which has been found to produce a sedative, pain-killing, and anticonvulsant effect.[1,2,3] Other named kavalactones include kavain, methysticin, and dihydromethysticin.

High dosages of kava extracts cause muscular relaxation, and at very high dosages paralysis without loss of consciousness develops.[4–7] Kava is also a local anesthetic, producing peculiar numbing sensations when held in the mouth.

The method of action of kava is not fully understood. Conventional tranquilizers in the Valium family interact with special binding sites in the brain called GABA receptors. Early studies of kava suggested that the herb does not affect these receptors.[8] However, more recent studies have found an interaction.[9] The early researchers may have missed the connection because kava appears to affect somewhat unusual parts of the brain.

## WHAT IS KAVA USED FOR TODAY?

In the words of Germany's Commission E, kava is useful for relieving "states of nervous anxiety, tension, and agitation." While it is not considered powerful enough to treat severe **anxiety** or **panic attacks** (page 8), kava is often used for milder symptoms. Its skeletal-muscle relaxing effects may make it particularly useful if you suffer from tension headaches. While prescription drugs for anxiety are generally more powerful, kava does not seem to impair mental functioning.[10,11]

The Commission E monograph recommends using kava for no more than 3 months, and accompanying its use with more curative treatments such as psychotherapy.

**Warning:** Various medical conditions, such as hyperthyroidism, can produce symptoms similar to anxiety. Medical evaluation is strongly recommended before self-treating with kava.

There is some evidence that kava can help **insomnia** (page 80).[12,13] It has also been proposed as a treatment for tension headaches and as an aid to alcohol withdrawal. For more information on kava, see *The Natural Pharmacist Guide to Kava and Anxiety.*

## WHAT IS THE SCIENTIFIC EVIDENCE FOR KAVA?

There have been five meaningful studies of kava, involving a total of about 400 participants. The best of these was a 6-month double-blind study that tested kava's effectiveness in 100 people with various forms of anxiety.[14] Over the course of the trial, they were evaluated with a list of questions called the Hamilton Anxiety Scale (HAM-A). The HAM-A assigns a total score based on such symptoms as restlessness, nervousness, heart palpitations, stomach discomfort, dizziness, and chest pain. Lower scores indicate reduced anxiety. Participants who were given kava showed significantly improved scores beginning at 8 weeks and continuing throughout the duration of the treatment.

This study is notable for the long delay before kava was effective. Previous studies had showed a good response in 1 week.[15,16,17] The reason for this discrepancy is unclear.

Besides these placebo-controlled studies, one 6-month, double-blind study compared kava against two standard anxiety drugs (oxazepam and bromazepam) in 174 people with anxiety symptoms.[18] Improvement in HAM-A scores was about the same in all groups. However, physicians who use kava state that prescription treatments are usually more powerful in real life. The HAM-A rating scale can only roughly document changes in mood and may not always be able to distinguish between excellent and modest improvement.

## DOSAGES

Kava is usually sold in a standardized form where the total amount of kavalactones per pill is listed. For use as an antianxiety agent, the dose of kava should supply about 40 to 70 mg of kavalactones 3 times daily. The total daily dosage should not exceed 300 mg. People who use kava frequently report that effects begin to be obvious in a week or less, but that full benefits require 4 to 8 weeks to manifest.

The proper dosage for insomnia is 210 mg of kavalactones 1 hour before bedtime.

## SAFETY ISSUES

When used appropriately, kava appears to be safe. Animal studies have shown that dosages of up to four times that of normal cause no problems at all, and 13 times the normal dosage causes only mild problems in rats.[19]

A study of 4,049 people who took a rather low dose of kava (70 mg of kavalactones daily) for 7 weeks found side effects in 1.5% of cases. These were mostly mild gastrointestinal complaints and allergic rashes.[20] A 4-week study of 3,029 individuals given 240 mg of kavalactones daily showed a 2.3% incidence of basically the same side effects.[21] However, long-term use (months to years) of kava in excess of 400 mg kavalactones per day can create a distinctive generalized dry, scaly rash.[22] It disappears promptly when the kava use stops.

Kava does not appear to produce mental cloudiness.[23,24,25] Nonetheless, I wouldn't recommend driving after using kava until you discover how strongly it affects you. It makes some people quite drowsy.

Contrary to many reports in the media, there is no evidence that kava actually improves mental function. Two studies are commonly cited as if to prove this, but actually there was only one study performed: It was described in two separate articles.[26,27] This tiny study found that kava does not impair mental function; however, it doesn't show that kava improves it. A slight improvement was seen on a couple of tests, but it was statistically insignificant (too small to mean anything).

High doses of kava are known to cause inebriation. For this reason, there is some concern that it could become an herb of abuse. There have been reports of young people trying to get high by taking products they thought contained kava. One of these products, fX, turned out to contain dangerous drugs but no kava at all. European physicians have not reported any problems with kava addiction.[28] However, one study in mice suggests that it might be possible.[29]

The German Commission E monograph warns against the use of kava during pregnancy and nursing.

Kava should not be taken along with alcohol, prescription tranquilizers or sedatives, or other depressant drugs as there have been reports of lethargy and disorientation caused by such combinations.[30] It also might interfere with the activity of the anti-Parkinson's drug levodopa.[31]

Safety in young children and those with severe liver or kidney disease has not been established.

## TRANSITIONING FROM MEDICATIONS TO KAVA

If you're taking Xanax or other drugs in the benzodiazepine family, switching to kava will be very

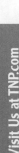

hard. You must seek a doctor's supervision, because withdrawal symptoms can be severe and even life-threatening.

It's easier to make the switch from milder antianxiety drugs, such as BuSpar and antidepressants. Nonetheless, a doctor's supervision is still strongly advised.

## ⚠ INTERACTIONS
## YOU SHOULD KNOW ABOUT

If you are taking

- **Medications for insomnia or anxiety:** Do not take kava in addition to them.

- **Levodopa** for Parkinson's disease: Kava might reduce its effectiveness.

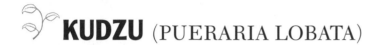

# KUDZU (PUERARIA LOBATA)

*Principal Proposed Uses*
  Alcoholism

*Other Proposed Uses*
  Cold with pain in the neck

**K**udzu is cooked as food in China, and also is used as an herb in traditional Chinese medicine. However, in the United States, kudzu has become an invasive pest. It was deliberately planted earlier this century for use as animal fodder and to control soil erosion. It turned out to be incredibly prolific and soon spread throughout the South like an alien invader. The problem is that kudzu can grow a foot a day during the summer, and as much as 60 feet a year, giving it the folk name "mile-a-minute vine." It swallows telephone poles, chokes trees, and takes over yards. The only defense may be to find a use for it.

## WHAT IS KUDZU USED FOR TODAY?

Besides cooking with it, feeding it to animals, and weaving baskets out of its rubbery vines, kudzu may also be useful in treating alcoholism. In Chinese folk medicine, a tea brewed from kudzu root is believed to be useful in "sobering up" a drunk. Taking the hint, a 1993 study evaluated the effects of kudzu in a species of hamsters known to enjoy drinking alcohol to intoxication.[1] Ordinarily, if given a choice, the Syrian golden hamster will prefer alcohol to water, but administration of kudzu reversed that preference. This has led to widespread speculation (but no proof

thus far) that kudzu may be useful in the treatment of human alcoholism.

The antialcohol effects of kudzu were initially attributed to the presence of the substances daidzin and daidzein, but later research cast doubt on this explanation.[2] At present, we do not know how kudzu may work.

In academic Chinese herbology (as opposed to Chinese folk medicine), kudzu is used for other purposes. One classic herbal formula containing kudzu is recommended for the treatment of **colds** (page 44) accompanied by pain in the neck, and modern Chinese herbalists frequently use it for this purpose.

## DOSAGES

The standard dosage of kudzu ranges from 9 to 15 g daily, in tea or tablets. The proper length of treatment for alcoholism has not been determined.

## SAFETY ISSUES

Based on its extensive food use, kudzu is believed to be reasonably safe. However, safety in young children, pregnant or nursing women, or those with severe kidney or liver disease has not been established.

# LAPACHO A.K.A. PAU D'ARCO, TAHEEBO
## (TABEBUIA IMPESTIGINOSA)

*Principal Proposed Uses*
  Yeast, respiratory, and bladder infections

*Other Proposed Uses*
  Diarrhea, cancer?

The inner bark of the lapacho tree plays a central role in the herbal medicine of several South American indigenous peoples. They use it to treat cancer as well as a great variety of infectious diseases. There is intriguing, but far from conclusive, scientific evidence for some of these traditional uses. One of lapacho's major ingredients, lapachol, definitely possesses antitumor properties, and for a time was under active investigation as a possible chemotherapy drug. Unfortunately, when given in high enough dosages to kill cancer cells, lapachol causes numerous serious side effects. Another component, b-lapachone, continues to be investigated as an anticancer agent since it may have a better side-effect profile and acts similarly to a new class of prescription antitumor drugs.[1]

Herbalists believe that the whole herb can produce equivalent benefits with fewer side effects, but this claim has never been properly investigated.

Various ingredients in lapacho can also kill bacteria and fungi in the test tube.[2] However, it is not yet clear how well the herb works for this purpose when taken orally.

## WHAT IS LAPACHO USED FOR TODAY?

Based on its traditional use and the fledgling scientific evidence, some herbalists recommend lapacho as a treatment for cancer. However, I do not endorse this usage. There is no good evidence that lapacho is an effective cancer treatment, and cancer is clearly not a disease to trifle with! Furthermore, the mechanism by which lapacho possibly works may cause it to interfere with the action of prescription anticancer drugs. Definitely do not add it to a conventional chemotherapy regimen without consulting your physician.

Lapacho is also sometimes used to treat **Candida** (page 33) yeast infections, respiratory infections such as **colds and flus** (page 44), infectious diarrhea, and **bladder infections** (page 23).

**Note:** Do not count on lapacho to treat serious infections.

## DOSAGES

Lapacho contains many components that don't dissolve in water, so making tea from the herb is not the best idea. It's better to take capsulized powdered bark, at a standard dosage of 300 mg 3 times daily. For the treatment of yeast and other infections, it is taken until symptoms resolve.

The inner bark of the lapacho tree is believed to be the most effective part of the plant. Unfortunately, inferior products containing only the outer bark and the wood are sometimes misrepresented as "genuine inner-bark lapacho."

## SAFETY ISSUES

Full safety studies of lapacho have not been performed. When taken in normal dosages, it does not appear to cause any significant side effects.[3] However, because its constituent lapachol is somewhat toxic, the herb is not recommended for pregnant or nursing mothers. Safety in young children or those with severe liver or kidney disease has also not been established.

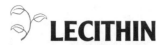

# LECITHIN

### Principal Proposed Uses
There are no well-documented uses for lecithin.

### Other Proposed Uses
High cholesterol, liver disease, psychological and neurological disorders (e.g., Tourette's syndrome, Alzheimer's disease, bipolar disorder)

### Supplement Forms/Alternative Names
Egg lecithin, soy lecithin, phosphatidylcholine in lecithin

For decades, lecithin has been a popular treatment for high cholesterol (although there is surprisingly little evidence that it works). More recently, lecithin has been proposed as a remedy for various psychological and neurological diseases, such as Tourette's syndrome, Alzheimer's disease, and bipolar disorder (also known as manic depression).

Lecithin contains a substance called *phosphatidylcholine* (PC) that is presumed to be responsible for its medicinal effects. Phosphatidylcholine is a major part of the membranes surrounding our cells. However, when you consume phosphatidylcholine it is broken down into the nutrient *choline* rather than being carried directly to cell membranes. Choline acts like folic acid, TMG (trimethylglycine), and SAMe (S-adenosylmethionine) to promote methylation (see the chapter on TMG [page 310] for further discussion of this subject). It is also used to make *acetylcholine,* a nerve chemical essential for proper brain function.

## SOURCES

Neither lecithin nor its ingredient phosphatidylcholine is an essential nutrient. For use as a supplement or a food additive, lecithin is often manufactured from soy.

## THERAPEUTIC DOSAGES

Ordinary lecithin contains about 10 to 20% phosphatidylcholine. However, European research has tended to use products concentrated to contain 90% phosphatidylcholine in lecithin, and the following dosages are based on that type of product. For psychological and neurological conditions, doses as high as 5 to 10 g taken 3 times daily have been used in studies. For liver disease, a typical dose is 350 to 500 mg taken 3 times daily; and for high cholesterol, 500 to 900 mg taken 3 times daily is common.

## THERAPEUTIC USES

For a while, lecithin/phosphatidylcholine was one of the most commonly recommended natural treatments for high **cholesterol** (page 39). This idea, however, appears to rest entirely on preliminary studies that lacked control groups.[1,2] A recent small, double-blind study of 23 men with high blood cholesterol levels found that lecithin had *no* significant effects on blood levels of total cholesterol, HDL ("good") cholesterol, LDL ("bad") cholesterol, or lipoprotein(a) and triglycerides (two harmful fats found in the blood).[3]

In Europe, phosphatidylcholine is also used to treat liver diseases, such as alcoholic fatty liver and viral **hepatitis** (page 71).[4] While there is some evidence from animal and human studies that it may be helpful, other studies found no benefit.[5–13]

Finally, because phosphatidylcholine plays a role in nerve function, it has also been suggested as a treatment for various psychological and neurological disorders, such as **Alzheimer's disease** (page 4), bipolar disorder, Tourette's syndrome, and tardive dyskinesia (a late-developing side effect of drugs used for psychosis). However, the evidence that it works is limited to small studies with somewhat conflicting results.[14–21]

## SAFETY ISSUES

Lecithin is believed to be generally safe. However, some people taking high dosages (several grams daily) experience minor but annoying side effects, such as abdominal discomfort, diarrhea, and nausea. Maximum safe dosages for young children, pregnant or nursing women, or those with severe liver or kidney disease have not been determined.

 # LICORICE (GLYCYRRHIZA GLABRA)

*Principal Proposed Uses*

Oral uses (DGL form): Ulcers, mouth sores, heartburn (esophageal reflux)

*Topical uses (whole herb):*
Eczema, psoriasis, herpes

*Oral uses (whole herb):*
Cough, asthma, chronic fatigue syndrome

A member of the pea family, licorice root has been used since ancient times both as food and as medicine. In Chinese herbology, licorice is an ingredient in nearly all herbal formulas for the traditional purpose of "harmonizing" the separate herbs involved.

Licorice possesses a variety of active ingredients. The most analyzed is glycyrrhizin, which has been found to possess anti-inflammatory, cough-suppressant, antiviral, estrogen-like, and aldosterone-like activities.[1] The natural hormone aldosterone can cause fluid retention, increased blood pressure, and potassium loss. Glycyrrhizin can produce similar effects, which may cause a problem (see the discussion under Safety Issues). To avoid the aldosterone-like effects, manufacturers have found a way to remove glycyrrhizin from licorice, producing the much safer product deglycyrrhizinated licorice, or DGL. However, it is not clear that DGL provides all the same benefits as whole licorice.

## WHAT IS LICORICE USED FOR TODAY?

Licorice appears to have a general healing effect on mucous membranes, perhaps by stimulating repair processes and activating the body's defenses against further injury.[2,3] For this reason, licorice or DGL was once a standard European treatment for **ulcers** (page 112).[4] Although it has been replaced by synthetic medications, there is a significant amount of evidence that DGL can be helpful. Animal studies suggest that DGL might help prevent ulcers caused by aspirin.[5]

DGL is also used for heartburn (esophageal reflux), but we don't know if it simply relieves symptoms or actually protects the esophagus from damage. Licorice (primarily DGL) is also used to relieve the discomfort of **canker sores** (page 35) and other mouth sores, based on its mucous membrane–healing capacity.

Creams containing whole licorice (often combined with chamomile extract) are often used for **eczema** (page 66), **psoriasis** (page 106), and **herpes** (page 73).

Whole licorice, not DGL, is used as an expectorant for respiratory problems such as coughs and **asthma** (page 11).

Recently, licorice has been suggested as a treatment for chronic fatigue syndrome (CFS), based on the observation that people with CFS appear to suffer from low levels of certain adrenal hormones. The glycyrrhizin portion of licorice may relieve symptoms by mimicking the effects of these hormones. However, this is a fairly dangerous approach to treatment that should be tried only under medical supervision.

Licorice has also been suggested as a treatment for numerous other conditions, including **hepatitis** (page 71) and **menopausal symptoms** (page 87), and for the prevention of **can-**

cer (page 26), but there is as yet little evidence that it really works.

## WHAT IS THE SCIENTIFIC EVIDENCE FOR LICORICE?

Several controlled, but not double-blind, studies suggest that regular use of DGL can heal ulcers as effectively as drugs in the Zantac family.[6,7,8] However, DGL must be taken continuously or the ulcer can be expected to return. Modern medical treatment tries to prevent the recurrence of ulcers permanently by eradicating the bacteria *Helicobacter pylori*. There is no evidence that DGL can do the same.

There is no solid evidence for the other proposed uses of licorice.

## DOSAGES

For supportive treatment of ulcer pain along with conventional medical care, chew two to four 380-mg tablets of DGL before meals and at bedtime.

Sucking on these tablets can substantially relieve the discomfort of mouth sores, although some people find the taste unpleasant.

For respiratory problems, take 1 to 2 g of licorice root 3 times daily for no more than 1 week.

For eczema, psoriasis, or herpes, apply licorice cream twice daily to the affected area.

When treating chronic fatigue syndrome, whole licorice must be taken at a sufficiently high dosage so that significant side effects are possible, and thus a physician's supervision is necessary.

## SAFETY ISSUES

Due to its aldosterone-like effects, whole licorice can cause fluid retention, high blood pressure, and potassium loss when taken at dosages exceeding 3 g daily for more than 6 weeks. These effects can be especially dangerous if you take digitalis, or if you have high blood pressure, heart disease, diabetes, or kidney disease.

Licorice may also increase both the positive and negative effects of treatment with corticosteroids, such as prednisone.[9]

DGL is believed to be safe, although extensive safety studies have not been performed. Side effects are rare.

Safety for either form of licorice in young children, pregnant or nursing women, or those with severe liver or kidney disease has not been established.

## ⚠ INTERACTIONS YOU SHOULD KNOW ABOUT

If you are taking

- **Digitalis:** Long-term use of licorice can be dangerous.

- **Thiazide** or **loop diuretics:** Use of licorice might lead to excessive potassium loss.

- **Corticosteroid treatment:** Licorice could increase both its effects and its side effects.

- **Aspirin** or other **anti-inflammatory drugs:** Regular use of DGL might help lower the risk of ulcers.

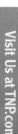

# 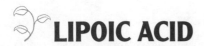 LIPOIC ACID

*Principal Proposed Uses*
  Diabetic peripheral neuropathy, diabetic autonomic neuropathy

*Other Proposed Uses*
  Diabetes (in general), liver disease, prevention of cancer, cataracts, and heart disease

*Supplement Forms/Alternative Names*
  Alpha-lipoic acid, thioctic acid

Lipoic acid, also known as alpha-lipoic acid, is a sulfur-containing fatty acid that has recently become very popular as a dietary supplement. It is found inside every cell of the body, where it helps generate the energy that keeps us alive and functioning. Lipoic acid is a key part of the metabolic machinery that turns glucose (blood sugar) into energy for the body's needs.

Lipoic acid is an antioxidant, which means it neutralizes naturally occurring, but harmful, chemicals known as free radicals. Unlike other antioxidants, which work only in water or fatty tissues, lipoic acid is unusual in that it functions in both water and fat.[1,2] By comparison, vitamin E works only in fat and vitamin C works only in water. This gives lipoic acid an unusually broad spectrum of action.

Different antioxidants work together to keep free radicals under control (for more information, see the chapter on **vitamin E** [page 337]). Antioxidants are a bit like kamikaze pilots, sacrificing themselves to knock out free radicals. One of the more interesting findings about lipoic acid is that it may help regenerate other antioxidants that have been used up. Some research also suggests that lipoic acid may do the work of other antioxidants in which the body is deficient.[3,4]

Thanks to its fat solubility, lipoic acid can get inside nerve cells, where it helps prevent free radical damage. Studies performed in Germany have shown success with lipoic acid in treating diabetic neuropathy, a condition in which nerve damage causes pain and numbness in the hands and feet.

## SOURCES

Because a healthy body makes enough lipoic acid to supply its energy requirements, there is no daily requirement for this supplement. However, several medical conditions appear to be accompanied by low levels of lipoic acid—specifically, diabetes, liver cirrhosis, and heart disease—which suggests (but definitely does not prove) that supplementation would be helpful.

Liver and yeast contain some lipoic acid. However, supplements are necessary to obtain therapeutic dosages.

## THERAPEUTIC DOSAGES

The typical dosage of lipoic acid for treating diabetes is 300 to 600 mg daily. Be patient, as the results take weeks to develop. For use as a general antioxidant, a lower dosage of 20 to 50 mg daily is commonly recommended.

## THERAPEUTIC USES

Lipoic acid has been widely used in Germany for more than 20 years to treat diabetic peripheral neuropathy, and there is some good evidence that it works.[5,6,7] Diabetic peripheral neuropathy is a condition caused by **diabetes** (page 60) in which nerves leading to the arms and legs become damaged, leading to numbness, pain, and other symptoms.

Lipoic acid may also be beneficial for another type of nerve damage caused by diabetes: autonomic neuropathy. This is a condition in which the nerves that control internal organs become damaged. When this occurs in the heart, the condition is called cardiac autonomic neuropathy, and it leads to irregularities of heart rhythm. There is some evidence that lipoic acid may be helpful for this condition.[8] When autonomic neuropathy occurs in the intestines, it causes extreme constipation. Based on its other effects, it appears possible that lipoic acid could help this condition as well, although there is no direct evidence to turn to.

Preliminary and sometimes contradictory evidence suggests that lipoic acid may improve other aspects of diabetes as well, including circulation in small blood vessels, metabolism of sugar and protein, and the body's response to insulin.[9–12]

Lipoic acid has been proposed as a treatment for liver conditions as well as for preventing **cancer** (page 26), **cataracts** (page 37), and **heart disease** (page 14). However, there is little to no real evidence that it is effective for these purposes.

## WHAT IS THE SCIENTIFIC EVIDENCE FOR LIPOIC ACID?

### Diabetic Peripheral Neuropathy

Lipoic acid's ability to prevent nerve cells from destruction by free radicals could explain the positive therapeutic results reported in Germany. In several studies, lipoic acid has produced noticeable improvement in the pain and numbness of diabetic peripheral neuropathy. The benefits develop gradually over weeks to months.

In one study, 328 subjects were randomly assigned to four groups. One group received placebo; the other three were given daily doses of 1,200, 600, or 100 mg of intravenous alpha-lipoic acid for 3 weeks.[13] A rating scale was used to measure the changes in the intensity of pain experienced by participants in all four groups. All three treatment groups improved, with the greatest benefit observed in the 600-mg group: 82.5% showed a good response (compared with only 57.6% in the placebo group).

This study employed a different form of lipoic acid than most people use—injected lipoic acid. The most common type of lipoic acid supplement is a capsule or tablet taken by mouth. This study, then, can't tell us how well oral lipoic acid

works. However, good results have also been seen in a number of small studies that used oral lipoic acid.[14]

**Warning:** You should *never* attempt taking any drug or supplement intravenously except under the care of a doctor.

Another study compared lipoic acid to less expensive antioxidants. Eighty people with diabetes were divided into four groups and were treated with oral lipoic acid (660 mg daily), selenium (100 mcg daily), vitamin E (1,200 IU daily), or placebo. They were followed for 3 months.[15] All three treatment groups improved about the same amount, and all three antioxidants were significantly more effective than the placebo.

These results suggest that cheaper antioxidants could be substituted for lipoic acid. However, lipoic acid still has the most evidence behind it for treating diabetic neuropathy.

Lipoic acid may work particularly well for diabetic peripheral neuropathy when it is combined with **GLA** (gamma linolenic acid) (page 210).[16,17]

### Diabetic Autonomic Neuropathy

Not only does diabetes damage the nerves in the arms and legs, but it can also affect deep nerves that control organs such as the heart and digestive tract. The DEKAN (Deutsche Kardiale Autonome Neuropathie) study followed 73 people with diabetes who had symptoms caused by nerve damage affecting the heart. Treatment with 800 mg daily of oral lipoic acid showed statistically significant improvement compared to placebo and caused no significant side effects.[18]

## SAFETY ISSUES

Oral lipoic acid appears to have no side effects at dosages up to about 800 mg daily. However, gastrointestinal side effects have been seen at a dosage of 1,200 mg daily, given intravenously.[19]

The maximum safe dosages for young children, women who are pregnant or nursing, or those with severe liver or kidney disease have not been established.

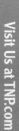

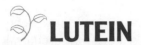

# LUTEIN

*Principal Proposed Uses*
There are no well-documented uses for lutein.

*Other Proposed Uses*
Cataracts, macular degeneration, atherosclerosis

Lutein, a chemical found in green vegetables, is a member of a family of substances known as *carotenoids*. **Beta-carotene** (page 131) is the most famous nutrient in this class. Like beta-carotene, lutein is an antioxidant that protects our cells against damage caused by dangerous, naturally occurring chemicals known as free radicals.

Recent evidence has found that lutein may play an important role in protecting our eyes and eyesight. It may work in two ways: by acting directly as a kind of natural sunblock, and also by neutralizing free radicals that can damage the eye.

## SOURCES

Lutein is not an essential nutrient. However, it may be very important for optimal health. We're learning more all the time about nutrients like lutein that aren't required for life, but protect us in various ways. At present, an intake of about 6 mg daily of lutein is considered adequate.

Green vegetables are the best source of lutein, especially spinach, kale, collard greens, romaine lettuce, leeks, and peas. Unlike beta-carotene, lutein is *not* found in high concentrations in yellow and orange vegetables such as carrots.

## THERAPEUTIC DOSAGES

We don't know how much lutein is necessary for a therapeutic effect, but estimates range from 5 to 30 mg daily.

## THERAPEUTIC USES

Evidence suggests that people who eat foods containing lutein are less likely to develop **macular degeneration** (page 85) or **cataracts** (page 37), the two most common causes of vision loss in adults.[1,2] However, these were observational studies, in which people simply eat what they please and researchers follow them to see what illnesses they develop. Because lutein is found in vegetables that may also contain other helpful substances, we don't know for sure if it is the lutein itself that is providing the benefit. We really need studies in which some people are given pure lutein and others a placebo, but as yet they have not been performed.

However, there are reasons to believe that lutein may indeed play an important role in protecting the eyes. Lutein is the main pigment (coloring chemical) in the center of the retina, the region of maximum visual sensitivity known as the *macula*. Macular degeneration consists of damage to the macula, and leads to a severe loss in vision.

Lutein appears to act as a natural eyeshade, protecting the retina against too much light.[3] As we age, our eyes gradually lose lutein.[4] Some researchers have theorized that this loss allows sunlight to damage the retina, leading to macular degeneration. This may explain why higher dietary intake of lutein appears to reduce the risk of this common cause of blindness in adults.

Besides protecting the macula, lutein may also shield the lens of the eye from light damage, slowing down the development of cataracts.

Furthermore, lutein fights free radicals. These chemicals can also damage the retina and the lens.

**Note:** Lutein may help prevent macular degeneration, but it has not been proven to treat the condition once it has developed. If you already have macular degeneration, medical supervision is essential.

Lutein might also help prevent **atherosclerosis** (page 14).[5]

## SAFETY ISSUES

Although lutein is a normal part of the diet, there has not been a formal evaluation of lutein's safety when taken as a concentrated supplement. Maximum safe dosages for young children, pregnant or nursing women, or those with severe liver or kidney disease have not been established.

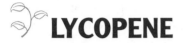

# LYCOPENE

*Principal Proposed Uses*
Cancer prevention

*Other Proposed Uses*
Prevention of macular degeneration and cataracts

Lycopene is a powerful antioxidant found in tomatoes and pink grapefruit. Like the better-known supplement beta-carotene, lycopene belongs to the family of chemicals known as *carotenoids* (for more information about carotenoids, see the chapter on **beta-carotene** [page 131]). As an antioxidant, it is about twice as powerful as beta-carotene.

There is some evidence that a diet high in lycopene may reduce the risk of cancer of the prostate as well as other cancers. Lycopene may also help prevent macular degeneration and cataracts.

## SOURCES

Lycopene is not a necessary nutrient. However, like other substances found in fruits and vegetables, it may be very important for optimal health.

Tomatoes are the best source of lycopene. Happily, cooking doesn't destroy lycopene, so pizza sauce is just as good as a fresh tomato. In fact, some studies indicate that cooking tomatoes in oil may provide lycopene in a way that the body can use better,[1,2] although not all studies agree.[3] Lycopene is also found in watermelon, guava, and grapefruit.

## THERAPEUTIC DOSAGES

The optimum dosage for lycopene has not been established. An important study on lycopene and prostate cancer suggested that about 6.5 mg was an effective daily intake.[4] However, another study suggested that a much higher dose was needed—75 mg, about 12 times as much![5] Clearly, more study is needed to determine the best dosage.

## THERAPEUTIC USES

Lycopene may help prevent **cancer** (page 26), particularly cancer of the prostate.[6–10] However, the evidence we have for this idea comes from *observational* studies in which researchers analyze people's diets, rather than the more definitive *intervention* trials, in which people are actually given lycopene supplements. In observational trials, it is always possible that other unrecognized factors are at work.

Weak evidence also suggests that lycopene can reduce the risk of **cataracts** (page 37) and **macular degeneration** (page 85).[11]

## WHAT IS THE SCIENTIFIC EVIDENCE FOR LYCOPENE?

### Cancer Prevention

Although there are no double-blind studies on lycopene, the results of observational studies are impressive.

One study followed 47,894 men for 4 years.[12] Subjects who ate large amounts of tomatoes or tomato sauce (including that on pizza) had lower rates of prostate cancer. In an evaluation that compared these foods to others that were studied, lycopene appeared to be the common denominator.[13]

In another study, elderly Americans who ate a diet high in tomatoes had 50% fewer cancers than those who did not.[14] Animal studies have also found some cancer-preventative benefits with lycopene.[15,16]

However, other observational studies have not found lycopene to be the key cancer-fighting ingredient in fruits and vegetables.[17,18] What we really need are large double-blind studies in which people are given either pure lycopene supplements or placebo treatment. Unfortunately, none have yet been performed.

## SAFETY ISSUES

Although lycopene is a normal part of the diet, there has not been a formal evaluation of lycopene's safety when it is taken as a concentrated supplement. Maximum safe dosages for young children, pregnant or nursing women, or those with severe liver or kidney disease have not been established.

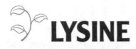 # LYSINE

### Principal Proposed Uses
Herpes simplex (e.g., cold sores, genital herpes)

### Supplement Forms/Alternative Names
L-lysine, lysine hydrochloride

Lysine is an essential amino acid, one that you need to get from food. Evidence suggests that supplemental lysine may be able to help herpes infections (cold sores and genital herpes), especially when combined with certain dietary changes.

## REQUIREMENT/SOURCES

Most people need about 1 g of lysine per day. The requirement may be greater for athletes and people recovering from major injuries, especially burns. The richest sources of lysine are animal proteins such as meat and poultry, but it is also found in dairy products, eggs, and beans.

## THERAPEUTIC DOSAGES

A typical therapeutic dosage of lysine for herpes is 1 g 3 times daily. You can take this as a regular part of your diet in hopes of preventing herpes flare-ups or at the first sign of an attack. For best results, you should probably restrict your intake of foods that contain a lot of arginine (see Therapeutic Uses).

## THERAPEUTIC USES

Some small studies suggest that regular use of lysine supplements can reduce the number of **herpes** (page 73) flare-ups, although other studies have not found the same benefit.[1–5] Lysine may also help you get over a herpes attack when it has just started.

Both cold sores and genital herpes are caused by a virus called *herpes simplex*. After you are first infected, this virus hides in certain nerve cells, and reemerges under times of stress. Test-tube research suggests that lysine fights this virus by blocking arginine, an amino acid the virus needs in order to replicate.[6]

For this reason, lysine may be most effective when used in conjunction with a low-arginine diet. Foods that you should avoid include chocolate, peanuts and other nuts, seeds, and, to a lesser extent, wheat. (See the chapter on **arginine** [page 126] for more information about this amino acid.)

## WHAT IS THE SCIENTIFIC EVIDENCE FOR LYSINE?

### Herpes Simplex

Although the evidence is still preliminary, it does appear that lysine supplements can reduce the incidence and severity of herpes infections.[7]

One double-blind placebo-controlled study enrolled 27 participants with a history of herpes flare-ups.[8] While receiving 3 g of L-lysine every day for 6 months, the treatment group experienced an average of 2.4 fewer herpes flare-ups than the placebo group—a significant difference. The lysine group's flare-ups were also significantly less severe and healed faster.

Another double-blind placebo-controlled study on 41 subjects also found good results with lysine.[9] Interestingly, this study found that 1,250 mg of lysine daily worked, but 624 mg did not.

However, two other small studies found lysine to have no effect on herpes simplex.[10,11]

All of these studies are too small to give conclusive answers. At this point, more evidence is needed to prove that lysine is an effective treatment for herpes simplex.

## SAFETY ISSUES

Although lysine is an essential part of the diet, the safety of concentrated lysine supplements has not been well studied. In animal studies, high dosages have caused gallstones and elevated cholesterol levels,[12,13] so you may want to use caution when using lysine if you have either of these problems. Maximum safe dosages for young children, pregnant or nursing women, or those with severe liver or kidney disease have not been established.

# MAGNESIUM

### Principal Proposed Uses

Migraine headaches, noise-related hearing loss, kidney stones, hypertension (high blood pressure)

### Other Proposed Uses

Premenstrual syndrome, painful menstruation, diabetes, osteoporosis, low blood sugar, glaucoma, fibromyalgia, fatigue, stroke, low HDL ("good") cholesterol, autism, various forms of heart disease (e.g. mitral valve prolapse, congestive heart failure), asthma

### Supplement Forms/Alternative Names

Magnesium is available in many chemical forms: magnesium sulfate, magnesium gluconate, magnesium fumarate, magnesium citrate, magnesium malate, magnesium oxide, and magnesium chloride.

Magnesium is an essential nutrient mineral, meaning that your body needs it for healthy functioning. It is found in significant quantities throughout the body and used for numerous purposes, including muscle relaxation, blood clotting, and the manufacture of ATP (adenosine triphosphate, the body's main energy molecule).

It has been called "nature's calcium channel–blocker." The idea refers to magnesium's ability to block calcium from entering muscle and heart cells. A group of prescription heart medications work in a similar way, although much more powerfully. This may be the basis for magnesium's effects on migraine headaches and high blood pressure.

Magnesium is one of the few essential nutrients for which deficiencies are fairly common. For this reason, it is probably reasonable for most people to take magnesium on general principle, regardless of particular therapeutic use.

## REQUIREMENTS/SOURCES

Requirements for magnesium increase as we grow and age. The U.S. Recommended Dietary Allowance is as follows

- Infants under 6 months, 30 mg
  6 months to 1 year, 75 mg

- Children 1 to 3 years, 80 mg

- Males 4 to 8 years, 130 mg
  9 to 13 years, 240 mg
  14 to 18 years, 410 mg
  19 to 30 years, 400 mg
  31 years and older, 420 mg

- Females 4 to 8 years, 130 mg
  9 to 13 years, 240 mg
  14 to 18 years, 360 mg
  19 to 30 years, 310 mg
  31 years and older, 320 mg

- Pregnant women 18 years and younger, 400 mg
  19 to 30 years, 350 mg
  31 to 50 years, 360 mg

- Nursing women 18 years and younger, 360 mg
  19 to 30 years, 310 mg
  31 to 50 years, 320 mg

In the United States, the average dietary intake of magnesium is significantly lower than it should be.[1,2] Alcohol, surgery, digoxin, diabetes, diuretics ("water pills"), oral contraceptives, **zinc** (page 348), and excessive intake of **calcium** (page 146) can all reduce your body's level of magnesium.[3,4] If you are taking **potassium** (page 282) or **manganese** (page 254), you may need extra magnesium as well. [5]

Kelp is very high in magnesium, as are wheat bran, wheat germ, almonds, and cashews. Other good sources include blackstrap molasses, brewer's yeast (not to be confused with nutritional yeast), buckwheat, and nuts and whole grains. You can also get appreciable amounts of magnesium from collard greens, dandelion greens, avocado, sweet corn, Cheddar cheese, sunflower seeds, shrimp, dried fruit (figs, apricots, and prunes), and many other common fruits and vegetables.

## THERAPEUTIC DOSAGES

A typical supplemental dosage of magnesium ranges from the nutritional needs described above to as high as 600 mg daily. For premenstrual syndrome (PMS) and dysmenorrhea (painful menstruation), an alternative approach is to start taking 500 to 1,000 mg daily, beginning on day 15 of the menstrual cycle and continuing until menstruation begins.

Magnesium may interfere with the absorption of various other minerals. For this reason it's suggested that those taking magnesium should also take a multimineral supplement.

## THERAPEUTIC USES

Several preliminary studies suggest that regular use of magnesium can help prevent **migraine headaches** (page 89).[6,7,8]

Magnesium may also be useful for protecting the ears against hearing loss caused by exposure to loud noises,[9] reducing the incidence of kidney stones,[10] and perhaps reducing **hypertension** (page 75).[11,12,13]

Weak evidence suggests that magnesium may be useful for **PMS (premenstrual syndrome)** (page 104)[14,15] and menstrual cramps or **dysmenorrhea** (page 65).[16,17]

Although there is no direct evidence that magnesium directly helps people with **diabetes** (page 60), such individuals are known to be deficient in magnesium,[18,19,20] and magnesium supplementation may be a good idea on general principle. (However, individuals with severe kidney disease should take magnesium supplements only on their physician's advice.)

Magnesium has also been suggested as a treatment for **osteoporosis** (page 100), low blood sugar, glaucoma, fibromyalgia, fatigue, stroke, low HDL ("good") cholesterol, autism, **Alzheimer's disease** (page 4), **angina** (page 7), **attention deficit disorder** (page 19), **periodontal disease** (page 103), **rheumatoid arthritis** (page 109), and various forms of heart disease including mitral valve prolapse and **congestive heart failure** (page 50). However, there is little to no real evidence that it is effective for these purposes.

Finally, alternative medicine literature frequently mentions magnesium as a treatment for **asthma** (page 11). However, this idea seems to be based entirely on the outdated practice of using intravenous magnesium as an emergency treatment for asthma. When you take something by mouth, it's a very different matter from having it injected into your veins. There is no evidence that oral magnesium helps asthma and even some evidence that it does not help.[21]

**Warning:** Do not self-inject magnesium! See your doctor for such treatment.

## WHAT IS THE SCIENTIFIC EVIDENCE FOR MAGNESIUM?

### Migraine Headaches

A recent double-blind study found that regular use of magnesium helps prevent migraine headaches. In this 12-week trial, 81 people with recurrent migraines were given either 600 mg of magnesium daily or placebo.[22] By the last 3 weeks of the study, the treated group's migraines had been reduced by 41.6%, compared to a reduction of 15.8% in the placebo group. The only side effects observed were diarrhea (in about one-fifth of the participants) and, less often, digestive irritation.

Similar results have been seen in other, smaller double-blind studies.[23,24] One study found no benefit,[25] but it has been criticized on many significant points, including using an excessively strict definition of what constituted benefit.[26]

### Noise-Related Hearing Loss

One double-blind placebo-controlled study on 300 military recruits suggests that 167 mg of magnesium daily can prevent hearing loss due to exposure to high-volume noise.[27]

### Kidney Stones

For reasons that are not entirely clear, magnesium may help reduce the incidence of kidney stones. One placebo-controlled study on 89 individuals with kidney stones found that 74% of those taking magnesium had no stones during the treatment period, compared with just 43% in the nontreated (placebo) group.[28]

### Hypertension (High Blood Pressure)

Magnesium works with calcium and potassium to regulate blood pressure. Several studies suggest that magnesium supplements can reduce blood pressure in people with hypertension,[29–32] although some have not.

## SAFETY ISSUES

In general, magnesium appears to be quite safe when taken at recommended dosages. The most common complaint is loose stools. However, people with severe kidney or heart disease should not take magnesium (or any other supplement) except on the advice of a physician. Maximum safe dosages have not been established for young children or women who are pregnant or nursing.

Magnesium can interfere with the absorption of antibiotics in the tetracycline family.[33] Also, when combined with oral diabetes drugs in the sulfonylurea family (Tolinase, Micronase, Orinase, Glucotrol, Diabinese, DiaBeta) magnesium may cause blood sugar levels to fall more than expected.[34]

## ⚠ INTERACTIONS YOU SHOULD KNOW ABOUT

If you are taking

- **Calcium** (including calcium antacids), **potassium supplements, manganese, corticosteroids, digoxin** (for heart problems), **diuretics, oral contraceptives, estrogen-replacement therapy, Prilosec, Prevacid:** You may need extra magnesium.

- **ACE inhibitors, antibiotics** in the tetracycline or quinolone (e.g., **Cipro**) family, **Dilantin (phenytoin), $H_2$ blockers** (e.g., **Zantac or Pepcid), macrodantin,** or **zinc:** You should take magnesium at a different time of day to avoid absorption problems.

- **Oral diabetes medications** in the sulfonylurea family: Work closely with your physician when taking magnesium to avoid hypoglycemia.

Magnesium

Visit Us at TNP.com

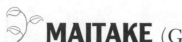

# MAITAKE (GRIFOLA FRONDOSA)

### Principal Proposed Uses
Adaptogen (improve resistance to stress), strengthen immunity

### Other Proposed Uses
High cholesterol, high blood pressure, diabetes

**M**aitake is a medicinal mushroom used in Japan as a general promoter of robust health. Like the similarly described **reishi** (page 291) fungus, innumerable healing powers have been attributed to maitake, ranging from curing cancer to preventing heart disease. Unfortunately, there hasn't been enough reliable research yet to determine whether any of these ancient beliefs are really true.

## WHAT IS MAITAKE USED FOR TODAY?

Contemporary herbalists classify maitake as an adaptogen, a substance said to help the body adapt to stress and resist infection (see the chapter on **ginseng** [page 206] for further explanation about adaptogens). However, as for other adaptogens, we lack definitive scientific evidence to show us that maitake really functions in this way.

Most investigation has focused on the polysaccharide constituents of maitake. This family of substances is known to affect the human immune system in complex ways, and one in particular,

beta-D-glucan, has been studied for its potential benefit in treating cancer and AIDS.[1,2] Highly preliminary studies also suggest that maitake may be useful in treating **diabetes** (page 60), **hypertension** (page 75) (high blood pressure), and high **cholesterol** (page 39). However, there is no real evidence as yet that maitake is effective for these or any other illnesses.

## DOSAGES

Maitake is an edible mushroom that can be eaten as food or made into tea. A typical dosage of dried maitake in capsule or tablet form is 3 to 7 g daily.

## SAFETY ISSUES

Maitake is widely believed to be safe, although formal safety studies have not been performed. Safety in young children, pregnant or nursing women, or those with severe liver or kidney disease has not been established.

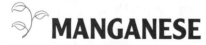

# MANGANESE

### Principal Proposed Uses
Osteoporosis, dysmenorrhea (menstrual pain)

### Other Proposed Uses
Rheumatoid arthritis, muscle sprains/strains, epilepsy, diabetes

### Supplement Forms/Alternative Names
Manganese sulfate, manganese chloride, manganese picolinate, manganese gluconate

**O**ur bodies contain only a very small amount of manganese, but this metal is important as a constituent of many key enzymes. The chemical structure of these enzymes is interest-

ing: large protein molecules cluster around a tiny atom of metal.

Manganese plays a particularly important role as part of the natural antioxidant enzyme superoxide dismutase (SOD), which helps fight damaging free radicals. It also helps energy metabolism, thyroid function, blood sugar control, and normal skeletal growth.

## REQUIREMENTS/SOURCES

Manganese is thought to be an essential nutrient, but the precise daily requirement isn't known. The following daily amounts are considered safe and adequate

- Infants under 6 months, 0.3 to 0.6 mg

  6 to 12 months, 0.6 to 1 mg

- Children 1 to 3 years, 1 to 1.5 mg

  4 to 6 years, 1.5 to 2.0 mg

  7 to 10 years, 2.0 to 3.0 mg

- Adults (and children 11 years and older), 2 to 5 mg

Antacids and oral contraceptives as well as **calcium** (page 146), **iron** (page 234), **copper** (page 169), **magnesium** (page 251), and **zinc** (page 348) supplements can reduce the body's absorption of manganese.[1,2] The best sources of dietary manganese are whole grains, legumes, avocados, grape juice, chocolate, seaweed, egg yolks, nuts, seeds, boysenberries, blueberries, pineapples, spinach, collard greens, peas, and green vegetables.

## THERAPEUTIC DOSAGES

A typical dosage used in studies on manganese is 3 to 6 mg daily. It is sometimes recommended at a much higher dose of 50 to 200 mg daily for 2 weeks following a muscle sprain or strain, but the safety of this dosage is not known.

## THERAPEUTIC USES

Because manganese plays a role in bone metabolism, it has been suggested as a treatment for **osteoporosis** (page 100), a condition in which bone mass deteriorates with age.[3] However, we have no direct evidence that manganese is helpful, except in combination with other minerals.

Manganese has also been suggested for **dysmenorrhea** (page 65) (painful menstruation),[4] muscle strains and sprains, and **rheumatoid arthritis** (page 109), but the evidence that it works is very weak.

People with epilepsy have lower-than-normal levels of manganese in their blood.[5] This suggests (but doesn't prove) that manganese supplements might be helpful for epilepsy. Unfortunately, the studies that could prove or disprove this idea haven't been performed. A similar situation exists regarding **diabetes** (page 60), where manganese deficiencies have been noted, but no trials that used manganese supplements have been reported.[6]

## WHAT IS THE SCIENTIFIC EVIDENCE FOR MANGANESE?

### Osteoporosis

Although manganese is known to play a role in bone metabolism, there is no direct evidence that manganese supplements can help prevent osteoporosis. However, one double-blind placebo-controlled study suggests that a combination of minerals including manganese may be helpful.[7] Fifty-nine women took either placebo, calcium (1,000 mg daily), or calcium plus a daily mineral supplement consisting of 5 mg of manganese, 15 mg of zinc, and 2.5 mg of copper. After 2 years, the group receiving calcium plus minerals showed better bone density than the group receiving calcium alone. But this study doesn't tell us whether it was the manganese or the other minerals that made the difference.

### Dysmenorrhea (Menstrual Pain)

One very small double-blind study suggested that 5.6 mg of manganese daily might ease menstrual discomfort.[8] In the same study, a lower dosage of 1 mg daily *wasn't* effective.

## SAFETY ISSUES

Manganese appears to be safe when taken at the usual recommended dosage of 6 mg or less daily. However, the safety of higher doses is not known. Very high exposure to manganese (due either to environmental pollution or manganese mining) has resulted in a serious psychiatric disorder known as "manganese madness."

Manganese

Visit Us at TNP.com

## ⚠ INTERACTIONS
## YOU SHOULD KNOW ABOUT

If you are taking

- **Iron, copper, zinc, magnesium,** or **calcium:** You may need extra manganese, and vice versa.

- **Antacids** or **oral contraceptives:** You may also need extra manganese.

# MARSHMALLOW (ALTHAEA OFFICINALIS)

*Principal Proposed Uses*

Cough, colds, asthma, ulcers, diarrhea, Crohn's disease, skin inflammation, sore throat

The similarity in name between the herb marshmallow and the sweet treat is more than a coincidence, although the modern sugar puff ball no longer bears much relationship to the old-fashioned candy flavored with marshmallow herb.

Besides inspiring makers of campfire food, the marshmallow has also been used medicinally since ancient Greece. Hippocrates spoke of it as a treatment for bruises and blood loss, and subsequent Roman physicians recommended marshmallow for toothaches, insect bites, chilblains, and irritated skin. In medieval Europe, herbalists used marshmallow to soothe toothaches, coughs, sore throats, chapped skin, indigestion, and diarrhea.

## WHAT IS MARSHMALLOW USED FOR TODAY?

Modern herbalists recommend marshmallow primarily for relieving digestive and respiratory problems, such as coughs, **colds** (page 44), and **asthma** (page 11). The herb contains very high levels of large sugar molecules called mucilage, which appear to exert a soothing effect on mucous membranes. While marshmallow is more a symptomatic treatment than a cure, its ability to soothe a raw throat can be very welcome. It is also sometimes recommended for Crohn's disease or **ulcers** (page 112) to reduce discomfort. No double-blind studies have been reported at this time.

## DOSAGES

Marshmallow can be made into a soothing tea by steeping roots overnight in water and diluting to taste. This tea can be drunk as desired for symptomatic relief. Alternatively, you can take marshmallow in capsules (5 to 6 g daily) or in tincture according to label directions.

Marshmallow ointments can be applied directly to soothe inflamed or irritated skin.

## SAFETY ISSUES

Marshmallow is believed to be entirely safe. It is approved for use in foods, and its chemical makeup does not suggest any but benign effects.[1] However, detailed safety studies have not been performed. One study suggests that marshmallow can slightly lower blood sugar levels.[2] For this reason, people with diabetes should use caution when taking marshmallow. Safety in young children, pregnant or nursing women, or those with severe liver or kidney disease has not been established.

# MEDIUM-CHAIN TRIGLYCERIDES

*Principal Proposed Uses*
  Difficulty digesting fat (malabsorption), athletic performance

*Other Proposed Uses*
  Weight loss, epilepsy

*Supplement Forms/Alternative Names*
  MCTs

Medium-chain triglycerides (MCTs) are fats with an unusual chemical structure that allows the body to digest them easily. Most fats are broken down in the intestine and remade into a special form that can be transported in the blood. But MCTs are absorbed intact and taken to the liver, where they are used directly for energy. In this sense, they are processed very similarly to carbohydrates.

MCTs are different enough from other fats that they can be used as fat substitutes by people (such as those with AIDS), who need calories but are unable to absorb or metabolize normal fats. Also, individuals who develop digestive distress from eating ordinary fats may do better by cooking with MCTs instead.

MCTs are also popular among athletes as a proposed performance enhancer, although there is little evidence as yet that they really work.

## SOURCES

There is no dietary requirement for MCTs. Coconut oil, palm oil, and butter contain up to 15% MCTs (plus a lot of other fats). You can also buy MCTs as purified supplements.

## THERAPEUTIC DOSAGES

MCTs can be eaten as salad oil or used in cooking. When taken as an athletic supplement, dosages in the neighborhood of 85 mg daily are common.

## THERAPEUTIC USES

Preliminary evidence suggests that MCTs are a useful fat substitute for those who have trouble digesting fat. This includes people with serious diseases such as AIDS who need to find a way to gain weight, as well as those who experience diarrhea from eating fatty foods because they lack the proper enzymes (pancreatic insufficiency).[1,2,3]

MCTs are also popular among athletes as a concentrated source of easily utilized energy.[4,5,6]

More controversially, MCTs have been used to promote ketosis, a fat-burning state that can cause weight loss[7] and also improve certain symptoms of epilepsy. In ketosis, the body burns its stored fat for energy. It ordinarily occurs in starvation, but it can be produced on purpose by eating few or no carbohydrates and consuming protein and fat instead. However, intentional ketosis has potential health risks and it is controversial.

## WHAT IS THE SCIENTIFIC EVIDENCE FOR MCTS?

### Fat Malabsorption/ Pancreatic Insufficiency

A double-blind placebo-controlled study on 23 men and women with AIDS suggests that MCTs can help improve AIDS-related fat malabsorption.[8] In this disorder, fat is not digested; it passes unchanged through the intestines, and the body is deprived of calories as well as fat-soluble vitamins.

The study subjects were split into two groups: One received a liquid diet containing normal fats, whereas the other group received mostly MCTs. After 12 days, the participants on the MCT formula showed significantly less fat in their stool and better fat absorption than the other group.

Another double-blind study found similar results in 24 men with AIDS-related fat malabsorption.[9]

A very small study (only 6 subjects) suggested that MCTs could be used in cases in which the pancreas was not producing enough lipase, a fat-digesting enzyme.[10]

## Athletic Performance

MCTs have been proposed as an "ergogenic aid," an energy-boosting supplement to enhance athletic performance. During intense exercise, your body first burns up available energy from the blood (in the form of glucose) and then starts to use energy stored in the form of a larger carbohydrate called *glycogen*. When the glycogen is depleted, exhaustion begins to set in.

One solution to this is *carbo-loading*, the practice of taking large doses of carbohydrates prior to exercise in order to increase glycogen stores. Athletes can also sip carbohydrate-loaded drinks during exercise.

MCTs may provide an alternative. Like other fats, they provide more energy per ounce than carbohydrates; but unlike normal fats, this energy can be released rapidly.[11]

A very small study compared MCTs and carbohydrates as performance boosters for 6 trained cyclists. The athletes took a 4.3% MCT beverage, a 10% carbohydrate beverage, or a drink containing both 4.3% MCTs and 10% carbohydrate.[12] Researchers found a slight advantage to the combination drink. Another study on 12 cyclists also suggested that MCTs plus carbohydrates enhanced performance.[13] However, a recent small study found no benefit with MCTs.[14] Larger studies are necessary to discover whether MCTs are really as useful for athletes as some of its proponents claim.

## SAFETY ISSUES

MCTs are thought to be quite safe, but the safety of using them as a general fat substitute has not been established. Some people who consume high doses of MCTs, especially on an empty stomach, experience annoying (but not severe) abdominal cramps and bloating.

People with diabetes should not use MCTs (or any other supplement) without a doctor's supervision. The safety of MCTs in young children, pregnant or nursing women, or people with serious kidney or liver disease has not been established.

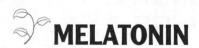

# MELATONIN

*Principal Proposed Uses*

Sleep disorders (e.g., insomnia, jet lag)

*Other Proposed Uses*

Cancer (as an addition to conventional therapy), strengthening the immune system, preventing heart disease, fighting aging

Melatonin is a natural hormone that regulates sleep. During daylight, the pineal gland in the brain produces an important neurotransmitter called serotonin. (A neurotransmitter is a chemical that relays messages between nerve cells.) But at night, the pineal gland stops producing serotonin and instead makes melatonin. This melatonin release helps trigger sleep.

The production of melatonin varies according to the amount of light you're exposed to; for example, your body produces more melatonin in a completely dark room than in a dimly lit one.

Melatonin hit the news in 1995. Not only was it recommended as a treatment for insomnia and jet lag, but for various theoretical reasons it was also described as a "wonder hormone" that could fight cancer, boost the immune system, prevent heart disease, and generally make you live longer. But all we really know is that it helps people whose natural sleep cycle has been disturbed, such as travelers suffering from jet lag and swing-shift workers.

## SOURCES

Melatonin is not a nutrient. However, your body makes less melatonin as you age, which might explain why some people sleep less (or less deeply) as they get older. Travelers and workers on rotating or late shifts can also experience sleep disturbances that seem to be caused by decreased melatonin levels.

You can boost your melatonin production naturally by getting thicker blinds for the bedroom windows or wearing a night mask. You can also take melatonin tablets.

## THERAPEUTIC DOSAGES

Melatonin is typically taken half an hour before bedtime for the first 4 days after traveling; however, the optimum dose is not clear. According to some studies, 0.5 mg is sufficient, while other studies have found benefits for insomnia only at 10 times the dose (5 mg).[1]

Melatonin is available in two forms: quick-release and slow-release. There is some debate as to which one is better.

## THERAPEUTIC USES

Reasonably good evidence tells us that melatonin can help people with jet lag or other similar sleep disturbances adjust to a new schedule.[2] We don't know for sure whether it is helpful for people with other types of **insomnia** (page 80), although there is some reason to believe that it may be.[3]

Highly preliminary evidence suggests that melatonin may be useful for some forms of cancer when combined with conventional anticancer treatment.[4–7] The explanation for this possible effect is unknown, and it may not be true for certain forms of chemotherapy. It is strongly recommended that you consult with your oncologist if you wish to take melatonin during chemotherapy.

Suggestions that melatonin can boost the immune system, prevent heart disease, and help you live longer are entirely hypothetical.

## WHAT IS THE SCIENTIFIC EVIDENCE FOR MELATONIN?

### Sleep Disorders

There is good evidence that melatonin can help you fall asleep when your bedtime rhythm has been disturbed. For example, one double-blind placebo-controlled study enrolled 320 people and followed them for 4 days after plane travel. The participants were divided into four groups and given a daily dose of 5 mg of standard melatonin, 5 mg of slow-release melatonin, 0.5 mg of standard melatonin, or placebo.[8] The group that received 5 mg of standard melatonin slept better, took less time to fall asleep, and felt more energetic and awake during the day than the other three groups.

Good results have been seen in other studies involving travelers, swing-shift workers, and people with insomnia.[9–12] According to one review of the literature, melatonin treatment for sleep disorders is most effective for those who have crossed a significant number of time zones, perhaps eight.[13] Only one study on travelers found *no* benefit, but it may be that the change in time zones experienced by these travelers wasn't great enough to require melatonin.[14]

### Cancer

Melatonin has been used with conventional anticancer therapy in more than a dozen clinical studies. Results have been surprisingly good, although this research must be considered preliminary. For example, a double-blind study on 30 people with advanced brain tumors suggested that melatonin might prolong life and also improve the quality of life.[15] Participants received standard radiation treatment with or without 20 mg daily of melatonin. After 1 year, 6 of 14 individuals in the melatonin group were still alive, compared with just 1 of 16 from the control group. The melatonin group also had fewer side effects due to the radiation treatment—a notable improvement in their quality of life.

Improvements in symptoms and a possible reduction of mortality were also seen in other studies.[16,17] Melatonin appears to work by increasing levels of the body's own tumor-fighting proteins, known as *cytokines*.[18]

## SAFETY ISSUES

Melatonin is probably safe for occasional use, but there are some real concerns about using it on a regular basis. Keep in mind that melatonin is not truly a food supplement but a hormone. Because the body's own production of melatonin probably equals about *one-tenth* of a milligram per day, taking melatonin as a supplement involves dosages that go far beyond normal levels. The consequences of doing so on a regular basis are completely unknown.[19]

As we know from other hormones used in medicine, such as estrogen and cortisone, harmful effects can take years to appear. Hormones are powerful substances that have many subtle effects in the body, and we're far from understanding them fully.

Because melatonin promotes sleep, you should not drive or operate machinery for several hours after taking it. Also, based on theoretical ideas of how melatonin works, some authorities specifically recommend against using it in people with depression, schizophrenia, autoimmune diseases, and other serious illnesses. Maximum safe dosages for young children, pregnant or nursing women, or those with serious liver or kidney disease have not been established.

 # MELISSA A.K.A. LEMON BALM (MELISSA OFFICINALIS)

*Principal Proposed Uses*

*Topical uses:*
    Oral and genital herpes

*Oral uses:*
    Insomnia, anxiety, nervous stomach

Better known in the United States as lemon balm, *Melissa officinalis* is a native of southern Europe, commonly planted in gardens to attract bees. Its leaves give off a delicate lemon odor when bruised.

Medical authorities of ancient Greece and Rome mentioned topical melissa as a treatment for wounds. The herb was later used orally as a treatment for influenza, insomnia, anxiety, depression, and nervous stomach.

## WHAT IS MELISSA USED FOR TODAY?

Modern German researchers have focused on the ability of melissa creams and ointments to inhibit the **herpes** (page 73) virus, as well as the stomach-calming and anti-insomnia benefits of the herb when taken by mouth.

Numerous test-tube studies have found that extracts of melissa possess antiviral properties.[1-4] We don't really know how it works, but the predominant theory is that the herb blocks viruses from attaching to cells.[5]

Melissa cream is used at the first sign of genital or oral herpes. It appears to make flare-ups less intense and last for a shorter period of time, but it doesn't completely eliminate them. There is no evidence that melissa reduces the chances that you can infect someone else. The cream is also applied on a daily basis to prevent flare-ups.

Oral melissa is often used for **insomnia** (page 80), **anxiety** (page 8), and nervous stomach.

## WHAT IS THE SCIENTIFIC EVIDENCE FOR MELISSA?

Besides the clinical research described here, see also the description of how melissa cream is made (under Dosage). It, too, provides indirect evidence for melissa's antiviral effect.

### Herpes

Early studies of melissa ointments showed a significant reduction in the duration and severity of herpes symptoms (both genital and oral) and, when the cream was used regularly, a marked reduction in the frequency of recurrences.[6,7] In one study, the melissa-treated participants recovered in 5 days, while participants receiving non-specific creams required 10 days.[8] Researchers also described a "tremendous reduction" in the frequency of recurrence. However, because these studies weren't double-blind, the results can't be taken as reliable.

A subsequent double-blind study followed 116 individuals at two dermatology centers.[9] Treated subjects recovered somewhat more rapidly than those taking placebo. The largest improvement was seen among the participants with oral herpes.

Although the benefits of melissa were less than dramatic, standard drugs for herpes, such as Zovirax, aren't super-powerful either. In fact, some studies have been unable to show any measurable benefit.[10,11] Zovirax probably does work, but the herb may be just as effective.

### Insomnia

Melissa extracts have also been found to produce a sedative effect in mice.[12] The benefits of combined melissa/valerian extracts in insomnia have been evaluated in one controlled study, discussed in the chapter on **valerian** (page 315).[13]

## DOSAGES

For treatment of an active flare-up of herpes, the proper dosage is four thick applications daily of a standardized melissa (70:1) cream. The dosage may be reduced to twice daily for preventive purposes.

The best melissa extracts are standardized by their capacity to inhibit the growth of herpes virus in a petri dish.[14] To make sure the extract has been properly prepared, manufacturers place cells in such a growing medium, and then add herpes virus. Normally, the virus will gradually destroy all the cells. But when little disks containing melissa are added, cells in the immediate vicinity are protected. Although manufacturers use this method as a form of quality control, it also provides evidence that melissa really works.

When taken orally for its calming effect, the standard dosage of melissa is 1.5 to 4.5 g of dried herb daily.

## SAFETY ISSUES

Topical melissa is not associated with any significant side effects, although allergic reactions are always possible. Oral melissa is on the FDA's GRAS (generally regarded as safe) list. There are no known drug interactions. However, there are theoretical concerns that if melissa is taken at the same time as standard sedative drugs, excessive sedation might occur.

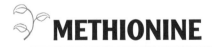

# METHIONINE

*Principal Proposed Uses*
   Urinary tract infection

*Other Proposed Uses*
   "Liver support"

*Supplement Forms/Alternative Names*
   L-methionine

---

**M**ethionine is an essential amino acid—one of the building blocks of proteins and peptides that your body cannot manufacture from other chemicals. The body uses methionine to manufacture **creatine** (page 171) and uses the sulfur in methionine for normal metabolism and growth.

One study suggests that methionine can prevent bacteria from sticking to urinary tract cells,[1] which may make it useful for preventing bladder infections. **Cranberry** (page 170) juice is thought to help reduce the incidence of bladder infections in a similar fashion.

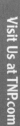

## REQUIREMENTS/SOURCES

Depending on your body weight, you need between 800 and 1,000 mg of methionine daily for normal health. Deficiency is unlikely, because enough methionine is generally available from the diet.

Meat, fish, dairy products, and other high-protein foods are good sources of methionine.

## THERAPEUTIC DOSAGES

A proper therapeutic dosage of methionine has not been determined. One study relating to urinary tract infections used a dosage of 500 mg 3 times daily.

## THERAPEUTIC USES

Because it seems to discourage bacteria from sticking to the wall of the bladder, methionine has been suggested as a treatment for chronic **bladder infections** (page 23).[2] However, there is as yet little direct evidence that it works.

One study on rats suggests that methionine might protect the liver against acetaminophen (e.g., Tylenol) poisoning.[3] Based on this, it has been proposed as a generally helpful substance—what our great-grandparents might have called a "tonic"—for the liver. However, in this particular study the action of methionine was more to fight acetaminophen specifically than to protect the liver in general. There is much better evidence that the herb **milk thistle** (page 262) is a general liver protectant.

## WHAT IS THE SCIENTIFIC EVIDENCE FOR METHIONINE?

### Bladder Infection

The clinical evidence for this use of methionine is based primarily on one study, a double-blind placebo-controlled trial that tested methionine against placebo in 33 women with chronic urinary tract infections. The dosage used in this study was 500 mg 3 times daily. Researchers found *no* infections in the methionine group during the 26-month study period.[4] Although methionine did not reduce the number of bacteria in the urinary tract, it appeared to lessen the bacteria's ability to latch on to cells.

## SAFETY ISSUES

Methionine is thought to be generally safe. However, the maximum safe dosages for young children, pregnant or nursing women, or those with serious liver or kidney disease have not been established.

## ⚠ INTERACTIONS YOU SHOULD KNOW ABOUT

If you are taking **methionine,** make sure to get enough **folic acid** (page 194), **vitamin B$_6$** (page 326), and **vitamin B$_{12}$** (page 329).[5]

# MILK THISTLE (SILYBUM MARIANUM)

*Principal Proposed Uses*

Chronic viral hepatitis, acute viral hepatitis, alcoholic liver disease, liver cirrhosis, mushroom poisoning (special intravenous form only), protection from liver-toxic medications

**M**ilk thistle, a spiny-leafed plant with reddish-purple, thistle-shaped flowers, has a long history of use both as a food and a medicine. English gardeners at the turn of the century grew milk thistle and used the leaves like lettuce, the stalks like asparagus, the roasted seeds like coffee, and the roots (soaked overnight) like oyster plant.

The seeds, fruit, and leaves of milk thistle are used for medicinal purposes. Over 2,000 years ago, Pliny the Elder reported that the juice of milk thistle could "carry off bile," an insight that foreshadowed its modern uses. In Europe, the herb was widely used through the early twentieth century for the treatment of jaundice as well as for insufficient breast milk.

## WHAT IS MILK THISTLE USED FOR TODAY?

Based on the extensive folk use of milk thistle in cases of jaundice, European medical researchers began to investigate its medicinal effects. The results led Germany's Commission E to approve an oral extract of milk thistle as a treatment for liver disease in 1986. It is widely used to treat alcoholic hepatitis, alcoholic fatty liver, liver cirrhosis, liver poisoning, and **viral hepatitis** (page 71), as well as to protect the liver from the effects of liver-toxic medications. Milk thistle is one of the few herbs that have no real equivalent in the world of conventional medicine.

According to reports and some research evidence that we'll review in the next section, treatment produces a modest improvement in symptoms of chronic liver disease, such as nausea, weakness, loss of appetite, fatigue, and pain. Liver enzymes as measured by blood tests frequently improve, and if a liver biopsy is performed, there may be improvements on the cellular level. Some studies have shown a reduction in death rate among those with serious liver disease.

The active ingredients in milk thistle appear to be four substances known collectively as silymarin, of which the most potent is named silibinin.[1] When injected intravenously, silibinin is one of the few known antidotes to poisoning by the deathcap mushroom, *Amanita phalloides*. Animal studies suggest that milk thistle extracts can also protect against many other poisonous substances, from toluene to the drug acetaminophen.[2–8]

Silymarin appears to function by displacing toxins trying to bind to the liver as well as by causing the liver to regenerate more quickly.[9] It may also scavenge free radicals and stabilize liver cell membranes.[10,11]

However, milk thistle is not effective in treating advanced liver cirrhosis, and only the intravenous form can counter mushroom poisoning.

In Europe, milk thistle is often added as extra protection when patients are given medications known to cause liver problems.

Milk thistle is also used in a vague condition known as minor hepatic insufficiency, or "sluggish liver."[12] This term is mostly used by European physicians and American naturopathic practition-

ers—conventional physicians don't recognize it. Symptoms are supposed to include aching under the ribs, fatigue, unhealthy skin appearance, general malaise, constipation, premenstrual syndrome, chemical sensitivities, and allergies.

Milk thistle is also sometimes recommended for **gallstones** (page 68) and **psoriasis** (page 106), but there is little to no evidence as yet that it really works for these conditions.

## WHAT IS THE SCIENTIFIC EVIDENCE FOR MILK THISTLE?

There is considerable evidence from studies in animals that milk thistle can protect the liver from numerous toxins. However, human studies of people suffering from various liver diseases have yielded mixed results.

### Deathcap Poisoning

In *Amanita* mushroom poisoning, silibinin appears to dramatically reduce death rates, which are typically from 30 to 50%, down to less than 10%.[13] This mushroom destroys the liver if left untreated. In conditions like this one, it isn't ethical to perform double-blind studies. However, milk thistle seems to be so dramatically effective that its value is not disputed.

### Chronic Viral Hepatitis

Preliminary double-blind studies of people with chronic viral hepatitis have found that milk thistle can produce significant improvement in symptoms such as fatigue, reduced appetite, and abdominal discomfort, as well as results on blood tests for liver inflammation.[14,15,16]

### Acute Viral Hepatitis

While good results have been reported in one study of 57 people with acute viral hepatitis,[17] another study of 151 participants showed no benefit.[18]

### Alcoholic Liver Disease

A 1981 double-blind study followed 106 Finnish soldiers with mild alcoholic liver disease. In the treated group, there was a significant improvement in liver function as measured by blood tests and biopsy.[19]

Another study reported similar results.[20] However, a study of 116 participants showed little to no benefit,[21] as did another study of 72 people followed for 15 months.[22]

### Liver Cirrhosis

A controlled study followed 170 people with liver cirrhosis for 3 to 6 years. In the treated group, the 4-year survival rate was 58% as compared to only 38% in the placebo group.[23] However, a recently reported 2-year double-blind study of 200 alcoholics with cirrhosis found no benefit.[24]

### Protection from Medications That Damage the Liver

Numerous medications can injure or inflame the liver. Preliminary evidence suggests that milk thistle might protect against liver toxicity caused by such drugs as acetaminophen, Dilantin, alcohol, and phenothiazines.[25]

## DOSAGES

The standard dosage of milk thistle is 200 mg 2 to 3 times a day of an extract standardized to contain 70% silymarin.

There is some evidence that silymarin bound to phosphatidylcholine may be better absorbed.[26,27] This form should be taken at a dosage of 100 to 200 mg twice a day.

**Warning:** Considering the severe nature of liver disease, a doctor's supervision is essential. Also, do not inject milk thistle preparations that are designed for oral use!

## SAFETY ISSUES

Milk thistle is believed to possess very little toxicity. Animal studies have not shown any negative effects even when high doses were administered over a long period of time.[28]

A study of 2,637 participants reported in 1992 showed a low incidence of side effects, limited mainly to mild gastrointestinal disturbance.[29]

On the basis of its extensive use as a food, milk thistle is believed to be safe for pregnant or nursing women and researchers have enrolled pregnant women in studies.[30] However, safety in young children, pregnant or nursing women, and individuals with severe renal disease has not been formally established.

No drug interactions are known. However, one report has noted that silibinin (a constituent of silymarin) can inhibit a bacterial enzyme called beta-glucuronidase, which plays a role in the activity of certain drugs, such as oral contraceptives.[31] This could reduce their effectiveness.

## ⚠ INTERACTIONS YOU SHOULD KNOW ABOUT

If you are taking

- **Oral contraceptives:** Milk thistle may reduce their effectiveness.
- **Medications that could damage the liver:** Milk thistle might be protective.

 # MULLEIN (VERBASCUM THAPSUS)

*Principal Proposed Uses*
    Asthma, colds, cough, ear infections, sore throat

Also called "grandmother's flannel" for its thick, soft leaves, mullein is a common wildflower that can grow almost anywhere. It reaches several feet in height and puts up a spike of densely packed tiny yellow flowers. Mullein has served many purposes over the centuries, from making candlewicks to casting out evil spirits, but as medicine it was primarily used to treat diarrhea, respiratory diseases, and hemorrhoids.

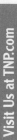

## WHAT IS MULLEIN USED FOR TODAY?

Contemporary herbalists sometimes recommend hot mullein tea for **asthma** (page 11), **colds** (page 44), coughs, and sore throats. Mullein seldom produces dramatic effects, but its soothing qualities will be appreciated. You can also breathe the steam from a boiling pot of mullein tea.

Like marshmallow, mullein contains a high proportion of mucilage (large sugar molecules that appear to soothe mucous membranes). It also contains saponins that may help loosen mucus.[1] However, there has not been very much scientific investigation into this popular herb. Mullein is said to be most effective when combined with other herbs of similar qualities, such as **yerba santa** (page 346), **marshmallow** (page 256), cherry bark, and **elecampane** (page 182).

Mullein is also often made into an oily eardrop solution to soothe the pain of ear infections.

## DOSAGES

To make mullein tea, add 1 to 2 teaspoons of dried leaves and flowers to 1 cup of boiling water and steep for 10 minutes. Make sure to strain the tea before drinking it because fuzzy bits of the herb can stick in your throat and cause an irritating tickle.

For painful ear infections, you can squeeze several drops of room-temperature mullein oil into the ear canal, so long as you are sure that the eardrum isn't punctured. But don't expect mullein oil to heal an ear infection: It only relieves the symptoms.

## SAFETY ISSUES

Mullein leaves and flowers are on the FDA's GRAS (generally regarded as safe) list. Side effects are rare. Nonetheless, safety in young children, pregnant or nursing women, or those with severe liver or kidney disease has not been established.

 # N-ACETYL CYSTEINE (NAC)

*Principal Proposed Uses*
Angina pectoris (in combination with conventional treatment)

*Other Proposed Uses*
Acute respiratory distress syndrome, bronchitis, emphysema, chemotherapy aid

N-acetyl cysteine (NAC) is a specially modified form of the dietary amino acid cysteine. NAC may help break up mucus, which is the basis for using it in respiratory conditions. It also helps the body make the important antioxidant enzyme glutathione. However, the only well-documented uses of NAC are for conditions too serious for self-treatment.

## SOURCES

There is no daily requirement for NAC, and it is not found in food.

## THERAPEUTIC DOSAGES

Optimal levels of NAC have not been determined. The amount used in studies has varied from 250 to 1,500 mg daily.

## THERAPEUTIC USES

Evidence suggests that NAC may be helpful for people who take the drug nitroglycerin for **angina** (page 7), the chest pain associated with heart disease.[1,2] However, severe headaches may develop as a side effect. NAC may also be helpful in a life-threatening condition called acute respiratory distress syndrome.[3] Finally, very high dosages of NAC are used in hospitals as a conventional treatment for acetaminophen poisoning.

**Note:** Do not attempt to self-treat angina, acute respiratory distress syndrome, or acetaminophen poisoning! Medical supervision is absolutely essential because of the very real risk of death in these conditions.

NAC is sometimes recommended as a treatment for bronchitis and emphysema, based on its mucus-thinning effects, and as an aid for enduring chemotherapy. However, there is no solid scientific evidence that it is effective for these conditions.

## WHAT IS THE SCIENTIFIC EVIDENCE FOR NAC?

### Angina Pectoris

Angina pectoris is a squeezing feeling in the chest caused by inadequate blood supply to the heart. It can be a precursor of heart attacks. People with angina often use the drug nitroglycerin to relieve symptoms. One 4-month, double-blind placebo-controlled study of 200 individuals with heart disease found that the combination of nitroglycerin and NAC significantly reduced the incidence of heart attacks and other severe heart problems.[4] NAC alone and nitroglycerin alone were not as effective. The only problem was that the combination of nitroglycerin and NAC caused severe headaches in many participants.

NAC may also help in cases of nitroglycerin tolerance, a condition in which the drug becomes less effective over time. In a small double-blind study of 32 people with angina, tolerance developed in 15 of 16 individuals who took nitroglycerin only, but in just 5 of 16 individuals who took nitroglycerin plus 2 g of NAC daily.[5]

### Acute Respiratory Distress Syndrome

A double-blind placebo-controlled clinical trial compared the effectiveness of NAC, Procysteine (a synthetic cysteine building-block drug), and placebo in 46 people with a condition called acute respiratory distress syndrome.[6] This catastrophic lung condition can be caused when an unconscious person inhales his or her own vomit. Both NAC and Procysteine reduced the severity of the condition in some people (as compared with placebo). However, overall it did not reduce the number of deaths.

## SAFETY ISSUES

NAC appears to be a very safe supplement when taken alone, although one study in rats suggests that 60 to 100 times the normal dose can cause liver injury.[7]

As mentioned earlier, the combination of nitroglycerin and NAC causes severe headaches. Safety in young children, women who are pregnant or nursing, and individuals with severe liver or kidney disease has not been established.

## ⚠ INTERACTIONS YOU SHOULD KNOW ABOUT

If you are taking **nitroglycerin,** NAC may cause severe headaches.

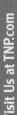

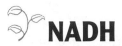

# NADH

*Principal Proposed Uses*
There are no well-documented uses for NADH.

*Other Proposed Uses*
Alzheimer's disease, Parkinson's disease, depression, exercise performance enhancement

*Supplement Forms/Alternative Names*
Nicotinamide adenine dinucleotide

NADH, short for *nicotinamide adenine dinucleotide,* is an important cofactor ("assistant") that helps enzymes in the work they do throughout the body. NADH particularly plays a role in the production of energy. It also participates in the production of L-dopa, which the body turns into the important neurotransmitter dopamine.

Based on these basic biochemical facts, NADH has been suggested as a treatment for Alzheimer's disease, Parkinson's disease, and depression and as a sports supplement. However, there isn't enough scientific evidence to prove or disprove its usefulness for any of these conditions.

## SOURCES

Healthy bodies make all the NADH they need, using **vitamin B₃** (page 323) (also known as niacin, or nicotinamide) as a starting point. The highest concentration of NADH in animals is found in muscle tissues, which means that meat might be a good source—were it not that most of the NADH in meat is destroyed during processing, cooking, and digestion. In reality, we don't get much NADH from our food.

## THERAPEUTIC DOSAGES

The typical dosage for supplemental NADH ranges from 5 to 50 mg daily.

## THERAPEUTIC USES

Supplemental NADH has been proposed as a treatment for **Alzheimer's disease** (page 4), Parkinson's disease, and **depression** (page 54). It has also been tried as an athletic performance enhancer. However, although a few studies have been performed on these uses,[1,2,3] none were designed in such a way as to produce scientifically meaningful results.

## SAFETY ISSUES

NADH appears to be quite safe when taken at a dosage of 5 mg daily or less. However, formal safety studies have not been completed, and safety in young children, pregnant or nursing women, or those with severe liver or kidney disease has not been established.

# NEEM (AZADIRACHTA INDICA)

*Principal Proposed Uses*
Fevers, respiratory diseases, skin diseases, and other conditions too numerous to list

The neem tree has been called "the village pharmacy," because its bark, leaves, sap, fruit, seeds, and twigs have so many diverse uses in the traditional medicine of India. This member of the mahogany family has been used medicinally for at least 4,000 years, and is held in such esteem that Indian poets called it *Sarva Roga Nivarini:* The One That Can Cure All Ailments.

Neem

Mohandas Gandhi encouraged scientific investigation of the neem tree as part of his program to revitalize Indian traditions, eventually leading to over 2,000 research papers and intense commercial interest.

At least 50 patents have been filed on neem, and neem-based products are licensed in the United States for control of insects in food and ornamental crops. However, the Indian government and many nongovernmental organizations have united to overthrow some patents of this type, which they regard as "folk-wisdom piracy." One fear is that if neem is patented, indigenous people who already use it will lose the right to continue to do so. Another point is the fundamental question: Who owns the genetic diversity of plants: the nations where the plants come from or the transnational corporations that pay for the research into those plants? Although this area of international law is rapidly evolving, a patent on the spice **turmeric** (page 311) has already been overturned, and neem may follow soon.

At least 100 bioactive substances have been found in neem, including nimbidin, azadiracthins, and other triterpenoids and limonoids. Although the scientific evidence for all of neem's uses in health care remains preliminary, the intense interest in the plant will eventually lead to proper double-blind clinical trials.

## WHAT IS NEEM USED FOR TODAY?

The uses of neem are remarkably diverse. In India, the sap is used for treating fevers, general debilitation, digestive disturbances, and skin diseases; the bark gum for respiratory diseases and other infections; the leaves for digestive problems, intestinal parasites, and viral infections; the fruit for debilitation, malaria, skin diseases, and intestinal parasites; and the seed and kernel oil for **diabetes** (page 60) fevers, fungal infections, bacterial infections, inflammatory diseases, and fertility prevention, and as an insecticide.[1,2] Which, if any, of these uses will be verified when proper research is performed remains unclear.

## DOSAGES

Because of the numerous parts of the neem tree used, and the many different ways these can be prepared, the only advice I can give at this time is to follow the directions on the label of the neem product you purchase.

## SAFETY ISSUES

Based on its extensive traditional use, neem seems to be quite safe. This is particularly remarkable considering that the oil of neem is a powerful insecticide! However, there has not yet been a full scientific evaluation of the toxicity and side effects of neem and its many constituents.

A somewhat worrisome recent report suggests that neem might damage chromosomes.[3] Although this information is still highly preliminary, at the present time neem is not recommended for use by young children, pregnant or nursing women, or those with severe liver or kidney disease.

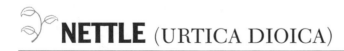

# NETTLE (URTICA DIOICA)

*Principal Proposed Uses*
  Benign prostatic hyperplasia (nettle root), allergies (nettle leaf)

Anyone who lives in a locale where nettle grows wild will eventually discover the powers of this dark-green plant. Depending on the species, the fine hairs on its leaves and stem cause burning pain that lasts from hours to weeks. But this well-protected herb can also serve as medicine. Nettle juice was used in Hippocrates' time to treat bites and stings, and European herbalists recommended nettle tea for lung disorders. Nettle tea was used by Native Americans as an aid in pregnancy, childbirth, and nursing.

## WHAT IS NETTLE USED FOR TODAY?

In Europe, nettle root is widely used for the treatment of **benign prostatic hyperplasia (BPH)** (page 20), or prostate enlargement. Like saw palmetto, pygeum, and beta-sitosterols, nettle appears to reduce obstruction to urinary flow and decrease the need for nighttime urination. However, the evidence is not as strong for nettle as it is for these other treatments. For more information on nettle and its use for prostate problems, see *The Natural Pharmacist Guide to Saw Palmetto and the Prostate*.

**Note:** Before self-treating with nettle, be sure to get a proper medical evaluation to rule out prostate cancer.

Nettle leaf has recently become a popular treatment for **allergies (hay fever)** (page 3) based on one preliminary study at the National College of Naturopathic Medicine in Portland.

Nettle leaf is also highly nutritious, and in cooked form may be used as a general dietary supplement.

## WHAT IS THE SCIENTIFIC EVIDENCE FOR NETTLE?

The evidence is much better for nettle root and prostatic enlargement than for nettle leaf and allergies.

### Nettle Root

The use of nettle root for treating benign prostatic hyperplasia has not been as well studied as saw palmetto, but the evidence is at least moderately convincing.

Nettle root contains numerous biologically active chemicals that may influence the function of the prostate, interact with sex hormones, and reduce inflammation.[1–4]

Open studies involving a total of over 2,000 men have found significant improvements in prostate size, nighttime urination, urination frequency, urine flow, and residual urine.[5] However, open studies are not necessarily reliable in this case because up to 60% of men with BPH show good responses to placebo.

In a 4- to 6-week double-blind study of 67 men, treatment with nettle produced a 14% improvement in urine flow and a 53% decrease in residual urine.[6] Another double-blind study of 40 men found a significant decrease in frequency of urination after 6 months.[7] A double-blind study of 50 men over 9 weeks found a significant improvement in urination volume.[8]

### Nettle Leaf

A preliminary double-blind placebo-controlled study following 69 individuals suggests that freeze-dried nettle leaf may at least slightly improve allergy symptoms.[9]

## DOSAGES

According to Commission E, the proper dosage of nettle root is 4 to 6 g daily of the whole root, or a proportional dose of concentrated extract.

For allergies, the proper dosage is 300 mg twice a day of freeze-dried nettle leaf.

## SAFETY ISSUES

Because nettle leaf has a long history of food use, it is believed to be safe.

Nettle root does not have as extensive a history to go by. Although detailed safety studies have not been reported, no significant adverse effects have been noted in Germany where nettle root is widely used. In practice, it is nearly side-effect free. In one study of 4,087 people who took 600 to 1,200 mg of nettle root daily for 6 months, less than 1% reported mild gastrointestinal distress and only 0.19% experienced allergic reactions (skin rash).[10]

For theoretical reasons, there are some concerns that nettle may interact with diabetes, blood pressure, anti-inflammatory, and sedative medications, although there are no reports of any problems occurring in real life.

The safety of nettle root or leaf for pregnant or nursing mothers has not been established. However nettle leaf tea is a traditional drink for pregnant and nursing women.

## ⚠ INTERACTIONS YOU SHOULD KNOW ABOUT

If you are taking **anti-inflammatory, anti-hypertensive, sedative,** or **blood sugar–lowering medications,** nettle might conceivably interact with them, although it is unlikely.

Nettle

Visit Us at TNP.com

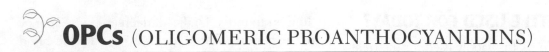

# OPCs (OLIGOMERIC PROANTHOCYANIDINS)

### Principal Proposed Uses
Strengthening blood vessels and reducing inflammation (e.g., varicose veins, hemorrhoids, swelling after injury or surgery, easy bruising)

### Other Proposed Uses
Poor night vision, aging skin, macular degeneration, cancer prevention, diabetic neuropathy, allergies, atherosclerosis prevention, diabetic retinopathy, liver cirrhosis

### Supplement Forms/Alternative Names
Procyanidolic oligomers (PCOs), grape seed extract, pine bark extract

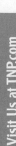

One of the bestselling herbal products of the early 1990s was an extract of the bark of French maritime pine. This substance consists of a family of chemicals known scientifically as oligomeric proanthocyanidin complexes (OPCs) or procyanidolic oligomers (PCOs). Similar substances are also found in grape seed.

The modern use of OPCs is closely linked to an event in 1534, when a French explorer and his crew were trapped by ice in the Saint Lawrence River. Many of the men were saved from scurvy by a Native American who suggested they make tea from the needles and bark of a local pine tree. Over 400 years later, Jacques Masquelier of the University of Bordeaux came across this story and decided to investigate the constituents of pine trees. In 1951, he extracted OPCs from the bark of the maritime pine, and found that they could duplicate many of the functions of vitamin C. Later, he found an even better source of OPCs in grape seed, which is their major source in France today.

Like the anthocyanosides found in **bilberry** (page 135) (to which they are closely related), OPCs appear to stabilize the walls of blood vessels, reduce inflammation, and generally support tissues containing collagen and elastin.[1–4] OPCs are also strong antioxidants. Vitamin E defends against fat-soluble oxidants and vitamin C neutralizes water-soluble ones, but OPCs are active against both types.[5,6,7]

Evidence suggests that OPCs can reduce the discomfort and swelling of varicose veins and decrease the edema (swelling) that often follows injury or surgery. On the basis of much weaker evidence, OPCs are also popular for preventing heart disease, revitalizing aging skin, and reducing the tendency toward easy bruising.

## SOURCES

Like other flavonoids, OPCs aren't necessary for life, although they may prove to be important for optimal health.

OPCs aren't a single chemical, but a group of closely related compounds. Several food sources contain similar chemicals: red wine, cranberries, blueberries, bilberries, tea (green and black), black currant, onions, legumes, parsley, and the herb hawthorn. However, most OPC supplements are made from either grape seed or the bark of the maritime pine. Grape seed is the preferred source in France, where this supplement was originally popularized, and is a more economical source than pine bark.

## THERAPEUTIC DOSAGES

For use as a general antioxidant—much as you might use **vitamin E** (page 337) or **vitamin C** (page 331)—50 mg of OPCs daily are sufficient. A higher dosage of 150 to 300 mg daily is generally used for treating specific diseases such as varicose veins. Grape seed OPCs are just as good and much less expensive than the maritime pine source.

## THERAPEUTIC USES

The best-documented use of OPCs is to treat venous insufficiency, a condition closely related to varicose veins (page 113). It refers to the situation when blood pools in the legs, causing aching, pain, heaviness, swelling, fatigue, and unsightly visible veins. There is good evidence that OPCs relieve the pain and swelling of venous insufficiency.[8,9,10] OPCs probably cannot make visible varicose veins disappear, but regular use might help prevent new ones from developing. Other approaches to varicose veins, include **horse chestnut** (page 228), **gotu kola** (page 218), and **bromelain** (page 144).

There is also some evidence that OPCs can be useful for the swelling that often follows injuries or surgery.[11,12,13] OPCs appear to speed the disappearance of swelling, presumably by strengthening damaged blood and lymph vessels that are leaking fluid.

For similar reasons, OPCs may also be helpful for people who bruise easily due to fragile blood vessels. Note: Keep in mind that there may be medical causes for easy bruising that require more specific treatment.

OPCs in cream form are a popular treatment for aging skin, on the theory that by repairing elastin and collagen they will return skin to a more youthful appearance. However, there is no solid evidence as yet that they are effective for this purpose.

On the basis of preliminary evidence, regular use of OPCs has been proposed as a measure to prevent **cancer** (page 26), **heart disease** (page 14), **macular degeneration** (page 85) (the major cause of age-related blindness), diabetic neuropathy and diabetic retinopathy (side effects of **diabetes** [page 60]), as well as a treatment for **allergies** (page 3) (hay fever), impaired **night vision** (page 94), and liver cirrhosis. However, much more research needs to be performed to discover whether these potential benefits are real.

## WHAT IS THE SCIENTIFIC EVIDENCE FOR OPCs?

Considerable evidence tells us that OPCs protect and strengthen collagen and elastin—proteins found in cartilage, tendons, blood vessels, and muscle.[14–19] There is also no question that OPCs are strong antioxidants, more powerful than either **vitamin E** (page 337) or **vitamin C** (page 331) by some measures.[20] The medicinal effects of OPCs are believed to be due to some combination of these properties.

## Venous Insufficiency (Varicose Veins)

There is good evidence for the use of OPCs to treat people with symptoms of venous insufficiency. A double-blind placebo-controlled study of 92 subjects found that OPCs, taken at a dose of 100 mg 3 times daily, significantly improved major symptoms, including heaviness, swelling, and leg discomfort.[21] Over a period of 1 month, 75% of the participants treated with OPCs improved substantially. This result doesn't seem quite so impressive when you note that significant improvement was also seen in 41% of the placebo group; nonetheless, OPCs still did significantly better than placebo.

According to sketchy information provided by one manufacturer, a controlled but not blinded study of 291 individuals with varicose veins also found significant benefit.[22] Finally, a double-blind study of 50 people with varicose veins of the legs found that doses of 150 mg per day of OPCs were more effective in reducing symptoms and signs than another natural treatment: the bioflavonoid diosmin, widely used in Europe for this condition.[23]

## Edema After Surgery or Injury

Breast cancer surgery often leads to swelling of the arm. A double-blind placebo-controlled study of 63 post-operative breast cancer patients found that 600 mg of OPCs daily for 6 months reduced edema, pain, and peculiar sensations known as paresthesias.[24] Also, in a double-blind placebo-controlled study of 32 "face-lift" patients who were followed for 10 days, edema disappeared much faster in the treated group.[25]

Another 10-day double-blind placebo-controlled study enrolling 50 participants found that OPCs improved the rate at which edema disappeared following sports injuries.[26]

## Night Vision

One interesting 6-week study evaluated the ability of grape seed OPCs to improve night vision in normal subjects.[27,28] In this trial of 100 healthy

OPCs

Visit Us at TNP.com

volunteers, those who received 200 mg per day of OPCs showed improvements in night vision and glare recovery as compared to placebo-treated subjects.

### Atherosclerosis

Although there are no reliable human studies, animal evidence suggests that OPCs can slow or reverse atherosclerosis.[29–32] This suggests (but definitely does not prove) that OPCs might be helpful for preventing heart disease.

### SAFETY ISSUES

OPCs have been extensively tested for safety and are generally considered to be essentially nontoxic.[33] Side effects are rare, but when they do occur they are limited to occasional allergic reactions and mild digestive distress. However, maximum safe dosages for young children, pregnant or nursing women, or those with severe liver or kidney disease have not been established.

OPCs may have some anticoagulant properties when taken in high doses, and should be used only under medical supervision by individuals on blood-thinner drugs such as Coumadin (warfarin) and heparin.

### ⚠ INTERACTIONS YOU SHOULD KNOW ABOUT

If you are taking **Coumadin (warfarin)** or **heparin,** high doses of OPCs might cause a risk of excessive bleeding.

# ORNITHINE ALPHA-KETOGLUTARATE

*Principal Proposed Uses*
There are no documented uses for ornithine alpha-ketoglutarate.

*Other Proposed Uses*
Athletic performance enhancer

O rnithine alpha-ketoglutarate (OKG) is manufactured from two amino acids, ornithine and glutamine. OKG is not found in food, although its two building blocks are.

Animal studies suggest that OKG may prevent the breakdown of muscle, which has led to the suggestion that it may be helpful for athletes in training.

### SOURCES

The amino acids that make up OKG are found in high-protein foods such as meat, fish, and dairy, but OKG itself is not found in foods. Supplements are available in tablet or pill form.

### THERAPEUTIC DOSAGES

Athletes have taken up to 35 g daily of OKG.

### THERAPEUTIC USES

OKG is widely used by athletes in the hope that it will increase their muscle development in training. However, there is practically no foundation for this belief, other than two rather theoretical studies in rats.[1,2]

### SAFETY ISSUES

OKG appears to be safe. However, as with all supplements used in multigram doses, it is important to purchase a reputable product, because a contaminant present even in small percentages could add up to a real problem. The maximum safe dosages for young children, women who are pregnant or nursing, or those with serious liver or kidney disease have not been established.

# 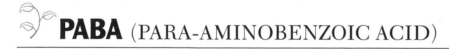OSHA (LIGUSTICUM PORTERI)

## Principal Proposed Uses
Coughs, respiratory infections, digestive disorders

Native to high altitudes in the Southwest and Rocky Mountain states, the root of the osha plant is a traditional Native American remedy for respiratory infections and digestive problems. A related plant, *Ligusticum wallichii,* has a long history of use in Chinese medicine, and most of the scientific studies on osha were actually performed on this species.

## WHAT IS OSHA USED FOR TODAY?

Osha is frequently recommended for use at the first sign of a respiratory infection. Like a sauna, it will typically induce sweating, and according to folk wisdom this may help avert the development of a full-blown **cold** (page 44). Osha is also taken during respiratory infections as a cough suppressant and expectorant, hence the common name "Colorado cough root."

Although there have not been any double-blind studies to verify these proposed uses, Chinese research suggests that *Ligusticum wallichii* can relax smooth muscle tissue (perhaps thereby moderating the cough reflex) and inhibit the growth of various bacteria.[1] Whether these findings apply to osha as well is unknown.

Like other bitter herbs, osha also tends to improve symptoms of indigestion and increase appetite.

## DOSAGES

Osha products vary in their concentration and should be taken according to directions on the label.

## SAFETY ISSUES

Osha is believed to be safe, although the scientific record is far from complete. Traditionally, it is not recommended for use in pregnancy. Safety in young children, nursing women, or those with severe liver or kidney disease has also not been established.

One potential risk with osha is contamination with hemlock parsley, a deadly plant with a similar appearance.[2]

# PABA (PARA-AMINOBENZOIC ACID)

## Principal Proposed Uses
There are no well-documented uses for PABA.

## Other Proposed Uses
Scleroderma, Peyronie's disease, male infertility, vitiligo

Para-aminobenzoic acid (PABA) is best known as the active ingredient in sunblock. This use of PABA is not really medicinal: like a pair of sunglasses, PABA physically blocks ultraviolet rays when it is applied to the skin.

There are, however, some proposed medicinal uses of oral PABA supplements. PABA is sometimes suggested as a treatment for various diseases of the skin and connective tissue, as well as for male infertility. However, most of the clinical

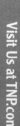

data on PABA comes from very old studies, some from the early 1940s.

## SOURCES

PABA is not believed to be an essential nutrient. Nonetheless, it is found in foods, mainly in grains and meat. Small amounts of PABA are usually present in B vitamin supplements as well as in some multiple vitamins.

## THERAPEUTIC DOSAGES

A typical therapeutic dosage of PABA is 300 to 400 mg daily. Some studies have used much higher dosages. However, serious side effects have been found in dosages above 8 g daily (see Safety Issues). You probably shouldn't take more than 400 mg daily except on medical advice.

## THERAPEUTIC USES

PABA has been suggested as a treatment for scleroderma, a disease that creates fibrous tissue in the skin and internal organs.[1,2] However, a small double-blind study found it ineffective.[3]

PABA has also been suggested for other diseases in which abnormal fibrous tissue is involved, such as Peyronie's disease, a condition in which the penis becomes bent owing to the accumulation of such tissue.[4,5,6] However, no double-blind studies have yet been performed.

Based on one small World War II–era study, PABA has been suggested for treating **infertility in men** (page 78) as well as vitiligo, a condition in which patches of skin lose their pigment, re-sulting in pale blotches. However, this study didn't have a control group, so its results aren't meaningful.[7] Ironically, a recent study suggests that high dosages of PABA can *cause* vitiligo (see Safety Issues).

## SAFETY ISSUES

PABA is probably safe when taken at a dosage up to 400 mg daily. Possible side effects at this dosage are minor, including skin rash and loss of appetite.[8]

Higher doses are a different story, however. There has been one reported case of severe liver toxicity in a woman taking 12 g daily of PABA.[9] Fortunately, her liver recovered completely after she discontinued her use of this supplement. Also, a recent study suggests that 8 g daily of PABA can cause vitiligo, the patchy skin disease described previously.[10]

Clearly, there are questions that need to be answered about the safety of high-dose PABA therapy. You shouldn't take more than 400 mg daily except under medical supervision.

PABA can interfere with certain medications, including sulfa antibiotics.[11]

Safety in young children, pregnant or nursing women, or those with serious liver or kidney disease has not been determined.

## ⚠ INTERACTIONS YOU SHOULD KNOW ABOUT

If you are taking **sulfa antibiotics** such as **Bactrim** or **Septra,** do not take PABA supplements except on medical advice.

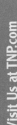

# PANTOTHENIC ACID AND PANTETHINE

*Principal Proposed Uses*
High triglycerides/high cholesterol

*Other Proposed Uses*
Rheumatoid arthritis, athletic performance, stress

*Supplement Forms/Alternative Names*
Pantothenic acid is often sold as calcium pantothenate. Pantethine, a special form of pantothenic acid, appears to have some unique properties. Regular pantothenic acid cannot be used as a substitute for pantethine.

The body uses pantothenic acid (better known as vitamin B5) to make proteins as well as other important chemicals needed to metabolize fats and carbohydrates. Pantothenic acid is also used in the manufacture of hormones, red blood cells, and *acetylcholine,* an important neurotransmitter (signal carrier between nerve cells). As a supplement, pantothenic acid has been proposed as a treatment for rheumatoid arthritis, an athletic performance enhancer, and an "antistress" nutrient.

In the body, pantothenic acid is converted to a related chemical known as pantethine. For reasons that are not clear, pantethine supplements (but not pantothenic acid supplements) appear to reduce levels of both triglycerides and cholesterol in the blood.

The supplement niacin, also called **vitamin B₃** (page 323), is generally more effective at lowering cholesterol than pantethine and far cheaper as well. However, whereas niacin can inflame the liver and possibly raise blood sugar in people with diabetes, pantethine has not been associated with these side effects.

## REQUIREMENTS/SOURCES

The word *pantothenic* comes from the Greek word meaning "everywhere," and pantothenic acid is indeed found in a wide range of foods. For this reason, pantothenic acid deficiency is rare. Although an exact daily requirement is not known, the Estimated Safe and Adequate Daily Dietary Intake is as follows

- Infants under 6 months, 2 mg
  6 to 12 months, 3 mg
- Children 1 to 3 years, 3 mg
  4 to 6 years, 3 to 4 mg
  7 to 10 years, 4 to 5 mg
- Adults (and children 11 years and older),
  4 to 7 mg

Brewer's yeast, torula (nutritional) yeast, and calf liver are excellent sources of pantothenic acid. Peanuts, mushrooms, soybeans, split peas, pecans, oatmeal, buckwheat, sunflower seeds, lentils, rye flour, cashews, and other whole grains and nuts are good sources as well, as are red chili peppers and avocados. Pantethine is not found in foods in appreciable amounts.

## THERAPEUTIC DOSAGES

For lowering cholesterol and triglycerides, the typical recommended dosage of pantethine is 300 mg 3 times daily. Dosages of pantothenic acid as high as 660 mg 3 times daily are sometimes recommended for people with arthritis.

## THERAPEUTIC USES

Quite a few small studies suggest that pantethine may lower blood levels of triglycerides and, to a lesser extent, **cholesterol** (page 39).[1,2,3] In general, elevated cholesterol is more harmful than elevated triglycerides. However, some people have only modestly elevated cholesterol but very high triglycerides, so pantethine may be especially useful for them. It also may be particularly helpful for people with diabetes who need to lower their triglyceride and/or cholesterol levels.[4–7]

Pantothenic acid has been proposed as a treatment for **rheumatoid arthritis** (page 109), but the evidence for this use is quite weak.[8,9]

Pantothenic acid is also recommended as an athletic performance enhancer, but there is no good evidence at all that it works. It is also sometimes referred to as an antistress nutrient because it plays a role in the function of the adrenal glands, but whether it really helps the body withstand stress is not known.

## WHAT IS THE SCIENTIFIC EVIDENCE FOR PANTOTHENIC ACID?

### High Triglycerides/High Cholesterol

Several small studies suggest (but do not prove) that pantethine can reduce total blood triglycerides and perhaps cholesterol as well.[10,11,12] For example, a double-blind placebo-controlled study followed 29 people with high cholesterol and triglycerides for 8 weeks.[13] The dosage used was 300 mg 3 times daily, for a total daily dose of 900 mg. In this study, subjects taking pantethine experienced a 30% reduction in blood triglycerides, a 13.5% reduction in LDL ("bad") cholesterol, and a 10% rise in HDL ("good") cholesterol. However, for reasons that are unclear, some studies have found no benefit.[14,15]

Several other studies have specifically studied the use of pantethine to improve cholesterol and triglyceride levels in people with diabetes and found it effective.[16–19]

These findings are supported by experiments in rabbits, which show that pantethine may prevent the buildup of plaque in major arteries.[20] We don't know how pantethine works in the body.

### Rheumatoid Arthritis

There is weak evidence for using pantothenic acid to treat rheumatoid arthritis. One observational study found 66 people with rheumatoid arthritis had less pantothenic acid in their blood than 29 healthy people. The more severe the arthritis, the lower the blood levels of pantothenic acid were.[21] However, this result doesn't prove that pantothenic acid supplements can effectively reduce any of the symptoms of rheumatoid arthritis.

To follow up on this finding, researchers then conducted a small placebo-controlled trial involving 18 subjects to see whether pantothenic acid would help. This study found that 2 g daily of pantothenic acid (in the form of calcium pantothenate) reduced morning stiffness, pain, and disability significantly better than placebo.[22] However, a study this small doesn't mean much on its own. More research is needed.

## SAFETY ISSUES

No significant side effects have been reported for pantothenic acid or pantethine, used by themselves or with other medications. However, maximum safe dosages for young children, pregnant or nursing women, or people with serious liver or kidney disease have not been established.

# PASSIONFLOWER (PASSIFLORA INCARNATA)

*Principal Proposed Uses*
Anxiety, insomnia, nervous stomach

The passionflower vine is a native of the Western hemisphere, named for symbolic connections drawn between its appearance and the crucifixion of Jesus. Native North Americans used passionflower primarily as a mild sedative. It quickly caught on as a folk remedy in Europe and was thereafter adopted by professional herbalists as a sedative and digestive aid.

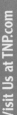

## WHAT IS PASSIONFLOWER USED FOR TODAY?

In 1985, Germany's Commission E officially approved passionflower as a treatment for "nervous unrest." The herb is considered to be a mildly effective treatment for **anxiety** (page 8) and **insomnia** (page 80), less potent than **kava** (page 239) and **valerian** (page 315), but nonetheless useful. Like **melissa** (page 260) (lemon balm), **chamomile** (page 156), and valerian, it is also used for nervous stomach.

Animal studies suggest that passionflower extracts can reduce agitation and prolong sleep. There have been no controlled double-blind studies of passionflower in humans, except in combination with other herbs.[1]

Several constituents of passionflower have been credited with causing its sedative effect. However, each has been proven ineffective when used alone. At the current state of knowledge, the best we can say is that we don't yet know how the herb works.

## DOSAGES

The proper dosage of passionflower is 1 cup 3 times daily of a tea made by steeping 1 teaspoon of dried leaves for 10 to 15 minutes. Passionflower tinctures and powdered extracts should be taken according to the label instructions.

## SAFETY ISSUES

Passionflower is on the FDA's GRAS (generally regarded as safe) list. Although the alkaloids harman and harmaline found in passionflower may increase the effects of drugs known as MAO inhibitors and also stimulate the uterus,[2] it seems unlikely that the normal use of passionflower produces the same effects. Passionflower might, however, increase the effect of sedative medications.[3]

Safety has not been established for pregnant or nursing mothers, very young children, or those with severe liver or kidney disease.

## ⚠ INTERACTIONS YOU SHOULD KNOW ABOUT

If you are taking

- **MAO inhibitors:** It is conceivable (but not likely) that passionflower could cause problems.

- **Sedative medications:** Passionflower might exaggerate their effect.

# PEPPERMINT (MENTHA PIPERITA)

*Principal Proposed Uses*
   Irritable bowel syndrome, coughs, colds, gallstones, candida

**P**eppermint is a relative of numerous wild mint plants, deliberately bred in the late 1600s in England to become the delightful tasting plant so well known today. It is widely used as a beverage tea and as a flavoring or scent in a wide variety of products.

Peppermint tea also has a long history of medicinal use, primarily as a digestive aid and for the symptomatic treatment of cough, colds, and fever. Peppermint oil is used for chest congestion (Vicks VapoRub), as a local anesthetic (Solarcaine, Ben-Gay), and most recently in the treatment of irritable bowel disease, also known as spastic colon.

## WHAT IS PEPPERMINT USED FOR TODAY?

Germany's Commission E authorizes the use of peppermint oil for treating colicky pain in the digestive tract, specifically **irritable bowel syndrome** (page 85), as well as for relieving mucus congestion of the lungs and sinuses caused by **colds and flus** (page 44).

Peppermint

Visit Us at TNP.com

There is also some evidence that it might be helpful for **gallstones** (page 68).[1] Peppermint is sometimes recommended for the treatment of **candida** (page 33) yeast infections, but there is as yet no real evidence that it works.

## WHAT IS THE SCIENTIFIC EVIDENCE FOR PEPPERMINT OIL?

The scientific record for peppermint oil in treating irritable bowel syndrome is contradictory.

Menthol is the primary ingredient in peppermint oil. Studies have found that it relaxes the muscles of the small intestine in dilutions as low as 1:20,000 and counters the effect of other drugs that cause intestinal spasm.[2,3,4]

Two preliminary double-blind studies, involving a total of 45 individuals with irritable bowel syndrome, found that peppermint can provide significant relief from crampy abdominal pain.[5,6] However, other studies, involving a total of more than 90 people, have found no significant improvement in symptoms.[7,8,9]

The most probable reason for these contradictory results is that peppermint oil is not terrifically effective. Also, the placebo effect is fairly strong in irritable bowel syndrome, making it hard to detect small improvements due to the actual effects of a medicine.

## DOSAGE

The proper dosage of peppermint oil when treating irritable bowel syndrome is 0.2 to 0.4 ml 3 times a day of an enteric-coated capsule. The capsule has to be enteric-coated to prevent stomach distress.

## SAFETY ISSUES

At the normal dosage, enteric-coated peppermint oil is believed to be reasonably safe in healthy adults.[10,11]

However, if you take too much, peppermint oil can be toxic, causing kidney failure and even death. Excessive intake of peppermint oil can also cause nausea, loss of appetite, heart problems, loss of balance, and other nervous system problems.

Safety in young children, pregnant or nursing women, or those with severe liver or kidney disease has not been established. In particular, peppermint can cause jaundice in newborn babies, so don't try to use it for colic.

A total of at least 200 people have participated in studies of peppermint oil, without any significant problems other than the usual occasional mild gastrointestinal distress or allergic reactions.[12]

# PHENYLALANINE

*Principal Proposed Uses*
    Depression

*Other Proposed Uses*
    Chronic pain (e.g., muscle pain, osteoarthritis, rheumatoid arthritis), vitiligo, attention deficit disorder

*Supplement Forms/Alternative Names*
    L-phenylalanine, D-phenylalanine, DL-phenylalanine

**P**henylalanine occurs in two chemical forms: *L-phenylalanine,* a natural amino acid found in proteins; and its mirror image, *D-phenylalanine,* a form synthesized in a laboratory. Some research has involved the L-form, others the D-form, and still others a combination of the two known as DL-phenylalanine.

In the body, phenylalanine is converted into another amino acid called tyrosine. Tyrosine in turn is converted into L-dopa, norepinephrine, and epinephrine, three key neurotransmitters (chemicals that transmit signals between nerve cells). Because some antidepressants work by raising levels of norepinephrine, various forms of phenylalanine have been tried as a possible treatment for depression.

D-phenylalanine (but not L-phenylalanine) has been proposed to treat chronic pain. It blocks *enkephalinase*, an enzyme that may act to increase pain levels in the body. Phenylalanine (various forms) has also been suggested as a treatment for vitiligo, a disease characterized by abnormal white blotches of skin due to loss of pigmentation.

## REQUIREMENTS/SOURCES

L-phenylalanine is an essential amino acid, meaning that we need it for life and our bodies can't manufacture it from other chemicals. It is found in protein-rich foods such as meat, fish, poultry, eggs, dairy products, and beans. Provided you eat enough protein, you are likely to get enough L-phenylalanine for your nutritional needs. There is no nutritional need for D-phenylalanine.

## THERAPEUTIC DOSAGES

When used as a treatment for depression, L-phenylalanine is typically started at a dosage of 500 mg daily, and then gradually increased to 3 to 4 g daily.[1] However, side effects may develop at dosages above 1,500 mg daily (see Safety Issues).

D- or DL-phenylalanine may be used for depression as well, but the typical dosage is much lower: 100 to 400 mg daily.[2]

For the treatment of chronic pain, usual recommended dosages of D-phenylalanine are as high as 2,500 mg daily.

It is best not to take your phenylalanine supplement at the same time as a high-protein meal, as it may not be absorbed well.

## THERAPEUTIC USES

Preliminary studies suggest that both the L- and D-forms of phenylalanine may be helpful for **depression** (page 54).[3,4]

Weak evidence suggests that D-phenylalanine may be useful for chronic pain,[5] such as **rheumatoid arthritis** (page 109), muscle pain, and **osteoarthritis** (page 95), but this conclusion has been contested.[6,7,8]

Phenylalanine is sometimes proposed as a treatment for vitiligo, but a double-blind study found *no* significant effect.[9]

Although it is sometimes proposed as a treatment for attention deficit disorder, phenylalanine taken alone does not appear to be helpful for **attention deficit disorder** (page 19).[10,11] Some proponents claim that it works better when combined with **tyrosine** (page 312), **glutamine** (page 215), and gamma-aminobutyric acid (GABA), but this has not been proven.

## WHAT IS THE SCIENTIFIC EVIDENCE FOR PHENYLALANINE?

### Depression

A pair of double-blind studies have found that D- or DL-phenylalanine is as effective as imipramine, a standard antidepressant drug, and that it may take effect much more quickly. The larger of the two studies compared the effectiveness of D-phenylalanine at 100 mg daily against the same daily dose of imipramine.[12] Sixty people with depression were randomly assigned to take either imipramine or D-phenylalanine for 30 days. The results in both groups were statistically equivalent, meaning that phenylalanine was about as effective as imipramine. D-phenylalanine worked more rapidly, however, producing significant improvement in only 15 days. Like most antidepressant drugs, imipramine requires several weeks to take effect.

The other double-blind study followed 27 individuals, half of whom received DL-phenylalanine (150 to 200 mg daily) and the other half imipramine (100 to 150 mg daily).[13] When they were reevaluated after 30 days, both groups had improved by a statistically equal amount. Very preliminary studies have also found benefits with L-phenylalanine.[14,15]

Unfortunately, there have been no good studies comparing any form of phenylalanine against placebo. This is too bad, since without such evidence we can't be sure that the supplement is actually effective.

### Chronic Pain

The use of D-phenylalanine to treat pain is primarily based on a study involving 43 individuals with chronic pain, mostly due to arthritis.[16]

However, this was not a double-blind study, and it suffered from other flaws as well.[17]

A small double-blind study reportedly found evidence for the effectiveness of D-phenylalanine,[18] but a careful look at the math involved undermined that conclusion.[19] Another small study found no benefits.[20]

## SAFETY ISSUES

Although most people do not report side effects from any type of phenylalanine, daily doses near or above 1,500 mg of L-phenylalanine can reportedly cause anxiety, headache, and even mildly elevated blood pressure.[21]

The long-term safety of phenylalanine in any of its forms is not known. Both L- and D-phenyl- alanine must be avoided by those with the rare metabolic disease phenylketonuria (PKU).

The safety of high dosages of L-phenylalanine, or any dosage of D-phenylalanine, has not been established for young children, pregnant or nursing women, or those with severe liver or kidney disease.

There are some indications that the combined use of phenylalanine with antipsychotic drugs might increase the risk of developing the long-term side effect known as tardive dyskinesia.[22,23]

## ⚠ INTERACTIONS YOU SHOULD KNOW ABOUT

If you are taking **antipsychotic medications,** do not use phenylalanine.

# PHOSPHATIDYLSERINE

*Principal Proposed Uses*
  Alzheimer's disease, age-related memory loss

*Other Proposed Uses*
  General improvement of mental performance, depression, enhancement of athletic training

Phosphatidylserine (fos-fah-TIDE-ul-ser-een), or PS for short, is a member of a class of chemical compounds known as *phospholipids*. PS is an essential component in all our cells; specifically, it is a major component of the cell membrane. The cell membrane is a kind of "skin" that surrounds living cells. Besides keeping cells intact, this membrane performs vital functions such as moving nutrients into cells and pumping waste products out of them. PS plays an important role in many of these functions.

Good evidence suggests that PS can help declining mental function and depression in the elderly, and it is widely used for this purpose in Italy, Scandinavia, and other parts of Europe. PS has also been marketed as a "brain booster" for people of all ages, said to sharpen memory and increase thinking ability.

Recently, PS has been marketed as a sports supplement, said to help bodybuilders and power athletes develop larger and stronger muscles.

## SOURCES

Your body makes all the PS it needs. However, the only way to get a therapeutic dosage of PS is to take a supplement.

PS was originally manufactured from the brains of cows, and all the studies described here used this form. However, because animal brain cells can harbor viruses, that form is no longer available, and most PS today is made from soybeans.

According to some experts, soy-based PS is just as effective as PS made from cows' brains.[1–5] However, not everyone agrees.[6]

Phosphatidylserine can also be manufactured from cabbage, but in one study the results with this form of the supplement were not impressive.[7]

## THERAPEUTIC DOSAGES

For the purpose of improving mental function, PS is usually taken in dosages of 100 mg 2 to 3 times daily. After maximum effect is achieved, the dosage can

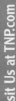

sometimes be reduced to 100 mg daily without losing benefit. PS can be taken with or without meals.

When taking PS for sports purposes, athletes may use as much as 800 mg daily.

## THERAPEUTIC USES

Impressive evidence from numerous double-blind studies suggests that PS is an effective treatment for **Alzheimer's disease** (page 4) and other forms of age-related mental decline.[8–17]

PS is widely marketed as a treatment for ordinary age-related memory loss, and there is some evidence that it might work. Keep in mind that in studies of severe mental decline, PS was equally effective whether the cause was Alzheimer's disease or something entirely unrelated (multiple small strokes). This certainly suggests that PS may have a positive impact on the brain that is not specific to any one condition. From this observation, it is not a great leap to suspect that it might make it useful for much less severe problems with memory and mental function, such as those that seem to occur in nearly all of us who are older than 40. Indeed one double-blind study did find that PS could improve mental function in individuals with relatively mild age-related memory loss.[18]

PS may also be helpful for **depression** (page 54).[19,20,21]

Recently, PS has become popular among athletes who hope it can help them build muscle more efficiently. This use is based on modest evidence that PS slows the release of cortisol following heavy exercise.[22,23] Cortisol is a hormone that causes muscle tissue to break down. For reasons that are unclear, the body produces increased levels of cortisol after heavy exercise. Strength athletes believe that this natural cortisol release works against their efforts to rapidly build muscle mass and hope that PS will help them advance more quickly. However, this idea has not been proven.

## WHAT IS THE SCIENTIFIC EVIDENCE FOR PHOSPHATIDYLSERINE?

### Alzheimer's Disease and Other Forms of Dementia

Overall, the evidence for PS is quite strong. Double-blind studies involving a total of over 1,000 people suggest that phosphatidylserine (at least the type from cow's brain) is an effective treatment for Alzheimer's disease and other forms of dementia.

The largest of these studies followed 494 elderly subjects in northeastern Italy over a course of 6 months.[24] All suffered from moderate to severe mental decline, as measured by standard tests. Treatment consisted of either 300 mg daily of PS or placebo. The group that took PS did significantly better in both behavior and mental function than the placebo group. Symptoms of depression also improved.

These results agree with those of numerous smaller double-blind studies involving a total of over 500 people with Alzheimer's and other types of age-related dementia.[25–32]

### Ordinary Age-Related Memory Loss

There is also some evidence that PS can help people with ordinary age-related memory loss. In one double-blind study that enrolled 149 individuals with memory loss but not dementia, PS provided significant benefits as compared to placebo.[33] Individuals with the most severe memory loss showed the most improvement.

### Athletic Performance

Weak evidence suggests that PS might decrease the release of the hormone cortisol after intense exercise.[34] Among its many effects, cortisol acts to break down muscle tissue—exactly the opposite of the effect desired by a strength athlete or bodybuilder. This double-blind placebo-controlled study on 11 intensely trained athletes found that 800 mg of PS taken daily reduced the cortisol rise by 20% as compared with placebo.[35] Another small study on 9 nonathletic males found that daily doses of 400 and 800 mg of PS reduced cortisol levels after exercise by 16% and 30%, respectively.[36]

However, there is as yet no direct evidence to support the claims that PS actually helps athletes build muscles more quickly and with less training effort.

### SAFETY ISSUES

Phosphatidylserine is generally regarded as safe when used at recommended dosages. Side ef-

Phosphatidylserine

Visit Us at TNP.com

fects are rare, and when they do occur they usually consist of nothing much worse than mild gastrointestinal distress.[37] However, the maximum safe dosages for young children, pregnant or nursing women, or those with severe liver or kidney disease have not been established.

PS is sometimes taken with **ginkgo** (page 204) because they both appear to enhance mental function. However, some caution might be in order: Ginkgo is a "blood thinner," and PS might be one as well. Together, the two supplements might interfere with normal blood clotting enough to cause problems. Although this is still hypothetical, we do have reason to believe that PS can enhance the effect of heparin, a very strong prescription blood thinner.[38]

Keep in mind, too, that Alzheimer's disease and other types of severe age-related mental impairment are too serious to treat on your own with PS or any other supplement. In some cases, the symptoms of these diseases may be a sign of other serious conditions. If you suspect that you or a loved one may have a severe age-related mental impairment, see your doctor for diagnosis and treatment.

## ⚠ INTERACTIONS YOU SHOULD KNOW ABOUT

If you are taking

- **Prescription blood thinners,** such as **heparin** or **Coumadin (warfarin):** Do not use phosphatidylserine except on a physician's advice.

- **Ginkgo:** Taking phosphatidylserine at the same time might conceivably "thin" the blood too much.

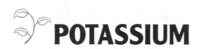

# POTASSIUM

*Principal Proposed Uses*
    Hypertension (high blood pressure)

*Supplement Forms/Alternative Names*
    Potassium chloride, potassium bicarbonate, chelated potassium (potassium aspartate, potassium citrate)

Potassium is a mineral found in many foods and supplements. But you will never see pure potassium in a health food store or pharmacy—it's a highly reactive metal that bursts into flame when exposed to water! The potassium you eat, or take as a supplement, is composed of potassium atoms bound to other nonmetallic substances—less exciting, perhaps, but chemically stable.

Potassium is one of the major *electrolytes* in your body, along with sodium and chloride. Potassium and sodium work together like a molecular seesaw: When the level of one goes up, the other goes down. All together, these three dissolved minerals play an intimate chemical role in every function of your body.

The most common use of potassium supplements is to make up for potassium depletion caused by diuretic drugs. These medications are often used to help regulate blood pressure, but by depleting the body of potassium they may inadvertently make blood pressure harder to control.

## REQUIREMENTS/SOURCES

Potassium is an essential mineral that we get from many common foods. A safe and adequate intake of potassium ranges from 1.9 g (for children) to 5.6 g (for adults) daily.

True potassium deficiencies are rare except in cases of prolonged vomiting or diarrhea, or with the use of diuretic drugs. Long-term use of corticosteroid drugs (such as prednisone) or colchicine can cause potassium depletion as well.

However, in one sense potassium deficiency is common, at least when compared to the amount of sodium we receive in our diets. It is probably healthy to take in at least five times as much potassium as sodium (and perhaps 50 to 100 times as much). But the standard American diet contains twice as much sodium as potassium. Therefore, taking extra potassium may be a good idea in order to balance the sodium we consume to such excess.

Bananas, orange juice, potatoes, avocados, lima beans, cantaloupes, peaches, tomatoes, flounder, salmon, and cod all contain more than 300 mg of potassium per serving. Other good sources include chicken, meat, and various other fruits, vegetables, and fish.

Over-the-counter potassium supplements typically contain 99 mg of potassium per tablet. There is some evidence that, of the different forms of potassium supplements, potassium citrate may be most helpful for those with high blood pressure.[1]

Research indicates that it is important to get enough **magnesium** (page 251), too, when you are taking potassium.[2] It might be wise to take extra **vitamin B$_{12}$** (page 329) as well.[3]

## THERAPEUTIC DOSAGES

When used by physicians, potassium is usually measured according to meqs (milliequivalents) rather than the more common mg (milligrams). A typical therapeutic dosage of potassium is between 10 and 20 meq (about 200 to 400 mg), taken 3 to 4 times daily.

## THERAPEUTIC USES

Potassium appears to be helpful for **hypertension** (page 75), especially among individuals who eat too much salt.[4,5]

Contrary to some reports, potassium supplements have not been found useful for preventing kidney stones. The substance potassium citrate might help for this purpose, but it is the citrate (not the potassium) that is believed to be active.[6,7]

## WHAT IS THE SCIENTIFIC EVIDENCE FOR POTASSIUM?

### High Blood Pressure

According to a review of 33 double-blind studies, potassium supplements can produce a slight but definite drop in blood pressure.[8] However, two large studies found *no* benefit.[9,10] The explanation is probably that potassium is only slightly helpful. When a treatment has only a small effect, it's not unusual for some studies to show no effect while others find a modest benefit. It's possible that potassium may only help people who are at least a bit deficient in this mineral.

Evidence suggests that potassium supplements may be most effective for people who eat too much salt.[11]

## SAFETY ISSUES

As an essential nutrient, potassium is safe when taken at appropriate dosages. If you take a bit too much, your body will simply excrete it in the urine. However, people who have severe kidney disease or are taking a type of medication called a "potassium-sparing diuretic" cannot excrete potassium normally, and should consult a physician before taking a potassium supplement. (For other drug interactions, see Interactions You Should Know About.)

Potassium pills can cause injury to the esophagus if they get stuck on the way down, so make sure to take them with plenty of water.

## ⚠ INTERACTIONS YOU SHOULD KNOW ABOUT

If you are taking

- **Diuretics** (other than potassium-sparing), **corticosteroids** (e.g., **prednisone**), **colchicine,** or **haloperidol:** You may need more potassium.

Potassium

Visit Us at TNP.com

- **ACE inhibitors** (e.g., **captopril, lisinopril, enalapril**), **potassium-sparing diuretics** (e.g., **triamterene,** or **spironolactone**): You should not take potassium except on the advice of a physician.

- **Tetracycline antibiotics:** You should take potassium supplements at a different time of day to avoid absorption problems.

- **Potassium:** You may need extra magnesium and vitamin B$_{12}$.

# PREGNENOLONE

## Principal Proposed Uses

There are no well-documented uses for pregnenolone.

## Other Proposed Uses

Memory enhancement, age-related hormone decline, Alzheimer's disease, menopausal symptoms, adrenal disease, Parkinson's disease, osteoporosis, fatigue, stress, depression, rheumatoid arthritis, nerve injury, weight loss

Pregnenolone has been called "the grandmother of all steroid hormones." The body manufactures it from cholesterol, and then uses it to make testosterone, cortisone, progesterone, estrogen, **DHEA** (page 176), **androstenedione** (page 124), aldosterone, and all other hormones in the "steroid" family.

One reason given for using pregnenolone is that the level of many of these hormones declines with age. By taking pregnenolone supplements, proponents say, you can keep all your hormones at youthful levels. However, pregnenolone levels themselves don't decline with age,[1] and there is no indication that taking extra pregnenolone will increase the levels of any other hormones. Furthermore, even if it did, that doesn't mean using pregnenolone is a great idea.

Steroid hormones are powerful substances, and they can cause harm as well as benefit. Long-term use of cortisone causes severe osteoporosis; estrogen can increase the risk of cancer; and anabolic steroids (used by athletes) may cause liver problems and stress the heart. We really have very little idea what long-term consequences the use of pregnenolone might entail.

Actually, it is ironic that pregnenolone is legally classified as a "dietary supplement" at all. Pregnenolone is not a nutrient. It is a drug, just as estrogen, cortisone, and aldosterone are drugs. I recommend not using it until we know more about what it really does.

## SOURCES

Pregnenolone is not normally obtained from foods. Your body manufactures it from cholesterol. Supplemental pregnenolone is made synthetically in a chemical laboratory from substances found in soybeans.

## THERAPEUTIC DOSAGES

A typical recommended dosage of pregnenolone is 30 mg daily, but some studies have used as much as 700 mg.

## THERAPEUTIC USES

If you browse the Internet or read health magazines, you'll find pregnenolone described as a treatment for an enormous list of health problems, including memory loss, **Alzheimer's disease** (page 4), **menopausal symptoms** (page 87), adrenal disease, Parkinson's disease, **osteoporosis** (page 100), fatigue, stress, **depression** (page 54), **rheumatoid arthritis** (page 109), and nerve injury. It is also supposed to help you lose weight, improve your brain power, and make you feel young again. However, like so many overhyped new supplements, there is very little scientific evidence for any of these uses.

Studies involving rats suggest that pregnenolone may enhance memory,[2,3] but there have been no human studies.

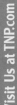

## SAFETY ISSUES

Pregnenolone is a powerful hormone, not a nutrient we would naturally get in our food. You should approach this supplement with caution, as if it were a drug—for all intents and purposes, it *is* a drug. It would be best to consult your doctor before taking it. Pregnenolone is definitely not recommended for children, pregnant or nursing women, or those with liver or kidney disease.

# PROTEOLYTIC ENZYMES

*Principal Proposed Uses*
Sports injuries, digestive aid

*Other Proposed Uses*
Food allergies, rheumatoid arthritis, autoimmune diseases, shingles (herpes zoster)

*Supplement Forms/Alternative Names*
Bromelain, papain, trypsin, chymotrypsin, pancreatin, "digestive enzymes"

Proteolytic enzymes help you digest the proteins in food. Although your body produces these enzymes in the pancreas, certain foods also contain proteolytic enzymes.

Papaya and pineapple are two of the richest plant sources, as attested by their traditional use as natural "tenderizers" for meat. Papain and **bromelain** (page 144) are the respective names for the proteolytic enzymes found in these fruits. The enzymes made in your body are called trypsin and chymotrypsin.

The primary use of proteolytic enzymes is as a digestive aid for people who have trouble digesting proteins. However, for reasons that are not clear, they also seem to help bruises and other traumas heal faster, which has made them popular in Europe as a treatment for sports injuries.

Many practitioners of alternative medicine believe that proteolytic enzymes can be helpful for a wide variety of other health conditions, especially food allergies and autoimmune diseases. However, there is little to no scientific evidence as yet that they really work for these problems.

## SOURCES

You don't need to get proteolytic enzymes from food, because the body manufactures them (primarily trypsin and chymotrypsin). However, deficiencies in proteolytic enzymes do occur, usually resulting from diseases of the pancreas. Symptoms include abdominal discomfort, gas, indigestion, poor absorption of nutrients, and passing undigested food in the stool.

For use as a supplement, trypsin and chymotrypsin are extracted from the pancreas of various animals. You can also purchase bromelain extracted from pineapple stems and papain made from papayas.

## THERAPEUTIC DOSAGES

When you purchase an enzyme, the amount is expressed not only in grams or milligrams but also in *activity units* or *international units*. These terms refer to the enzyme's potency (i.e., its digestive power). There is more than one way to measure this.

Bromelain dosages are measured in MCUs (milk-clotting units) or GDUs (gelatin-dissolving units). High-potency bromelain preparations contain at least 2,000 MCUs (or 1,333 GDUs) per gram. Some health authorities recommend taking 3,000 MCUs of bromelain 3 times daily.

Dosages of pancreatic extract are rated by an "X" factor: 5X pancreatin is five times stronger than a certain standard pancreatin preparation. If you use pancreatic enzyme extract, a dosage of 0.5 to 1.5 g of 9X pancreatin with each meal is probably sufficient. If you take a lower-strength formulation, you will need a higher dosage.

Proteolytic enzymes can be broken down by stomach acid. To prevent this from happening, supplemental enzymes are often coated with a substance that doesn't dissolve until it reaches the intestine. Such a preparation is called "enteric coated."

## THERAPEUTIC USES

The most obvious use of proteolytic enzymes is to assist digestion. In addition, some evidence suggests that they might be able to improve the rate of healing of sports injuries.[1,2] Other approaches include **OPCs (oligomeric proanthocyanidins)** (page 270) and **horse chestnut** (page 228). We don't really know how they work, but it probably isn't by affecting digestion. There is some evidence that proteolytic enzymes can be absorbed whole[3] and may produce a variety of effects in the body.

Proteolytic enzymes may also help reduce symptoms of food allergies, presumably by digesting the food so well that there is less to be allergic to.

Proteolytic enzymes have also been proposed as a treatment for **rheumatoid arthritis** (page 109) and other autoimmune diseases. Theoretically, these diseases may be made worse by whole proteins from foods leaking into the blood and causing an immune reaction. Digestive enzymes may help foil this so-called leaky gut problem. However, there is no real evidence as yet to substantiate this use. Another natural approach for this condition is the amino acid **glutamine** (page 215).

Finally, proteolytic enzymes are sometimes suggested for the treatment of the painful condition known as shingles (herpes zoster), but there is some evidence that they do not work.[4]

## WHAT IS THE SCIENTIFIC EVIDENCE FOR PROTEOLYTIC ENZYMES?

### Sports Injuries

Two small double-blind studies, involving a total of more than 50 athletes, found that treatment with proteolytic enzymes significantly speeded healing of bruises and other mild athletic injuries, as compared to placebo.[5,6]

## SAFETY ISSUES

Proteolytic enzymes are believed to be quite safe, although there are some concerns that they might further damage the exposed tissue in an ulcer (by partly digesting it). One proteolytic enzyme, pancreatin, may interfere with **folic acid** (page 194) absorption.[7]

## ⚠ INTERACTIONS YOU SHOULD KNOW ABOUT

If you take the proteolytic enzyme **pancreatin,** you may need extra folic acid.

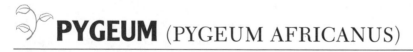

# PYGEUM (PYGEUM AFRICANUS)

*Principal Proposed Uses*
    Benign prostatic hyperplasia (prostate enlargement)

*Other Proposed Uses*
    Prostatitis (prostate infection), male impotence, infertility

The pygeum tree (pronounced pie-jee-um) is a tall evergreen native to central and southern Africa. Its bark has been used since ancient times to treat problems with urination.

## WHAT IS PYGEUM USED FOR TODAY?

Today, pygeum is primarily used as a treatment for **benign prostatic hyperplasia (BPH)** (page

20), or prostate enlargement, for which purpose it appears to be almost but not quite as effective as **saw palmetto** (page 295). It is more popular in France and Italy than in Germany.

However, saw palmetto is probably the better treatment to use. More is known about it, and furthermore the pygeum tree has been so devastated by collection for use in medicine that some regard it as a threatened species. Saw palmetto is cultivated rather than collected in the wild.

Like other herbs used for prostate problems, pygeum contains many active constituents that are believed to interact with hormones and also inhibit inflammation.[1]

Pygeum is also sometimes used to treat prostatitis, as well as **impotence** (page 77) and **infertility in men** (page 78).

**Note:** Before self-treating with pygeum, be sure to get a proper medical evaluation to rule out prostate cancer.

## WHAT IS THE SCIENTIFIC EVIDENCE FOR PYGEUM?

At least nine double-blind trials of pygeum have been performed, involving a total of over 600 people, and ranging in length from 45 to 90 days.[2] Overall, the results make a reasonably strong case that pygeum can reduce such symptoms as nighttime urination, urinary frequency and residual urine volume.

However, a comparison study with saw palmetto found that saw palmetto was more effective than pygeum.[3]

## DOSAGES

The proper dosage of pygeum is 50 to 100 mg twice a day of an extract standardized to contain 14% triterpenes and 0.5 percent n-docosanol. It is often sold at a lower dosage in combination with saw palmetto.

## SAFETY ISSUES

Pygeum appears to be essentially nontoxic, both in the short and long term.[4] The most common side effect is mild gastrointestinal distress. However, safety in young children, pregnant or nursing women, or those with severe liver or kidney disease has not been established.

# 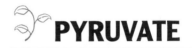 PYRUVATE

*Principal Proposed Uses*
  Weight reduction

*Other Proposed Uses*
  Enhancing athletic endurance

*Supplement Forms/Alternative Names*
  Sodium pyruvate, calcium pyruvate, potassium pyruvate, magnesium pyruvate, dihydroxyacetone pyruvate (DHAP)

Pyruvate supplies the body with pyruvic acid, a natural compound that plays important roles in the manufacture and use of energy. Pyruvate supplements have become popular with bodybuilders and other athletes, based on claims that pyruvate can reduce body fat and enhance the ability to use energy efficiently. However, there is very little evidence at the present time that it really works.

## SOURCES

Pyruvate is not an essential nutrient, since your body makes all it needs. But it can be found in food, with an average diet supplying anywhere from 100 mg to 2 g daily. Apples are the best source: A single apple contains about 450 mg of pyruvate. Beer and red wine contain about 75 mg per serving.

Therapeutic dosages are usually much higher than what you can get from food: You'd have to eat almost 70 apples a day to get the proper amount! To use pyruvate for therapeutic purposes, you must take a supplement.

Although most products on the market contain only (or almost only) pyruvate, some also contain small amounts of a related compound, dihydroxyacetone, which the body converts to pyruvate. The combination of the two products is known as DHAP.

## THERAPEUTIC DOSAGES

A typical therapeutic dosage of pyruvate is 30 g daily.

## THERAPEUTIC USES

Weak evidence (all from one group of researchers) suggests that pyruvate may enhance weight loss.[1,2,3] Even weaker evidence from the same researchers suggests that pyruvate may slightly increase an athlete's capacity for endurance exercise.[4,5] Unfortunately, these studies were all too small (mostly 10 people or less) for the results to mean very much.

## WHAT IS THE SCIENTIFIC EVIDENCE FOR PYRUVATE?

### Weight Reduction

In one double-blind placebo-controlled study, 34 people trying to lose weight were given either placebo or a dosage of pyruvate ranging from 22 to 44 g daily.[6] The treatment group lost significantly more weight.

Smaller studies have shown similar benefits.[7,8]

## SAFETY ISSUES

Both pyruvate and dihydroxyacetone appear to be quite safe, aside from mild side effects such as occasional stomach upset and diarrhea. However, maximum safe dosages for children, women who are pregnant or nursing, or those with liver or kidney disease have not been established.

Keep in mind that, because such enormous doses of pyruvate are used, if a contaminant were present even in very small percentages there could be harmful results. For this reason, you should make sure to use a high-quality product.

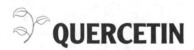

# QUERCETIN

*Principal Proposed Uses*
There are no well-documented uses for quercetin.

*Other Proposed Uses*
Allergies (hay fever), asthma, eczema, hives, heart disease prevention, stroke prevention, cancer prevention

*Supplement Forms/Alternative Names*
Quercetin chalcone

You may have heard of the "French paradox." The French diet is very high in fat and cholesterol (just think of *pâté de fois gras* and croissants), yet France has one of the world's lowest rates of heart disease. One theory for this discrepancy is that another major player in the French diet—red wine—protects the arteries of the heart.

A natural antioxidant found in red wine, quercetin protects cells in the body from damage by free radicals (naturally occurring but harmful substances). Heart disease and high cholesterol are thought to be at least partly caused by free radical damage to blood vessels, so it makes sense that quercetin might help protect against heart attacks and strokes. For information about a more proven antioxidant, see the chapter on **vitamin E** (page 337).

Quercetin belongs to a class of water-soluble plant coloring agents called *bioflavonoids,* a type of nutrient that we're learning more about all the time. Although they don't seem to be essential to life, it's likely that we need them for optimal health.

Another intriguing finding is that quercetin may help prevent immune cells from releasing *histamine,* the chemical that initiates the itching, sneezing, and swelling of an allergic reaction. Based on this very preliminary research, quercetin is often recommended as a treatment for allergies and asthma.

## SOURCES

Quercetin is not an essential nutrient. It is found in red wine, grapefruit, onions, apples, black tea and, in lesser amounts, in leafy green vegetables and beans. However, to get a therapeutic dosage, you'll have to take a supplement.

Quercetin supplements are available in pill and tablet form. One problem with them, however, is that they don't seem to be well absorbed by the body. A special form called quercetin chalcone appears to be better absorbed.

## THERAPEUTIC DOSAGES

A typical dosage is 200 to 400 mg 3 times daily. Quercetin may be better absorbed if taken on an empty stomach.

## THERAPEUTIC USES

The most popular use of quercetin is as a treatment for allergic conditions such as **asthma** (page 11), **hay fever** (page 3), **eczema** (page 66), and hives. This use is based on test-tube research showing that quercetin prevents certain

immune cells from releasing histamine, the chemical that triggers an allergic reaction.[1] It also may block other substances involved with allergies.[2] But we have no evidence as yet that taking quercetin supplements will reduce your allergy symptoms.

Very preliminary evidence also suggests that quercetin might help prevent **heart disease** (page 14) and strokes.[3–7]

Test-tube and animal research also suggests that quercetin might be able to help prevent tumors in hamsters[8] or enhance the effects of cancer-fighting drugs.[9,10] An animal study found that quercetin might protect rodents with diabetes from forming cataracts.[11] Another intriguing finding of test-tube research is that quercetin seems to prevent a wide range of viruses from infecting cells and reproducing once they are inside cells. One study found that quercetin produced this effect against herpes simplex, polio virus, flu virus, and respiratory viruses.[12,13] However, none of this research tells us whether humans taking quercetin supplements can hope for the same benefits. Much more research needs to be done on the use of quercetin for these conditions.

## SAFETY ISSUES

Quercetin appears to be quite safe. However, at one point concerns were raised that it might cause cancer. Quercetin "fails" a standard laboratory test called the Ames test, which is designed to identify chemicals that might be carcinogenic. However, a bad showing on the Ames test does not definitely mean a chemical causes cancer. Other evidence suggests that quercetin does *not* cause cancer, and may in fact help prevent cancer.[14,15] Maximum safe dosages for young children, women who are pregnant or nursing, or those with serious liver or kidney disease have not been established.

Quercetin

Visit Us at TNP.com

# RED CLOVER (TRIFOLIUM PRATENSE)

**Principal Proposed Uses**
Menopausal symptoms

**Other Proposed Uses**
Eczema, acne, psoriasis, cancer?

Red clover has been cultivated since ancient times, primarily to provide a favorite grazing food for animals. But, like many other herbs, red clover was also a valued medicine. Although it has been used for many purposes worldwide, the one condition most consistently associated with red clover is cancer. Chinese physicians and Russian folk healers also used it to treat respiratory problems.

In the nineteenth century, red clover became popular among herbalists as an "alterative" or "blood purifier." This medical term, long since defunct, refers to an ancient belief that toxins in the blood are the root cause of many illnesses. Cancer, eczema, and the eruptions of venereal disease were all seen as manifestations of toxic buildup.

Red clover was considered one of the best herbs to "purify" the blood. For this reason, it is included in many of the famous treatments for cancer, including the Hoxsey cancer cure (see Burdock) and Jason Winter's cancer-cure tea.

## WHAT IS RED CLOVER USED FOR TODAY?

Recently, an Australian product made from red clover has been marketed as a treatment for **menopausal symptoms** (page 87). It contains high concentrations of four major estrogen-like substances called **isoflavones** (page 236). Studies not yet published at the time of this writing have reportedly found good results.

There is no evidence that red clover can help cancer. However, its usage in many parts of the world as a traditional cancer remedy has prompted scientists to take a close look at the herb. It turns out that the isoflavones in red clover may possess antitumor activity.[1,2] However, such preliminary research does not prove that red clover can treat cancer.

Red clover is sometimes recommended for the treatment of **acne** (page 2), **eczema** (page 66), **psoriasis** (page 106), and other skin diseases.

## DOSAGES

A typical dosage of red clover is 2 to 4 g of dried flowers 3 times per day, until symptoms resolve.

## SAFETY ISSUES

Red clover is on the FDA's GRAS (generally regarded as safe) list, and is included in many beverage teas. However, detailed safety studies have not been performed. Concentrated extracts of red clover may possess dangers not present in beverage teas made from the raw herb. Because of their estrogen-like and blood-thinning constituents, red clover extracts should not be used by pregnant or nursing women, or women who have had breast or uterine cancer. Safety in young children, or those with severe liver or kidney disease also has not been established.

Based on their constituents, red clover extracts may conceivably interfere with hormone treatments and anticoagulant drugs.

## ⚠ INTERACTIONS YOU SHOULD KNOW ABOUT

If you are taking **hormones** (such as **oral contraceptives**) or **anticoagulants** (such as **Coumadin** or **heparin**), red clover should be used only under physician supervision.

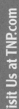

# RED RASPBERRY (RUBUS IDAEUS)

## Principal Proposed Uses
Prevent complications of pregnancy

Herbalists have long believed that raspberry leaf tea taken regularly during pregnancy can prevent complications and make delivery easier. Raspberry has also been used to reduce excessive menstruation and relieve symptoms of diarrhea.

## WHAT IS RED RASPBERRY USED FOR TODAY?

Red raspberry tea is still commonly recommended for pregnant women.

An interesting study suggests that red raspberry inhibits uterine contractions during pregnancy but not outside of pregnancy.[1] This naturally leads one to wonder whether raspberry leaf first stabilizes the uterus to prevent miscarriages and then somehow turns around and allows the uterus to relax for delivery. However, this is just speculation at the present time. If you take red raspberry during pregnancy, you are doing so based on long tradition, not on science.

## DOSAGES

To make raspberry leaf tea, pour 1 cup of boiling water over 1 or 2 teaspoons of dried leaf, steep for 10 minutes, and then sweeten to taste. Unlike many medicinal herbs, raspberry leaf actually has a pleasant taste! During pregnancy, drink 2 to 3 cups daily.

## SAFETY ISSUES

Strangely enough, the safety of red raspberry during pregnancy and nursing has not been established. Yet years of traditional use and the widespread availability of the beverage make it difficult to get very concerned. Safety in young children or those with severe liver or kidney disease has also not been established.

 # REISHI (GANODERMA LUCIDUM)

## Principal Proposed Uses
Adaptogen (improve resistance to stress), strengthen immunity against colds and other infections, improve mental function, prevent altitude sickness

## Other Proposed Uses
Asthma, bronchitis, viral hepatitis, cardiovascular disease, ulcers, cancer?

The tree fungus known as reishi has a long history of use in China and Japan as a semi-magical healing herb. More revered than ginseng and, up until recently, more rare, many stories tell of people with severe illnesses journeying immense distances to find it. Presently, reishi is artificially cultivated and widely available in stores that sell herb products.

## WHAT IS REISHI USED FOR TODAY?

Reishi is marketed as a cure-all, said to prevent and treat cancer, strengthen immunity against infection, restore normal immune function in autoimmune diseases (such as myasthenia gravis), improve symptoms of **asthma** (page 11) and bronchitis, overcome viral **hepatitis** (page 71), prevent and treat cardiovascular disease, improve mental function, heal ulcers (page 112), and prevent altitude sickness. However, there is no real evidence that reishi is effective for any of these conditions.

Contemporary herbalists regard it as an adaptogen, a substance believed to be capable of helping the body to resist stress of all kinds. For more information on adaptogens, see the discussion about them in the chapter on **ginseng** (page 206). However, while there has been a great deal of basic scientific research into the chemical constituents of reishi, reliable double-blind studies are lacking.

## DOSAGES

The proper dosage of reishi is 2 to 6 g per day of raw fungus, or an equivalent dosage of concentrated extract, taken with meals. Reishi is often combined with related fungi, such as shiitake, hoelen, or polyporus. Results may develop after about 1 to 2 weeks. It is often taken continually for its presumed overall health benefits.

## SAFETY ISSUES

Reishi appears to be extremely safe. Occasional side effects include mild digestive upset, dry mouth, and skin rash. Reishi can "thin" the blood slightly, and therefore should not be combined with drugs such as Coumadin (warfarin) or heparin. Safety in young children, pregnant or nursing women, or those with severe liver or kidney disease has not been established.

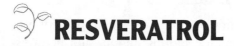

# RESVERATROL

*Principal Proposed Uses*
  There are no well-documented uses for resveratrol.

*Other Proposed Uses*
  Heart disease, cancer prevention

*Supplement Forms/Alternative Names*
  Grape skin

You may have heard of the "French paradox." The national diet of France includes a lot of butter, cream, meat, and other high-fat, high-cholesterol foods suspected to be bad for the heart. Yet France has one of the world's *lowest* rates of heart disease. The leading theory attempting to explain this puzzle suggests that the French are somehow protected from cardiovascular disease because they drink red wine.

Resveratrol is an ingredient of red wine that may be at least partly responsible for this beneficial effect. (**Quercetin** [page 288] is another such ingredient.) Resveratrol is a *polyphenol,* a natural antioxidant that protects cells against dangerous, naturally occurring substances known as free radicals.

Test-tube and observational studies have linked resveratrol to reduced rates of heart disease and cancer. Unfortunately, there hasn't been any clinical research on human beings yet, but the attention resveratrol has been getting via news stories on the "French Paradox" might lead to clinical studies in the near future.

## SOURCES

Resveratrol is not an essential nutrient. It is found in red wine as well as in red grape skins and seeds and purple grape juice. Peanuts also contain a small amount of resveratrol. Resveratrol supplements are available as well.

## THERAPEUTIC DOSAGES

Because there haven't been any clinical studies, the optimal therapeutic dosage hasn't been established for resveratrol. Based on animal studies, a reasonable therapeutic dosage of resveratrol might be about 500 mg daily.

## THERAPEUTIC USES

Very preliminary evidence suggests that resveratrol may help prevent **heart disease** (page 14),[1–4] although some studies have not been favorable.[5,6,7]

Test-tube studies also suggest that resveratrol might have a number of properties[8–12] that might make it helpful for preventing **cancer** (page 26).

## SAFETY ISSUES

Resveratrol appears to be quite safe according to the research done thus far, but full safety studies have not been performed. Maximum safe dosages for children, pregnant or nursing women, or those with severe liver or kidney disease have not been determined.

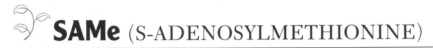

# SAMe (S-ADENOSYLMETHIONINE)

*Principal Proposed Uses*
Osteoarthritis, depression

*Other Proposed Uses*
Liver diseases, fibromyalgia

*Supplement Forms/Alternative Names*
Ademetionine, S-adenosylmethionine, SAM

**S**-*adenosylmethionine* is quite a mouthful; the abbreviation *SAMe* (pronounced "Sam") is easier to say. Its chemical structure and name are derived from two materials you may have heard about already: methionine, a sulfur-containing amino acid; and adenosine triphosphate (ATP), the body's main energy molecule.

SAMe was discovered in Italy in 1952. It was first investigated as a treatment for depression, but along the way it was accidentally noted to improve arthritis symptoms—a kind of positive "side effect." SAMe is presently classed with **glucosamine** (page 213) and **chondroitin** (page 159) as a potential "chondroprotective" agent, one that can go beyond treating symptoms to actually slowing the progression of arthritis. However, this exciting possibility has not yet been proven.

SAMe is also sometimes used by Italian physicians in the first weeks of conventional treatment for depression, because it is thought to act more quickly than certain antidepressant drugs.

Unfortunately, SAMe is at present an extraordinarily expensive supplement. Full dosages can easily cost more than $200 per month.

## SOURCES

The body makes all the SAMe it needs, so there is no dietary requirement. However, deficiencies in **methionine** (page 261), **folic acid** (page 194), or **vitamin B$_{12}$** (page 329) can reduce SAMe levels. SAMe is not found in appreciable quantities in foods, so it must be taken as a supplement. It's been suggested that the supplement **TMG** (page 310) might indirectly increase SAMe levels and provide similar benefits, but this effect has not been proven.

## THERAPEUTIC DOSAGES

A typical full dosage of SAMe is 400 mg taken 3 to 4 times per day. If this dosage works for you, take it for a few weeks and then try reducing the dosage. As little as 200 mg twice daily may suffice to keep you feeling better once the full dosage has "broken through" the symptoms.

However, some people develop mild stomach distress if they start full dosages of SAMe at once. To get around this, you may need to start low and work up to the full dosage gradually.

## THERAPEUTIC USES

A substantial amount of evidence suggests that SAMe can be an effective treatment for **osteoarthritis** (page 95), the "wear and tear" type of arthritis that many people develop as they get older.[1] However, the supplements glucosamine and chondroitin are much less expensive and just as well documented.

Several small studies also suggest that SAMe can be helpful for **depression** (page 54).[2]

This supplement may be helpful for certain liver conditions such as the jaundice of pregnancy and Gilbert's syndrome.[3–6]

SAMe may also help the painful muscle condition known as fibromyalgia.[7,8]

Intriguing new evidence suggests that SAMe might help medications for Parkinson's disease work better or with fewer side effects.[9]

## WHAT IS THE SCIENTIFIC EVIDENCE FOR SAMe?

Although there have been many studies of SAMe, a substantial percentage of them involved intravenous use of the supplement instead of the oral form. Here we discuss only the evidence for SAMe when it is taken orally.

### Osteoarthritis

A great deal of good scientific evidence supports the use of SAMe to treat osteoarthritis.[10] Double-blind studies involving a total of more than a thousand participants suggest that SAMe is about as effective as standard anti-inflammatory drugs.

For example, a double-blind placebo-controlled Italian study tracked 732 people taking SAMe, naproxen (a standard anti-inflammatory drug), or placebo.[11] After 4 weeks, participants taking SAMe or naproxen showed about the same level of benefit as compared with those in the placebo group.

However, it should be noted that the dosage of naproxen used in this study was definitely on the low side, only 750 mg daily. This is about half the amount most people would use for arthritis. If a normal dosage of naproxen had been used, the therapeutic effect would probably have been greater, and the drug might have proven more effective. Therefore, this study alone does not prove that SAMe is as effective as conventional treatment when taken in proper doses.

Another double-blind study compared SAMe with a full dosage of a different anti-inflammatory drug, piroxicam.[12] A total of 45 individuals were followed for 84 days. The two treatments proved equally effective. However, the SAMe-treated individuals maintained their improvement long after the treatment was stopped, whereas those on piroxicam quickly started to hurt again. Similarly long-lasting results have been seen with glucosamine and chondroitin, and suggest that these treatments are somehow making a deeper impact on osteoarthritis than simply relieving symptoms.

In other double-blind studies, oral SAMe has also shown equivalent benefits to various doses of indomethacin, ibuprofen, and naproxen.[13,14,15]

### Depression

SAMe's antidepressant activity was first reported in 1976.[16] Since then, several small double-blind studies involving a total of about 175 individuals have found oral SAMe to be an effective treatment for depression.[17–22] Some of these studies compared SAMe with placebo, while others used a control group given another antidepressant drug. Unfortunately, none enrolled enough participants to provide definitive evidence that SAMe is effective.

We need some large, long-term, placebo-controlled studies to know for sure whether this expensive supplement really works.

## SAFETY ISSUES

SAMe appears to be quite safe, according to both human and animal studies.[23–26] The most common side effect is mild digestive distress. However, SAMe does not actually damage the stomach.[27]

Like other substances with antidepressant activity, SAMe might trigger a manic episode in those with bipolar disease (manic-depressive illness).[28,29,30]

Safety in young children, pregnant or nursing women, or those with severe liver or kidney disease has not been established.

There may be risks involved in combining SAMe with standard antidepressants.[31] Consult your doctor before combining SAMe with any antidepressant medication.

## ⚠ INTERACTIONS YOU SHOULD KNOW ABOUT

If you are taking

- **Standard antidepressants:** Do not take SAMe except on a physician's advice.

- **Medications for manic-depressive disease:** Do not take SAMe except on a physician's advice.

- **Drugs that are "excreted by conjugation":** It is possible that use of SAMe may require you to increase your medication dose.[32] Ask your pharmacist for advice.

- **Levodopa** for Parkinson's disease: SAMe might help it work better.

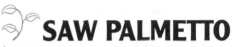

# SAW PALMETTO
## (SERENOA REPENS OR SABAL SERRULATA)

*Principal Proposed Uses*
Benign prostatic hyperplasia (prostate enlargement)

*Other Proposed Uses*
Prostatitis (prostate infection)

Saw palmetto is a native plant of North America, and although Europeans are its principal consumers, it is still primarily grown in the United States.

The saw palmetto tree grows only about 2 to 4 feet high, with fan-shaped serrated leaves and abundant berries. Native Americans used these berries for the treatment of various urinary problems in men, as well as for women with breast disorders. European and American physicians took up saw palmetto as a treatment for benign prostatic hyperplasia (BPH), but in the United States the herb ultimately fell out of favor, along with all other herbs.

European interest endured, and in the 1960s, French researchers discovered that by concentrating the oils of saw palmetto berry they could maximize the herb's effectiveness.

Saw palmetto contains many biologically active chemicals. Unfortunately, we don't know which ones are the most important. We also don't really know how saw palmetto works, although it appears to interact with various sex hormones.

## WHAT IS SAW PALMETTO USED FOR TODAY?

Saw palmetto oil is an accepted medical treatment for **benign prostatic hyperplasia** (page 20) in New Zealand, France, Germany, Austria, Italy, Spain, and other European countries. In some countries it is regarded as the "gold standard" against which new prostate drugs must prove themselves!

Typical symptoms of BPH include difficulty starting urination, weak urinary stream, frequent urination, dribbling after urination, and waking up several times at night to urinate. Research suggests that saw palmetto can markedly improve all these symptoms. Benefits require approximately 4 to 6 weeks of treatment to develop and endure for at least 3 years. It appears that about two-thirds of men respond reasonably well.

Furthermore, while the prostate tends to continue to grow when left untreated,[1] saw palmetto causes a small but definite shrinkage.[2,3] In other words, it isn't just relieving symptoms, but may actually be retarding prostate enlargement. The drug

Saw Palmetto

Visit Us at TNP.com

Proscar does this too (and to even a greater extent than saw palmetto) but other standard medications for BPH have no effect on prostate size.

Research tells us that saw palmetto is equally effective to Proscar, but it has one great advantage: It leaves PSA (prostate-specific antigen) levels unchanged. Cancer raises PSA levels, and lab tests that measure PSA are used to screen for prostate cancer. Because Proscar lowers PSA measurements, its use may have the unintended effect of masking prostate cancer. Saw palmetto won't do this. On the other hand, Proscar has been shown to reduce the need for surgery, unlike saw palmetto or any of the other drugs used for BPH.

**Note:** Before self-treating with saw palmetto, be sure to get a proper medical evaluation to rule out prostate cancer.

Saw palmetto is also widely used to treat chronic prostatitis, but its effectiveness in this regard has not been documented.

For more information on saw palmetto, see *The Natural Pharmacist Guide to Saw Palmetto and the Prostate.*

## WHAT IS THE SCIENTIFIC EVIDENCE FOR SAW PALMETTO?

The science for the effectiveness of saw palmetto in treating prostate enlargement is quite strong, although it could stand to improve.

At least seven double-blind studies involving a total of about 500 people have compared the benefits of saw palmetto against placebo over a period of 1 to 3 months.[4–10] In these studies, the herb significantly improved urinary flow rate and most other measures of prostate disease.[11] Only one study failed to find any benefit. This is fairly impressive, but it would be nice to have a long-term (6 months to 1 year) study of saw palmetto versus placebo.

A double-blind study followed 1,098 men who received either saw palmetto or the drug Proscar over a period of 6 months (unfortunately, there was no placebo group).[12] The treatments were equally effective, but while Proscar lowered PSA levels and caused a slight worsening of sexual function on average, saw palmetto caused no significant side effects.

A recent study involving 435 men found that the benefits of saw palmetto endure for at least 3 years.[13,14] However, there was no control group in this study, making the results unreliable.

## DOSAGES

The standard dosage of saw palmetto is 160 mg twice a day of an extract standardized to contain 85 to 95% fatty acids and sterols. A single daily dose of 320 mg seems to be just as effective.[15] However, taking more than this amount does not seem to produce better results.[16]

## SAFETY ISSUES

Saw palmetto appears to be essentially non-toxic.[17] It is also nearly side-effect free. In a 3-year study only 34 of the 435 participants complained of side effects—primarily the usual mild gastrointestinal distress.[18] There are no known drug interactions.

Safety for those with severe kidney or liver disease has not been established.

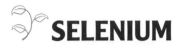

# SELENIUM

## Principal Proposed Uses
Cancer prevention

## Other Proposed Uses
AIDS, acne, cataracts, heart disease, multiple sclerosis, cervical dysplasia, asthma, rheumatoid arthritis, anxiety, gout, infertility in men, psoriasis, ulcers, osteoarthritis

## Supplement Forms/Alternative Names
Selenite, selenomethionine, selenized yeast, selenium dioxide

**S**elenium is a trace mineral that our bodies use to produce *glutathione peroxidase,* an enzyme that serves as a natural antioxidant. Glutathione peroxidase works with vitamin E to protect cell membranes from damage caused by dangerous, naturally occurring substances known as free radicals.

You may have heard that China has very low rates of colon cancer, presumably because of the nation's lowfat diet. However, in some parts of China where the soil is depleted of selenium, the incidence of various types of cancer is much higher than in the rest of the country. This fact has given rise to a theory that selenium deficiency is a common cause of cancer, and that selenium supplements can reduce this risk.

As we will see, there is some real evidence that selenium supplements can provide some protection against several types of cancer. This "chemopreventive" effect isn't fully understood. It might be due to the protective effects of the antioxidant glutathione peroxidase, but other explanations have also been suggested.[1,2]

## REQUIREMENTS/SOURCES

The U.S. Recommended Dietary Allowance for selenium is as follows

- Infants under 6 months, 10 mcg
  6 to 12 months, 15 mcg

- Children 1 to 6 years, 20 mcg
  7 to 10 years, 30 mcg

- Males 11 to 14 years, 40 mcg
  15 to 18 years, 50 mcg
  19 years and older, 70 mcg

- Females 11 to 14 years, 45 mcg
  15 to 18 years, 50 mcg
  19 years and older, 55 mcg

- Pregnant women, 65 mcg

- Nursing women, 75 mcg

Studies suggest that many people in developed countries do not get enough selenium in their diets.[3]

Foods containing significant amounts of selenium include wheat germ, Brazil nuts, other nuts, oats, whole-wheat bread, bran, red Swiss chard, brown rice, turnips, garlic, barley, and orange juice.

However, even these foods won't give you an adequate intake if the soil they were grown in was poor in selenium. Unfortunately, most of us have no way of knowing what kind of soil our food was grown in, so supplements may be a good idea.

The two general types of selenium supplements available to consumers are organic and inorganic. These terms have a very specific chemical meaning and have nothing to do with "organic" foods. In chemistry, organic means a substance's chemical structure includes carbon. Inorganic chemicals have no carbon atoms.

The inorganic form of selenium, selenite, is essentially selenium atoms bound to oxygen. Some research suggests that selenite is harder for the body to absorb than organic forms of selenium, such as selenomethionine (selenium bound to methionine, an essential amino acid) or high-selenium yeast (which contains selenomethionine).[4,5] However, other research on both animals and humans suggests that selenite supplements are almost as good as organic forms of selenium.[6,7]

Treatment with corticosteroids may induce selenium deficiency.[8]

## THERAPEUTIC DOSAGES

In controlled trials of selenium, a typical dosage was 100 to 200 mcg daily, in the same ballpark as nutritional doses.

## THERAPEUTIC USES

Impressive evidence indicates that supplemental selenium may help prevent **cancer** (page 26).[9–14] Based on what science knows about antioxidants in general, selenium has been proposed as a preventive measure or treatment for AIDS, **acne** (page 2), **cataracts** (page 37), **heart disease** (page 14), multiple sclerosis, **cervical dysplasia** (page 38), **asthma** (page 11), and **rheumatoid arthritis** (page 109). Besides the antioxidant rationale, people with these conditions often have lower-than-normal tissue levels of selenium. This suggests that selenium supplements might be a good treatment for these conditions. However, it is definitely not proof, and in the case of rheumatoid arthritis at least, there's some evidence that selenium supplements *don't* help.[15]

Selenium has also been recommended for many other conditions, including **anxiety** (page 8), **gout** (page 69), **infertility in men** (page 78), **psoriasis** (page 106), and **ulcers** (page 112), and **osteoarthritis** (page 95), but there is no real evidence as yet that it really works.

## WHAT IS THE SCIENTIFIC EVIDENCE FOR SELENIUM?

### Cancer Prevention

A large body of evidence has found that increased intake of selenium is tied to a reduced risk of cancer. The most important blind study on selenium and cancer was a double-blind intervention trial conducted by researchers at the University of Arizona Cancer Center. In this trial, which began in 1983, 1,312 individuals were divided into two groups. One group received 200 mcg of yeast-based selenium daily;

the other received placebo.[16] The researchers were trying to determine whether selenium could lower the incidence of skin cancers.

Although they found no benefit for skin cancer, they saw dramatic declines in the incidence of several other cancers in the selenium group. For ethical reasons, researchers felt compelled to stop the study after several years and allow all participants to take selenium.

When all the results were tabulated, it became clear that the selenium-treated group developed almost 66% fewer prostate cancers, 50% fewer colorectal cancers, and about 40% fewer lung cancers as compared with the placebo group. (All these results were statistically significant.) Selenium-treated subjects also experienced a statistically significant (17%) decrease in overall mortality, a greater than 50% decrease in lung cancer deaths, and nearly a 50% decrease in total cancer deaths.

Further evidence for the anticancer benefits of selenium comes from large-scale Chinese studies showing that giving selenium supplements to people who live in selenium-deficient areas reduces the incidence of cancer.[17]

Also, observational studies have indicated that cancer deaths rise when dietary intake of selenium is low.[18,19]

The results of animal studies corroborate these results. One recent animal study examined whether two experimental organic forms of selenium would protect laboratory rats against chemically induced cancer of the tongue.[20] Rats were given one of three treatments: 5 parts per million of selenium in their drinking water, 15 parts per million of selenium, or placebo. The study was blinded so that the researchers wouldn't know until later which rats received which treatment. Whereas 47% of rats in the placebo group developed tongue tumors, none of the rats that were given the higher selenium dosage developed tumors.

Another study examined whether selenium supplements could stop the spread (metastasis) of cancer in mice. In this study, a modest dosage of supplemental selenium reduced metastasis by 57%.[21] Even more significant was the decrease in the number of tumors that had spread to the lungs: Mice in the control group had an average

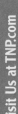

of 53 tumors *each,* whereas mice fed supplemental selenium had an average of *one* lung tumor.

Putting all this information together, it definitely appears that selenium can help reduce the risk of developing cancer.

## SAFETY ISSUES

Selenium is safe when taken at the recommended dosages. However, very high selenium dosages, above 900 mcg daily, are known to cause selenium toxicity. Signs of selenium toxicity include depression, nervousness, emotional instability, nausea, vomiting, and in some cases loss of hair and fingernails.

## ⚠ INTERACTIONS YOU SHOULD KNOW ABOUT

If you are taking **corticosteroids** (such as **prednisone**), you may need extra selenium.

# SITOSTEROL (FROM *HYPOXIS ROOPERI*)

*Principal Proposed Uses*
  Benign prostatic hyperplasia (prostate enlargement)

*Other Proposed Uses*
  General health benefits

The South African plant *Hypoxis rooperi* has a long history of native use for treating bladder and prostate problems. Its tubers contain a family of cholesterol-like compounds called beta-sitosterols, of which the most important is believed to be beta-sitosterolin. It binds to prostate tissue and affects the metabolism of prostaglandins, substances found in the body that affect pain and inflammation.[1] However, it is not clear whether this is the correct explanation of how sitosterol works or merely an interesting finding.

## WHAT IS SITOSTEROL USED FOR TODAY?

For some reason, there seem to be more useful herbal treatments for **benign prostatic hyperplasia** (page 20) (BPH), or prostate enlargement, than any other disease (except perhaps varicose veins)! Sitosterol joins saw palmetto, nettles, and pygeum as a documented treatment for BPH.

Based on preliminary evidence, it has been suggested that sitosterols may also offer general health benefits, in particular strengthening the immune system.[2] Sitosterols may eventually take their place alongside flavonoids and carotenes as beneficial substances found in food that aren't essential for life but may enhance overall health. However, more research needs to be done.

## WHAT IS THE SCIENTIFIC EVIDENCE FOR SITOSTEROL?

One well-designed double-blind placebo-controlled study followed 200 men with BPH for a period of 6 months.[3] Those treated with sitosterol showed significant improvement in many symptoms of prostate enlargement. Smaller studies corroborate these results.[4]

## DOSAGES

The daily dosage of sitosterols should supply 60 to 130 mg of beta-sitosterol. Full effects may take 6 months to develop.

## SAFETY ISSUES

Although detailed safety studies have not been performed, sitosterol is believed to be safe. No significant side effects or drug interactions have been reported.[5]

# SKULLCAP (SCUTELLARIA LATERIFLORA)

## Principal Proposed Uses

Anxiety, insomnia, drug and alcohol withdrawal

Native Americans as well as traditional European herbalists used skullcap to induce sleep, relieve nervousness, and moderate the symptoms of epilepsy, rabies, and other diseases related to the nervous system. In other words, skullcap was believed to function as an herbal sedative.

A relative of skullcap, *Scutellaria baicalensis*, is a common Chinese herb. However, the root instead of the above-ground plant is used, and overall effects appear to be far different. The discussion below addresses European skullcap (*Scutellaria lateriflora*) only.

## WHAT IS SKULLCAP USED FOR TODAY?

Skullcap is still popular as a sedative. Unfortunately, there has been virtually no scientific investigation of how well the herb really works. In practice, skullcap seems to produce a mild calming effect, generally not as strong as that of the herb **kava** (page 239), but enough to be helpful at times. It appears to take the edge off mild **anxiety** (page 8) and make falling asleep easier for those troubled by **insomnia** (page 80). Skull-cap is also sometimes used to ease drug or alcohol withdrawal.

## DOSAGES

When taken by itself, the usual dosage of skullcap is approximately 1 to 2 g, 3 times a day. However, skullcap is more often taken in combination with other sedative herbs such as **valerian** (page 315), **passionflower** (page 276), **hops** (page 227), and **melissa** (page 260), also called lemon balm. When using an herbal combination, follow the label instructions for dosage. Skullcap is usually not taken long term.

## SAFETY ISSUES

Not much is known about the safety of skullcap. However, if you take too much, it can cause confusion and stupor.[1] There have been reports of liver damage following consumption of products labeled skullcap; however, since skullcap has been known to be adulterated with germander, an herb toxic to the liver, it may not have been the skullcap that was at fault. Safety in young children, pregnant or nursing women, or those with severe liver or kidney disease has not been established.

# SLIPPERY ELM (ULMUS RUBRA, ULMUS FULVA)

## Principal Proposed Uses

Coughs, irritated digestion, irritable bowel syndrome, hemorrhoids

The dried inner bark of the slippery-elm tree was a favorite of many Native American tribes, and was subsequently adopted by European colonists. Like **marshmallow** (page 256) and **mullein** (page 264), slippery elm was used as a treatment for sore throat, coughs, dryness of the lungs, wounds, skin inflammations, and irritations of the digestive tract.[1] It was also made into a kind of porridge to be taken by weaned infants and during convalescence from illness: Various heroes of the Civil War are said to have credited slippery elm with their recovery from war wounds.

## WHAT IS SLIPPERY ELM USED FOR TODAY?

Slippery elm has not been scientifically studied to any significant extent. It's primarily used today as a cough lozenge, widely available in pharmacies. Based on its soothing properties, slippery elm is also sometimes recommended for treating **irritable bowel syndrome** (page 85), inflammatory bowel disease (such as Crohn's disease and ulcerative colitis), gastritis, esophageal reflux (heartburn), and **hemorrhoids** (page 70).

## DOSAGE

Suck cough lozenges as needed. For digestive disorders, make a porridge of slippery elm sweetened with honey and eat as desired, or take 500 to 1,000 mg of capsulized powder 3 times daily.

## SAFETY ISSUES

Other than occasional allergic reactions, slippery elm has not been associated with any toxicity. However, its safety has never been formally studied. Safety in young children, pregnant or nursing women, or those with severe liver or kidney disease has not been established.

 # SOY PROTEIN (SEE ALSO ISOFLAVONES)

*Principal Proposed Uses*
High cholesterol

*Other Proposed Uses*
Menopausal symptoms, reducing breast cancer risk

*Supplement Forms/Alternative Names*
Soy protein extract, hydrolyzed soy protein

The soybean has been prized for centuries in Asia as a nutritious, high-protein food with myriad uses, and today it's popular in the United States not only in Asian food but also as a cholesterol-free meat and dairy substitute in traditional American foods. Soy burgers, soy yogurt, tofu hot dogs, and tofu cheese can be found in a growing number of grocery stores alongside the traditional white blocks of tofu.

Several elements in soybeans, including soy protein, have been studied for possible health benefits. Soy protein appears to reduce blood cholesterol levels, and the U.S. Food and Drug Administration has proposed allowing soy protein foods to carry a "heart-healthy" label.

In addition to protein, soybeans contain chemicals that are similar to estrogen. These may be the active ingredient in soy protein formulations,[1] although we don't know for sure. They are described in the chapter on **isoflavones** (page 236).

## SOURCES

If you like Japanese, Chinese, Thai, or Vietnamese food, it's easy to get a healthy dose of soy protein. Tofu is one of the world's most versatile foods. It can be stir-fried, steamed, or added to soup. You can also mash a cake of tofu and use it in place of ricotta cheese in your lasagna. If you don't like tofu, there are many other soy products to try: plain soybeans, soy cheese, soy burgers, soy milk, or tempeh. Or you can use a soy protein supplement instead.

## THERAPEUTIC DOSAGES

The FDA has proposed a daily intake of 25 g of soy protein to reduce cholesterol. This amount is typically found in about 2½ cups of soy milk or ½ pound of tofu. Studies have used dosages of up to 40 g daily.

## THERAPEUTIC USES

According to the combined evidence of 38 controlled studies, soy protein can reduce blood **cholesterol** (page 39) levels and improve the ratio of LDL ("bad") versus HDL ("good") cholesterol.[2] At an average dosage of 47 g daily, total cholesterol falls by about 9%, LDL cholesterol by 13%, and triglycerides by 10%. Soy protein's effects on HDL cholesterol itself are less impressive.

Soy protein also seems to reduce the common **menopausal symptom** (page 87) known as "hot flashes."[3] Unlike estrogen, soy appears to reduce the risk of uterine **cancer** (page 26).[4] Its effect on breast cancer is not as well established, but there are reasons to believe that soy can help reduce breast cancer risk as well.[5] The **isoflavones** (page 236) in soy are very likely responsible for these benefits.

## WHAT IS THE SCIENTIFIC EVIDENCE FOR SOY PROTEIN?

### High Cholesterol

In 1995, a review of all studies performed to date on soy protein and heart disease concluded that soy is definitely effective at reducing total cholesterol, LDL ("bad") cholesterol, and triglycerides.[6]

A more recent double-blind study involving 66 older women found improvements in HDL ("good") cholesterol as well.[7] The women were divided into three groups. The first group received 40 g of skim milk protein daily. The second group was given the same amount of soy protein, and the third received 40 g of soy protein with extra soy isoflavones. Compared with the skim milk (placebo) group, both soy groups showed significant improvements in both total cholesterol and HDL cholesterol.

One benefit from eating soy protein is that, unlike most other sources of protein, it contains no fat. However, soy produces benefits above and beyond substituting for less healthful forms of protein.[8]

### Menopausal Symptoms ("Hot Flashes")

Soy protein seems to relieve "hot flashes," a common symptom of menopause. A double-blind placebo-controlled study involving 104 women found that soy protein provided significant relief compared to placebo (milk protein). After 3 weeks, the women taking daily doses of 60 g of soy protein were having 26% fewer hot flashes.[9] By week 12, the reduction was 45%. Women taking placebo also experienced a big improvement by week 12 (30% fewer hot flashes), but soy gave significantly better results.

For more information on soy and menopausal symptoms, see *The Natural Pharmacist Guide to Menopause*.

## SAFETY ISSUES

As a food that has been eaten for centuries, soy protein is believed to be quite safe. However, the isoflavones in soy could conceivably have some potentially harmful hormonal effects in certain specific situations. In particular, we don't know if high doses of soy are safe for women who have already had breast cancer (for more information, see the chapter on isoflavones). They may also interact with hormone medications.

## ⚠ INTERACTIONS YOU SHOULD KNOW ABOUT

If you are taking

- **Zinc, iron,** or **calcium supplements:** It may be best to eat soy at a different time of day to avoid absorption problems.[10,11,12]

- **Oral contraceptives:** It is possible that soy might interfere with their effects.

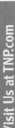

# STEVIA (STEVIA REBAUDIANA)

## Principal Proposed Uses
Sweetener

This member of the *Aster* family has a long history of native use in Paraguay as a sweetener for teas and foods. It contains a substance known as stevioside that is 100 to 300 times sweeter than sugar, but provides no calories.[1]

In the early 1970s, a consortium of Japanese food manufacturers developed stevia extracts for use as a zero-calorie sugar substitute. Subsequently, stevia extracts became a common ingredient in Asian soft drinks, desserts, chewing gum, and many other food products. Extensive Japanese research has found stevia to be extremely safe. However, there have not been enough U.S. studies for the FDA to approve stevia as a sugar substitute. Without identifying it as such, stevia is nonetheless widely used by savvy manufacturers to sweeten commercial beverage teas and other products.

## WHAT IS STEVIA USED FOR TODAY?

Although some people have claimed that stevia can help regulate blood sugar, the evidence for such an effect is negligible. This dietary supplement is primarily useful as a sweetening agent.

## DOSAGES

Stevia is sold as a powder to be added to foods as needed for appropriate sweetening effects. It tastes slightly bitter if placed directly in the mouth, but in liquids this is generally not noticeable, and most people find the taste delightfully unique.

## SAFETY ISSUES

Neither animal tests nor the extensive Japanese experience with stevia have uncovered any significant adverse effects.[2,3] However, safety in young children, pregnant or nursing women, or those with severe liver or kidney disease has not been established.

St. John's Wort

# ST. JOHN'S WORT (HYPERICUM PERFORATUM)

## Principal Proposed Uses
Mild to moderate depression

## Other Proposed Uses
Anxiety associated with depression, insomnia associated with depression, seasonal affective disorder (SAD)

## Probably Ineffective Uses
Viral diseases

St. John's wort is a common perennial herb of many branches and bright yellow flowers that grows wild in much of the world. Its name derives from the herb's tendency to flower around the feast of St. John. (A "wort" is simply a plant in Old English.) The species name *perforatum* derives from the watermarking of translucent dots that can be seen when the leaf is held up to the sun.

St. John's wort has a long history of use in treating emotional disorders. During the Middle Ages, St. John's wort was popular for "casting out demons," conceivably an archaic description of curing mental illness. In the 1800s, the herb was classified as a "nervine," or a treatment for "nervous disorders." It began to be considered a treatment for depression in the early 1900s, and when pharmaceutical antidepressants were invented, German researchers began to look for similar properties in St. John's wort.

Today, St. John's wort is one of the best-documented herbal treatments, with a scientific record approaching that of many prescription drugs. Indeed, this herb *is* a prescription antidepressant in Germany, covered by the national health-care system, and is prescribed more frequently for depression than any synthetic drug.

The active components in St. John's wort are found in the buds, flowers, and newest leaves. Extracts are usually standardized to the substance hypericin, which has led to the widespread misconception that hypericin is the active ingredient. However, there is no evidence that hypericin itself is an antidepressant. Recent attention has focused on another ingredient of St. John's wort named hyperforin as the potential active ingredient.

Hyperforin was first identified as a constituent of *Hypericum perforatum* in 1971 by Russian researchers, but it was incorrectly believed to be too unstable to play a major role in the herb's action.[1] However, recent evidence has corrected this view. It now appears that standard St. John's wort extract contains about 1 to 6% hyperforin.[2]

We don't really know how St. John's wort works. Early research suggested that St. John's wort works like the oldest class of antidepressants, the MAO inhibitors.[3] However, later research essentially discredited this idea.[4,5] More recent research suggests that St. John's wort may raise levels of serotonin, norepinephrine, and dopamine.[6,7]

Evidence from animal and human studies suggests that hyperforin is the ingredient in St. John's wort that raises these neurotransmitters.[8,9,10] However, there may be other active ingredients in St. John's wort also at work.[11]

## WHAT IS ST. JOHN'S WORT USED FOR TODAY?

St. John's wort is primarily used to treat mild to moderate **depression** (page 54). Typical symptoms include depressed mood, lack of energy, sleep problems, anxiety, appetite disturbance, difficulty concentrating, and poor stress tolerance. Irritability can also be a sign of depression.

Research suggests that St. John's wort is effective in about 55% of cases. As with other antidepressants, the full effect takes approximately 4 to 6 weeks to develop. Although St. John's wort appears to be somewhat less powerful than standard antidepressants, it has one great advantage: It scarcely, if ever, causes side effects.

However, St. John's wort should never be relied on for the treatment of severe depression. If you or a loved one are feeling suicidal, unable to cope with daily life, paralyzed by anxiety, incapable of getting out of bed, unable to sleep, or uninterested in eating, see a physician at once. Drug therapy may save your life.

Furthermore, various systemic diseases may masquerade as depression, such as hypothyroidism, chronic hepatitis, and anemia. Make sure to find out whether you have an undiagnosed medical illness before treating yourself with St. John's wort.

Like other antidepressants, St. John's wort is also used in the treatment of chronic **insomnia** (page 80) and **anxiety** (page 8) when they are related to depression. It may be effective in relieving seasonal affective disorder (SAD) as well.

Early reports suggested that St. John's wort might be active against viruses such as HIV, but these haven't panned out because unrealistically high concentrations are required.

## WHAT IS THE SCIENTIFIC EVIDENCE FOR ST. JOHN'S WORT?

None of the double-blind studies of St. John's wort have been particularly large, but taken together they make a convincing case that the herb is an effective antidepressant. There have been two main kinds of studies: those that compared St. John's wort to placebo, and others that compared it to prescription antidepressants.

### St. John's Wort Versus Placebo

Probably the best-designed St.-John's-wort-versus-placebo study was reported in 1993 by the German physician K. D. Hansgen and his colleagues.[12] In this 4-week trial, 72 moderately depressed individuals were randomly assigned to receive either placebo or 300 mg 3 times a day of an extract of St. John's wort standardized to contain 0.3% hypericin.

Participants were evaluated using a set of questions called the Hamilton Depression Index (HAM-D). This scale rates the extent of depression, with higher numbers indicating more serious symptoms. Over 80% of the participants taking St. John's wort improved significantly based on this index, while only 26% of the placebo group responded. Later, 36 additional people were added to the trial, with essentially identical results.

A recent double-blind study examined the effectiveness of a new kind of St. John's wort extract standardized to its content of hyperforin rather than to hypericin.[13] It followed 147 people with mild to moderate depression for a period of 42 days. Participants were given either a placebo or one of two forms of St. John's wort: a low-hyperforin product (0.5%) or a high-hyperforin product (5%).

The results showed that the St. John's wort containing 5% hyperforin was successful in controlling depression symptoms in about 50% of cases, a better result than placebo. Although identical to the high hyperforin product in every respect other than hyperforin content, the low hyperforin product did not do any better than the placebo. This study provides strong evidence that hyperforin is at least one of the active ingredients in St. John's wort.

There have been over 13 other double-blind placebo-controlled studies as well.[14] A review that evaluated most of the published studies up through 1994 found that nine of them were performed according to adequate scientific standards, involving a total of over 600 participants.[15] Adding in the hyperforin study just mentioned, the combined results make a compelling case for St. John's wort as an effective antidepressant.

This body of research has been criticized by some authorities who point out that none of the studies exceeded 8 weeks in length. However, as it states in the *Physician's Desk Reference*, Prozac was approved on the basis of studies no longer than 6 weeks. It isn't fair to apply a higher standard to herbs than to drugs.

## St. John's Wort Versus Medications

To date, about 10 trials have compared St. John's wort against old-fashioned but tried-and-true antidepressants such as imipramine, maprotiline, and amitriptyline.[16,17,18] Although these studies found generally equal benefits, the dosages of the drugs used were too low to prove much. Instead of the typical 150 to 250 mg a day, participants were only given 50 to 75 mg of the drugs. At these dosages, the drugs didn't really stand a chance of working.

One recent study did use a realistic dose of the drug imipramine, and compared it against double the usual dose of St. John's wort.[19] Interestingly, it followed 209 individuals whose depression was severe rather than mild to moderate. According to the study authors, the results showed that St. John's wort at a double dose was almost as effective as imipramine. However, this seems to be an incorrect reading of the results. St. John's wort was less effective than imipramine, and its performance was not much better than what is usually seen with a placebo. St. John's wort, even at double strength, is probably not an effective treatment for severe depression.

## Depression-Related Symptoms

In many of the studies described above, anxiety and insomnia associated with depression were noted to improve with St. John's wort treatment.

## Seasonal Affective Disorder

One small, controlled study found St. John's wort to be effective in the treatment of seasonal affective disorder (SAD), a form of depression that occurs primarily during the winter.[20]

## DOSAGES

The standard dosage of St. John's wort is 300 mg 3 times a day of an extract standardized to contain 0.3% hypericin. A few new products on the market are standardized to hyperforin content (usually 3 to 5%) instead of hypericin. These are taken at the same dosage.

Some people take 500 mg twice a day, or 600 mg in the morning and 300 mg in the evening. If the herb bothers your stomach, take it with food.

St. John's Wort

Visit Us at TNP.com

Remember that the full effect takes 4 weeks to develop. Don't give up too soon!

## SAFETY ISSUES

St. John's wort is essentially side-effect free. Strangely, this good news has an unfortunate consequence: Some people who try St. John's wort decide that it must not be very powerful since it doesn't make them feel ill, and quit. Be patient! When St. John's wort works, it is very smooth.

In a study designed to look for side effects, 3,250 people took St. John's wort for 4 weeks.[21] Overall, about 2.4% experienced side effects. The most common were mild stomach discomfort (0.6%), allergic reactions—primarily rash—(0.5%), tiredness (0.4%), and restlessness (0.3%).

In the extensive German experience with St. John's wort as a treatment for depression, there have been no published reports of serious adverse consequences or drug interactions.[22] Animal studies involving enormous doses for 26 weeks have not shown any serious effects.[23]

Cows and sheep grazing on St. John's wort have sometimes developed severe and even fatal sensitivity to the sun. However, this has never occurred in humans taking St. John's wort at normal dosages.[24] In one study, highly sun-sensitive people were given twice the normal dose of the herb.[25] The results showed a mild but measurable increase in reaction to ultraviolet radiation. The moral of the story is that if you are especially sensitive to the sun, don't exceed the recommended dose of St. John's wort and continue to take your usual precautions against burning. Nonetheless, there might be problems if you combine St. John's wort with other medications that cause increased sun sensitivity.

A recent report suggests that regular use of St. John's wort might increase the risk of cataracts.[26] While this is preliminary information, it might make sense to wear sunglasses when outdoors if you are taking this herb on a long-term basis.

Older reports suggested that St. John's wort works like the class of drugs known as MAO inhibitors.[27] This led to a number of warnings, including avoiding cheese and decongestants while taking St. John's wort. However, this concern is no longer considered realistic.[28,29]

For some time, herbal experts have warned that combining St. John's wort with drugs in the Prozac family (SSRIs) might raise serotonin too much and cause a number of serious problems. Recently, case reports of such events have begun to trickle in.[30,31] This is a potentially serious risk. Do not combine St. John's wort with prescription antidepressants except on the specific advice of a physician. Since some antidepressants, such as Prozac, linger in the blood for quite some time, you also need to exercise caution when switching from a drug to St. John's wort. (See Transitioning from Medications to St. John's Wort.)

There has also recently been an informal report of St. John's wort lowering blood levels of theophylline, an asthma medication. Preliminary investigation carried out at the University of Colorado suggests that the hypericin in St. John's wort may increase the activity of an enzyme called cytochrome P-450.[32] Throughout evolution, our bodies have developed over 25 different types of this enzyme in our livers and kidneys to break down many naturally occurring chemicals in our diet. Because these enzymes evolved to metabolize many different kinds of natural chemicals, it just so happens that these enzymes break down modern drugs and chemicals, too. Cytochrome P-450 is one of these enzymes. By increasing P-450 activity, St. John's wort may cause the body to speed the breakdown of various drugs (such as theophylline), thereby decreasing their effectiveness. Before taking St. John's wort, it might be a good idea to ask your doctor if any of your medications would be affected by "cytochrome P-450 CYP 1A1 and 1A2 induction."

Finally, preliminary reports from the University of Colorado suggest that St. John's wort may interfere with the action of the antitumor drugs etoposide (VePesid), teniposide (Vumon), mitoxantrone (Novantrone), and doxorubicin (Adriamycin).[33]

Safety in young children, pregnant or nursing women, or those with severe liver or kidney disease has not been established.

## TRANSITIONING FROM MEDICATIONS TO ST. JOHN'S WORT

If you are taking a prescription drug for mild to moderate depression, switching to St. John's wort may be a reasonable idea if you would prefer taking an herb. Since no one knows whether it is absolutely safe to combine the herb with medications, the safest approach is to stop taking the drug and allow it to wash out of your system before starting St. John's wort. Consult with your doctor on how much time is necessary.

However, if you are taking medication for severe depression, switching over to St. John's wort is *not* a good idea. The herb probably won't work well enough, and you may sink into a dangerous depression.

## ⚠ INTERACTIONS YOU SHOULD KNOW ABOUT

If you are taking

- Standard **antidepressant drugs,** especially those in the Prozac family: Do not take St. John's wort at the same time. Actually, you need to let the medication flush out of your system for a while (perhaps weeks) before you start the herb.

- **Medications** affected by "cytochrome P-450 CYP 1A1 and 1A2 induction:" St. John's wort might cause problems. Ask your pharmacist or physician.

- The anticancer drugs **etoposide (VePesid), teniposide (Vumon), mitoxantrone (Novantrone),** or **doxorubicin (Adriamycin):** Don't take St. John's wort.

- **Medications** that cause sun sensitivity: Keep in mind that St. John's wort might have an additive effect.

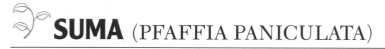

# SUMA (PFAFFIA PANICULATA)

### Principal Proposed Uses
Adaptogen (improve resistance to stress), strengthen immunity (against colds, flus, and other infections), enhance exercise ability

### Other Proposed Uses
Chronic fatigue syndrome, menopausal symptoms, ulcer disease, anxiety, menstrual problems, impotence, aphrodisiac

Suma is a large ground vine native to Central and South America. Sometimes called "Brazilian ginseng," native peoples have long used suma to promote robust health as well as to treat practically all illnesses. They called it *Para Toda,* which means "for all things."[1]

## WHAT IS SUMA USED FOR TODAY?

Suma's ancient reputation has generated worldwide interest. However, there has been little formal scientific investigation at this time.

According to most contemporary herbalists, suma is best understood as an adaptogen, a substance that helps one adapt to stress and fight infection. See the chapter on **ginseng** (page 206) for a more in-depth discussion about adaptogens. Along with other adaptogens, Russian Olympic athletes have used suma in the belief that it will enhance sports performance. In the United States,

suma is often recommended as a general strengthener of the body, as well as for the treatment of chronic fatigue syndrome, **menopausal symptoms** (page 87), **ulcers** (page 112), **anxiety** (page 8), menstrual problems, **impotence** (page 77), and low resistance to illness. The herb also enjoys a considerable reputation as an aphrodisiac.

## DOSAGES

A typical dosage of suma is 500 mg twice daily. It is usually taken for an extended period of time.

## SAFETY ISSUES

Suma has not been associated with any serious adverse reactions. However, comprehensive safety studies have not been undertaken. Safety in young children, pregnant or nursing women, or those with severe liver or kidney disease has not been established.

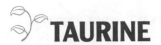

# TAURINE

*Principal Proposed Uses*
   Congestive heart failure, viral hepatitis

*Other Proposed Uses*
   Stroke, hypertension (high blood pressure), epilepsy, gallbladder disease, alcoholism, cataracts, multiple sclerosis, psoriasis, diabetes

*Supplement Forms/Alternative Names*
   L-taurine

Taurine is an amino acid, one of the building blocks of proteins. Found in the nervous system and muscles, taurine is one of the most abundant amino acids in the body. It is thought to help regulate heartbeat, maintain cell membranes, and affect the release of neurotransmitters (chemicals that carry signals between nerve cells) in the brain.

Taurine's best-established use is to treat congestive heart failure (CHF), a condition in which the heart muscle progressively weakens. It may also be useful for hepatitis.

**Warning:** Please keep in mind that CHF is too serious for self-treatment. If you're interested in trying taurine or any other supplement for CHF, you should first consult your doctor.

## SOURCES

There is no dietary requirement for taurine, since the body can make it out of **vitamin B$_6$** (page 326) and the amino acids **methionine** (page 261) and cysteine. Deficiencies occasionally occur in vegetarians, whose diets may not provide the building blocks for making taurine.

People with diabetes have lower-than-average blood levels of taurine, but whether this means they should take extra taurine is unclear.

Meat, poultry, eggs, dairy products, and fish are good sources of taurine. Legumes and nuts don't contain taurine, but they do contain methionine and cysteine.

## THERAPEUTIC DOSAGES

A typical therapeutic dosage of taurine is 2 g 3 times daily.

## THERAPEUTIC USES

Preliminary evidence suggests that taurine might be helpful in **congestive heart failure** (page 50), a condition in which the heart has trouble pumping blood, which leads to fluid accumulating in the legs and lungs.[1]

There is also some evidence that taurine may be helpful for acute viral **hepatitis** (page 71).[2]

Taurine has additionally been proposed as a treatment for numerous other conditions, including stroke, **hypertension** (page 75), epilepsy, gallbladder disease, alcoholism, **cataracts** (page 37), multiple sclerosis, **psoriasis** (page 106), and **diabetes** (page 60), but the evidence for these uses is weak and, in some cases, contradictory.[3–7] Taurine is also sometimes combined in an "amino acid cocktail" with other amino acids for the treatment of **attention deficit disorder** (page 19), but there is no evidence as yet that it works for this purpose.

## WHAT IS THE SCIENTIFIC EVIDENCE FOR TAURINE?

### Congestive Heart Failure

Several studies (primarily by one researcher) suggest that taurine may be useful for congestive heart failure (CHF). For example, in one double-blind trial, 58 people with CHF took either placebo or 2 g of taurine 3 times daily for 4 weeks.[8] Then the groups were switched. During taurine treatment, the study participants showed highly significant improvement in breathlessness, heart palpitations, fluid buildup, and heart x ray, as well as standard scales of heart failure severity. Animal research as well as other, small blinded or open studies in humans have also found positive effects.[9–13] Interestingly, one very small study compared taurine with another supplement commonly used for congestive heart failure, **coenzyme Q$_{10}$** (page 164). The results suggest that taurine is more effective.[14]

### Viral Hepatitis

There are several viruses that can cause acute hepatitis, a disabling and sometimes dangerous infection of the liver. The most common are hepatitis A and B, although there are others (with such imaginative names as C and D).

One double-blind study suggests that taurine supplements might be useful for acute viral hepatitis. In this double-blind placebo-controlled study, 63 people with hepatitis were given either 12 g of taurine daily or placebo.[15] (The report does not state what type of viral hepatitis they had.) According to blood tests, the taurine group experienced significant improvements in liver function as compared to the placebo group.

Acute hepatitis can also develop into a long-lasting or permanent condition known as chronic hepatitis. One small double-blind study suggests that taurine does not help chronic hepatitis.[16]

For this purpose, the herb **milk thistle** (page 262) may be better.

## SAFETY ISSUES

As an amino acid found in food, taurine is thought to be quite safe. However, maximum safe dosages of taurine supplements for children, pregnant or nursing women, or those with severe liver or kidney disease have not been determined.

As with any supplement taken in multigram doses, it is important to purchase a reputable product, because a contaminant present even in small percentages could add up to a real problem.

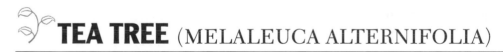

# TEA TREE (MELALEUCA ALTERNIFOLIA)

*Principal Proposed Uses*

Wound healing, acne, body odor, fungal infections of the skin, vaginal infections, periodontal disease

Captain Cook named this tree, after finding that its aromatic, resinous leaves made a satisfying substitute for proper tea. One hundred and fifty years later, an Australian government chemist named A. R. Penfold studied tea tree leaves and discovered their strong antiseptic properties. Tea tree oil subsequently became a standard treatment in Australia for the prevention and treatment of wound infections. During World War II, the Australian government classi-

fied tea tree oil as an essential commodity and exempted producers from military service.

However, tea tree oil fell out of favor when antibiotics became widely available.

## WHAT IS TEA TREE USED FOR TODAY?

There is little question that tea tree oil is an effective antiseptic, active against many bacteria and fungi.[1] It also possesses a penetrating quality that may make it particularly useful for treating infected wounds. However, it is probably not effective as an oral antibiotic.

Like other topical antibiotics, tea tree oil may help control **acne** (page 2) when applied to the skin directly.[2] Preliminary studies also hint that it could be useful for treating vaginal infections caused by **candida** (page 33) or other organisms, as well as fungal infections of the feet and nails. Australian dentists frequently use tea tree oil mouthwash prior to dental procedures and as a daily preventive against **periodontal disease** (page 103).

Tea tree oil also appears to possess deodorant properties, probably through suppressing odor-causing bacteria.

## DOSAGES

Tea tree preparations contain various percentages of tea tree oil. For treating acne, the typical strength is 5 to 15%; for fungal infections, 70 to 100% is usually used; and for use as a vaginal douche (with medical supervision), 1 to 40% concentrations have been used. It is usually applied 2 to 3 times daily, until symptoms resolve. However, tea tree oil can be irritating to the skin, so start with low concentrations until you know your tolerance.

The best tea tree products contain oil from the *alternifolia* species of *Melaleuca* only, standardized to contain not more than 10% cineole (an irritant) and at least 30% terpinen-4-ol.

## SAFETY ISSUES

Like other essential oils, tea tree oil can be toxic if taken orally in excessive doses. Since the maximum safe dosage has not been determined, I recommend using it only topically, where it is believed to be quite safe. However, don't get it in your eye or it will sting badly. Safety in young children, pregnant or nursing women, or those with severe liver or kidney disease has not been established.

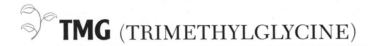

# TMG (TRIMETHYLGLYCINE)

*Principal Proposed Uses*
 There are no documented uses for trimethylglycine.

*Other Proposed Uses*
 Reducing homocysteine levels, liver protection, substitute for SAMe, enhancing athletic performance

*Supplement Forms/Alternative Names*
 Betaine (similar to betaine hydrochloride, but not identical)

TMG (trimethylglycine) has been available for decades. Recently, it has drawn attention as a possible treatment for elevated homocysteine levels.

Homocysteine is a naturally occurring chemical that may be as harmful to blood vessels as cholesterol. **Folic acid** (page 194) and **vitamin B$_6$** (page 326) destroy homocysteine by "methylating" it—attaching one carbon atom and three hydrogen atoms to it. This makes homocysteine harmless. Recent studies have found that vitamin B$_6$ and folic acid can help prevent heart disease, apparently by lowering homocysteine levels in the blood.

After this discovery, great interest developed in other substances that can methylate homocysteine. Chemicals of this type are called "methylating agents." **SAMe** (page 293), or S-adenosylmethionine, is one; TMG is another. However, research into this subject is still in its infancy.

After TMG has done its work on homocysteine, it is turned into another substance, dimethylglycine (DMG). In Russia, DMG is used extensively as an athletic performance enhancer; however, TMG is cheaper and may have the same effects (if any).

## SOURCES

TMG is not required in the diet because the body can manufacture it from other nutrients. Grains, nuts, seeds, and meats contain small amounts of TMG. However, most TMG in food is destroyed during cooking or processing, so food isn't a reliable way to get a therapeutic dosage.

Some manufacturers will tell you that DMG is identical to TMG, but this isn't true. DMG is not a methylating agent, so it can't have any effect on homocysteine.

## THERAPEUTIC DOSAGES

There hasn't been enough research to establish the optimal therapeutic dosage of TMG. One manufacturer recommends using between 375 and 1,000 mg daily.

## THERAPEUTIC USES

One small study suggests that TMG may lower homocysteine levels, which might be helpful for those with **atherosclerosis** (page 14).[1]

TMG may also help protect the liver against the effects of alcohol, perhaps by stimulating the formation of SAMe.[2,3] Additionally, it may be useful for other purposes for which SAMe is used, although this has not been proven.

DMG (the substance TMG changes into in the body) has been extensively used as a performance enhancer by Russian athletes, and has recently become popular among American athletes. However, one small study suggests that it does not work.[4]

## SAFETY ISSUES

TMG appears to be safe. However, the maximum safe dosages for young children, pregnant or nursing mothers, or those with severe liver or kidney disease have not been established.

 # TURMERIC (CURCUMA LONGA)

*Principal Proposed Uses*
Rheumatoid arthritis, osteoarthritis, digestive problems

*Other Proposed Uses*
Heart disease prevention, cancer prevention, cataracts, dysmenorrhea, gallstones

Turmeric is a widely used tropical herb in the ginger family. Its stalk is used both in food and medicine, yielding the familiar yellow ingredient that colors and adds flavor to curry. In the traditional Indian system of herbal medicine known as Ayurveda, turmeric is believed to strengthen the overall energy of the body, relieve gas, dispel worms, improve digestion, regulate menstruation, dissolve gallstones, and relieve arthritis, among other uses.

Modern interest in turmeric began in 1971 when Indian researchers found evidence that whole turmeric possesses anti-inflammatory properties. Much of this observed activity seems to be due to the presence of a con-stituent called curcumin.[1] Curcumin is also a powerful antioxidant.[2]

## WHAT IS TURMERIC USED FOR TODAY?

Turmeric's antioxidant abilities make it a good food preservative, provided that the food is already yellow in color! It is also reasonable to suppose that turmeric might provide benefits similar to those of other antioxidants, such as **vitamin E** (page 337), in the prevention of **heart disease** (page 14), and **cancer** (page 26). However, this has not been proven.

Based on its anti-inflammatory properties, curcumin is commonly recommended as a natural treatment for arthritis as well. One small and highly preliminary double-blind study suggests that curcumin may be helpful in the treatment of **rheumatoid arthritis** (page 109).[3] It also has been suggested for **osteoarthritis** (page 95).

Unlike anti-inflammatory drugs, curcumin does not appear to cause stomach ulcers. (In fact, it might even help prevent them!)[4] But much more and better evidence will be necessary before curcumin can be described as an effective treatment for arthritis. Curcumin is also sometimes recommended for **gallstones** (page 68), **cataracts** (page 37), and menstrual pain or **dysmenorrhea** (page 65), but there is as yet no real evidence that it works.

## DOSAGES

For medicinal purposes, turmeric is frequently taken in a form standardized to curcumin con-

tent, to provide 400 to 600 mg of curcumin 3 times daily.

Unfortunately, curcumin is not absorbed well by the body.[5] It is often sold in combination with **bromelain** (page 144) for the supposed purpose of enhancing absorption. While there is no evidence or even sensible reason to believe that this strategy works, bromelain possesses some anti-inflammatory powers of its own that may add to those of curcumin.

## SAFETY ISSUES

Turmeric is on the FDA's GRAS (generally recognized as safe) list, and curcumin, too, is believed to be extremely nontoxic.[6,7] Side effects are rare and are generally limited to the usual mild stomach distress. However, safety in young children, pregnant or nursing women, or those with severe liver or kidney disease has not been established.

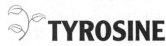

# TYROSINE

*Principal Proposed Uses*
   There are no well-documented uses for tyrosine.

*Other Proposed Uses*
   Sleep deprivation, depression, attention deficit disorder

*Supplement Forms/Alternative Names*
   L-tyrosine

Tyrosine is an amino acid found in meat proteins. Your body uses it as a starting material to make several neurotransmitters (chemicals that help the brain and nervous system function). Based on this fact, tyrosine has been proposed as a treatment for various conditions in which mental function is impaired or slowed down, such as sleep deprivation and depression. It has also been tried for attention deficit disorder (ADD).

## SOURCES

Your body makes tyrosine from another common amino acid, **phenylalanine** (page 278), so deficiencies are rare; however, they can occur in certain forms of severe kidney disease as

well as in phenylketonuria (PKU), a metabolic disorder that requires complete avoidance of phenylalanine.

Good sources of tyrosine include dairy products, meats, fish, and beans.

## THERAPEUTIC DOSAGES

The typical recommended dosage of tyrosine is 7 to 30 g daily.

## THERAPEUTIC USES

According to very preliminary evidence, tyrosine supplements may help fight fatigue and increase alertness in people who are deprived of sleep.[1]

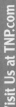

Tyrosine may also provide some temporary benefit for **attention deficit disorder** (page 19), but the benefits appear to wear off in a couple of weeks.[2,3,4] Tyrosine is said to work better for this purpose when it is combined in an "amino acid cocktail" along with gamma-aminobutyric acid (GABA), **phenylalanine** (page 278), and **glutamine** (page 215); however, there is no scientific evidence to support this use.

Although one extremely tiny study found tyrosine helpful for **depression** (page 54),[5] a recent larger study found it not effective.[6]

## WHAT IS THE SCIENTIFIC EVIDENCE FOR TYROSINE?

### Sleep Deprivation

A placebo-controlled study that enrolled 20 U.S. Marines suggests that tyrosine can improve alertness during periods of sleep deprivation. In this study, the participants were deprived of sleep for a night and then tested frequently for their alertness throughout the day as they worked. Compared to placebo, 10 to 15 g of tyrosine given twice daily seemed to provide a "pick-up" for about 2 hours.[7]

### Depression

A study that enrolled nine individuals is widely quoted as evidence that tyrosine can help depression.[8] However, a recent double-blind placebo-controlled study of 65 people with depression found *no* benefit.[9]

## SAFETY ISSUES

Tyrosine seems to be generally safe, though at high dosages some people have reported nausea, diarrhea, vomiting, or nervousness. As with any other supplement taken in multigram doses, it is important to use a high-quality product; even a very small percentage of contaminant in the product might add up to a dangerous amount.

Maximum safe dosages for young children, women who are pregnant or nursing, or those with severe liver or kidney disease have not been established.

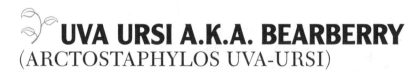

# UVA URSI A.K.A. BEARBERRY
## (ARCTOSTAPHYLOS UVA-URSI)

*Principal Proposed Uses*
Treatment of urinary tract infection (not recommended for prevention of urinary tract infections)

The uva ursi plant is a low-lying evergreen bush whose berries are a favorite of bears; hence the name "bearberry." However, it is the leaves that are used medicinally.

Uva ursi has a long history of use for treating urinary conditions in both America and Europe. Up until the development of sulfa antibiotics, its principal active component, arbutin, was frequently prescribed as a urinary antiseptic.

Although we don't know for sure how uva ursi works, it appears that the arbutin contained in uva ursi leaves is broken down in the intestine to another chemical, hydroquinone. This chemical is altered a bit by the liver and then sent to the kidneys for excretion.[1] In the bladder, it acts as an antiseptic.

Uva ursi appears to be most effective in an alkaline urine, so taking vitamin C with uva ursi probably hampers its work.[2,3]

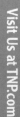

## WHAT IS UVA URSI USED FOR TODAY?

The European Scientific Cooperative on Phytotherapy recommends uva ursi for "uncomplicated infections of the urinary tract such as cystitis when antibiotic treatment is not considered essential."[4] This herb is most useful for women who can tell when they are just starting to develop a **bladder infection** (page 23) and can start treatment early. Once you have a severe bladder infection, uva ursi probably won't work very well.

**Warning:** The herb is definitely not appropriate for kidney infections. If you develop symptoms such as high fever, chills, nausea, vomiting, diarrhea, or severe back pain, get medical assistance immediately.

Furthermore, because hydroquinone can be toxic (discussed under Safety Issues), it isn't a good idea to take uva ursi for a long period of time.

## WHAT IS THE SCIENTIFIC EVIDENCE FOR UVA URSI?

The research foundation for uva ursi is surprisingly weak considering the popularity of this herb.[5]

### Treatment

No double-blind studies have evaluated the clinical effectiveness of uva ursi. However, two studies have evaluated the antibacterial power of the urine of people given uva ursi, and have found activity against most major bacteria that infect the urinary tract.[6,7] This doesn't prove much, however.

### Prevention

One double-blind study followed 57 women for one year. Half were given a standardized dose of uva ursi, while the others received placebo treatment. Over the course of the study, none of the women taking uva ursi developed a bladder infection, while five of the untreated women did.[8]

However, most experts do not believe that continuous treatment with uva ursi is a good idea (see Safety Issues).

## DOSAGES

The dosage of uva ursi should be adjusted to provide 400 to 800 mg of arbutin daily.[9,10,11] This dosage should not be exceeded, and if the herb is not successful within a week you should definitely seek medical attention. No more than 2 weeks of treatment with uva ursi is recommended, and it should not be used more than five times a year.

Uva ursi should be taken with meals to minimize gastrointestinal upset. Because uva ursi is most effective in alkaline urine, it should not be combined with **vitamin C** (page 331) or cranberry juice. You might try taking it along with calcium citrate to alkalinize the urine instead.

Uva ursi is also frequently sold in combination with other herbs believed to treat bladder infections, including cleavers, **juniper berry** (page 238), buchu, and parsley.

## SAFETY ISSUES

Unfortunately, hydroquinone is a liver toxin, carcinogen, and irritant.[12–15] For this reason uva ursi is not recommended for young children, pregnant or nursing women, or those with severe liver or kidney disease.

However significant problems are rare among individuals using prepared uva ursi products in appropriate doses for a short period of time. Gastrointestinal distress (ranging from mild nausea and diarrhea to vomiting) can occur, especially with prolonged use.[16]

## ⚠ INTERACTIONS YOU SHOULD KNOW ABOUT

If you are taking **drugs** or **supplements that acidify the urine,** such as **cranberry juice,** uva ursi may not work very well.

# VALERIAN (VALERIANA OFFICINALIS)

**Principal Proposed Uses**
Insomnia

**Other Proposed Uses**
Anxiety

Over 200 plant species belong to the genus *Valeriana,* but the one most commonly used as an herb is *Valeriana officinalis.* The root is used for medicinal purposes.

Galen recommended valerian for insomnia in the second century A.D. From the sixteenth century onward, this herb became popular as a sedative in Europe (and later, the United States). Scientific studies on valerian in humans began in the 1970s, leading to its approval as a sleep aid by Germany's Commission E in 1985.

As for most herbs, we are not exactly sure which ingredients in valerian are most important.[1,2] Early research focused on a group of chemicals known as valepotriates, but they are no longer considered candidates. A constituent called valerenic acid is presently under study, but its role is far from clear.

Our understanding of how valerian functions is similarly incomplete. Several studies suggest that valerian affects GABA, a naturally occurring amino acid that appears to be related to the experience of anxiety. Conventional tranquilizers in the Valium family are known to bind to GABA receptors in the brain, and valerian may work similarly. Studies suggest that it either stimulates GABA receptors[3,4] or increases GABA concentrations.[5] However, these hypotheses have been disputed.[6]

## WHAT IS VALERIAN USED FOR TODAY?

Valerian is commonly recommended as a mild treatment for occasional **insomnia** (page 80). It appears to be somewhat more effective than herbs such as **hops** (page 227), **skullcap** (page 300), and **passionflower** (page 276), but less effective than pharmaceutical sleeping pills such as Ambien.

Interestingly, a recent German herbal text suggests that valerian is most useful when taken over an extended period of time.[7] The authors suggest combining valerian extract with a comprehensive sleep-management program for people with chronic sleeping troubles.

Valerian is used to treat **anxiety** (page 8) as well, although there is much more scientific evidence for the herb **kava** (page 239).

## WHAT IS THE SCIENTIFIC EVIDENCE FOR VALERIAN?

The research basis for valerian is growing. The well-designed 28-day study described below still appears to be little known in the United States.

### Insomnia

The best study to date of valerian's effectiveness in treating insomnia involved 121 people followed for 28 days.[8] Half of the participants took 600 mg of an alcohol-based valerian extract 1 hour before bedtime, the other half placebo.

At first, placebo and valerian were running neck and neck. But by the end of the study, the participants treated with valerian were definitely sleeping better.

Although positive, these results are a bit confusing because earlier studies showed immediate effects.[9,10] For example, an early double-blind study followed 128 subjects who had no sleeping problems.[11] On three consecutive nights they took either valerian or placebo. The valerian pills significantly reduced the time needed to fall asleep, without affecting dreams or nighttime waking. It is possible that different subspecies of valerian with differing medicinal effects have been used in the various trials.

Finally, a recent double-blind crossover study of 20 people with insomnia compared the benefits

Valerian

of the sleeping drug Halcion (0.125 mg) against placebo and a combination of valerian and lemon balm.[12] Both valerian and Halcion seemed equally effective, but with so few participants, the results can't be taken as a reliable indication that this herbal combination is equally effective to Halcion.

### Anxiety

Forty-eight participants were placed under situations of "social stress" in a double-blind study of valerian.[13] Individuals in the treated group reported less anxiety.

### Animal Studies

Both valerenic acid and whole valerian have been found to produce calming, sleepiness, and reduced activity in laboratory mice.[14–17] Both substances also help prevent seizures. Since most pharmaceutical tranquilizers also reduce seizures, the latter result can be taken as additional indirect evidence of valerian's tranquilizing powers.

**Warning:** Do not try to substitute valerian for your antiseizure medication. The herb is not powerful enough.

## DOSAGES

For insomnia, the standard dosage of valerian is 2 to 3 g of dried herb, 270 to 450 mg of an aqueous valerian extract, or 600 mg of an ethanol extract, taken 30 to 60 minutes before bedtime.[18]

According to the study mentioned previously that used this dosage, valerian may require weeks to reach its full effects. The same amount, or a reduced dose, can be taken twice daily for anxiety.

Because of valerian's unpleasant odor, European manufacturers have created odorless valerian products. However, these are not yet widely available in the United States.

Valerian is not recommended for children under 3 years old.

## SAFETY ISSUES

Valerian is on the FDA's GRAS (generally regarded as safe) list, and is approved for use as a food. In animals, even very high doses have not produced serious effects.[19]

There are some safety concerns about valepotriates, constituents of valerian, because they can cause DNA-altering and other toxic effects. However, valepotriates are unstable and not present to a significant extent in any commercial preparations.[20,21]

Except for the unpleasant odor, valerian generally causes no side effects.[22] A few people experience mild gastrointestinal distress, and there have been rare reports of people developing a paradoxical mild stimulant effect from valerian.

Valerian does not appear to impair driving ability or produce morning drowsiness when it is taken at night.[23,24,25] However, there does appear to be some impairment of attention for a couple of hours after taking valerian.[26] For this reason, it isn't a good idea to drive immediately after taking it.

There have been no reported drug interactions with valerian. A 1995 study found no interaction between alcohol and valerian as measured by concentration, attentiveness, reaction time, and driving performance.[27] However, one Japanese study found that valerian extracts prolong drug-induced sleeping time in mice.[28] Thus, it is possible that valerian could compound the effects of other central-nervous-system depressants.

Safety in young children, pregnant or nursing women, or those with severe liver or kidney disease has not been established.

## ⚠ INTERACTIONS YOU SHOULD KNOW ABOUT

If you are taking **medications for insomnia or anxiety,** don't take valerian in addition to them.

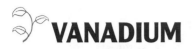

# VANADIUM

***Principal Proposed Uses***
There are no well-documented uses for vanadium, and there are serious safety concerns regarding its use.

***Other Proposed Uses***
Diabetes, bodybuilding, osteoporosis

***Supplement Forms/Alternative Names***
Vanadyl sulfate, vanadate

Vanadium, a mineral, is named after the Scandinavian goddess of beauty, youth, and luster. Taking vanadium will not make you beautiful, youthful, and lustrous, but evidence from animal studies suggests it may be an essential micronutrient. That is, your body may need it, but in *very* low doses.

Based on promising animal studies, high doses of vanadium have been tested as an aid to controlling blood sugar levels in people with diabetes. Like **chromium** (page 161), another trace mineral used in diabetes, vanadium has also been recommended as an aid in bodybuilding. However, animal studies suggest that taking high doses of vanadium can be harmful.

## REQUIREMENTS/SOURCES

We don't know exactly how much vanadium people require, but estimates range from 10 to 30 mcg daily. (To realize how tiny this amount is, consider that it's about *one millionth* of the amount of calcium you need.) Human deficiencies have not been reported, but goats fed a low-vanadium diet have developed birth defects.[1]

Vanadium is found in very small amounts in a wide variety of foods, including breakfast cereals, canned fruit juices, wine, beer, buckwheat, parsley, soy, oats, olive oil, sunflower seeds, corn, green beans, peanut oil, carrots, cabbage, and garlic. The average daily American diet provides between 10 and 60 mcg of vanadium.[2]

## THERAPEUTIC DOSAGES

In various studies, vanadium has been used at doses thousands of times higher than is present in the diet, as high as 125 mg per day. However, there are serious safety concerns about taking vanadium at such high doses (see Safety Issues). I do not recommend exceeding the nutritional dose of 10 to 30 mcg daily.

## THERAPEUTIC USES

Vanadium has been proposed as a treatment for **diabetes** (page 60), based on promising studies in animals and a few small human trials.[3,4]

Vanadium is also sometimes used by bodybuilders, but there is no evidence that it is effective.[5]

Because studies in mice have found that vanadium is deposited in bone,[6] some practitioners of nutritional medicine have suggested that it may be helpful for **osteoporosis** (page 100). However, since many toxic metals also accumulate in the bones—without strengthening them—this doesn't prove that vanadium is good for bones.

## WHAT IS THE SCIENTIFIC EVIDENCE FOR VANADIUM?

### Diabetes

Studies in rats with and without diabetes suggest that vanadium may have an insulin-like effect, reducing blood sugar levels.[7–17] Based on these findings, preliminary studies involving human subjects have been conducted, with promising results.[18–21] However, they were all too small to be taken as definitive proof. More research is needed to definitely establish whether vanadium is effective (not to mention safe) for the treatment of diabetes.

### Bodybuilding

A double-blind placebo-controlled study involving 31 weight-trained athletes found *no* benefit at a dosage more than 1,000 times the nutritional dose.[22]

## SAFETY ISSUES

Studies of diabetic rats suggest that, at high dosages, vanadium can accumulate in the body until it reaches toxic levels.[23–26] Based on these results, high dosages of vanadium can't be considered safe for human use. If you wish to take it, stick to the 10 to 30 mcg a day mentioned earlier.

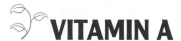 **VITAMIN A**

*Principal Proposed Uses*

Viral infections in children in developing countries

*Other Proposed Uses*

Diabetes, skin disorders (e.g., acne and psoriasis), menorrhagia (heavy menstruation), Crohn's disease, ulcerative colitis, impaired night vision, ulcers, ear infections, eating disorders, lupus, AIDS, gout, glaucoma, multiple sclerosis, kidney stones, Down's syndrome

*Supplement Forms/Alternative Names*

Retinol

**Note:** Beta-carotene is sometimes used interchangeably with vitamin A, because the body can turn beta-carotene into vitamin A.

Vitamin A is a fat-soluble antioxidant that protects your cells against damaging free radicals and plays other vital roles in the body. However, it is potentially more dangerous than most other vitamins because it can build up to toxic levels, causing liver damage and birth defects. Because of this risk, vitamin A supplements have few therapeutic uses.

In general, **beta-carotene** (page 131) supplements taken at nutritional doses are a safer way to get the vitamin A you need. Sometimes called "provitamin A," beta-carotene is transformed into vitamin A as your body needs it, and presents much less risk of toxicity.

## REQUIREMENTS/SOURCES

Vitamin A is an essential nutrient—meaning you must get it in the diet. The U.S. Recommended Dietary Allowance is as follows

- Infants under 1 year, 1,250 IU; 375 mcg (or retinol equivalent, RE)

- Children 1 to 3 years, 1,333 IU; 400 mcg

  4 to 6 years, 1,667 IU; 500 mcg

  7 to 10 years, 2,333 IU; 700 mcg

- Males 11 years and older, 3,333 IU; 1,000 mcg

- Females 11 years and older, 2,667 IU; 800 mcg

- Pregnant women, 2,667 IU; 800 mcg

- Nursing women, 4,000 to 4,338 IU; 1,200 to 1,300 mcg

These amounts can be obtained safely by taking beta-carotene instead of vitamin A. The proper dose may be calculated by keeping in mind that 1 IU of beta-carotene is equivalent to 1 IU of vitamin A; 1 mg of beta-carotene is equivalent to 500 mcg of vitamin A.

**Warning:** Pregnant women should not take vitamin A supplements. Instead they should take beta-carotene.

We get vitamin A from many foods, in the form of either vitamin A or beta-carotene. Liver and dairy products are excellent sources of vitamin A. Carrots, apricots, collard greens, kale, sweet potatoes, parsley, and spinach are good sources as well.

Deficiency in vitamin A is common in developing countries.[1] In the developed world, deficiency is relatively rare, except among teenagers and those in lower socioeconomic groups. Also, the older cholesterol-lowering drugs cholestyramine and colestipol can reduce vitamin A levels.[2]

## THERAPEUTIC DOSAGES

Doses of vitamin A above the basic nutritional requirement is not recommended.

## THERAPEUTIC USES

There is some evidence that vitamin A supplements reduce deaths from measles and other causes among children in developing countries,[3] presumably because they correct a deficiency in the children's diets. This doesn't mean that vitamin A supplements above and beyond the basic nutritional requirement are a useful treatment for measles or any other childhood disease.

Vitamin A may be helpful for **diabetes** (page 60) as well. However, there are concerns that people with diabetes may be especially vulnerable to liver damage from excessive amounts of vitamin A (see Safety Issues). Therefore, if you have diabetes, you should take vitamin A only on the advice of a physician.

Vitamin A has been used in the past for a variety of skin diseases such as **acne** (page 2) and **psoriasis** (page 106), but since you need to use large amounts (which could cause toxicity) to achieve benefits, standard medications are safer. High-dose vitamin A may also be helpful for menorrhagia (heavy menstruation),[4] but again it is not safe.

In addition, vitamin A has been proposed as a treatment for a wide variety of other conditions, some of them quite serious, including ulcerative colitis, impaired **night vision** (page 94), **ulcers** (page 112), ear infections, eating disorders, lupus, AIDS, **gout** (page 69), glaucoma, multiple sclerosis, kidney stones, and Down's syndrome. There is little to no evidence that it is effective for any of these conditions. One study suggests that vitamin A is not effective for Crohn's disease.[5]

## WHAT IS THE SCIENTIFIC EVIDENCE FOR VITAMIN A?

### Viral Infections (in Children Living in Developing Countries)

Vitamin A has been tried as a treatment for various viral infections, including measles, respiratory syncytial virus (RSV, a common childhood viral disease of the respiratory tract), chicken pox, and AIDS.

Most of the research on vitamin A has concentrated on children in developing countries. A review article examining 12 studies suggested that vitamin A supplements can protect such children from dying, and should be used more widely.[6]

Success with measles led researchers to study its use in another childhood viral disease, respiratory syncytial virus (RSV).[7,8] However, the results were not impressive.

### Diabetes

According to many,[9,10] but not all studies,[11,12] people with diabetes tend to be deficient in vitamin A.

An observational study suggests that vitamin A supplements may improve blood sugar control in people with diabetes.[13] However, due to safety concerns, they should not supplement with vitamin A except under medical supervision (see Safety Issues).

### Skin Disorders

Vitamin A has been tried for various skin disorders, including acne, psoriasis, rosacea, seborrhea, and eczema.[14–17] However, the benefits have not been great, and generally vitamin A has to be taken in potentially toxic dosages to produce good effects.

### Menorrhagia (Heavy Menstruation)

One study suggests that women with heavy menstrual bleeding can benefit from taking 25,000 IU daily of vitamin A.[18] But vitamin A cannot be recommended as an ongoing treatment for menorrhagia, since women who menstruate can become pregnant, and even low doses of supplemental vitamin A may cause birth defects.

### Crohn's Disease

According to a double-blind study of 86 people with Crohn's disease, vitamin A does *not* help prevent flare-ups.[19]

## SAFETY ISSUES

Dosages of vitamin A above 50,000 IU per day taken for several years can cause liver injury, bone problems, fatigue, hair loss, headaches, and dry skin. If you already have liver disease, check with your doctor before taking vitamin A supplements, because even small doses may be harmful for you. Also, it is thought that people with diabetes may have trouble releasing vitamin A

stored in the liver. This may mean that they are at greater risk for vitamin A toxicity.

Women should avoid supplementing with vitamin A during pregnancy, because at toxic levels it may increase the risk of birth defects.

**Warning:** Be sure to store vitamin A supplements where children cannot reach them!

## ⚠ INTERACTIONS YOU SHOULD KNOW ABOUT

If you are taking

- The older cholesterol-lowering drugs **cholestyramine** or **colestipol:** You may need more vitamin A (preferably as beta-carotene).

- **Isotretinoin (Accutane):** Don't take vitamin A as they enhance each other's toxicity.

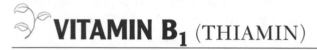

# VITAMIN B₁ (THIAMIN)

*Principal Proposed Uses*
There are no well-documented uses for vitamin B₁ except to correct a deficiency.

*Other Proposed Uses*
Alzheimer's disease, epilepsy, canker sores, fibromyalgia

Vitamin B₁, also called *thiamin*, was the first B vitamin ever discovered. Your body uses it to process fats, carbohydrates, and proteins. Every cell in your body needs thiamin to make adenosine triphosphate, or ATP, the body's main energy-carrying molecule.

Severe deficiency results in beriberi, a disease common among sailors through the nineteenth century, but rare today. Beriberi is still seen, however, in developing countries as well as in alcoholics and people with diseases that significantly impair the body's ability to absorb vitamin B₁.

There is little evidence that vitamin B₁ supplements have any therapeutic use beyond correcting a nutritional deficiency.

## REQUIREMENTS/SOURCES

Your need for vitamin B₁ varies with age. The U.S. Recommended Dietary Allowance is as follows

- Infants under 6 months, 0.3 mg
  6 months to 1 year, 0.4 mg

- Children 1 to 3 years, 0.7 mg
  4 to 6 years, 0.9 mg
  7 to 10 years, 1.0 mg

- Males 11 to 14 years, 1.3 mg
  15 to 50 years, 1.5 mg
  51 years and older, 1.2 mg

- Females 11 to 50 years, 1.1 mg
  51 years and older, 1.0 mg

- Pregnant women, 1.5 mg

- Nursing women, 1.6 mg

Alcoholism, Crohn's disease, diabetes, anorexia, kidney dialysis, folic acid deficiency, and multiple sclerosis may all lead to a vitamin $B_1$ deficiency, and people with these conditions should consider taking $B_1$ supplements. Certain foods may impair your body's absorption of $B_1$ as well, including fish, shrimp, clams, mussels, and the herb horsetail.

Brewer's and nutritional yeast are the richest sources of $B_1$. Peas, beans, nuts, seeds, and whole grains also provide fairly good amounts.

## THERAPEUTIC DOSAGES

Very high dosages of $B_1$—up to 8 g daily—have been recommended for a variety of conditions.

Since the B vitamins tend to work together, many nutritional experts recommend taking $B_1$ with other B vitamins in the form of a B-complex supplement.

## THERAPEUTIC USES

Weak and contradictory evidence suggests that vitamin $B_1$ may be helpful for **Alzheimer's disease** (page 4).[1–5] Vitamin $B_1$ has also been proposed as a treatment for epilepsy, **canker sores** (page 35), and fibromyalgia, but the evidence for these uses is too weak to cite.

## SAFETY ISSUES

Vitamin $B_1$ appears to be quite safe even when taken in very high doses.

## ⚠ INTERACTIONS YOU SHOULD KNOW ABOUT

If you are taking **oral contraceptives** or **loop diuretics** (e.g., **furosemide**), you may need extra vitamin $B_1$.[6]

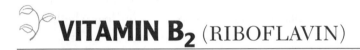

# VITAMIN B₂ (RIBOFLAVIN)

*Principal Proposed Uses*
There are no well-documented uses for vitamin $B_2$.

*Other Proposed Uses*
Migraine headaches, cataracts, sickle-cell anemia, canker sores, athletic performance

*Supplement Forms/Alternative Names*
Riboflavin-5-phosphate

Riboflavin, also known as vitamin $B_2$, is an essential nutrient required for life. This vitamin works with two enzymes critical to the body's production of adenosine triphosphate, or ATP, its main energy source. Vitamin $B_2$ is also used to process amino acids and fats, and to activate vitamin $B_6$ and folic acid.

Preliminary evidence suggests that riboflavin supplements may offer benefits for two illnesses: migraine headaches and cataracts.

## REQUIREMENTS/SOURCES

The U.S. Recommended Dietary Allowance for riboflavin is as follows

- Infants under 6 months, 0.4 mg
  6 to 12 months, 0.5 mg
- Children 1 to 3 years, 0.8 mg
  4 to 6 years, 1.1 mg
  7 to 10 years, 1.2 mg
- Males 11 to 14 years, 1.5 mg
  15 to 18 years, 1.8 mg
  19 to 50 years, 1.7 mg
  51 years and older, 1.4 mg
- Females, 11 to 50 years, 1.3 mg
  51 years and older, 1.2 mg
- Pregnant women, 1.6 mg
- Nursing women, 1.7 to 1.8 mg

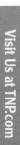

Riboflavin is found in organ meats (such as liver, kidney, and heart) and in many vegetables, nuts, legumes, and leafy greens. The richest sources are torula (nutritional) yeast, brewer's yeast, and calf liver. Almonds, wheat germ, wild rice, and mushrooms are good sources as well.

Although serious riboflavin deficiencies are rare, slightly low levels can occur in children, the elderly, and those in poverty.[1–4]

## THERAPEUTIC DOSAGES

For migraine headaches, the typical recommended dosage of riboflavin is much higher than nutritional needs: 400 mg daily. For cataract prevention, riboflavin may be taken at the nutritional dosages described. Since the B vitamins tend to work together, many nutritional experts recommend taking B$_2$ with other B vitamins, perhaps in the form of a B-complex supplement.

## THERAPEUTIC USES

There are no well-documented uses of riboflavin. However, preliminary evidence suggests that riboflavin supplements taken at high dosages may reduce the frequency of **migraine headaches** (page 89).[5]

One very large study suggests that riboflavin at nutritional doses may be helpful for **cataracts** (page 37), but in this study it was combined with another B vitamin, niacin or **vitamin B$_3$** (page 323), so it's hard to say which vitamin was responsible for the effect.[6]

Riboflavin has also been proposed as a treatment for sickle-cell anemia[7] and **canker sores** (page 35),[8] and as a performance enhancer for athletes, but there is no real evidence that it is effective for these uses.

## WHAT IS THE SCIENTIFIC EVIDENCE FOR RIBOFLAVIN?

### Migraine Headaches

According to a recent 3-month double-blind study of 55 people with migraines, 400 mg of riboflavin daily can reduce the frequency of migraine headaches by 50%.[9]

### Cataracts

Riboflavin supplements may help prevent cataracts, but the evidence isn't yet clear. In a large, double-blind placebo-controlled study, 3,249 people were given either placebo or one of four nutrient combinations (vitamin A/zinc, riboflavin/niacin, vitamin C/molybdenum, or selenium/beta-carotene/vitamin E) for a period of 6 years.[10] Those receiving the niacin/riboflavin supplement showed a significant (44%) reduction in the incidence of cataracts. Strangely, there was a small, but statistically significantly *higher* incidence of a special type of cataract (called a subcapsular cataract) in the niacin/riboflavin group. However, it is unclear whether the effects seen in this group were due to niacin, riboflavin, or the combination of the two.

## SAFETY ISSUES

Riboflavin seems to be an extremely safe supplement.

## ⚠ INTERACTIONS YOU SHOULD KNOW ABOUT

If you are taking **oral contraceptives,** you may need extra riboflavin.

# VITAMIN B₃ (NIACIN, NIACINAMIDE)

### Principal Proposed Uses

High cholesterol/triglycerides (niacin), diabetes prevention and treatment (niacinamide), intermittent claudication (inositol hexaniacinate), osteoarthritis (niacinamide), Raynaud's phenomenon (inositol hexaniacinate)

### Other Proposed Uses

Bursitis, cataracts, pregnancy support

### Supplement Forms/Alternative Names

Niacin, niacinamide, nicotinamide, inositol hexaniacinate

Vitamin $B_3$ is required for the proper function of more than 50 enzymes. Without it, your body would not be able to release energy or make fats from carbohydrates. Vitamin $B_3$ is also used to make sex hormones and other important chemical signal molecules.

Vitamin $B_3$ comes in two principal forms: niacin (nicotinic acid) and niacinamide (nicotinamide). When taken in low doses for nutritional purposes, they are essentially identical. However, each has its own particular effects when taken in high doses. High-dose niacin is principally used for lowering cholesterol. High-dose niacinamide may be helpful in preventing type 1 (childhood-onset) diabetes and reducing symptoms of osteoarthritis. However, there are concerns regarding liver inflammation when any form of niacin is taken at high dosages.

Additionally, good evidence suggests that a special form of niacin, *inositol hexaniacinate*, can improve walking distance in intermittent claudication. It may also reduce symptoms of Raynaud's phenomenon.

## REQUIREMENTS/SOURCES

The U.S. Recommended Dietary Allowance for niacin is

- Infants under 6 months, 5 mg

  6 to 12 months, 6 mg

- Children 1 to 3 years, 9 mg

  4 to 6 years, 12 mg

  7 to 10 years, 13 mg

- Males 11 to 14 years, 17 mg

  15 to 18 years, 20 mg

  19 to 50 years, 19 mg

  51 years and older, 15 mg

- Females 11 to 50 years, 15 mg

  51 years and older, 13 mg

- Pregnant women, 17 mg

- Nursing women, 20 mg

Because the body can make niacin from the common amino acid tryptophan, niacin deficiencies are rare in developed countries. However, the antituberculosis drug isoniazid (INH) impairs the conversion of tryptophan to niacin, and may produce symptoms of niacin deficiency (see Interactions You Should Know About).[1]

Good food sources of niacin are seeds, yeast, bran, peanuts (especially with skins), wild rice, brown rice, whole wheat, barley, almonds, and peas. Tryptophan is found in protein foods (meat, poultry, dairy products, fish). Turkey and milk are particularly excellent sources of tryptophan.

## THERAPEUTIC DOSAGES

When used as therapy for a specific disease, niacin, niacinamide, and inositol hexaniacinate are taken in dosages much higher than nutritional needs, about 1 to 4 g daily. Because of the risk of liver inflammation at these doses, medical supervision is essential.

For prevention of diabetes in children, the usual dosage of niacinamide is 25 mg per kilogram

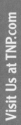

body weight per day. There are 2.2 pounds in a kilogram, so a 40-pound child would get about 450 mg daily.

**Warning:** Medical supervision is essential before giving your child long-term niacinamide treatment.[2]

Many people experience an unpleasant flushing sensation and headache when they take niacin. These symptoms can usually be reduced by gradually increasing the dosage over several weeks or by using slow-release niacin. However, slow-release niacin appears to be more likely to cause liver inflammation than other forms. Inositol hexaniacinate may also cause less flushing than plain niacin, and if you take an aspirin along with niacin, the flushing reaction will usually decrease.

## THERAPEUTIC USES

There is no question that niacin (but not niacinamide) can significantly lower total **cholesterol** (page 39) and LDL ("bad") cholesterol and raise HDL ("good") cholesterol.[3–7] However, unpleasant flushing reactions and the risk of liver inflammation have kept niacin from being widely used (see Safety Issues).

Intriguing evidence suggests that regular use of niacinamide (but not niacin) may help prevent **diabetes** (page 60) in children at special risk of developing it.[8] Risk can be determined by measuring the ratio of antibodies to islet cells (ICA antibody test).

Niacinamide may improve blood sugar control in both children and adults who already have diabetes.[9,10]

According to several good-size, double-blind studies, inositol hexaniacinate may be able to improve walking distance in **intermittent claudication** (page 83) (severe leg cramps caused by hardening of the arteries).[11] Other treatments that may help intermittent claudication include **carnitine** (page 151) and **ginkgo** (page 204).

Preliminary evidence suggests that inositol hexaniacinate may be able to reduce symptoms of **Raynaud's phenomenon** (page 108) as well.[12] This condition includes an extreme response to cold, usually most severely in the hands.

Preliminary evidence suggests that niacinamide may be able to reduce symptoms of **osteoarthritis** (page 95).[13]

Very weak evidence suggests one of the several forms of niacin may be helpful in bursitis,[14] **cataracts** (page 37),[15] and pregnancy.[16]

## WHAT IS THE SCIENTIFIC EVIDENCE FOR NIACIN?

Niacin is one of the best researched of all the vitamins, and the evidence for using it to treat at least one condition—high cholesterol—is strong enough that it has become an accepted mainstream treatment.

### High Cholesterol/Triglycerides

Niacin has been used since the 1950s to lower harmful blood lipids (cholesterol, triglycerides, and lipoproteins) and to raise levels of HDL ("good") cholesterol. According to numerous studies, niacin can lower total cholesterol and LDL ("bad") cholesterol by 15 to 25%, lower triglycerides by 2 to 50%, and raise HDL ("good") cholesterol by about 15 to 25%.[17–20] Furthermore, long-term use of niacin has been shown to significantly reduce death rates from cardiovascular disease.[21]

### Preventing Diabetes

Exciting evidence from a huge study conducted in New Zealand suggests that niacinamide can prevent high-risk children from developing diabetes.[22] In this study, more than 20,000 children were screened for diabetes risk by measuring ICA antibodies. It turned out that 185 of these children had detectable levels. About 170 of these children were then given niacinamide for 7 years (not all parents agreed to give their children niacinamide or stay in the study for that long). About 10,000 other children were not screened, but they were followed to see whether they developed diabetes.

The results were very impressive. In the group in which children were screened and given niacinamide if they were positive for ICA antibodies, the incidence of diabetes was reduced by as much as 60%.

These findings suggest that niacinamide is a very effective treatment for preventing diabetes. (It also shows that tests for ICA antibodies can very accurately identify children at risk for diabetes.)

At present, an enormous-scale, long-term trial called the European Nicotinamide Diabetes Intervention Trial is being conducted to definitively determine whether regular use of niacinamide can prevent diabetes. Results from the German portion of the study have been released at press time, and they were not positive.[23] However, until the entire study is complete, it is not possible to draw conclusions.

### Treating Diabetes

If your child has just developed diabetes, niacinamide may prolong what is called the honeymoon period.[24] This is the interval in which the pancreas can still make some insulin, and insulin needs are low. By giving your child niacinamide, you may be able to buy some time to allow him or her to adjust to a life of insulin injections.

A recent study suggests that niacinamide may also improve blood sugar control in type 2 (adult-onset) diabetes, but it did not use a double-blind design.[25]

### Intermittent Claudication

Double-blind studies involving a total of over 500 individuals have found that inositol hexaniacinate can improve walking distance for people with intermittent claudication.[26–30] For example, in one study, 120 individuals were given either placebo or 2 g of inositol hexaniacinate daily. Over a period of 3 months, walking distance improved significantly in the treated group.[31] The effect was roughly comparable to that of L-carnitine.

### Osteoarthritis

There is some evidence that niacinamide may provide some benefits for those with osteoarthritis. In a double-blind study, 72 individuals with arthritis were given either 3,000 mg daily of niacinamide (in 5 equal doses) or placebo for 12 weeks.[32] The results showed that treated participants experienced a 29% improvement in symptoms, whereas those given placebo worsened by 10%. However, at this dose, liver inflammation is a concern that must be taken seriously.

### Raynaud's Phenomenon

According to one small double-blind study, the inositol hexaniacinate form of niacin may be help-ful for Raynaud's phenomenon.[33] The dosage used was 4 g daily, again a dosage high enough for liver inflammation to be a real possibility.

## SAFETY ISSUES

When taken at a dosage of more than 100 mg daily, niacin frequently causes annoying skin flushing, especially in the face. This reaction may be accompanied by stomach distress, itching, and headache. In studies, as many as 43% of individuals taking niacin quit because of unpleasant side effects.[34]

A more dangerous effect of niacin is liver inflammation. Although most commonly seen with slow-release niacin, it can occur with any type of niacin when taken at a daily dose of more than 500 mg (usually 3 g or more). Regular blood tests to evaluate liver function are therefore mandatory when using high-dose niacin (or niacinamide or inositol hexaniacinate). This side effect almost always goes away when niacin is stopped.

If you have liver disease, ulcers (presently or in the past), gout, or diabetes, do not take high-dose niacin except on medical advice.

Maximum safe dosages for young children and pregnant or nursing women have not been established.

## ⚠ INTERACTIONS YOU SHOULD KNOW ABOUT

If you are taking

- **Cholesterol-lowering drugs** in the statin family, or if you drink **alcohol** excessively: Do not take niacin.[35]

- Older cholesterol-lowering drugs such as **cholestyramine** or **colestipol**: You should take niacin at a different time of day to avoid absorption problems.[36]

- **Oral contraceptives:** You may need extra niacin.

- The antituberculosis drug **isoniazid (INH):** You may need extra niacin.

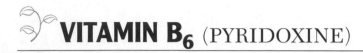

# VITAMIN B$_6$ (PYRIDOXINE)

### *Principal Proposed Uses*

Heart disease prevention, morning sickness, asthma, premenstrual syndrome (PMS)

### *Other Proposed Uses*

MSG sensitivity, carpal tunnel syndrome, diabetic neuropathy, depression, epilepsy, kidney stones, autism (B$_6$ combined with magnesium)

### *Supplement Forms/Alternative Names*

Pyridoxine hydrochloride, pyridoxal-5-phosphate

---

Vitamin B$_6$ plays a major role in making proteins, hormones, and neurotransmitters (chemicals that carry signals between nerve cells). Because mild deficiency of vitamin B$_6$ is common, this is one vitamin that is probably worth taking as insurance.

There's good evidence that adequate intake of vitamin B$_6$ can help prevent heart disease and reduce symptoms of morning sickness. This vitamin is also widely recommended for premenstrual syndrome (PMS) and asthma, but there is little evidence that it is effective for either use. When combined with magnesium, vitamin B$_6$ may be helpful for autism.

## REQUIREMENTS/SOURCES

Vitamin B$_6$ requirements increase with age. The U.S. Recommended Dietary Allowance is as follows

- Infants under 6 months, 0.3 mg

  6 months to 1 year, 0.6 mg

- Children 1 to 3 years, 1.0 mg

  4 to 6 years, 1.1 mg

  7 to 10 years, 1.4 mg

- Males 11 to 14 years, 1.7 mg

  15 years and older, 2.0 mg

- Females 11 to 14 years, 1.4 mg

  15 to 18 years, 1.5 mg

  19 years and older, 1.6 mg

- Pregnant women, 2.2 mg

- Nursing women, 2.1 mg

Severe deficiencies of vitamin B$_6$ are rare, but mild deficiencies are extremely common. In a survey of 11,658 adults, 71% of men and 90% of women were found to have diets deficient in B$_6$.[1] Vitamin B$_6$ is the most commonly deficient water-soluble vitamin in the elderly,[2] and children, too, don't get enough.[3]

Dietary deficiency can be worsened by use of corticosteroids (such as prednisone), hydralazine (for high blood pressure), penicillamine (used for rheumatoid arthritis and certain rare diseases), theophylline (an older drug for asthma), and the antituberculosis drug isoniazid (INH), all of which are thought to interfere with B$_6$ to some degree.[4–11] (But see Interactions You Should Know About for special information regarding isoniazid and epilepsy drugs.) Good sources of B$_6$ include nutritional (torula) yeast, brewer's yeast, sunflower seeds, wheat germ soybeans, walnuts, lentils, lima beans, buckwheat flour, bananas, and avocados.

## THERAPEUTIC DOSAGES

When used therapeutically, B$_6$ is commonly recommended at a daily dose of 10 to 300 mg daily, much higher than the basic nutritional requirement. However, it's probably not wise to take more than 50 mg daily, except on a physician's advice (see Safety Issues).

Since the B vitamins tend to work together, many nutritional experts recommend taking B$_6$ with other B vitamins, perhaps in the form of a B-complex supplement.

## THERAPEUTIC USES

There is convincing evidence that an adequate nutritional intake of vitamin $B_6$ (as low as 2 to 4 mg daily) can significantly reduce the risk of **heart disease** (page 14).[12]

A large double-blind study suggests that a higher dose (30 mg daily) of vitamin $B_6$ can reduce the **nausea** (page 92) of morning sickness.[13] For another approach, see the chapter on **ginger** (page 202).

Other common uses of $B_6$ are not very well established. For example, vitamin $B_6$ is widely recommended by conventional physicians as a treatment for carpal tunnel syndrome.[14,15] However, there is little to no evidence that it actually works. Similarly, although $B_6$ is frequently suggested as a treatment for **PMS** (page 104) (premenstrual syndrome), there is some fairly good evidence that it *doesn't* work for this purpose.[16]

Some natural medicine authorities state that vitamin $B_6$ is a useful treatment for diabetic neuropathy. This idea is based on the fact that $B_6$ deficiency can cause neuropathy, and people with diabetes may be low in $B_6$. However, there is clinical evidence that $B_6$ supplements do *not* help diabetic neuropathy.[17–19]

Very weak evidence suggests that $B_6$ may be helpful for **depression** (page 54),[20] allergy to monosodium glutamate (MSG, a highly allergenic food additive used to enhance flavor), **asthma** (page 11),[21,22] diabetes caused by pregnancy (gestational diabetes),[23] and kidney stones.[24,25,26] Finally, an interesting series of studies suggests (but certainly doesn't prove) that the combination of vitamin $B_6$ and magnesium can be helpful in autism.[27]

## WHAT IS THE SCIENTIFIC EVIDENCE FOR VITAMIN $B_6$?

### Prevention of Heart Disease

According to data gathered in the Nurses' Health Study, one of the largest long-term medical studies ever performed, vitamin $B_6$ supplements can significantly reduce a woman's risk of developing heart disease.[28] A total of 80,000 women with no history of heart disease were studied for possible links between vitamin $B_6$, folic acid, and the development of heart disease. The results showed that adequate intake of $B_6$ (3 to 4 mg daily) could significantly reduce the risk of heart disease. **Folic acid** (page 194) was also effective.

Vitamin $B_6$ reduces blood levels of *homocysteine,* a chemical that has been linked to hardening of the arteries and heart disease. At first, it was assumed that the benefits of vitamin $B_6$ were all due to reducing homocysteine. However, a subsequent study found *no* association between high homocysteine levels and the risk of heart disease.[29] Instead, researchers found a connection between heart disease and low levels of vitamin $B_6$. People with the highest vitamin $B_6$ levels were 28% less likely to develop heart disease than those with the lowest $B_6$ levels. This study has led to the hypothesis that it is vitamin $B_6$ itself that reduces heart disease risk, and the reduction of homocysteine seen at the same time is simply incidental. However, the matter remains controversial.

Vitamin $B_6$ may help the heart in several ways. Preliminary studies suggest that it can reduce the tendency of platelets in the blood to form clots,[30] and also lower blood pressure to some extent.[31]

## Morning Sickness (Nausea and Vomiting in Pregnancy)

Vitamin $B_6$ supplements have been used for years by conventional physicians as a treatment for morning sickness. In 1995, a large double-blind study validated this use.[32] A total of 342 pregnant women were given placebo or 30 mg of vitamin $B_6$ daily. Subjects then graded their symptoms by noting the severity of their nausea and recording the number of vomiting episodes. The women in the $B_6$ group experienced significantly less nausea than those in the placebo group, suggesting that regular use of $B_6$ can be helpful for morning sickness. However, vomiting episodes were not significantly reduced.

## Premenstrual Syndrome

More than a dozen double-blind studies investigated the effectiveness of vitamin $B_6$ for

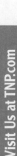

premenstrual syndrome (PMS). Many of these studies reported positive results, but a careful review of the literature found serious flaws in nearly all of them, so the results can't be taken as reliable.[33]

A recent properly designed double-blind trial of 120 women found *no* benefit.[34] In this study, three prescription antidepressants were compared against vitamin $B_6$ (pyridoxine, at 300 mg daily) and placebo. All study participants received 3 months of treatment and 3 months of placebo. Although the antidepressants were effective, vitamin $B_6$ proved to be no better than placebo.

## Autism

According to four double-blind controlled trials, the combination of $B_6$ and magnesium may be helpful in autism.[35] Sixty autistic children were treated with either $B_6$ alone, $B_6$ plus magnesium, or magnesium alone. Researchers found a modest benefit in behavior among the children taking both magnesium and $B_6$, but not in either of the other groups.

## Asthma

A double-blind study of 76 children with asthma found significant benefit after 1 month.[36] Children in the vitamin $B_6$ group were able to reduce their doses of asthma medication (bronchodilators and steroids). However, a recent double-blind study of 31 adults who used either inhaled or oral steroids did *not* show any benefit.[37] The dosages of $B_6$ used in these studies were quite high, in the range of 200 to 300 mg daily. Be-

cause of the risk of nerve injury, it is not advisable to take this much $B_6$ without medical supervision (see Safety Issues).

## SAFETY ISSUES

Vitamin $B_6$ appears to be completely safe for adults at dosages up to 50 mg daily. However, at higher dosages (especially above 2 g daily) there is a very real risk of nerve damage. Nerve-related symptoms have even been reported at doses as low as 200 mg.[38] (This is a bit ironic, given that $B_6$ deficiency *also* causes nerve problems.)

In addition to the risk of nerve damage, there have been a few reports of liver inflammation when $B_6$ was taken daily at more than 50 mg in a single dose.[39] In some cases, very high doses of vitamin $B_6$ can cause or worsen acne symptoms.[40,41]

Maximum safe dosages for children, pregnant or nursing women, or those with severe liver or kidney disease have not been established.

## ⚠ INTERACTIONS YOU SHOULD KNOW ABOUT

If you are taking

- **Isoniazid (INH), corticosteroids, penicillamine, hydralazine, oral contraceptives, phenelzine,** or **theophylline:** You may need extra vitamin $B_6$.

- **Levodopa** (for Parkinson's disease): Do not take more than 5 mg of vitamin $B_6$ daily except on medical advice.[42]

# VITAMIN B$_{12}$ (COBALAMIN)

### Principal Proposed Uses
Pernicious anemia

### Other Proposed Uses
Male infertility, asthma, AIDS, diabetic neuropathy, multiple sclerosis, tinnitus, Alzheimer's disease, depression, osteoporosis, periodontal disease

### Supplement Forms/Alternative Names
Methylcobalamin, cyanocobalamin, hydrocobalamin

Vitamin B$_{12}$, an essential nutrient, is also known as cobalamin. The "cobal" in the name refers to the metal cobalt contained in B$_{12}$. Vitamin B$_{12}$ is required for the normal activity of nerve cells, and works with folic acid and vitamin B$_6$ to lower blood levels of *homocysteine,* a chemical in the blood that is thought to contribute to heart disease. For more information about homocysteine, see the chapter on **atherosclerosis** (page 14).

Vitamin B$_{12}$ also plays a role in the body's manufacture of S-adenosylmethionine, or **SAMe** (page 293).

Anemia is usually the first sign of B$_{12}$ deficiency. Earlier in this century, doctors coined the name "pernicious anemia" for a stubborn anemia that didn't improve even when the patient was given iron supplements. Today we know that pernicious anemia is usually caused by a condition in which the stomach fails to excrete a special substance called intrinsic factor. The body needs the intrinsic factor for efficient absorption of vitamin B$_{12}$. In 1948, vitamin B$_{12}$ was identified as the cure for pernicious anemia.

More recent evidence suggests that B$_{12}$ supplements may improve sperm count and mobility, possibly enhancing fertility. Vitamin B$_{12}$ has also been proposed as a treatment for numerous other conditions, but as yet there is no definitive evidence that it is effective.

## REQUIREMENTS/SOURCES

Extraordinarily small amounts of vitamin B$_{12}$ suffice for nutritional needs. The U.S. Recommended Dietary Allowance is as follows

- Infants under 6 months, 0.3 mcg
  6 months to 1 year, 0.5 mcg
- Children 1 to 3 years, 0.7 mcg
  4 to 6 years, 1.0 mcg
  7 to 10 years, 1.4 mcg
- Adults (and children 11 years and older), 2 mcg
- Pregnant women, 2.2 mcg
- Nursing women, 2.6 mcg

Vitamin B$_{12}$ deficiency is rare in the young, but it's not unusual in older people: Probably 10 to 20% of the elderly are deficient in B$_{12}$.[1–4] This may be because older people have lower levels of stomach acid. The vitamin B$_{12}$ in our food comes attached to proteins, and must be released by acid in the stomach in order to be absorbed. When stomach acid levels are low, we don't absorb as much vitamin B$_{12}$ from our food. Fortunately, vitamin B$_{12}$ supplements don't need acid for absorption. For this reason, people who take medications that greatly reduce stomach acid, such as Prilosec or Zantac, should probably also take B$_{12}$ supplements.[5,6,7]

Stomach surgery and other conditions affecting the digestive tract can also lead to B$_{12}$ deficiency. Vitamin B$_{12}$ absorption is impaired by corticosteroids, colchicine (for gout), metformin and phenformin (for diabetes), colestipol and cholestyramine (for high cholesterol), and methotrexate (for cancer as well as some inflammatory diseases).[8–12] Slow-release **potassium** (page 282) supplements can also impair B$_{12}$ absorption.[13]

Severe B$_{12}$ deficiency can cause anemia and, potentially, nerve damage. The latter may become permanent if the deficiency is not corrected in time. Anemia usually develops first, leading to treatment before permanent nerve damage develops. However, **folic acid** (page 194) supplements can get in the way of this "early warning system." This is why people are cautioned against taking high doses of folic acid without medical supervision. When taken at a dosage of higher than 800 IU daily, folic acid can prevent anemia caused by B$_{12}$ deficiency, thereby allowing permanent nerve damage to develop without any warning. Therefore, you should not take folic acid at high dosages without first getting a blood test to evaluate your B$_{12}$ levels.

Vitamin B$_{12}$ is found in most animal foods. Beef, liver, clams, and lamb provide a whopping 80 to 100 mcg of B$_{12}$ per 3.5-ounce serving, at least 40 times the daily requirement. Sardines, chicken liver, beef kidney, and calf liver are also good sources, providing between 25 and 60 mcg per serving. Trout, salmon, tuna, eggs, whey, and many cheeses provide at least the recommended daily intake. Nondairy, or total, vegetarians can eventually become B$_{12}$-deficient, unless they take B$_{12}$ supplements or eat B$_{12}$-enriched yeast.

Vitamin B$_{12}$ is available in three forms: cyanocobalamin, hydrocobalamin, and methylcobalamin. The first is the most widely available and least expensive, but some experts think that the other two forms are preferable.

## THERAPEUTIC DOSAGES

Although the actual daily requirement of vitamin B$_{12}$ is very low, enormously higher daily doses—ranging from 100 to 2,000 mcg—are sometimes recommended for various conditions.

Because the B vitamins tend to work together, many nutritional experts recommend taking B$_{12}$ with other B vitamins in the form of a B-complex supplement.

## THERAPEUTIC USES

Traditionally, B$_{12}$ injections are used to treat pernicious anemia, but research has shown that oral B$_{12}$ works just as well, provided you take enough of it (between 300 and 1,000 mcg daily).[14–17]

Evidence also suggests that B$_{12}$ supplements can improve sperm activity and perhaps help treat **infertility in men** (page 78).[18,19] However, there is as yet no direct evidence that the vitamin can make men more fertile.

Vitamin B$_{12}$ is widely recommended as a treatment for **asthma** (page 11),[20] but there is little real evidence that it is effective. Very weak evidence suggests that B$_{12}$ may be helpful in AIDS,[21,22] diabetic neuropathy,[23,24] multiple sclerosis (MS),[25,26] and tinnitus.[27]

Although vitamin B$_{12}$ has been proposed as a treatment for **Alzheimer's disease** (page 4), this recommendation is based solely on the results of one small, poorly designed study.[28] More recent and better-designed studies found little to no benefit.[29,30]

Vitamin B$_{12}$ is also sometimes recommended for numerous other problems, including **depression** (page 54), **osteoporosis** (page 100), and **periodontal disease** (page 103), but there is little to no evidence as yet that it really works.

## WHAT IS THE SCIENTIFIC EVIDENCE FOR VITAMIN B$_{12}$?

### Male Infertility

Vitamin B$_{12}$ deficiencies in men can lead to reduced sperm counts and lowered sperm mobility. It makes sense, then, that B$_{12}$ supplements might improve fertility for men who are truly deficient in this vitamin. Furthermore, several small studies suggest that B$_{12}$ supplementation (1,000 mcg daily) can sometimes improve sperm counts and sperm activity even for men who have *no* deficiency.[31,32] Better sperm count and mobility doesn't necessarily mean higher fertility—but they can't hurt!

## SAFETY ISSUES

Vitamin B$_{12}$ appears to be extremely safe. However, in some cases very high doses of vitamin B$_{12}$ can cause or worsen acne symptoms.[33,34]

## ⚠ INTERACTIONS YOU SHOULD KNOW ABOUT

If you are taking

- **Medications that reduce stomach acid, colchicine, corticosteroids, methotrexate, metformin, phenformin, oral contraceptives, nitrous oxide, cholestyramine, colestipol,** or **clofibrate:** You may need extra B$_{12}$.

- **Potassium:** You may need extra B$_{12}$.
- High doses of **vitamin C:** Blood tests for vitamin B$_{12}$ may not be reliable.

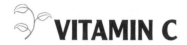

# VITAMIN C

*Principal Proposed Uses*
   Colds, cataracts, macular degeneration

*Other Proposed Uses*
   Cancer prevention and treatment, heart disease prevention, hypertension, asthma, low sperm count, bedsores, Alzheimer's disease, diabetes, hepatitis, herpes, insomnia, osteoarthritis, Parkinson's disease, periodontal disease, preeclampsia, rheumatoid arthritis, ulcers, allergies, general antioxidant, bladder infections, menopausal symptoms, migraine headaches, nausea

*Supplement Forms/Alternative Names*
   Ascorbic acid, ascorbate

Although most animals can make vitamin C from scratch, humans have lost the ability. We must get it from food, chiefly fresh fruits and vegetables. One of this vitamin's main functions is helping the body manufacture collagen, a key protein in our connective tissues, cartilage, and tendons.

From ancient times through the early nineteenth century, sailors and others deprived of fresh fruits and vegetables developed a disease called *scurvy.* Scurvy involves so-called scorbutic symptoms, which include nonhealing wounds, bleeding gums, bruising, and overall weakness. Now we know that scurvy is nothing more than vitamin C deficiency.

Scurvy was successfully treated with citrus fruit during the mid-1700s. In 1928, when Albert Szent-Gyorgyi isolated the active ingredient, he called it the "anti-scorbutic principle," or ascorbic acid. This, of course, is vitamin C.

Vitamin C is a powerful antioxidant that protects against damaging natural substances called free radicals. It works in water, both inside and outside of cells. Vitamin C complements another antioxidant vitamin, **vitamin E** (page 337), which works in lipid (fatty) parts of the body.

Vitamin C is the single most popular vitamin supplement in the United States, and perhaps the most controversial as well. In the 1960s, two-time Nobel Prize winner Dr. Linus Pauling claimed that vitamin C could effectively treat both cancer and the common cold. Research has been mixed on both counts, but that hasn't dampened enthusiasm for this essential nutrient. The vitamin C movement has led to hundreds of clinical studies testing the vitamin on dozens of illnesses.

Fair evidence supports using vitamin C supplements to help colds, slightly improve asthma, and reduce the risk of macular degeneration and cataracts. Evidence for its effectiveness in treating other conditions is highly preliminary at best.

## REQUIREMENTS/SOURCES

Vitamin C is an essential nutrient that must be obtained from food or supplements—the body cannot manufacture it. The U.S. Recommended Dietary Allowance is as follows

- Infants under 6 months, 30 mg
  6 to 12 months, 35 mg
- Children 1 to 3 years, 40 mg
  4 to 10 years, 45 mg
  11 to 14 years, 50 mg
- Adults (and teenagers 15 years and older),
  60 mg
- Pregnant women, 70 mg
- Nursing women, 90 to 95 mg

Scurvy, the classic vitamin C deficiency disease, is now a rarity in the developed world, although a more subtle deficiency of vitamin C is fairly common, especially among hospital patients.[1-5] Also, aspirin, other anti-inflammatory drugs, and corticosteroids can lower body levels of vitamin C.[6,7,8]

Most of us think of orange juice as the quintessential source of vitamin C, but many vegetables are actually even richer sources. Red chili peppers, sweet peppers, kale, parsley, collard, and turnip greens are excellent sources, as are broccoli, brussels sprouts, watercress, cauliflower, cabbage, and strawberries. (Oranges and other citrus fruits are good sources, too.)

One great advantage of getting vitamin C from foods rather than from supplements is that you will get many other healthy nutrients at the same time, such as bioflavonoids and carotenes. However, vitamin C in food is partially destroyed by cooking and exposure to air, so for maximum nutritional benefit you might want to try freshly made salads rather than dishes that require a lot of cooking.

Vitamin C supplements are available in two forms: ascorbic acid and ascorbate. The latter is less intensely sour.

## THERAPEUTIC DOSAGES

Ever since Linus Pauling, proponents have recommended taking vitamin C in enormous doses, as high as 20 to 30 g daily. However, some evidence suggests that there might not be any reason to take more than 200 mg of vitamin C daily (10 to 100 times less than the amount recommended by vitamin C proponents).[9] The reason is that if you consume more than 200 mg daily (researchers have tested up to 2,500 mg) your kidneys begin to excrete the excess at a steadily increasing rate, matching the increased dose. Your digestive tract also stops absorbing it well. The net effect is that no matter how much you take, your blood levels of vitamin C don't increase.

However, there are some gaps in this research as well as contradictory evidence.[10] Many nutritional experts recommend a total of 500 mg of vitamin C daily. This dose is almost undoubtedly safe. Others recommend that you take as much vitamin C as you can, up to 30,000 mg daily, cutting back only when you start to develop stomach cramps and diarrhea. This recommendation is not so much based on any evidence that such huge doses of vitamin C are good for you, but primarily on a semireligious enthusiasm.

## THERAPEUTIC USES

According to numerous double-blind studies, vitamin C supplements can reduce symptoms of **colds** (page 44), shorten the length of the illness, and, when taken regularly, perhaps slightly reduce your chance of catching a cold in the first place.[11,12,13]

Observational studies tell us that people who regularly use vitamin C supplements are less likely to develop either of two eye problems, **cataracts** (page 37) and **macular degeneration** (page 85) (for a definition of observational studies, see the introduction).[14-19]

Many studies have tried to evaluate whether vitamin C supplements can help **asthma** (page 11), and although the results have been mixed, on balance the evidence suggests that vitamin C may be slightly helpful.[20]

Small double-blind studies suggest that vitamin C may be able to speed recovery from bedsores[21] and increase sperm count.[22] In addition, vitamin C supplements have been recommended for **Alzheimer's disease** (page 4), **hypertension** (page 75), **diabetes** (page 60), **hepatitis** (page 71), **herpes** (page 73), **insomnia** (page 80), Parkinson's disease, **periodontal disease** (page 103), preeclampsia, **rheumatoid arthritis** (page 109), **bladder infections** (page 23), **menopausal symptoms** (page 87), **migraine headaches** (page 89), **nausea** (page 92), and **ulcers**

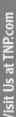

(page 112), but there is no solid scientific basis for any of these uses.

Vitamin C is often suggested as a treatment for **allergies** (page 3), but the research results are very preliminary and somewhat contradictory.[23,24,25]

Vitamin C in the diet appears to reduce the risk of **cancer** (page 26) and **heart disease** (page 14) and slow the progression of **osteoarthritis** (page 95).[26,27] However, there is little evidence that vitamin C *supplements* provide the same benefits. As noted earlier, foods containing vitamin C also contain many other healthful ingredients (such as bioflavonoids and carotenes), so it's not clear that pills containing vitamin C alone work just as well.

## WHAT IS THE SCIENTIFIC EVIDENCE FOR VITAMIN C?

### Colds

As the most famous of all natural treatments for colds, vitamin C has been subjected to irresponsible hype from both proponents and opponents. Enthusiasts claim that if you take vitamin C daily, you will never get sick, while enemies of the treatment insist that vitamin C has no benefit at all.

However, a cool-headed evaluation of the research indicates something in between. It appears that vitamin C supplements *can* significantly reduce symptoms of colds and help you get over a cold faster.[28,29] In 11 studies, during which participants took 1,000 mg daily or more, symptom severity was reduced by 40%, and the average length of colds was shorter by a day.

Vitamin C also seems to prevent colds, but not very well. The results of numerous studies suggest that regular use of vitamin C can slightly reduce the number of colds you get each year by perhaps 20%.[30] One particular type of cold may respond better than others: the "post-marathon sniffle." Heavy endurance exercise temporarily weakens the immune system, leading to a high incidence of infection following marathons and triathlons. There is some evidence that vitamin C can prevent such colds.[31,32]

Part of the confusion over vitamin C results from a misleading review article published in the 1970s. This article stated that vitamin C reduced the length of colds by a mere 2.5 hours, on average—not exactly an impressive finding![33] After this article was published, many physicians adopted a negative attitude toward vitamin C. A close look at the data, however, shows that the article's conclusions were biased. The reviewer included studies in which subjects took as little as 25 mg of vitamin C daily—less than what you'd get in half an orange.[34] You clearly need more vitamin C than that if you want to see any benefits.

### Cataracts

Regular use of vitamin C may reduce the risk of cataracts, probably by fighting free radicals that damage the lens of the eye. In an observational study of 50,800 nurses followed for 8 years, it was found that people who used vitamin C supplements for more than 10 years had a 45% lower rate of cataract development.[35] Interestingly, diets high in vitamin C were *not* found to be protective—only supplemental vitamin C made a difference. This is the opposite of what has been found with vitamin C in the prevention of other diseases, such as **cancer** (page 26).

A more recent study of 247 women suggests that vitamin C supplements taken for more than 10 years reduce the incidence of cataracts by 77%.[36] In this study, no benefit was found for shorter-term vitamin C supplementation.

It has been suggested that vitamin C may be particularly useful against cataracts in people with diabetes, because of its influence on *sorbitol*, a sugar-like substance that tends to accumulate in the cells of diabetics. Excess sorbitol is believed to play a role in the development of diabetes-related cataracts, and vitamin C appears to help reduce sorbitol buildup.[37]

### Macular Degeneration

After cataracts, injury to the macula (the most important part of the retina) is the second most common cause of vision loss in people 65 and older.

Observational studies involving a total of over 4,000 people suggest that regular use of vitamin C supplements may help prevent macular degeneration.[38,39] Vitamin C is thought to work by protecting the retina against damaging free radicals.

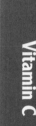

Vitamin C

According to one study, a combination of many antioxidants including vitamin C might be able to halt macular degeneration that has already begun. In this 18-month double-blind trial, a daily supplement containing 750 mg of vitamin C, 200 IU of vitamin E, 50 mcg of selenium, and 20,000 IU of beta-carotene actually stopped progression of macular degeneration.[40]

**Warning:** If you have macular degeneration, do not self-treat it without first seeing a physician. One particular type of macular degeneration must be treated with laser surgery.

## Cancer Prevention

While there is some evidence that dietary vitamin C from fruits and vegetables can reduce the risk of cancer, we don't know if vitamin C *supplements* are particularly helpful. This is a crucial distinction. When you get vitamin C from fruits and vegetables, you also receive myriad other substances such as bioflavonoids and carotenes that may provide health benefits. The studies involving vitamin C supplements and cancer prevention have not shown stellar results.

One study found that vitamin C supplementation at 500 mg or more daily was connected to a lower incidence of bladder cancer.[41] However, another study found *no* benefit.[42]

Supplemental vitamin C at 1 g daily failed to prevent new colon cancers after one had developed.[43] In another large observational study, 500 or more mg of vitamin C daily over a period of 6 years provided *no* significant protection against breast cancer.[44] Another study found similar results.[45]

## Cancer Treatment

Cancer treatment is one of the more controversial proposed uses of vitamin C. An early study tested vitamin C in 1,100 terminally ill cancer patients. One hundred patients received 10 g daily of vitamin C, while 1,000 other patients (the control group) received placebo. Those taking the vitamin survived more than 4 times longer on average (210 days) than those in the control group (50 days).[46] A large (1,826 subjects) follow-up study by the same researchers found a nearly doubled survival rate (343 days versus 180 days) in vitamin C–treated patients whose cancers were deemed "incurable."[47] However, other studies

have found no benefit of vitamin C in cancer.[48,49] At the present time, vitamin C cannot be regarded as a proven treatment for cancer.

It is also controversial whether any antioxidants should be taken *during* cancer chemotherapy. It is possible (but definitely not proven) that they may block the action of certain medications.[50] Since this is a very active area of research, cancer patients should talk with their oncologists about the wisdom of using *any* supplements while receiving chemotherapeutic drugs.

## Heart Disease Prevention

As with cancer prevention, there is some evidence that eating vitamin C–rich foods can reduce your risk of heart disease. However, it's less clear whether vitamin C supplements can do the same.[51,52,53]

In one major study, the combination of vitamin C and vitamin E supplements was better than vitamin E alone in preventing heart disease.[54] Vitamin C supplements alone, however, did not seem to be effective.

## Hypertension (High Blood Pressure)

Several studies suggest that 1,000 mg daily or more of vitamin C may modestly reduce blood pressure.[55] However, none of the major studies were double-blinded, so the results could have been influenced by the power of suggestion. One double-blind study found no difference between vitamin C and placebo.[56] A small double-blind study did find a slightly superior effect with vitamin C as compared to placebo.[57]

## SAFETY ISSUES

Vitamin C is indisputably safe at dosages up to 500 mg daily, and is probably not dangerous at much higher doses. Reports that vitamin C can cause DNA damage were based on an exaggerated interpretation of a fairly theoretical finding.[58]

If you take more than 1,000 to 2,000 mg daily, you may develop diarrhea. This side effect may go away with continued use of vitamin C, but you may have to cut down your dosage for a while, and then build up again gradually. At a high enough dosage, however, the diarrhea can continue indefinitely as long as you keep taking the vitamin C. Staying below this amount is called "taking vitamin C to bowel tolerance." However, as mentioned earlier, there may not be much point to taking more than 200 to 500 mg of vitamin C daily.

High-dose vitamin C can cause **copper** (page 169) deficiency and excessive **iron** (page 234) absorption. There have also been warnings that long-term vitamin C treatment can cause kidney stones,[59] but in a large-scale study the people who took the most vitamin C (over 1,500 mg daily) actually had a *lower* risk of kidney stones than those taking the least amounts.[60] Nonetheless, people with a history of kidney stones and those with kidney failure who have a defect in vitamin C or oxalate metabolism should probably restrict vitamin C intake to approximately 100 mg daily.[61]

You should also avoid high-dose vitamin C if you have glucose-6-phosphate dehydrogenase deficiency, iron overload, kidney failure, or a history of intestinal surgery. Vitamin C may also reduce the blood-thinning effects of Coumadin (warfarin) and heparin.[62,63]

The maximum safe dosages of vitamin C for young children, pregnant or nursing women, or those with severe liver or kidney disease have not been determined.

Vitamin C may raise blood levels of some drugs, such as aspirin and other salicylates.

## ⚠ INTERACTIONS YOU SHOULD KNOW ABOUT

If you are taking

- **Aspirin,** other **anti-inflammatory drugs, oral contraceptives, estrogen-replacement therapy,** or **phenobarbital:** You may need more vitamin C. (But see next bullet.)

- **Aspirin** or other **salicylates:** Vitamin C may raise blood levels of these drugs. Consult your physician to determine whether this could cause a problem for you.

- **Coumadin** or **heparin:** High-dose vitamin C might reduce their effectiveness.

- **Iron supplements:** High-dose vitamin C can cause you to absorb too much iron. This is especially a problem for people with diseases that cause them to store too much iron.

- **High doses of vitamin C:** Your ability to absorb copper may be impaired, and tests for vitamin $B_{12}$ levels may not be accurate.

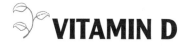

# VITAMIN D

*Principal Proposed Uses*
Preventing and treating osteoporosis

*Other Proposed Uses*
Cancer prevention, psoriasis

*Supplement Forms/Alternative Names*
Cholecalciferol (vitamin $D_3$), ergocalciferol (vitamin $D_2$)

**V**itamin D is both a vitamin and a hormone. It's a vitamin because your body cannot absorb calcium without it; it's a hormone because your body manufactures it in response to your skin's exposure to sunlight.

There are two major forms of vitamin D, and both have the word *calciferol* in their names. In Latin, calciferol means "calcium carrier." Vitamin $D_3$ (cholecalciferol) is made by the body and is found in some foods. Vitamin $D_2$ (ergocalciferol) is the form most often added to milk and other foods, and the form you're most likely to use as a supplement.

Reasonably good evidence tells us that the combination of vitamin D and calcium supplements can be quite helpful for preventing and treating osteoporosis.

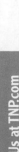

## REQUIREMENTS/SOURCES

As with **vitamin A** (page 318) and **vitamin E** (page 337), dosages of vitamin D are expressed in terms of *international units* (IU) rather than milligrams. The adequate intake (AI) for vitamin D is as follows

- Males and females up to 50 years, 200 IU daily

  51 to 70 years, 400 IU

  71 years and older, 600 IU

- Pregnant women, 200 IU

- Nursing women, 200 IU

However, some authorities think that the recommendations for adults are too low, and 800 IU may be more appropriate.[1]

Vitamin D is unusual in that you can get it by simply going outdoors and exposing your skin to moderate amounts of sunlight. However, in many parts of the world it's hard to get enough sunlight in winter. In the past, severe vitamin D deficiency was common in England due to coal smoke obscuring the sun. Cod liver oil, which is high in vitamin D, became popular as a children's supplement to help prevent rickets. Rickets is a disease in which developing bones soften and curve because they aren't receiving enough calcium.

Today, severe vitamin D deficiency is rare in the developed world. However, it is sometimes seen in elderly people who don't get enough sunlight.[2] Marginal vitamin D deficiency may also occur in people who live in northern latitudes and don't drink vitamin D–enriched milk. Additionally, phenytoin, primidone and phenobarbital (for seizures), corticosteroids, cimetidine (for ulcers), colestipol and cholestyramine (older drugs used for lowering cholesterol), and the antituberculosis drug isoniazid (INH) may interfere with vitamin D absorption or activity.[3–9]

Good food sources of vitamin D include cod liver oil, coldwater fish (such as mackerel, salmon, and herring), butter, and egg yolks. Milk and milk products are usually fortified with vitamin D. Vegetables provide little vitamin D, but dark-green leafy vegetables do contain some.

## THERAPEUTIC DOSAGES

For therapeutic purposes, vitamin D is taken at nutritional doses, as described in the Requirements/Sources section. Because of the risk of toxicity, this dosage should not be exceeded except under medical supervision (see Safety Issues).

## THERAPEUTIC USES

Without question, if you are concerned about **osteoporosis** (page 100), you should take **calcium** (page 146) and vitamin D. The combination definitely helps prevent bone loss.[10,11] This is true even if you are taking estrogen or any other treatment for osteoporosis; after all, you can't build bone without calcium, and you can't properly absorb and utilize calcium without adequate intake of vitamin D.

Other uses of vitamin D are less well documented. Some evidence suggests that vitamin D may help prevent **cancer** (page 26) of the breast, colon, pancreas, and prostate, but the research on this question has yielded mixed results.[12–18]

Vitamin D is sometimes mentioned as a treatment for **psoriasis** (page 106). However, this recommendation is based on Danish studies using calcipotriol, a variation of vitamin $D_3$ that is used externally (applied to the skin).[19] Calcipotriol does *not* affect your body's absorption of calcium, so it is really a very different substance from the vitamin D you can purchase at a store.

## WHAT IS THE SCIENTIFIC EVIDENCE FOR VITAMIN D?

### Osteoporosis

There is very little doubt that the combination of calcium plus vitamin D can slow down or even reverse osteoporosis, and reduce the risk of fractures.

One double-blind study followed 249 women in Boston for 1 year; the location of this study is important because your body can't produce significant amounts of vitamin D from sunlight during the winter in Boston.[20] These were postmenopausal women with an average age of 61, none of whom were taking estrogen or other medications for bone loss. Half of the women received a calcium citrate malate supplement (400 mg daily) plus a vitamin D supplement (400 IU daily), while the other half received placebo. The women in this study who were taking the vitamin D and calcium experienced a net increase in spinal bone mass (0.85%), while the placebo group showed no net change—a significant difference.

Another double-blind placebo-controlled study enrolling 3,270 women (nearly all of whom had never been on estrogen-replacement therapy) found that higher dosages of vitamin D produced even better results. For a period of 1½ years, participants received either placebo or 1,200 mg of calcium and 800 IU of vitamin D. At the end of the study period, the researchers found that the bone density in the hips of the women who had taken calcium and vitamin D had *increased* by 2.7%, while the hip bone density of the women who had taken placebo *decreased* by 4.6%. The calcium/vitamin D group also had 43% fewer hip fractures. A reduced fracture rate was also seen in another large, double-blind placebo-controlled study.[21]

However, vitamin D alone does not appear to be effective.[22] It must be combined with calcium to help.

## SAFETY ISSUES

When taken at recommended dosages, vitamin D appears to be safe. However, when taken to excess, vitamin D can build up in the body and cause severe symptoms of toxicity. Generally, toxic symptoms are seen when dosages above 1,200 IU daily are taken for long periods of time. These range from headaches, weight loss, and kidney stones to deafness, blindness, and death. Because you may be getting other sources of vitamin D as well, we do not recommend taking more than 800 IU daily except on physician advice.

People with sarcoidosis or hyperparathyroidism should never take vitamin D without first consulting a physician.

## ⚠ INTERACTIONS YOU SHOULD KNOW ABOUT

If you are taking **antiseizure drugs (phenobarbital, primidone, valproic acid or phenytoin), corticosteroids, H2 blockers** (e.g., **Zantac), heparin, isoniazid (INH), rifampin,** or the older cholesterol-lowering drugs **colestipol** and **cholestyramine,** you may need extra vitamin D.

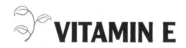

# VITAMIN E

*Principal Proposed Uses*
Heart disease prevention, cancer prevention

*Other Proposed Uses*
Tardive dyskinesia, impaired immunity, Alzheimer's disease, male infertility, diabetes, PMS, cataracts, osteoarthritis, cyclic mastalgia, asthma, menopausal symptoms, psoriasis, acne, gout, macular degeneration

*Supplement Forms/Alternative Names*
Alpha tocopherol, D-tocopherol, DL-tocopherol, DL-alpha tocopherol, tocopheryl acetate, tocopheryl succinate, D-alpha-tocopherol, D-delta-tocopherol, D-beta-tocopherol, D-gamma-tocopherol, and mixed tocopherols

Vitamin E is an antioxidant that fights damaging natural substances known as free radicals. It works in lipids (fats and oils), which makes it complementary to vitamin C, which fights free radicals dissolved in water.

Of all the antioxidants so much in the news today, vitamin E has the best evidence for its effectiveness. Impressive studies suggest that it can significantly reduce the risk of heart disease and various forms of cancer. Vitamin E has also

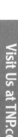

shown considerable promise for improving immunity, slowing the progression of Alzheimer's disease, and improving male fertility.

## REQUIREMENTS/SOURCES

The U.S. Recommended Dietary Allowance for vitamin E is measured not in milligrams but in *international units* (IU) and is as follows

- Infants under 6 months, 3 IU

  6 months to 1 year, 4 IU

- Children 1 to 3 years, 6 IU

  4 to 6 years, 7 IU

  7 to 10 years, 7 IU

- Males 11 years and older, 10 IU

- Females 11 years and older, 8 IU

- Pregnant women, 10 IU

- Nursing women, 11 to 12 IU

Vitamin E intake is commonly slightly deficient in developed countries.[1,2] Furthermore, various drugs can inhibit vitamin E absorption or utilization, including the older cholesterol drugs cholestyramine and colestipol.[3–6]

Vitamin E is actually a family of compounds called *tocopherols*. While there are many tocopherols, the most common form used in supplements is a synthetic form called *DL-alpha tocopherol*. However, there is some evidence that natural forms of vitamin E are more effective.[7,8,9] Natural-source vitamin E contains beta-, delta-, and gamma-tocopherols, as well as other compounds in the tocopherol family (such as tocotrienols). Natural vitamin E also differs from the synthetic kind in another way as well. Natural vitamin E comes in a form called a *D-isomer* (the "D" stands for *dextro,* or right-handed). Synthetic vitamin E contains a mixture of D- and L-isomers ("L" is for *levo,* or left-handed).

It has been suggested that the best vitamin E supplement would be a natural mixture of tocopherols including alpha-, delta-, and gamma- ("mixed tocopherols"), all of which should be in the "D" form. However, all the scientific evidence we have for the effectiveness of vitamin E supplements comes from studies using synthetic DL-alpha-tocopherol, so at this point we have

no direct confirmation that natural vitamin E is better.

The best food sources of vitamin E are polyunsaturated vegetable oils, seeds, nuts, and whole grains. To get a therapeutic dosage, though, you need to take a supplement.

## THERAPEUTIC DOSAGES

The optimal therapeutic dosage of vitamin E has not been established. Most studies have used between 50 and 800 IU daily, and some have used even higher doses.

If you wish to purchase natural vitamin E, look for a label that says "mixed tocopherols." However, some manufacturers use this term to mean the synthetic DL-alpha tocopherol, so you need to read the contents closely. Natural tocopherols come as D-alpha-, D-gamma-, D-delta-, and D-beta-tocopherol.

## THERAPEUTIC USES

There is fairly strong evidence that regular use of vitamin E can reduce the risk of **heart disease** (page 14).[10–13]

Also, vitamin E appears to help prevent various forms of **cancer** (page 26), especially prostate[14] and colon[15] cancer.

Vitamin E appears to reduce symptoms of tardive dyskinesia, an unpleasant movement disorder that can develop after years of taking antipsychotic drugs. [16–20]

Intriguing evidence suggests that vitamin E may also improve immunity,[21] slow the progression of **Alzheimer's disease** (page 4),[22] and be helpful in treating **infertility in men** (page 78).[23]

Weaker evidence suggests that vitamin E can improve blood sugar control in people with type 2 **diabetes** (page 60),[24,25,26] reduce symptoms of **PMS** (page 104),[27,28] prevent **cataracts** (page 37),[29–32] and slow the progression of **osteoarthritis** (page 95),[33] and help prevent or treat **macular degeneration** (page 85).

Vitamin E does *not* appear to be helpful for cyclic breast pain, sometimes called fibrocystic breast disease, cyclic mastitis, or **cyclic mastalgia** (page 52).[34]

Vitamin E and other antioxidants are frequently recommended for **asthma** (page 11), on the grounds that they may protect inflamed lung tissue, but there is no scientific evidence that they work. Similarly, although vitamin E has been suggested as a treatment for **menopausal symptoms** (page 87), **psoriasis** (page 106), **gout** (page 69), and **acne** (page 2) there is no real supporting evidence for any of these uses.

There is also some evidence that vitamin E might help reduce the lung-related side effects caused by the drug amiodarone (used to prevent abnormal heart rhythms).[35]

## WHAT IS THE SCIENTIFIC EVIDENCE FOR VITAMIN E?

### Heart Disease

Vitamin E is the best-documented antioxidant supplement for the prevention of heart disease. It seems to be able to reduce the risk of heart disease and heart attacks by 40 to 80%, depending on the dose.

In a double-blind intervention trial (see the Introduction for definition), 2,002 individuals with heart disease were given either placebo or vitamin E (400 or 800 IU daily) and followed for about 18 months.[36] The treated participants (at both dosages combined) showed almost an 80% drop in nonfatal heart attacks, a remarkable improvement. Curiously, fatal heart attacks were not reduced, for reasons that are not clear.

An enormous observational study (see the Introduction for definition) enrolling 39,910 American male health professionals followed for 4 years, vitamin E supplementation at a dosage of 100 IU daily or more was associated with a 37% reduced risk of heart disease.[37]

Vitamin E seems to be helpful for women too. An even larger (87,245 participants) and longer (8 years) study of female nurses, aged 34 to 59 years old with no previously diagnosed heart disease, found that women who took vitamin E supplements for at least 2 years had a 40% lower risk of developing heart disease.[38]

Finally, another large observational study (over 11,000 participants) suggests that if you take both vitamins E and C, the results will be even better.[39]

In two studies, vitamin E was *not* effective.[40,41] However, the dosage of vitamin E used

in these studies was small—about 50 IU daily—and the participants were smokers. It appears that low-dose vitamin E cannot counter the powerful negative influence of smoking.

Although we don't really know how vitamin E works to prevent heart disease, there are several theories. One points out that vitamin E protects fats and cholesterol from being converted by free radicals into an especially damaging form.[42] Another possible explanation hinges on vitamin E's effect on the formation of dangerous blood clots. Platelets stick to the walls of blood vessels damaged by atherosclerosis, forming blood clots that can then break off and cause heart attacks and strokes. Like aspirin, vitamin E interferes with the activity of blood platelets.[43]

### Cancer Prevention

Vitamin E appears to offer dramatic benefits for preventing prostate and colon cancer. In an intervention trial that involved 29,133 smokers, those who were given about 50 IU of vitamin E daily for 5 to 8 years showed a 32% lower incidence of prostate cancer, a 41% drop in prostate cancer deaths, and a 16% decrease in the incidence of colon cancer.[44]

Surprisingly, these benefits were seen fairly soon after the start of supplementation, even though prostate cancer is very slow growing. A cancer that shows up today had its start many years ago. The fact that vitamin E almost immediately lowered the incidence of prostate cancer suggests that it somehow blocks the step at which a hidden prostate cancer makes the leap into becoming detectable.

The dosage of vitamin E used in this study was lower than what is usually recommended. It is quite reasonable to assume that a higher dosage would be more effective, but this has not been proven.

Vitamin E may be even more effective in people who do not smoke. Researchers at the Fred Hutchinson Cancer Research Center in Seattle found that regular use of supplemental vitamin E (200 IU or more daily) cut colon cancer risk by 57%.[45] Another observational study found a 29 to 59% reduction, based on the length of time of using vitamin E.[46]

Vitamin E

Visit Us at TNP.com

## Tardive Dyskinesia

Tardive dyskinesia consists of involuntary movements of the face, arms, and head, usually caused by the long-term use of antipsychotic drugs. In a double-blind study, 50 subjects were given either placebo or 1,600 IU of vitamin E per day for a period of up to 36 weeks.[47] The vitamin E group did significantly better than those taking placebo. Good results have been seen in smaller, shorter-term studies,[48,49,50] although there have been negative studies too.[51,52] According to one study, 1,600 IU of vitamin E daily is much more effective than 600 IU.[53] However, physician supervision is necessary when using this much.

## Immunity

A recent double-blind study suggests that vitamin E may be able to strengthen immunity. In this study, 88 people over the age of 65 were given either placebo or vitamin E at 60 IU, 200 IU, or 800 IU daily.[54] The researchers then gave all participants immunizations against hepatitis B, tetanus, diphtheria, and pneumonia, and looked at subjects' immune response to these vaccinations. The researchers also used a skin test that evaluates the overall strength of the immune response.

The results were impressive. Vitamin E at all dosages significantly increased the strength of the immune response. However, a daily dosage of 200 IU produced the most marked benefits.

## Alzheimer's Disease

Preliminary evidence suggests that high-dose vitamin E may slow the progression of Alzheimer's disease.[55] In a double-blind placebo-controlled study, 341 subjects received either 2,000 IU daily of vitamin E, the antioxidant drug selegiline, or placebo. Those given vitamin E took nearly 200 days longer to reach a severe state of the disease than the placebo group. (Selegiline was even more effective.)

**Warning:** Such high dosages of vitamin E should not be taken except under a doctor's supervision (see Safety Issues).

## Low Sperm Count/Infertility

In one placebo-controlled study of 52 men whose sperm showed subnormal activity, treatment with 100 IU of vitamin E daily resulted in improved sperm activity and higher actual fertility (measured in pregnancies).[56] It is not known whether somewhat higher doses of vitamin E, such as are commonly used for general health purposes, would provide even greater benefit.

## SAFETY ISSUES

Vitamin E is generally regarded as safe when taken at the recommended dosage of 400 to 800 IU daily. However, vitamin E does have a "blood-thinning" effect that could lead to problems in certain situations. In one study, vitamin E supplementation at the low dose of about 50 IU per day was associated with an increase in hemorrhagic stroke, the kind of stroke caused by bleeding.[57]

Based on its blood-thinning effects, there are concerns that vitamin E could cause problems if it is combined with medications that also thin the blood, such as Coumadin (warfarin), heparin, Trental (pentoxifylline), and aspirin. Theoretically, the net result could be to thin the blood *too* much, causing bleeding problems. A study that evaluated vitamin E plus aspirin did in fact find an additive effect.[58] In contrast, the results of a study on vitamin E and Coumadin found no evidence of interaction, but it would still not be advisable to combine these treatments except under a physician's supervision.[59]

There is also at least a remote possibility that vitamin E could also interact with herbs that possess a mild blood-thinning effect, such as **garlic** (page 197) and **ginkgo** (page 204). Individuals with bleeding disorders such as hemophilia, and those about to undergo surgery or labor and delivery should also approach vitamin E with caution.

## ⚠ INTERACTIONS YOU SHOULD KNOW ABOUT

If you are taking

- Strong **blood-thinning drugs,** such as **Coumadin (warfarin)** or **heparin:** Seek medical advice before taking vitamin E.

- **Older cholesterol-lowering drugs (colestipol, cholestyramine):** You may need to take extra vitamin E.

- **Amiodarone:** Vitamin E may help protect you from lung-related side effects.

- **Iron** (page 234): Take vitamin E at a different time of day from when you take iron to avoid absorption problems.[60]

- **High doses of vitamin E:** You may need extra **vitamin K** (page 341).[61,62]

# 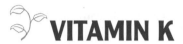 VITAMIN K

*Principal Proposed Uses*
Treating medication-induced vitamin K deficiency

*Other Proposed Uses*
Osteoporosis, menorrhagia (heavy menstrual bleeding), nausea

*Supplement Forms/Alternative names*
Vitamin $K_1$ (phylloquinone), vitamin $K_2$ (menaquinone), vitamin $K_3$ (menadione)

There's a good chance you haven't even heard of vitamin K. However, this obscure member of the vitamin clan is very important for good health. Without it, your blood wouldn't clot properly. There are three forms of vitamin K: $K_1$ (phylloquinone), found in plants; $K_2$ (menaquinone), produced by bacteria in your intestines; and $K_3$ (menadione), a synthetic form.

Vitamin K is used to reverse the effects of "blood-thinning" drugs such as Coumadin (warfarin). Its other proposed uses have little to no supporting evidence as yet.

## REQUIREMENTS/SOURCES

Vitamin K is an essential nutrient, but you need only a tiny amount of it. The U.S. Recommended Dietary Allowance is 1 mcg per kilogram body weight. This translates into the following

- Infants under 6 months, 5 mcg
  6 to 12 months, 10 mcg

- Children 1 to 3 years, 15 mcg
  4 to 6 years, 20 mcg
  7 to 10 years, 30 mcg

- Males 11 to 14 years, 45 mcg
  15 to 18 years, 65 mcg
  19 to 24 years, 70 mcg
  25 years and older, 80 mcg

- Females 11 to 14 years, 45 mcg
  15 to 18 years, 55 mcg
  19 to 24 years, 60 mcg
  25 years and older, 65 mcg

- Pregnant women, 65 mcg, preferably the $K_1$ variety (phylloquinone)

- Nursing women, 65 mcg, preferably the $K_1$ variety

However, a recent study suggests that a higher intake of vitamin K, in the range of 110 mcg daily, might be helpful for preventing osteoporosis.[1]

Vitamin K (in the form of $K_1$) is found in green leafy vegetables. Kale, green tea, and turnip greens are the best food sources, providing about 10 times the daily adult requirement in a single serving. Spinach, broccoli, lettuce, and cabbage are very rich sources as well, and you can get perfectly respectable amounts of vitamin K in such common foods as oats, green peas, whole wheat, and green beans, as well as watercress and asparagus.

Vitamin K (in the form of $K_2$) is also manufactured by bacteria in the intestines, and is a major source of vitamin K. Long-term use of antibiotics can cause a vitamin K deficiency by killing these bacteria. Pregnant women, newborn babies, and postmenopausal women are also sometimes deficient in this vitamin.[2,3,4]

Certain drugs can interfere with the action or absorption of vitamin K, including phenytoin (for seizures), cholestyramine (for high cholesterol), and even high doses of vitamin E.[5,6] The blood-thinning drug Coumadin (warfarin) works by antagonizing the effects of vitamin K. Conversely, vitamin K supplements, or intake of foods containing high levels of vitamin K, blocks the action of this medication, and can be used as an antidote.[7]

People with disorders of the digestive tract, such as chronic diarrhea, celiac sprue, ulcerative colitis, or Crohn's disease, may have trouble absorbing vitamin K.[8–11] Alcoholism can also lead to vitamin K deficiency.[12]

## THERAPEUTIC DOSAGES

For some purposes, vitamin K has been recommended at a daily dose of 150 to 500 mcg. Although such dosages are much higher than required for nutritional purposes, they are not out of the range of what can be reached through eating plenty of green leafy vegetables.

## THERAPEUTIC USES

There are no well-established therapeutic uses of vitamin K, other than its conventional use as an antidote for blood-thinning medications. However, vitamin K may be helpful when you are taking medications that can deplete your body's stores of vitamin K (see Interactions You Should Know About).

Recent evidence suggests that vitamin K supplements can be helpful for preventing osteoporosis.[13–22]

Based on its ability to help blood clot normally, vitamin K has been proposed as a treatment for excessive menstrual bleeding.[23] However, the last actual study testing this idea was carried out more than 55 years ago.[24] Vitamin K has also been recommended for **nausea** (page 92), although there is as yet little evidence that it really works.

## WHAT IS THE SCIENTIFIC EVIDENCE FOR VITAMIN K?

### Osteoporosis

Vitamin K plays a known biochemical role in the formation of new bone. This has led researchers to look for relationships between vitamin K intake and osteoporosis.

Research has found that people with osteoporosis have much lower blood levels of vitamin K than other people. For example, in a study of 71 postmenopausal women, participants with reduced bone mineral density showed lower serum vitamin $K_1$ levels than those with normal bone density.[25] Similar results have been seen in other studies.[26,27,28]

A recent report from 12,700 participants in the Nurse's Health Study found that higher dietary intake of vitamin K is associated with a significantly reduced risk of hip fracture.[29]

Interestingly, the most common source of vitamin K used by individuals in the study was iceberg lettuce, followed by broccoli, spinach, romaine lettuce, brussels sprouts, and dark greens. Women who ate lettuce each day had only 55% the risk of hip fracture as those who ate it only weekly. However, among women taking estrogen, no benefit was seen, probably because estrogen is so much more powerful.

Research also suggests that supplemental vitamin K can reduce the amount of **calcium** (page 146) lost in the urine.[30,31,32] This is indirect evidence of a beneficial effect on bone.

Taken together, these findings suggest that vitamin K supplements might help prevent osteoporosis.

## SAFETY ISSUES

Vitamin K is probably quite safe at the recommended therapeutic dosages, since those quantities are easily obtained from food.

Newborns are commonly given vitamin $K_1$ injections to prevent bleeding problems. Although some have suggested that this practice may increase the risk of cancer,[33] enormous observational studies have found no such connection (one such trial involved more than a million participants).[34,35]

## ⚠ INTERACTIONS YOU SHOULD KNOW ABOUT

If you are taking

■ **Coumadin (warfarin):** Do not take vitamin K supplements or eat foods high in vitamin K except under the supervision of a physician.

(You will need to have your medication dosage adjusted.)

■ **Phenytoin (Dilantin), phenobarbital, cholestyramine, colestipol,** long-term **antibiotic therapy,** or high doses of **vitamin E:** You may need more vitamin K.

# WHITE WILLOW (SALIX ALBA)

*Principal Proposed Uses*
Bursitis, tendinitis, headaches, back pain, osteoarthritis, rheumatoid arthritis, dysmenorrhea

White willow has been used as a treatment for pain and fever in China since 500 B.C. In Europe, it was primarily used for altogether different purposes, such as stopping vomiting, removing warts, and suppressing sexual desire(!). However, in 1828, European chemists made a discovery that would bring some of these different uses together. They extracted the substance salicin from white willow, which was soon purified to salicylic acid. Salicylic acid is an effective treatment for pain and fever, but it also is sufficiently irritating to do a good job of burning off warts.

Chemists later modified salicylic acid (this time from the herb meadowsweet) to create acetylsalicylic acid, or aspirin.

## WHAT IS WHITE WILLOW USED FOR TODAY?

As interest in natural medicine has grown, many people have begun to turn back to white willow as an alternative to aspirin. It is used for many of the same conditions as aspirin, such as bursitis, tendinitis, headaches, **osteoarthritis** (page 95), **dysmenorrhea** (page 65) and **rheumatoid arthritis** (page 109). Interestingly, this herb is reportedly not particularly hard on the stomach. This may be due to the fact that most of the salicylic acid in white willow is present in chemical forms that are only converted to salicylic acid after absorption into the body.[1]

## DOSAGES

White willow bark can be made into tea by boiling 1 to 2 g per cup of water for 10 minutes. Standardized tinctures and dry extracts are also available. They should be taken in a dose to provide 60 to 120 mg of salicin daily.[2]

## SAFETY ISSUES

Although white willow doesn't appear to upset the stomach as easily as aspirin, based on its chemical constituents it is almost certain that it can cause stomach irritation and even bleeding ulcers if used over the long term. All the other risks of aspirin therapy apply as well. For example, white willow should not be given to children, due to the risk of Reye's syndrome. It should also not be used by people with aspirin allergies, bleeding disorders, ulcers, kidney disease, liver disease, or diabetes, and it may interact adversely with alcohol, "blood thinners," other anti-inflammatories, methotrexate, metoclopramide, phenytoin, probenecid, spironolactone, and valproate.

Safety in pregnant or nursing women, or those with severe liver or kidney disease has not been established.

White Willow

Visit Us at TNP.com

# WILD CHERRY (PRUNUS SEROTINA)

## Principal Proposed Uses
Cough

The bark of the wild cherry tree is a traditional Native American remedy for two seemingly unrelated conditions: respiratory infections and anxiety. European settlers quickly adopted the herb for similar purposes.

## WHAT IS WILD CHERRY USED FOR TODAY?

Over time, wild cherry has come to be used primarily as a component of cough syrups. It is tempting to connect the two traditional uses of wild cherry by imagining that it functions like codeine to affect both the mind and the cough reflex. However, this is just speculation, as there has been very little scientific evaluation of this herb.

## DOSAGES

Syrups containing wild cherry should be taken as directed.

## SAFETY ISSUES

Wild cherry is generally regarded as safe when used at recommended dosages. However, since it contains small amounts of cyanide, it should not be taken to excess. It is not recommended for use by young children, pregnant or nursing women, or those with severe liver or kidney disease.

# WILD YAM A.K.A. MEXICAN YAM
## (DIOSCOREA SPECIES)

## Principal Proposed Uses
There are no well-documented uses for wild yam.

## Incorrect Proposed Uses
Source of women's hormones

Various species of wild yam grow throughout North and Central America and Asia. Traditionally, this herb has been used as a treatment for indigestion, coughs, morning sickness, gallbladder pain, menstrual cramps, joint pain, and nerve pain.[1,2] The main use of wild yam in the United States today, however, is based on a fundamental misconception: that it contains women's hormones such as progesterone and **DHEA** (page 176).

In reality, there is no progesterone, DHEA, or any other hormone in wild yam, nor are there any substances that the body can directly use to make such hormones.

To explain this widespread misunderstanding, I have to go back a number of years. When progesterone was first discovered, it was very expensive to produce. The first methods involved direct extraction of progesterone from cow ovaries, a process that required 50,000 cows to yield 20 mg of purified hormone![3] Other hormones such as estrogen and DHEA were also difficult to manufacture. Although doctors wanted to experiment with prescribing these treatments as medicine, until a simpler production method could be developed, it simply wasn't feasible.

The race to discover a more economical source of hormones was won by a scientist/businessman named Russell Marker. In the 1940s, he perfected a method of synthesizing progesterone from a constituent of wild yams called diosgenin. This process involves several chemical transformations carried out in the laboratory.

Marker focused his attention on two species of yam found in Mexico, *Dioscorea macrostachya* and *Dioscorea barabasco,* the latter of which is richer in diosgenin, while the former is much easier to harvest in the wild. He formed a manufacturing company in Mexico that produced progesterone and DHEA from these raw materials.

Unfortunately, corporate competition and difficult labor conditions eventually forced him to close his plant. But Marker's method of synthesizing progesterone continued to be used, bringing the price down drastically and helping to pave the way for the modern birth control pill. Progesterone continued to be manufac-

tured from wild yam for decades, until a cheaper source of raw material was found in cultivated soybeans.

But neither soybeans nor wild yam contain progesterone. They only contain chemicals that chemists can use as a starting point to manufacture progesterone. Furthermore, the body almost certainly can't turn diosgenin into progesterone, because the synthetic steps used by chemists to do so don't even remotely resemble natural processes.[4] Thus, any product that claims to contain "natural progesterone from wild yam" is misleading.

Nonetheless, some wild yam products do contain progesterone. Am I contradicting myself? Not at all: Manufacturers add synthetic progesterone to these creams. There may be a value to taking progesterone in cream form, but the Mexican yam part of the product is a red herring!

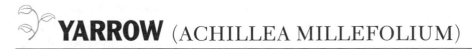

# YARROW (ACHILLEA MILLEFOLIUM)

## Principal Proposed Uses

*Topical uses:*
   Bleeding

*Oral uses:*
   Respiratory infections (prevention)

---

According to legend, the Greek general Achilles used yarrow to stop the bleeding of his soldiers' wounds during the Trojan War: hence the scientific name *Achillea* and the common names "soldier's wound-wort," "bloodwort," and *"herbe militaire."*

Yarrow has also been used traditionally as treatment for respiratory infections, menstrual pain, and digestive upsets.

## WHAT IS YARROW USED FOR TODAY?

Like osha, yarrow tea is commonly taken at the first sign of a **cold** (page 44) or flu to bring on sweating and, according to tradition, ward off infection. Crushed yarrow leaves and flower tops are also applied directly as first aid to stop nose-

bleeds and bleeding from minor wounds. However, there has not been any formal scientific study of how well yarrow works.

## DOSAGES

To make yarrow tea, steep 1 to 2 teaspoons of dried herb per cup of water. Combination products should be taken according to label instructions.

## SAFETY ISSUES

No clear toxicity has been associated with yarrow.[1] The FDA has expressed concern about a toxic constituent of yarrow known as thujone and permits only thujone-free yarrow

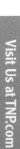Yarrow

Visit Us at TNP.com

extracts for use in beverages. Nonetheless, the common spice sage contains more thujone than yarrow, and the FDA lists sage as generally regarded as safe.

Yarrow seldom produces any side effects other than the occasional allergic reaction. Nonetheless, safety in young children, pregnant or nursing women, or those with severe liver or kidney disease has not been established.

# YERBA SANTA (ERIODICTYON CALIFORNICUM)

*Principal Proposed Uses*

*Oral uses:*
   Respiratory diseases (e.g., bronchitis, asthma)

*Topical uses:*
   Rash (e.g., poison ivy)

Yerba santa is a sticky-leafed evergreen that is native to the American Southwest. It was given its name ("holy weed") by Spanish priests impressed with its medicinal properties. The aromatic leaves were boiled to make a tea to treat coughs, colds, asthma, pleurisy, tuberculosis, and pneumonia, and a poultice of the leaves was applied to painful joints.

Unlike most medicinal herbs, yerba santa actually has a pleasant taste. It has been used as a general food flavoring and in cough syrups to disguise the bad taste of other ingredients.

## WHAT IS YERBA SANTA USED FOR TODAY?

Some modern herbalists regard yerba santa as one of the most effective natural treatments for chronic respiratory problems such as bronchitis and **asthma** (page 11). Unfortunately, scientific studies of this herb have not been carried out. About the most that can be said is that one of its constituents, eriodictyol, appears to be a mild expectorant.[1]

Yerba santa is occasionally used topically as a treatment for poison ivy.[2]

## DOSAGES

Yerba santa tea may be made by adding 1 teaspoon of crushed leaves to a cup of boiling water and steeping for half an hour. However, because many of its resinous constituents do not dissolve in water, alcoholic tinctures of yerba santa may be more effective. Such tinctures should be taken according to the directions on the label. Drink 3 cups a day until symptoms subside.

Yerba santa is often combined with the herbs **osha** (page 273) and grindelia.

## SAFETY ISSUES

Yerba santa is on the FDA's GRAS (generally regarded as safe) list for use as a food flavoring. There have been no reports of significant side effects or adverse reactions,[3] except for the inevitable occasional allergic reaction. Nonetheless, safety in young children, pregnant or nursing women, or those with severe liver or kidney disease has not been established.

# YOHIMBE (PAUSINYSTALIA YOHIMBE)

**Principal Proposed Uses**
Impotence (not recommended)

The bark of the West African yohimbe tree is a traditional aphrodisiac and the source of yohimbine, a prescription drug for impotence.

Yohimbine (the drug) is only modestly effective at best, better than placebo but only successful in about 30 to 45% of the men who use it.[1] However, it seems to work even in men whose impotence is caused by a serious illness such as diabetes.

We don't really know how yohimbine works, but recent thinking suggests that it operates by suppressing parts of the brain that keep sexual arousal under control.[2] In other words, it takes the brake off, which can be useful when the engine has lost some of its power.

## WHAT IS YOHIMBE USED FOR TODAY?

Like the drug yohimbine, the bark of the yohimbe tree is widely used to treat **impotence** (page 77). Many herbalists report that the herb is more effective than the purified drug, perhaps due to the presence of other unidentified active ingredients. However, there have been no good studies to prove this.

Yohimbe is also sometimes recommended as an antidepressant. However, its effectiveness is unknown and there are much safer herbs for this purpose, such as **St. John's wort** (page 303).

## DOSAGES

Yohimbe bark is best taken in a form standardized to yohimbine content. Most people take a dose that supplies 15 to 30 mg of yohimbine daily. However, higher doses are not necessarily better, and some people respond optimally to 10 or even 5 mg daily. Furthermore, while some people appear to respond immediately to a single dose, for others it takes 2 to 3 weeks of treatment to provide significant benefits.

Because yohimbine is a somewhat dangerous substance (see Safety Issues), I recommend a physician's supervision when taking it.

## SAFETY ISSUES

Yohimbe should not be used by pregnant or nursing women, or those with kidney, liver, or ulcer disease or high blood pressure. Dosages that provide more than 40 mg a day of yohimbine can cause a severe drop in blood pressure, abdominal pain, fatigue, hallucinations, and paralysis. (Interestingly, lower dosages can cause an increase in blood pressure.) Since 40 mg is not very far above the typical recommended dose, yohimbe has what is known as a narrow therapeutic index. This means that there is a relatively small dosing range, below which the herb doesn't work and above which it is toxic.

Even when taken in normal dosages, side effects of dizziness, anxiety, hyperstimulation, and nausea are not uncommon.

Yohimbine may also share some properties of a group of rather dangerous antidepressants called monoamine-oxidase inhibitors (MAOIs).[3] While the MAOI-like effects of yohimbine are believed to be weak and probably not significant, it may be prudent to use typical MAOI precautions, such as avoiding cheese, red wine, liver, and other tyramine-containing foods.

Yohimbe is not recommended for young children, pregnant or nursing women, or those with severe liver or kidney disease.

## ⚠ INTERACTIONS YOU SHOULD KNOW ABOUT

If you are taking **tricyclic antidepressants, phenothiazines, phentolamine, phenoxybenzamine, clonidine, MAO inhibitors, central nervous system stimulants,** or **naloxone,** don't use yohimbine.[4]

# YUCCA (YUCCA BREVIFOLIA AND OTHER SPECIES)

*Principal Proposed Uses*
Arthritis (both rheumatoid and osteoarthritis)

Various species of yucca plant were used as food by Native Americans and early California settlers. Yucca contains high levels of soapy compounds known as saponins that also made it a useful natural shampoo and soap.

## WHAT IS YUCCA USED FOR TODAY?

When taken for a long period of time, yucca is said to reduce osteo- and rheumatoid **arthritis** (page 95 and page 109) symptoms. However, the only scientific evidence for this claim comes from one preliminary study.[1]

Yucca extracts are also widely used to enhance the foaming effect of carbonated beverages.

## DOSAGES

The standard dosage is 2 to 4 tablets of concentrated yucca saponins daily.

## SAFETY ISSUES

Yucca is generally accepted as safe based on its long history of use as a food. However, it sometimes causes diarrhea if taken to excess. Safety in young children, pregnant or nursing women, or those with severe liver or kidney disease has not been established.

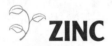

# ZINC

*Principal Proposed Uses*
Colds, general nutritional supplementation

*Other Proposed Uses*
Acne, sickle-cell anemia, male infertility, rheumatoid arthritis, macular degeneration, ulcers, attention deficit disorder, bladder infection, cataracts, eczema, periodontal disease, psoriasis, many others

*Supplement Forms/Alternative Names*
Zinc sulfate, zinc gluconate, zinc citrate, zinc picolinate, chelated zinc

Zinc is an important element that is found in every cell in the body. More than 300 enzymes in the body need zinc in order to function properly. Although the amount of zinc we need in our daily diet is tiny, it's very important that we get it. However, the evidence suggests that many of us do *not* get enough. Mild zinc deficiency seems to be fairly common.

Severe zinc deficiency can cause a major loss of immune function, and mild zinc deficiency might impair immunity slightly. For this reason, making sure to get enough zinc may help keep you from catching colds or other infections. But zinc may be helpful for colds in a completely different way, too, by directly killing viruses in the throat. When used in this way, it is taken in the form of lozenges every 2 hours from the first sign of cold symptoms.

Intriguing evidence suggests that zinc supplements may have other specific benefits as well, including helping stomach ulcers heal, relieving symptoms of rheumatoid arthritis, slightly improving acne symptoms, increasing sperm count, and preventing "sickle-cell crisis" (a serious condition in people with sickle-cell anemia).

## REQUIREMENTS/SOURCES

The U.S. Recommended Dietary Allowance for zinc is as follows

- Infants under 1 year, 5 mg
- Children 1 to 10 years, 10 mg
- Males 11 years and older, 15 mg
- Females 11 years and older, 12 mg
- Pregnant women, 15 mg
- Nursing women, 16 to 19 mg

However, the average diet in the developed world commonly provides less than two-thirds the recommended amount of zinc.[1,2] For this reason, it may be a wise idea to increase your intake of zinc on general principle.

Children, adolescents, pregnant women, and the elderly are particularly at risk for zinc deficiency, as are those with alcoholism, sickle-cell anemia, diabetes, and kidney disease. The drug AZT, used for AIDS, may impair zinc absorption;[3] the same is true for soy, manganese, and high intake of copper and iron.[4–8] Contrary to previous reports, folate does not affect zinc absorption.[9] However, calcium might interfere with zinc absorption under certain circumstances.[10,11] Loop and thiazide diuretics ("water pills") can cause excessive loss of zinc in the urine.[12]

Oysters are by far the best food source of zinc—a single serving will give you *10 times* the recommended daily intake! Seeds and nuts, peas, whole wheat, rye, and oats are not nearly as high in zinc, but you can get about 3 mg per serving of these foods.

Zinc can also be taken as a nutritional supplement, in one of many forms. Zinc citrate, zinc acetate, or zinc picolinate may be the best absorbed, although zinc sulfate is less expensive. When you purchase a supplement, you should be aware of the difference between the milligrams of actual zinc the product contains (so-called "elemental zinc") and the total milligrams of the zinc product. For example, 220 mg of zinc sulfate contains 50 mg of zinc. (The rest of the weight is the sulfate.) All figures given in this chapter refer to the amount of actual zinc to take.

## THERAPEUTIC DOSAGES

For most purposes, zinc should simply be taken at the recommended daily requirements listed previously. For best absorption, zinc supplements should not be taken at the same time as high fiber foods;[13,14] however, many high fiber foods provide zinc in themselves.

When taking zinc long term it is advisable to take 1 to 3 mg of **copper** (page 169) daily as well, because zinc supplements can cause copper deficiency.[15,16] Zinc also interferes with **magnesium** (page 251),[17] **calcium** (page 146),[18] and **iron** (page 234)[19] absorption.

For treatment of colds, much higher doses of zinc are used, although only for a short period of time. The usual dosage is 13 to 23 mg of zinc as zinc gluconate every 2 hours for a week or two (but no longer). The purpose is not to increase zinc levels in your body, but to kill viruses in the back of your throat. It appears that of the common forms of zinc, only zinc gluconate and zinc acetate have the required antiviral properties.[20,21] Also, some sweeteners and flavorings used in lozenges can block zinc's antiviral action. Dextrose, sucrose, mannitol, and sorbitol appear to be fine, but citric acid and tartaric acid are not. The information on glycine as a flavoring agent is a bit equivocal.

Long-term use of relatively high-dose zinc (90 mg daily or more) has been tried for various conditions such as acne, sickle-cell anemia, and rheumatoid arthritis, but medical supervision is essential because of the risk of toxicity (see Safety Issues).

## THERAPEUTIC USES

Good evidence suggests that if you take zinc lozenges every 2 hours at the beginning of a **cold** (page 44), you will recover much more quickly.[22] Long-term zinc supplementation at nutritional doses may also reduce the chance of getting sick, but probably only if you are deficient in zinc to begin with.[23]

Evidence also suggests that, when taken in relatively high dosages, zinc can reduce symptoms of **acne** (page 2).[24]

Zinc

Visit Us at TNP.com

Zinc

Zinc may also help prevent the development of sickle-cell crisis in sickle-cell anemia[25] and speed the healing of stomach **ulcers** (page 112).[26,27]

People with **rheumatoid arthritis** (page 109) have been found to have lower-than-average blood levels of zinc. Although this doesn't necessarily mean that zinc supplements will reduce symptoms of rheumatoid arthritis, several small studies suggest that they might help slightly.[28,29,30] However, others have shown no benefit at all.[31,32,33] It may be that zinc is only helpful for those who are zinc-deficient in the first place.[34]

One small study found that zinc supplements increased sperm counts and improved **fertility** (page 78) for men with low testosterone levels.[35] But no such effect was seen in men whose testosterone levels were normal to begin with.

Although the evidence that it works is not yet meaningful, zinc is sometimes recommended for the following conditions as well: **macular degeneration** (page 85),[36,37] **benign prostatic hyperplasia** (page 20),[38–46] prostatitis,[47] **impotence** (page 77),[48,49] Down's syndrome,[50,51,52] **Alzheimer's disease** (page 4),[53–56] wound healing,[57,58,59] inflammatory bowel disease (ulcerative colitis and Crohn's disease),[60–63] tinnitus,[64,65] **osteoporosis** (page 100),[66] **diabetes** (page 60),[67–69] AIDS,[70] anorexia nervosa,[71–74] **attention deficit disorder** (page 19), **bladder infection** (page 23), **cataracts** (page 37), **eczema** (page 66), **periodontal disease** (page 103), and **psoriasis** (page 106).

## WHAT IS THE SCIENTIFIC EVIDENCE FOR ZINC?

### Colds

Numerous studies have evaluated the effects of zinc lozenges for colds. All but one found that zinc lozenges can significantly improve cold symptoms, as long as the right form of zinc is used (zinc gluconate or acetate).[75,76] For example, in a recent double-blind study, 100 nursing home workers with early cold symptoms received either zinc gluconate lozenges or placebo.[77] They took the lozenges until their cold symptoms abated. Overall, the workers who took zinc had fewer days of coughing (2.2 days, compared to 4 for the placebo group), sore throat (1 day versus 3), nasal drainage (4 days versus 7), and headache (2 days versus 3) than the placebo group.

Good results have been seen in several other double-blind studies,[78] including one that used zinc acetate and enrolled about 100 participants.[79] A few studies found no benefit, but a close review of the evidence showed that these studies used forms of zinc lozenges that did not release virus-killing ions into the throat.[80] There has been only one study using the proper chemical form of zinc that did not find benefits, but a cherry flavoring added to the lozenges in that study might have interfered with ion release.[81]

Besides using zinc as a "virus killer," supplementation at nutritional dosages may also help reduce the frequency of colds by strengthening your overall health. In a 2-year study of nursing home residents, participants given zinc and selenium developed illnesses much less frequently than those given placebo.[82] Of course, it isn't clear from this study which was more helpful, the zinc or the selenium, but we do know that chronic zinc deficiency weakens the immune system.[83]

### Acne

Studies suggest that people with acne have lower-than-normal levels of zinc in their bodies.[84–87] This fact alone does not prove that taking zinc supplements will help acne, but several small double-blind studies involving a total of over 300 people have found generally positive results.

In one of these studies, 54 people were given either placebo or 135 mg of zinc as zinc sulfate daily. Zinc produced slight but measurable benefits.[88] Similar results have been seen in other studies using 90 to 135 mg of zinc daily.[89–93] In some studies, however, no benefits were seen.[94,95]

Two studies have compared zinc against a standard treatment for acne, the antibiotic tetracycline. One found that zinc was as effective as tetracycline,[96] but another found the antibiotic more effective.[97]

Keep in mind that the dosages of zinc used in these studies are rather high, and should be used only under a physician's supervision.

## Sickle-Cell Anemia

Zinc may also be helpful in preventing "sickle-cell crisis" in individuals with sickle-cell anemia.[98] A placebo-controlled double-blind study treated 145 sickle-cell subjects with either 220 mg of zinc sulfate 3 times daily or placebo. During 18 months of treatment, the zinc-treated subjects had an average of 2.5 crises, compared to 5.3 for the placebo group. However, zinc didn't seem to reduce the severity of a crisis, as measured by the number of days spent in the hospital for each crisis.

**Warning:** Sickle-cell anemia is far too serious a condition to self-treat, and the relatively high dosages of zinc used in this study should be taken only under the supervision of a doctor (see Safety Issues).

## Macular Degeneration

Macular degeneration is one of the most common causes of vision loss in the elderly. One double-blind study of 151 individuals followed for 1 to 2 years found that zinc supplements helped preserve vision.[99] However, another study of 112 individuals found no benefit.[100]

## SAFETY ISSUES

Zinc seldom causes any immediate side effects other than occasional stomach upset, usually when it's taken on an empty stomach. Some forms do have an unpleasant metallic taste.

However, long-term use of zinc at dosages of 100 mg or more daily can cause a number of toxic effects, including severe copper deficiency, impaired immunity, heart problems, and

anemia.[101,102,103] Unless a physician specifically advises you to take a higher dosage, you should stick to the nutritional dosage range described under Requirements/Sources.

Use of zinc can interfere with the absorption of **manganese** (page 254), **soy** (page 301), penicillamine, and antibiotics in the tetracycline or quinolone (Cipro, Floxin) family.[104,105,106]

## ⚠ INTERACTIONS YOU SHOULD KNOW ABOUT

If you are taking

- **Medications that reduce stomach acid, diuretics, ACE inhibitors, oral contraceptives, estrogen-replacement therapy, thiazide diuretics, loop diuretics, ethambutol, corticosteroids, copper,** or **iron:** You may need to take extra zinc.

- **Manganese, antacids, soy,** or **antibiotics** in the quinolone (e.g., **Cipro, Floxin**) or tetracycline family: Take zinc at a different time of the day.

- **Zinc supplements:** You should also take extra copper, calcium, and perhaps magnesium as well because zinc interferes with their absorption. These should be taken at a different time of day from when you take zinc. Zinc interferes with iron absorption, too, but you shouldn't take iron supplements unless you know you are deficient.

- **Penicillamine:** You may need extra zinc; however, zinc interferes with penicillamine's absorption, so it may be advisable to take zinc and penicillamine at least 2 hours apart.

# NOTES

## Acne

1. Pohit J, et al. Zinc status of acne vulgaris patients. *J Appl Nutr* 37(1): 18–25, 1985.

2. Amer M, et al. Serum zinc in acne vulgaris. *Int J Dermat* 21: 481, 1982.

3. Michaelsson G, et al. Serum zinc and retinol-binding protein in acne. *Br J Dermatol* 96(3): 283–286, 1977.

4. Michaelsson G and Ljunghall K. Patients with dermatitis herpetiformis, acne, psoriasis and Darier's disease have low epidermal zinc concentrations. *Acta Dermatovenereol* (Stockh) 70(4): 304–308, 1990.

5. Liden S, et al. Clinical evaluation of acne. *Acta Dermatovenereol* (Stockh) 89(Suppl.): 49–52, 1980.

6. Goransson K, et al. Oral zinc in acne vulgaris: a clinical and methodological study. *Acta Dermatovenereol* (Stockh) 58(5): 443–448, 1978.

7. Dreno B, et al. Low doses of zinc gluconate for inflammatory acne. *Acta Dermatovenereol* (Stockh) 69(6): 541–543, 1989.

8. Verma KC, et al. Oral zinc sulfate therapy in acne vulgaris: a double-blind trial. *Acta Dermatovenereol* (Stockh) 60: 337, 1980.

9. Weimar VM, et al. Zinc sulfate in acne vulgaris. *Arch Dermatol* 114(12): 1776–1778, 1978.

10. Hillstrom L, Pettersson L, Hellbe L, et al. Comparison of oral treatment with zinc sulphate and placebo in acne vulgaris. *Br J Dermatol* 97(6): 679–684, 1977.

11. Michaelsson G, Johlin L, and Ljunghall K. A double-blind study of the effect of zinc and vitamin A in acne vulgaris. *Arch Derm* 113: 31, 1977.

12. Weissman K, Wadskov S, and Sondergaard J. Oral zinc sulphate therapy for acne vulgaris. *Acta Derm Venereol* (Stockh) 57(4): 357–360, 1977.

13. Orris L, et al. Oral zinc therapy of acne. Absorption and clinical effect. *Arch Dermatol* 114(7): 1018–1020, 1978.

14. Michaelsson G, Johlin L, and Ljunghall K. A double-blind study of the effect of zinc and oxytetracycline in acne vulgaris. *Br J Dermatol* 97(5): 561–566, 1977.

15. Cunliffe WJ, et al. A double-blind trial of a zinc sulphate/citrate complex and tetracycline in the treatment of acne vulgaris. *Br J Dermatol* 101(3): 321–325, 1979.

## Allergies

1. Mittman P. Randomized, double-blind study of freeze-dried *Urtica dioica* in the treatment of allergic rhinitis. *Planta Medica* 56: 44–47, 1990.

2. Middleton E Jr, et al. The effects of citrus flavonoids on human basophil and neutrophil function. *Planta Medica* 53: 325–328, 1987.

3. Amellal M, Bronner C, Briancon F, et al. Inhibition of mast cell histamine release by flavonoids and bioflavonoids. *Planta Medica* 51: 16–20, 1985.

4. Gäbor M. Anti-inflammatory and anti-allergic properties of flavonoids. *Prog Clin Biol Res* 213: 471–480, 1986.

5. Middleton E Jr. Effect of flavonoids on basophil histamine release and other secretory systems. *Prog Clin Biol Res* 213: 493–506, 1986.

6. Ogasawara H and Middleton E Jr. Effect of selected flavonoids on histamine release (HR) and hydrogen peroxide ($H_2O_2$) generation by human leukocytes. *J Allergy Clin Immunol* 75: 184, 1985.

7. Middleton E Jr and Drzewiecki G. Flavonoid inhibition of human basophil histamine release stimulated by various agents. *Biochem Pharmacol* 33(21): 3333, 1984.

8. Pearce FL, et al. Mucosal mast cells III. Effect of quercetin and other flavonoids on antigen-induced histamine secretion from rat intestinal mast cells. *J Allergy Clin Immunol* 73: 819–823, 1984.

9. Middleton E Jr, Drzewiecki G, and Krishnarao D. Quercetin: an inhibitor of antigen-induced human basophil histamine release. *J Immunol* 127(2): 546–550, 1981.

10. Yoshimoto T, et al. Flavonoids: potent inhibitors of arachidonate 5-lipoxygenase. *Biochem Biophys Res Commun* 116: 612–618, 1983.

11. Bucca C, et al. Effect of vitamin C on histamine bronchial responsiveness of patients with allergic rhinitis. *Ann Allergy* 65: 311–314, 1990.

12. Bellioni P, et al. La provocazione istaminica in soggetti allergici. Il ruolo dell'acido ascorbico. *Eur Rev Med Pharmacol Sci* 9: 419–422, 1987.

13. Fortner BR Jr, et al. The effect of ascorbic acid on cutaneous and nasal response to histamine and allergen. *J Allergy Clin Immunol* 69(6): 484–488, 1982.

## Alzheimer's Disease (and Non-Alzheimer's Dementia)

1. Stoppe G, et al. Prescribing practice with cognition enhancers in outpatient care: are there differences regarding type of dementia? Results of a representative survey in lower Saxony, Germany. *Pharmacopsychiatry* 29(4): 150–155, 1996.

2. Kleijnen J and Knipschild P. *Ginkgo biloba. Lancet* 340: 1136–1139, 1992.

3. Hofferberth B. The efficacy of EGb 761 in patients with senile dementia of the Alzheimer type, a double-blind, placebo-controlled study on different levels of investigation. *Hum Psychopharmacol* 9: 215–222, 1994.

4. Kanowski S, et al. Proof of efficacy of the *Ginkgo biloba* special extract EGb 761 in outpatients suffering from mild to moderate primary degenerative dementia of the Alzheimer type or multi-infarct dementia. *Pharmacopsychiatry* 29: 47–56, 1996.

5. Schulz V, et al. Rational phytotherapy. New York: Springer-Verlag, 1998: 46–47.

6. LeBars PL, et al. A placebo-controlled, double-blind, randomized trial of an extract of *Ginkgo biloba* for dementia. *JAMA* 278: 1327–1332, 1997.

7. Winther K, Randlov C, Rein E, et al. Effect of *Ginkgo biloba* extract on cognitive function and blood pressure in elderly subjects. *Current Ther Res* 59: 881–888, 1998.

8. Schulz V, et al. Rational phytotherapy. New York: Springer-Verlag, 1998: 43.

9. Schulz V, et al. Rational phytotherapy. New York: Springer-Verlag, 1998: 41.

10. De Feudis FV. *Ginkgo biloba* extract (EGb 761): Pharmacological activity and clinical applications. Paris: Elsevier, 1991: 143–146.

11. Rosenblatt M and Mindel J. Spontaneous hyphema associated with ingestion of *Ginkgo biloba* extract. *N Engl J Med* 336(15): 1108, 1997.

12. Rowin J and Lewis SL. Spontaneous bilateral subdural hematomas associated with chronic *Ginkgo biloba* ingestion. *Neurology* 46: 1775–1776, 1996.

13. Cenacchi T, et al. Cognitive decline in the elderly: a double-blind, placebo-controlled multicenter study on efficacy of phosphatidylserine administration. *Aging* 5: 123–133, 1993.

14. Crook T, et al. Effects of phosphatidylserine in age-associated memory impairment. *Neurology* 41(5): 644–649, 1991.

15. Delwaide PJ, et al. Double-blind randomized controlled study of phosphatidylserine in senile demented patients. *Acta Neurol Scand* 73(2): 136–140, 1986.

16. Engel RR, et al. Double-blind cross-over study of phosphatidylserine vs. placebo in subjects with early cognitive deterioration of the Alzheimer type. *Eur Neuropsychopharmacol* 2: 149–155, 1992.

17. Fagioli S, et al. Phosphatidylserine administration during postnatal development improves memory in adult mice. *Neurosci Lett* 101(2): 229–233, 1989.

18. Funfgeld E, et al. Double-blind study with phosphatidylserine (PS) in Parkinsonian patients with senile dementia of Alzheimer's type (SDAT). *Prog Clin Biol Res* 317: 1235–1246, 1989.

19. Crook T, et al. Effects of phosphatidylserine in Alzheimer's disease. *Psychopharmacol Bull* 28: 161–166, 1992.

20. Amaducci L, et al. Phosphatidylserine in the treatment of Alzheimer's disease: results of a multicenter study. *Psychopharmacol Bull* 24(1): 130–134, 1988.

21. Villardita C, et al. Multicenter clinical trial of brain phosphatidylserine in elderly patients with intellectual deterioration. *Clin Trials J* 24(1): 84–89, 1987.

22. Palmieri G, et al. Double-blind controlled trial of phosphatidylserine in patients with senile mental deterioration. *Clin Trials J* 24(1): 73–83, 1987.

23. Van den Besselaar AM. Phosphatidylethanolamine and phosphatidylserine synergistically promote heparin's anticoagulant effect. *Blood Coagul Fibrinolysis* 6: 239–244, 1995.

24. Calvani M, et al. Action of acetyl-L-carnitine in neurodegeneration and Alzheimer's disease. *Ann N Y Acad Sci* 663: 483–486, 1992.

25. Cipolli C, et al. Effects of L-acetylcarnitine on mental deterioration in the aged: Initial results. *Clin Ther* 132: 479–510, 1990.

26. Garzya G, et al. Evaluation of the effects of L-acetylcarnitine on senile patients suffering from depression. *Drugs Exp Clin Res* 16: 101–106, 1990.

27. Passeri M, et al. Acetyl-L-carnitine in the treatment of mildly demented elderly patients. *Int J Clin Pharmacol Res* 10: 75–79, 1990.

28. Salvioli G and Neri M. L-acetylcarnitine treatment of mental decline in the elderly. *Drugs Exp Clin Res* 20: 169–176, 1994.

29. Spagnoli A, et al. Long-term acetyl-L-carnitine treatment in Alzheimer's disease. *Neurology* 41: 1726–1732, 1991.

30. Vecchi GP, et al. Acetyl-L-carnitine treatment of mental impairment in the elderly: Evidence from a multicenter study. *Arch Gerontol Geriatr* 2(Suppl): 159–168, 1991.

31. Thal LJ, et al. A 1-year multicenter placebo-controlled study of acetyl-L-carnitine in patients with Alzheimer's disease. *Neurology* 47(3): 705–711, 1996.

32. Sano M, et al. Double-blind parallel design pilot study of acetyl-levocarnitine in patients with Alzheimer's disease. *Arch Neurol* 49: 1137–1141, 1992.

33. Campi N, et al. Selegiline versus l-acetylcarnitine in the treatment of Alzheimer-type dementia. *Clin Ther* 12: 306–314, 1990.

34. Rai G, et al. Double-blind, placebo-controlled study of acetyl-l-carnitine in patients with Alzheimer's dementia. *Curr Med Res Opin* 11(10): 638–647.

35. Bonavita E. Study of the efficacy and tolerability of L-acetylcarnitine therapy in the senile brain. *Int J Clin Pharmacol Ther Toxicol* 24: 511–516, 1986.

36. Spagnoli A, Lucca U, Menasce G, et al. Long-term acetyl-L-carnitine treatment in Alzheimer's disease. *Neurology* 41(11): 1726–1732, 1991.

37. Thal LJ, Carta A, Clarke WR, et al. A 1-year multicenter placebo-controlled study of acetyl-L-carnitine in patients with Alzheimer's disease. *Neurology* 47: 705–711, 1996.

38. Goa KL, et al. L-carnitine—A preliminary review of its pharmacokinetics and its therapeutic use in ischemic cardiac disease and primary and secondary carnitine deficiencies in relationship to its role in fatty acid metabolism. *Drugs* 34: 1–24, 1987.

39. Sano M, Ernesto C, Thomas RG, et al. A controlled trial of selegiline, alpha-tocopherol, or both as treatment for Alzheimer's disease. *N Engl J Med* 336: 1216–1222, 1997.

## Angina

1. Cacciatore L, et al. The therapeutic effect of L-carnitine in patients with exercise-induced stable angina: a controlled study. *Drugs Exp Clin Res* 17: 225–335, 1991.

2. Bartels GL, et al. Anti-ischaemic efficacy of L-propionylcarnitine—A promising novel metabolic approach to ischaemia? *Eur Heart J* 17(3): 414–420, 1996.

3. Kamikawa T, et al. Effects of coenzyme $Q_{10}$ on exercise tolerance in chronic stable angina pectoris. *Am J Cardiol* 56: 247, 1985.

4. McLean RM. Magnesium and its therapeutic uses: a review. *Am J Med* 96: 63–76, 1994.

5. Pizzulli L, Hagendorff A, and Zirbes M. N-acetylcysteine attenuates nitroglycerin tolerance in patients with angina pectoris and normal left ventricular function. *Am J Cardiol* 79: 28–33, 1997.

6. Ardissino D, Merlini PA, Savonitto S, et al. Effect of transdermal nitroglycerin or N-acetylcysteine, or both, in the long-term treatment of unstable angina pectoris. *J Am Coll Cardiol* 29: 941–947, 1997.

7. Ornish D, et al. Can lifestyle changes reverse coronary heart disease? *Lancet* 336: 129–133, 1990.

## Anxiety and Panic Attacks

1. Meyer HJ, et al. Kawa-Pyrone-eine neuartige Substanzgruppe zentraler Muskelrelaxantien vom Typ des Mephenesins. *Klin Wochenschr* 44: 902–903, 1966.

2. Klohs MW, et al. A chemical and pharmacological investigation of *Piper methysticum forst*. *J Med Pharmacol Chem* 1: 95–103, 1959.

3. Bruggenmann F, et al. Die analgetische Wirkung der Kawa-Inhaltsstoffe Dihydrokawain und Dihydromethysticin. *Arzneimittelforschung* 13: 407–409, 1963.

4. Meyer HJ. Pharmakologie der Wirksamen Prinzipien des Kawa-Rhizoms (*Piper methysticum Forst*). *Arch Int Pharmacodyn Therapie* 138: 505–535, 1982.

5. Meyer HJ. Lokalanaesthetische Eigenschaften naturlicher Kawa-Pyrone. *Arzneimittelforschung* 42: 407, 1964.

6. Meyer HJ, et al. Kawa-Pyrone-eine neuartige Substanzgruppe zentraler Muskelrelaxantien vom Typ des Mephenesins. *Klin Wochenschr* 44: 902–903, 1966.

7. Singh YN. Effects of kava on neuromuscular transmission and muscle contractility. *Ethnopharmacology* 7: 267–276, 1983.

8. Volz HP, et al. Kava-kava extract WS 1490 versus placebo in anxiety disorders—A randomized placebo-controlled 25 week outpatient trial. *Pharmacopsychiatry* 30(1): 1–5, 1997.

9. Kinzler E, et al. Effect of a special kava extract in patients with anxiety, tension, and excitation states of nonpsychotic genesis. Double-blind study with placebos over 4 weeks. *Arzneimittelforschung* 41(6): 584–588, 1991.

10. Warnecke G, et al. Wirksamkeit von Kawa-Kawa-Extract beim klimakterischen Syndrom. *Z Phytother* 11: 81–86, 1990.

11. Warnecke G. Psychosomatic dysfunctions in the female climacteric. Clinical effectiveness and tolerance of kava extract WS 1490. *Fortschr Med* 109(4): 119–122, 1991.

12. Woelk H, et al. Behandlung von Angst-Patienten. *Z Allg* 69: 271–277, 1993.

13. Jussofie A, Schmiz A, and Hiemke C. Kavapyrone-enriched extract from *Piper methysticum* as modulator of the GABA binding site in different regions of rat brain. *Psychopharmacology* 116: 469–474, 1994.

14. Schulz V, et al. Rational phytotherapy. New York: Springer-Verlag, 1998.

15. Schulz V, et al. Rational phytotherapy. New York: Springer-Verlag, 1998.

16. Schulz V, et al. Rational phytotherapy. New York: Springer-Verlag, 1998.

17. Norton SA, et al. Kava dermopathy. *Am Acad Dermatol* 31(1): 89–97, 1994.

18. Munte TF, et al. Effects of oxazepam and an extract of kava roots (*Piper methysticum*) on event-related potentials in a word recognition task. *Neuropsychobiology* 27(1): 46–53, 1993.

19. Heinze HJ, et al. Pharmacopsychological effects of oxazepam and kava extract in a visual search paradigm assessed with event-related potentials. *Pharmacopsychiatry* 27(6): 224–230, 1994.

20. Herberg KW. Effect of Kava-Special Extract WS 1490 combined with ethyl alcohol on safety-relevant performance parameters. *Blutalkohol* 30(2): 96–105, 1993.

21. Cawte J. Parameters of kava used as a challenge to alcohol. *Aust N Z J Psychiatry* 20(1): 70–76, 1986.

22. Schulz V, et al. Rational phytotherapy. New York: Springer-Verlag, 1998: 72.

23. Duffield PH and Jamieson D. Development of tolerance to kava in mice. *Clin Exp Pharmacol Physiol* 18: 571–578, 1991.

24. Almeida JC and Grimsley EW. Coma from the health-food store: interaction between kava and alprazolam. *Ann Intern Med:* 1996.

25. Kohnen R, et al. The effects of valerian, propranolol, and their combination on activation, performance and mood of healthy volunteers under social stress conditions. *Pharmacopsychiatry* 21: 447–448, 1988.

## Asthma

1. Shivpuri DN, et al. Treatment of asthma with an alcoholic extract of *Tylophora indica:* a crossover, double-blind study. *Ann Allergy* 30: 407–412, 1972.

2. Shivpuri DN, et al. A crossover double-blind study on *Tylophora indica* in the treatment of asthma and allergic rhinitis. *J Allergy* 43: 145–150, 1969.

3. Gupta S, et al. *Tylophora indica* in bronchial asthma—A double-blind study. *Ind J Med Res* 69: 981–989, 1979.

4. Hatch GE. Asthma, inhaled oxidants, and dietary antioxidants. *Am J Clin Nutr* 61(Suppl. 3): 625S–630S, 1995.

5. Bielory L and Gandhi R. Asthma and vitamin C. *Ann Allergy* 73(2): 89–96, 1994.

6. Wright J. Vitamin $B_{12}$: Powerful protection against asthma. *Int Clin Nutr Rev* 9(4): 185–188, 1989.

7. Collipp PJ. Pyridoxine treatment of childhood bronchial asthma. *Ann Allergy* 35: 93–97, 1975.

8. Sur S, Camara M, Buchmeier A, et al. Double-blind trial of pyridoxine (vitamin $B_6$) in the treatment of steroid-dependent asthma. *Ann Allergy* 70: 147–152, 1993.

9. Dry J and Vincent D. Effects of a fish oil diet on asthma: results of a one-year double-blind study. *Int Arch Allergy Immunol* 95: 156–157, 1991.

10. Stenius-Aarniala B, Aro A, Hakaulinen A, et al. Evening primrose oil and fish oil are ineffective as supplementary treatment of bronchial asthma. *Ann Allergy* 62(6): 534–547, 1989.

11. Picado C, et al. Effects of a fish oil enriched diet on aspirin intolerant asthmatic patients: a pilot study. *Thorax* 43(2): 93–97, 1988.

12. Arm J, et al. The effects of dietary supplementation with fish oil on asthmatic responses to antigen. *J Clin Allergy* 81: 183, 1988.

13. Stenius-Aarniala B, et al. Symptomatic effects of evening primrose oil, fish oil, and olive oil in patients with bronchial asthma (Abstract). *Ann Allergy* 55: 330, 1985.

14. Thien FC, et al. Fish oils and asthma—A fishy story? *Med J Aust* 164: 135–136, 1996.

15. Arm JP, Thien FC, and Lee TH. Leukotrienes, fish oil, and asthma. *Allergy Proc* 15: 129–134, 1994.

16. Lee TH and Arm JP. Prospects for modifying the allergic response by fish oil diets. *Clin Allergy* 16(2): 89–100, 1986.

17. Monteleone CA and Sherman AR. Nutrition and asthma. *Arch Intern Med* 157: 23–24, 1997.

18. Rolla G, et al. Magnesium attenuates methacholine-induced bronchoconstriction in asthmatics. *Magnesium* 6(4): 201–204, 1987.

## Atherosclerosis

1. Stephens NG, Parsons A, Schofield PM, et al. Randomized controlled trial of vitamin E in patients with coronary disease: Cambridge Heart Antioxidant Study (CHAOS). *Lancet* 347: 781–786, 1996.

2. Rapola JM, Virtamo J, Ripatti S, et al. Randomized trial of alpha-tocopherol and beta-carotene supplements on incidence of major coronary events in men with previous myocardial infarction. *Lancet* 349: 1715–1720, 1997.

3. Albanes D, Heinonen OP, Huttunen JK, et al. Effects of alpha-tocopherol and beta-carotene supplements on

cancer incidence in the Alpha-Tocopherol Beta-Carotene Cancer Prevention Study. *Am J Clin Nutr* 62(Suppl.): 1427S–1430S, 1995.

4. Losonczy KG, Harris TB, and Havlik RJ. Vitamin E and vitamin C supplement use and risk of all-cause and coronary heart disease mortality in older persons: the established populations for epidemiologic studies of the elderly. *Am J Clin Nutr* 64: 190–196, 1996.

5. Rimm EB, Stampfer MJ, Ascherio A, et al. Vitamin E consumption and the risk of coronary heart disease in men. *N Engl J Med* 328(20): 1450–1456, 1993.

6. Stampfer M, Hennekens C, Manson J, et al. Vitamin E consumption and the risk of coronary heart disease in women. *N Engl J Med* 328: 1444–1449, 1993.

7. Jialal I and Fuller CJ. Effect of vitamin E, vitamin C, and beta-carotene on LDL oxidation and atherosclerosis. *Can J Cardiol* 1(Suppl. G): 97G–103G, 1995.

8. Morel DW, de la Llera-Moya M, and Friday KE. Treatment of cholesterol-fed rabbits with dietary vitamins E and C inhibits lipoprotein oxidation but not development of atherosclerosis. *J Nutr* 124: 2123–2130, 1994.

9. Calzada C, Bruckdorfer K, and Rice-Evans C. The influence of antioxidant nutrients on platelet function in healthy volunteers. *Atherosclerosis* 128(1): 97–105, 1997.

10. Albanes D, Heinonen OP, Huttunen JK, et al. Effects of alpha-tocopherol and beta-carotene supplements on cancer incidence in the Alpha-Tocopherol Beta-Carotene Cancer Prevention Study. *Am J Clin Nutr* 62(Suppl.): 1427S–1430S, 1995.

11. Bellizzi MC, Franklin MF, Duthie GG, et al. Vitamin E and coronary heart disease: the European paradox. *Eur J Clin Nutr* 48: 822–831, 1994.

12. Steiner M, Glantz M, and Lekos A. Vitamin E plus aspirin compared with aspirin alone in patients with transient ischemic attacks. *Am J Clin Nutr* 62(Suppl.): 1381S–1384S, 1995.

13. Ness AR. Vitamin C and cardiovascular disease. *Nutr Rep* 15(3): 1997.

14. Simon JA. Vitamin C and cardiovascular disease: a review. *J Am Coll Nutr* 11(2): 107–125, 1992.

15. Trout DL. Vitamin C and cardiovascular risk factors. *Am J Clin Nutr* 53: 322S–325S, 1991.

16. Kohlmeier L and Hastings SB. Epidemiologic evidence of a role of carotenoids in cardiovascular disease prevention. *Am J Clin Nutr* 62(Suppl.): 1370S–1376S, 1995.

17. Albanes D, et al. Alpha-Tocopherol, Beta-Carotene Cancer Prevention Study Group. The effect of vitamin E and beta-carotene on the incidence of lung cancer and other cancers in male smokers. *N Engl J Med* 330: 1029–1035, 1994.

18. Rapola JM, Virtamo J, Ripatti S, et al. Randomized trial of alpha-tocopherol and beta-carotene supplements on incidence of major coronary events in men with previous myocardial infarction. *Lancet* 349: 1715–1720, 1997.

19. Rapola JM, Virtamo J, Haukka JK, et al. Effect of vitamin E and beta-carotene on the incidence of angina pectoris. *JAMA* 275(9): 693–698, 1996.

20. Kohlmeier L and Hastings SB. Epidemiologic evidence of a role of carotenoids in cardiovascular disease prevention. *Am J Clin Nutr* 62(Suppl.): 1370S–1376S, 1995.

21. White WS, et al. Pharmacokinetics of beta-carotene and canthaxanthin after individual and combined doses by human subjects. *J Am Coll Nutr* 13: 665–671, 1994.

22. Efendi JL, et al. The effect of the aged garlic extract, "kyolic," on the development of experimental atherosclerosis. *Atherosclerosis* 132(1): 37–42, 1997.

23. Schulz V, et al. Rational phytotherapy. New York: Springer-Verlag, 1998: 112.

24. Breithaupt-Grogler K, et al. Protective effect of chronic garlic intake on the elastic properties of the aorta in the elderly. *Circulation* 96(7): 2649–2655, 1997.

25. Kubow S. Lipid oxidation products in food and atherogenesis. *Nutr Rev* 51(2): 3339, 1993.

26. Kromhout D, et al. Alcohol, fish, fibre and antioxidant vitamins intake do not explain population differences in coronary heart disease mortality. *Int J Epidemiol* 25: 753–759, 1996.

27. Pietinen P, et al. Intake of fatty acids and risk of coronary heart disease in a cohort of Finnish men: the Alpha-Tocopherol, Beta-Carotene Cancer Prevention Study. *Am J Epidemiol* 145(10): 876–887, 1997.

28. Pearson TA. Alcohol and heart disease. *Circulation* 94(11): 3023–3025, 1996.

29. Rimm EB and Ellison RC. Alcohol in the Mediterranean diet. *Am J Clin Nutr* 61(Suppl.): 1378S–1382S, 1995.

30. Hammar N, Romelsjo A, and Alfredsson L. Alcohol consumption, drinking pattern, and acute myocardial infarction: a case reference study based on the Swedish twin register. *J Intern Med* 241(2): 125–131, 1997.

31. Camargo CA Jr, et al. Moderate alcohol consumption and risk for angina pectoris or myocardial infarction in U.S. male physicians. *Ann Intern Med* 126(5): 372–375, 1997.

32. Kawachi K, Colditz GA, and Stone CB. Does coffee drinking increase the risk of coronary heart disease? Results from a meta-analysis. *Br Heart J* 72: 269–275, 1994.

33. Willett WC, Stampfer MJ, Manson JA, et al. Coffee consumption and coronary heart disease in women: a ten-year follow-up. *JAMA* 275(6): 458–462, 1996.

34. Nyg RD, et al. Coffee consumption and plasma total homocysteine: the Hordaland Homocysteine Study. *Am J Clin Nutr* 65: 136–143, 1997.

35. Dyerberg J. N-3 fatty acids and coronary artery disease: potentials and problems. *Omega-3, Lipoproteins Atherosclerosis* 27: 251–258, 1996.

36. Harris WS. N-3 fatty acids and serum lipoproteins: human studies. *Am J Clin Nutr* 65(Suppl.): 1645S–1654S, 1997.

37. Dyerberg J. N-3 fatty acids and coronary artery disease: potentials and problems. *Omega-3, Lipoproteins Atherosclerosis* 27: 251–258, 1996.

38. Whelton PK, Kumanyika SK, and Cook NR. Efficacy of nonpharmacologic interventions in adults with high-normal blood pressure: results from phase 1 of the Trials of Hypertension Prevention. Trials of Hypertension Prevention Collaborative Research Group. *Am J Clin Nutr* 65: 652S–660S, 1997.

39. Prichard BN, et al. Fish oils and cardiovascular disease. *BMJ* 310: 819–820, 1995.

40. Stone NJ. From the Nutrition Committee of the American Heart Association. Fish consumption, fish oil, lipids, and coronary heart disease. *Am J Clin Nutr* 65: 1083–1086, 1997.

41. Harris WS. Dietary fish oil and blood lipids. *Curr Opin Lipidol* 7: 3–7, 1996.

42. Harris WS. N-3 fatty acids and serum lipoproteins: human studies. *Am J Clin Nutr* 65(Suppl.): 1645S–1654S, 1997.

43. Laurora G, et al. Control of the progress of arteriosclerosis in high risk subjects treated with mesoglycan: measuring the intima media. *Minerva Cardioangiol* 46(3): 41–47, 1998.

44. Laurora G, Cesarone MR, De Sanctis MT, et al. Delayed arteriosclerosis progression in high-risk subjects treated with mesoglycan. Evaluation of intima-media thickness. *J Cardiovasc Surg* (Torino) 34(4): 313–318, 1993.

45. Tanganelli P, Bianciardi G, Carducci A, et al. Updating on in-vivo and in-vitro effects of heparin and other glycosaminoglycans (mesoglycan) on arterial endothelium: a morphometrical study. *Int J Tissue React* 14(3): 149–153, 1992.

## Attention Deficit Disorder

1. Kleijnen J and Knipschild P. Niacin and vitamin $B_6$ in mental functioning: a review of controlled trials in humans. *Biol Psychiatry* 29(9): 931–941, 1991.

## Benign Prostatic Hyperplasia

1. Emili E, et al. Clinical trial of a new drug for treating hypertrophy of the prostate (Permixon). *Urologia* 50: 1042–1048, 1983.

2. Champault G, et al. A double-blind trial of an extract of the plant *Serenoa repens* in benign prostatic hyperplasia. *Br J Clin Pharmacol* 18(3): 461–462, 1984.

3. Tasca A, et al. Treatment of obstructive symptomatology caused by prostatic adenoma with an extract of *Serenoa repens*. Double-blind clinical study vs. placebo. *Minerva Urol Nefrol* 37(1): 87–91, 1985.

4. Boccafoschi S et al. Comparison of *Serenoa repens* extract with placebo by controlled clinical trial in patients with prostatic adenomatosis. *Urologia* 50: 1257–1268, 1983.

5. Smith RH, et al. The value of Permixon in benign prostatic hypertrophy *Br J Urol* 58: 36–40, 1986.

6. Descotes JL, et al. Placebo-controlled evaluation of the efficacy and tolerability of Permixon in benign prostatic hyperplasia after exclusion of placebo responders. *Clin Drug Invest* 9: 291–297, 1995.

7. Mattei FM, et al. *Serenoa repens* extract in the medical treatment of benign prostatic hypertrophy. Urologia 55: 547–552, 1988.

8. Carraro J, et al. Comparison of phytotherapy (Permixon) with finasteride in the treatment of benign prostate hyperplasia: a randomized international study of 1,098 patients. *Prostate* 29(4): 231–240, 1996.

9. Plosker GL, et al., *Serenoa repens* (Permixon). A review of its pharmacology and therapeutic efficacy in benign prostatic hyperplasia. *Drugs Aging* 9(5): 379–395, 1996.

10. Plosker GL, et al., *Serenoa repens* (Permixon). A review of its pharmacology and therapeutic efficacy in benign prostatic hyperplasia. *Drugs Aging* 9(5): 379–395, 1996.

11. Bach D, et al. Phytopharmaceutical and synthetic agents in the treatment of benign prostatic hyperplasia (BPH). *Phytomedicine* 3(4): 309–313, 1997.

12. Duvia R, et al. Advances in the phytotherapy of prostatic hypertrophy. *Med Praxis* 4: 143–148, 1983.

13. Schulz V, et al. Rational phytotherapy. New York: Springer-Verlag, 1998: 233.

14. Schulz V, et al. Rational phytotherapy. New York: Springer-Verlag, 1998: 233.

15. Dathe G and Schmid H. Phytotherapy of benign prostate hyperplasia with *Serenoa repens* extract (Permixon(R)). *Urologe Ausg B* 31(5): 220–223, 1991.

16. ESCOP monographs. Fascicule 2: *Urticae radix*. Exeter, UK: European Scientific Cooperative on Phytotherapy, 1997: 4.

17. ESCOP monographs. Fascicule 2: *Urticae radix*. Exeter, UK: European Scientific Cooperative on Phytotherapy, 1997: 4.

18. Schulz V, et al. Rational phytotherapy. New York: Springer-Verlag, 1998: 229.

19. Berges RR, et al., Randomised, placebo-controlled, double-blind clinical trial of beta-sitosterol in patients with benign prostatic hyperplasia. *Lancet* 345: 1529–1532, 1995.

20. Schulz V, et al. Rational phytotherapy. New York: Springer-Verlag, 1998: 231.

21. Berges RR, et al., Randomised, placebo-controlled, double-blind clinical trial of beta-sitosterol in patients with benign prostatic hyperplasia. *Lancet* 345: 1529–1532, 1995.

22. Buck AC, et al. Treatment of outflow tract obstruction due to benign prostatic hyperplasia with the pollen extract, Cernilton: a double-blind placebo-controlled study. *Br J Urol* 66(4): 398–404, 1990.

23. Schulz V, et al. Rational phytotherapy. New York: Springer-Verlag, 1998: 229–230.

24. Ito R, Ishii M, Yamashita S, et al. Cernitin pollen extract (Cernilton); anti-prostatic hypertrophic action of Cernitin pollen extract. *Pharmacometrics* 31: 1–11, 1986.

25. Kimura M, Kumra I, Hanakse K, et al. Micturition activity of pollen extract: contractile effects on bladder and inhibitory effects on urethral smooth muscle of mouse and pig. *Planta Med* 2: 148–151, 1986.

26. Habib K, Ross M, Buck AC, et al. In vitro evaluation of the pollen extract, Cernitin T-60, in the regulation of prostate cell growth. *Br J Urol* 66: 393–397, 1990.

27. Buck AC, Rees RWM, and Ebeling L. Treatment of chronic prostatitis and prostodynia with pollen extract. *Br J Urol* 64: 496–499, 1989.

28. Rugendorff W, Weiner L, Ebeling L, et al. Results of treatment with pollen extract (Cernilton N) in chronic prostatitis and prostatodynia. *Br J Urol* 71: 433–438, 1993.

29. Yasumota R, Kawanishi H, Tsujino T, et al. Clinical evaluation of long-term treatment using Cernitin pollen extract in patients with benign prostatic hyperplasia. *Clin Ther* 17: 82–87, 1995.

30. Dutkiewicz S. Usefulness of Cernilton in the treatment of benign prostatic hyperplasia. *Int Urol Nephrol* 28(1): 49–53, 1996.

## Bladder Infection

1. Sobota AE. Inhibition of bacterial adherence by cranberry juice: potential use for the treatment of urinary tract infections. *J Urol* 131(5): 1013–1016, 1984.

2. Schmidt DR, et al. An examination of the anti-adherence activity of cranberry juice on urinary and nonurinary bacterial isolates. *Microbios* 55: 173–181, 224–225, 1998.

3. Zafriri D, et al. Inhibitory activity of cranberry juice on adherence of type 1 and type P fimbriated *Escherichia coli* to eucaryotic cells. *Antimicrob Agents Chemother* 33(1): 92–98, 1989.

4. Howell A, et al. Letter. *N Engl J Med* 339: 1085, 1998.

5. Schaefer AJ. Recurrent urinary tract infections in the female patient. *Urology* 32 (Suppl.): 12–15, 1988.

6. Avorn J, et al. Reduction of bacteriuria and pyuria after ingestion of cranberry juice. *JAMA* 271(10): 751–754, 1994.

7. Frohne V, et al. Untersuchungen zur Frage der harndesifizierenden Wirkungen von Barentraubenblatt-extracten. *Planta Med* 18: 1–25, 1970. As cited in ESCOP, Fascicule 5: *Uvae Ursi Folium* (bearberry leaf). Exeter, UK: European Scientific Cooperative on Phytotherapy, 1997: 2.

8. ESCOP monographs. Fascicule 5: *Uvae Ursi Folium* (bearberry leaf). Exeter, UK: European Scientific Cooperative on Phytotherapy, 1997: 1.

9. Schulz V, et al. Rational phytotherapy. New York: Springer-Verlag, 1998: 223.

10. ESCOP monographs. Fascicule 5: *Uvae Ursi Folium* (bearberry leaf). Exeter, UK: European Scientific Cooperative on Phytotherapy, 1997: 2.

11. Kedzia B, et al. Antibacterial action of urine containing arbutin metabolic products. *Med Dosw Mikrobiol* 27: 305–314, 1975.

12. Larsson B, et al. Prophylactic effect of UVA-E in women with recurrent cystitis: a preliminary report. *Curr Ther Res* 53: 441–443, 1993.

13. ESCOP monographs. Fascicule 5: *Uvae Ursi Folium* (bearberry leaf). Exeter, UK: European Scientific Cooperative on Phytotherapy, 1997.

14. Tyler V. Herbs of choice. New York: Pharmaceutical Production Press, 1994: 79.

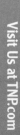

15. Schulz V, et al. Rational phytotherapy. New York: Springer-Verlag, 1998: 224.

16. Nowak AK, et al., Darkroom hepatitis after exposure to hydroquinone. *Lancet* 345: 1187, 1995.

17. U.S. Environmental Protection Agency. Extremely hazardous substances: Superfund chemical profiles. Park Ridge, NJ: Noyes Data Corporation, 1988: 1906–1907.

18. Lewis RJ. Sax's dangerous properties of industrial materials, 8th ed. New York: Van Nostrand Reinhold, 1989: 1906–1907.

19. Schulz V, et al. Rational phytotherapy. New York: Springer-Verlag, 1998: 223.

20. ESCOP monographs. Fascicule 5: *Uvae Ursi Folium* (bearberry leaf). Exeter, UK: European Scientific Cooperative on Phytotherapy, 1997: 2.

## Cancer Prevention: Reducing the Risk

1. Longo D. Approach to the patient with cancer (ch. 81) in Harrison's principles of internal medicine, 14th ed. New York: McGraw-Hill, 1998.

2. Welland D. Fifteen cancer-preventing strategies that stack the odds in your favor. *Environ Nutr* 21(3): 1, 1998.

3. Osborne M, et al. Cancer prevention. *Lancet* 349(Suppl. 2): SII27–SII30, 1997.

4. Heinonen OP, et al. Prostate cancer and supplementation with alpha-tocopherol and beta-carotene: incidence and mortality in a controlled trial. *J Natl Cancer Inst* 90(6): 440–446, 1998.

5. White E, et al. Relationship between vitamin and calcium supplement use and colon cancer. *Cancer Epidemiol Biomarkers Prev* 6(10): 769–774, 1997.

6. Macready N. Vitamins associated with lower colon-cancer risk. *Lancet* 350: 9089, 1997.

7. Losonczy KG, Harris TB, and Havlik RJ. Vitamin E and vitamin C supplement use and risk of all-cause and coronary heart disease mortality in older persons: the established populations for epidemiologic studies of the elderly. *Am J Clin Nutr* 64: 190–196, 1996.

8. Bostick RM, Potter JD, McKenzie DR, et al. Reduced risk of colon cancer with high intake of vitamin E: the Iowa Women's Health Study. *Cancer Res* 53: 4230–4237, 1993.

9. Zheng W, Sellers TA, Doyle TJ, et al. Retinol, antioxidant vitamins, and cancer of the upper digestive tract in a prospective cohort study of postmenopausal women. *Am J Epidemiol* 142: 955–960, 1995.

10. Esteve J, et al. Diet and cancers of the larynx and hypopharynx: the IARC multi-center study in southwestern Europe. *Cancer Causes Control* 7: 240–252, 1996.

11. Albanes D, Heinonen OP, Huttunen JK, et al. Effects of alpha-tocopherol and beta-carotene supplements on cancer incidence in the Alpha-Tocopherol Beta-Carotene Cancer Prevention Study. *Am J Clin Nutr* 62(Suppl.): 1427S–1430S, 1995.

12. Chen J, Geissler C, Parpia B, et al. Antioxidant status and cancer mortality in China. *Int J Epidemiol* 21: 625–635, 1992.

13. Ocke M, Bueno-deo-Mesquita H, Feskens E, et al. Repeated measurements of vegetables, fruits, beta-carotene, and vitamins C and E in relation to lung cancer. *Am J Epidemiol* 145(4): 358–365, 1997.

14. Bellizzi MC, Franklin MF, Duthie GG, et al. Vitamin E and coronary heart disease: the European paradox. *Eur J Clin Nutr* 48: 822–831, 1994.

15. Albanes D, Heinonen OP, Huttunen JK, et al. Effects of alpha-tocopherol and beta-carotene supplements on cancer incidence in the Alpha-Tocopherol Beta-Carotene Cancer Prevention Study. *Am J Clin Nutr* 62(Suppl.): 1427S–1430S, 1995.

16. National Research Council. Diet and health: implications for reducing chronic risk. Washington DC: National Academy Press, 1989: 376–379.

17. Clark LC, Combs GF Jr, Turnbull BW, et al. Effects of selenium supplementation for cancer prevention in patients with carcinoma of the skin. *JAMA* 276(24): 1957–1963, 1996.

18. Stewart MS, Spalholz JE, Neldner KH, and Pence BC. Selenium compounds have disparate abilities to impose oxidative stress and induce apoptosis. *Free Radic Biol Med* 26: 42–48, 1999.

19. Shiobara Y, Yoshida T, and Suzuki KT. Effects of dietary selenium species on Se concentrations in hair, blood, and urine. *Toxicol Appl Pharmacol* 152: 309–314, 1998.

20. Wen HY, Davis RL, and Shi B. Bioavailability of selenium from veal, chicken, beef, lamb, flounder, tuna, selenomethionine, and sodium selenite assessed in selenium-deficient rats. *Biol Trace Elem Res* 58: 43–53, 1997.

21. Neve J. Human selenium supplementation as assessed by changes in blood selenium concentration and glutathione peroxidase activity. *J Trace Elem Med Biol* 9: 65–73, 1995.

22. Fan AM, et al. Selenium: nutritional, toxicological, and clinical aspects. *West J Med* 153: 160–167, 1990.

23. Steinmetz KA, et al. Vegetables, fruit, and colon cancer in the Iowa Women's Health Study. *Am J Epidemiol* 139(1): 1–13, 1994.

24. Sumiyoshi H. New pharmacological activities of garlic and its constituents. *Nippon Yakurigaku Zasshi* 110(Suppl. 1): 93P–97P, 1997.

25. Agarwal KC. Therapeutic actions of garlic constituents. *Med Res Rev* 16(1): 111–124, 1996.

26. Popov I, et al. Antioxidant effects of aqueous garlic extract, 1st communication: direct detection using photochemoluminescence. *Arzneimittelforschung Drug Res* 44(1): 602–604, 1994.

27. Torok B, et al. Effectiveness of garlic on radical activity in radical generating systems. *Arzneimittelforschung Drug Res* 44(1): 608–611, 1994.

28. Das T, et al. Modification of clastogenicity of three known clastogens by garlic extract in mice in vivo. *Environ Mol Mutagen* 21(4): 383–388, 1993.

29. Ip C, et al. Efficacy of cancer prevention by high-selenium garlic is primarily dependent on the action of selenium. *Carcinogenesis* 16(11): 2649–2652, 1995.

30. Steinmetz KA and Potter JD. Vegetables, fruit, and cancer prevention: a review. *J Am Diet Assoc* 96(10): 1027–1039, 1996.

31. Ziegler RG. A review of epidemiologic evidence that carotenoids reduce the risk of cancer. *J Nutr* 119: 116–122, 1989.

32. Flagg EW, Coates RJ, and Greenberg RS. Epidemiologic studies of antioxidants and cancer. *J Am Coll Nutr* 14(5): 419–427, 1995.

33. Vena JE, Graham S, Freudenheim J, et al. Diet in the epidemiology of bladder cancer in western New York. *Nutr Cancer* 18(3): 255–264, 1992.

34. Rock CL, Saxe GA, Ruffin MT IV, et al. Carotenoids, vitamin A, and estrogen receptor status in breast cancer. *Nutr Cancer* 25(3): 281–296, 1996.

35. Zheng W, Sellers TA, Doyle TJ, et al. Retinol, antioxidant vitamins, and cancer of the upper digestive tract in a prospective cohort study of postmenopausal women. *Am J Epidemiol* 142: 955–960, 1995.

36. Zheng W, Sellers TA, Doyle TJ, et al. Retinol, antioxidant vitamins, and cancer of the upper digestive tract in a prospective cohort study of postmenopausal women. *Am J Epidemiol* 142: 955–960, 1995.

37. Santamaria L and Bianchi-Santamaria A. Carotenoids in cancer chemoprevention and therapeutic interventions. *J Nutr Sci Vitaminol* (Tokyo) *Spec* 321: 6, 1992.

38. Albanes D, Heinonen OP, Huttunen JK, et al. Effects of alpha-tocopherol and beta-carotene supplements on cancer incidence in the Alpha-Tocopherol Beta-Carotene Cancer Prevention Study. *Am J Clin Nutr* 62(Suppl.): 1427S–1430S, 1995.

39. Omenn GS, Goodman GE, Thornquist MD, et al. Effects of a combination of beta-carotene and vitamin A on lung cancer and cardiovascular disease. *N Engl J Med* 334: 1150–1155, 1996.

40. Hennekens CH, Buring JE, Manson JAE, et al. Lack of effect of long-term supplementation with beta-carotene on the incidence of malignant neoplasms and cardiovascular disease. *N Engl J Med* 334(18): 1145–1149, 1996.

41. White WS, et al. Pharmacokinetics of beta-carotene and canthaxanthin after individual and combined doses by human subjects. *J Am Coll Nutr* 13: 665–671, 1994.

42. Franceschi S, et al. Tomatoes and risk of digestive-tract cancers. *Int J Cancer* 59: 181–184, 1994.

43. Giovannucci E, Ascherio A, Rimm EB, et al. Intake of carotenoids and retinol in relation to risk of prostate cancer. *J Natl Cancer Inst* 87: 1767–1776, 1995.

44. Clinton SK, et al. Cis-trans lycopene isomers, carotenoids, and retinol in the human prostate. *Cancer Epidemiol Biomarkers Prevent* 5: 823–833, 1996.

45. Cohen M and Bhagavan HN. Ascorbic acid and gastrointestinal cancer. *J Am Coll Nutr* 14(6): 565–578, 1995.

46. Ocke M, Kromhout D, Menotti A, et al. Average intake of antioxidant (pro) vitamins and subsequent cancer mortality in the 16 cohorts of the Seven Countries Study. *Int J Cancer* 61(4): 480–484, 1995.

47. Kromhout D and Bueno-de-Mesquita HB. Antioxidant vitamins and stomach cancer: the role of ecologic studies. *Cancer Lett* 114: 333–334, 1997.

48. Shibata A, et al. Intake of vegetables, fruits, beta-carotene, vitamin C, and vitamin supplements and cancer incidence among the elderly: a prospective study. *Br J Cancer* 66(4): 673–679, 1992.

49. Cohen M and Bhagavan HN. Ascorbic acid and gastrointestinal cancer. *J Am Coll Nutr* 14(6): 565–578, 1995.

50. Esteve J, et al. Diet and cancers of the larynx and hypopharynx: the IARC multi-center study in southwestern Europe. *Cancer Causes Control* 7: 240–252, 1996.

51. Flagg EW, Coates RJ, and Greenberg RS. Epidemiologic studies of antioxidants and cancer. *J Am Coll Nutr* 14(5): 419–427, 1995.

52. Block G. Epidemiologic evidence regarding vitamin C and cancer. *Am J Clin Nutr* 54: 1310S–1314S, 1991.

53. Daviglus ML, et al. Dietary beta-carotene, vitamin C, and risk of prostate cancer: results from the Western Electric Study. *Epidemiology* 7(5): 472–477, 1996.

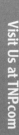

54. Bruemmer B, et al. Nutrient intake in relation to bladder cancer among middle-aged men and women. *Am J Epidemiol* 144(5): 485–495, 1996.

55. Otoole P and Lombard M. Vitamin C and gastric cancer: supplements for some or fruit for all. *Gut* 39(3): 345–347, 1996.

56. Greenberg ER, Baron JA, Tosteson TD, et al. A clinical trial of antioxidant vitamins to prevent colorectal adenoma. *N Engl J Med* 331: 141–147, 1994.

57. Kushi L, Fee R, Sellers T, et al. Intake of vitamins A, C, and E and postmenopausal breast cancer: the Iowa Women's Health Study. *Am J Epidemiol* 144(2): 165–174, 1996.

58. Hunter DJ, Manson JE, Colditz GA, et al. A prospective study of the intake of vitamins C, E, and A and the risk of breast cancer. *N Engl J Med* 329(4): 234–240, 1993.

59. Katiyar SK and Mukhtar H. Tea antioxidants in cancer chemoprevention. *J Cell Biochem* 27 (Suppl.): 59–67, 1997.

60. Wang ZY, et al. Inhibitory effects of black tea, green tea, decaffeinated black tea, and decaffeinated green tea on ultraviolet B light-induced skin carcinogenesis in 7,12-dimethylbenz[a]anthracene-initiated SKH-1 mice. *Cancer Res* 54(13): 3428–3435, 1994.

61. McCord H. More good news in tea leaves. *Prevention* 47(3): 51, 1995.

62. Yang CS and Wang ZY. Tea and cancer. *J Natl Cancer Inst* 85(13): 1038–1049, 1993.

63. Imai K, et al. Cancer-preventive effects of drinking green tea among a Japanese population. *Prev Med* 26(6): 769–775, 1997.

64. Ji BT, et al. Green tea consumption and the risk of pancreatic and colorectal cancers. *Int J Cancer* 70(3): 255–258, 1997.

65. Yu GP, et al. Green-tea consumption and risk of stomach cancer: A population-based case-control study in Shanghai, China. *Cancer Causes Control* 6(6): 532–538, 1995.

66. Stich HF. Teas and tea components as inhibitors of carcinogen formation in model systems and man. *Prev Med* 21: 377–384, 1992.

67. Komori A, et al. Anticarcinogenic activity of green tea polyphenols. *Jpn J Clin Oncol* 23(3): 186–190, 1993.

68. Messina MJ, et al. Soy intake and cancer risks: a review of the in vitro and in vivo data. *Nutr Cancer* 21: 113–131, 1994.

69. Adlercreutz H and Mazur W. Phyto-oestrogens and western diseases. *Ann Med* 29: 95–120, 1997.

70. Stoll BA. Eating to beat breast cancer: potential role for soy supplements. *Ann Oncol* 8: 223–225, 1997.

71. Day NE. Phyto-estrogens and hormonally dependent cancers. *Pathol Biol* 42(10): 1090, 1994.

72. Day NE. Phyto-estrogens and hormonally dependent cancers. *Pathol Biol* 42(10): 1090, 1994.

73. Adlercreutz H and Mazur W. Phyto-oestrogens and western diseases. *Ann Med* 29: 95–120, 1997.

74. Butterworth CE Jr. Effect of folate on cervical cancer: synergism among risk factors. *Ann N Y Acad Sci* 669: 293–299, 1992.

75. Kim Y-I, Mason JB, et al. Folate, epithelial dysplasia, and colon cancer. *Proc Assoc Am Physicians* 107: 218–227, 1995.

76. Tseng M, et al. Micronutrients and the risk of colorectal adenomas. *Am J Epidemiol* 144(11): 1005–1014, 1996.

77. Heimberger DC. Localized deficiencies of folic acid in aerodigestive tissues. *Ann N Y Acad Sci* 669: 87–96, 1992.

78. Heimberger DC. Localized deficiencies of folic acid in aerodigestive tissues. *Ann N Y Acad Sci* 669: 87–96, 1992.

79. Garland FC, et al. Geographic variation in breast cancer mortality in the United States: a hypothesis involving exposure to solar radiation. *Prev Med* 19(6): 614–622, November 1990.

80. Key SW and Marble M. Studies link sun exposure to protection against cancer. *Cancer Weekly Plus:* 5–6, November 17, 1997.

81. Martinez ME, et al. Calcium, vitamin D, and the occurrence of colorectal cancer among women. *J Natl Cancer Inst* 88(19): 1375–1382, 1996.

82. Kearney J, et al. Calcium, vitamin D, and dairy foods and the occurrence of colon cancer in men. *Am J Epidemiol* 143(9): 907–917, 1996.

83. James SY, et al. Effects of 1,25 dihydroxyvitamin $D_3$ and its analogues on induction of apoptosis in breast cancer cells. *J Steroid Biochem Mol Biol* 58(4): 395–401, July 1996.

84. Taylor JA, et al. Association of prostate cancer with vitamin D receptor gene polymorphism. *Cancer Res* 56(18): 4108–4110, 1996.

85. Douglas WC. Vitamin D scores again. *Second Opinion* 7(7): 4–5, July 1997.

86. Martinez ME, et al. Calcium, vitamin D, and the occurrence of colorectal cancer among women. *J Natl Cancer Inst* 88(19): 1375–1382, 1996.

87. Adlercreutz H and Mazur W. Phyto-oestrogens and western diseases. *Ann Med* 29: 95–120, 1997.

88. Serraino M and Thompson LU. The effect of flaxseed supplementation on the initiation and promotional stages of mammary tumorigenesis. *Nutr Cancer* 17: 153–159, 1992.

89. Bougnoix P, et al. Alpha-linolenic acid content of adipose breast tissue: a host determinant of the risk of early metastasis in breast cancer. *Br J Cancer* 70: 330–334, 1994.

90. Jang M, Cai L, Udeani GO, et al. Cancer chemopreventive activity of resveratrol, a natural product derived from grapes. *Science* 275: 218–220, 1997.

91. Kearney J, et al. Calcium, vitamin D, and dairy foods and the occurrence of colon cancer in men. *Am J Epidemiol* 143(9): 907–917, 1996.

92. Baron JA, Beach M, and Mandel JS. Calcium supplements for the prevention of colorectal adenomas. *New Engl J Med* 340: 101–107, 1999.

93. Hyman J, Baron JA, Dain BJ, et al. Dietary and supplemental calcium and the recurrence of colorectal adenomas. *Cancer Epidemiol Biomarkers Prev* 7: 291–295, 1998.

## Canker Sores

1. Das SK, et al. Deglycyrrhizinated liquorice in apthous ulcers. *J Assoc Physicians India* 37: 647, 1989.

## Cardiomyopathy

1. Langsjoen H, Langsjoen P, Langsjoen P, et al. Usefulness of coenzyme $Q_{10}$ in clinical cardiology: a long-term study. *Mol Aspects Med* 15(Suppl. PS): 165–175, 1994.

2. Langsjoen PH, et al. Response of patients in classes III and IV of cardiomyopathy to therapy in a blind and crossover trial with coenzyme $Q_{10}$. *Proc Natl Acad Sci* 82: 4240, 1985.

3. Pogessi L, Galanti G, Comeglio M, et al. Effect of coenzyme $Q_{10}$ on left ventricular function in patients with dilative cardiomyopathy. *Curr Ther Res* 49: 878–886, 1991.

4. Langsjoen PH, et al. A six-year clinical study of therapy of cardiomyopathy with coenzyme $Q_{10}$. *Int J Tissue React* 12(3): 169–171, 1990.

5. Langsjoen PH, et al. Response of patients in classes III and IV of cardiomyopathy to therapy in a blind and crossover trial with coenzyme $Q_{10}$. *Proc Natl Acad Sci* 82: 4240, 1985.

6. Permanetter B, et al. Ubiquinone (coenzyme $Q_{10}$) in the long-term treatment of idiopathic dilated cardiomyopathy. *Eur Heart J* 13: 1528–1533, 1991.

7. Winter S, Jue K, Prochazka J, et al. The role of L-carnitine in pediatric cardiomyopathy. *J Child Neurol* (Canada) 10(Suppl. 2): 2S45–2S51, 1995.

8. Pepine CJ. The therapeutic potential of carnitine in cardiovascular disorders. *Clin Ther* 13(1): 2–21, 1991.

9. Bertelli A, et al. Carnitine and coenzyme $Q_{10}$: biochemical properties and functions, synergism and complementary action. *Int J Tissue React* 15(Suppl.): 183–186, 1990.

## Cataracts

1. Hankinson S, Stampfer M, Seddon J, et al. Nutrient intake and cataract extraction in women: a prospective study. *BMJ* 305: 335–339, 1992.

2. Gerster H. No contribution of ascorbic acid to renal calcium oxalate stones. *Ann Nutr Metab* 41(5): 269–282, 1997.

3. Tavani A, et al. Food and nutrient intake and risk of cataract. *Ann Epidemiol* 6: 41–46, 1996.

4. Carson C, Lee S, De Paola C, et al. Antioxidant intake and cataract in the Melbourne Visual Impairment Project. *Am J Epidemiol* 139(11): S18, 1994.

5. Robertson JM, et al. Vitamin E intake and risk of cataracts in humans. *Ann N Y Acad Sci* 570: 372–382, 1989.

6. Rouhiainen P, Rouhiainen H, Salonen J, et al. Association between low plasma vitamin E concentration and progression of early cortical lens opacities. *Am J Epidemiol* 144(5): 496–500, 1996.

7. Vitale S, West S, Hallfrish H, et al. Plasma antioxidants and risk of cortical and nuclear cataract. *Epidemiology* 4: 195–203, 1993.

8. Vitale S, et al. Plasma vitamin C, E, and beta-carotene levels and risk of cataract. *Invest Ophthalmol Vis Sci* 32: 723, 1991.

9. Ross WM, Creighton MO, and Trevithick JR. Radiation cataractogenesis induced by neutron or gamma irradiation in the rat lens is reduced by vitamin E. *Scanning Microsc* 4: 641–650, 1990.

10. Albanes D, Heinonen OP, Huttunen JK, et al. Effects of alpha-tocopherol and beta-carotene supplements on cancer incidence in the Alpha-Tocopherol Beta-Carotene Cancer Prevention Study. *Am J Clin Nutr* 62(Suppl.): 1427S–1430S, 1995.

11. Bellizzi MC, Franklin MF, Duthie GG, et al. Vitamin E and coronary heart disease: the European paradox. *Eur J Clin Nutr* 48: 822–831, 1994.

12. Mares-Perlman JA, Brady WE, Klein BE, et al. Diet and nuclear lens opacities. *Am J Epidemiol* 141(4): 322–334, 1995.

13. Hankinson S, Stampfer M, Seddon J, et al. Nutrient intake and cataract extraction in women: a prospective study. *BMJ* 305: 335–339, 1992.

14. Carson C, Lee S, De Paola C, et al. Antioxidant intake and cataract in the Melbourne Visual Impairment Project. *Am J Epidemiol* 139(11): S18, 1994.

15. Vitale S, West S, Hallfrish H, et al. Plasma antioxidants and risk of cortical and nuclear cataract. *Epidemiology* 4: 195–203, 1993.

16. Bravetti G. Preventive medical treatment of senile cataract with vitamin E and anthocyanosides: clinical evaluation. *Ann Ottalmol Clin Ocul* 115: 109, 1989.

## Cervical Dysplasia

1. Butterworth CE Jr, Hatch KD, Gore H, et al. Improvement in cervical dysplasia associated with folic acid therapy in users of oral contraceptives. *Am J Clin Nutr* 35(1): 73–82, 1982.

2. Zarcone R, Bellini P, Carfora E, et al. Folic acid and cervix dysplasia. *Minerva Ginecol* 48: 397–400, 1996.

3. Childers JM, Chu J, Voigt LF, et al. Chemoprevention of cervical cancer with folic acid: a phase III Southwest Oncology Group Intergroup study. *Cancer Epidemiol Biomarkers Prev* 4(2): 155–159, 1995.

4. Butterworth CE Jr, Hatch KD, Soong SJ, et al. Oral folic acid supplementation for cervical dysplasia: a clinical intervention trial. *Am J Obstet Gynecol* 166(30): 803–809, 1992.

5. Orr J, et al. Nutritional status of patients with untreated cervical cancer I and II. *Am J Obstet Gynecol* 151: 625–635, 1985.

6. Romney SL, et al. Nutrient antioxidants in the pathogenesis and prevention of cervical dysplasia and cancer. *J Cell Biochem* 23: 96–103, 1995.

7. Butterworth CE Jr. Effect of folate on cervical cancer. Synergism among risk factors. *Ann N Y Acad Sci* 669: 293–299, 1992.

## Cholesterol

1. Mader FH. Treatment of hyperlipidaemia with garlic-powder tablets: evidence from the German Association of General Practitioners' multicentric placebo-controlled double-blind study. *Arzneimittelforschung* 40(10): 1111–1116, 1990.

2. Neil HA, et al. Garlic powder in the treatment of moderate hyperlipidaemia: a controlled trial and meta-analysis. *J R Coll Physicians Lond* 30(4): 329–334, 1990.

3. Simons LA, et al. On the effect of garlic on plasma lipids and lipoproteins in mild hypercholesterolaemia. *Atherosclerosis* 13(2): 219–225, 1995.

4. Silagy CA, et al. A meta-analysis of the effect of garlic on blood pressure. *J Hypertens* 12(4): 463–468, 1994.

5. Warshafsky S, et al. Effect of garlic on total serum cholesterol: a meta-analysis. *Ann Intern Med* 119(Pt. 1): 599–605, 1993.

6. Steiner M, et al. A double-blind crossover study in moderately hypercholesterolemic men that compared the effect of aged garlic extract and placebo administration on blood lipids. *Am J Clin Nutr* 64(6): 866–870, 1996.

7. Santos OS de A, et al. Effects of garlic powder and garlic oil preparations on blood lipids, blood pressure and well being. *Br J Clin Res* 6: 91–100, 1995.

8. Breithaupt-Grogler K, et al. Protective effect of chronic garlic intake on the elastic properties of the aorta in the elderly. *Circulation* 96(7): 2649–2655, 1997.

9. Schulz V, et al. Rational phytotherapy. New York: Springer-Verlag, 1998.

10. Agarwal KC, et al. Therapeutic actions of garlic constituents. *Med Res Rev* 16(1): 111–124, 1996.

11. Legnani C, et al. Effects of dried garlic preparation on fibrinolysis and platelet aggregation in healthy subjects. *Arzneimittelforschung* 43: 119–121, 1993.

12. Chutani SK, et al. The effect of dried vs. raw garlic on fibrinolytic activity in man. *Atherosclerosis* 38: 417–421, 1981.

13. Kiesewetter H, et al. Effect of garlic on thrombocyte aggregation, microcirculation, and other risk factors. *Int J Clin Pharmacol Ther Toxicol* 29: 151–155, 1991.

14. Reuter HD, et al. *Allium sativum* and *Allium ursinum:* chemistry, pharmacology and medical applications. *Econo Med Plant Res* 6: 56–108, 1994.

15. Popov I, et al. Antioxidant effects of aqueous garlic extract, 1st communication: direct detection using photochemoluminescence. *Arzneimittelforschung Drug Res* 44(1): 602–604, 1994.

16. Torok B, et al. Effectiveness of garlic on radical activity in radical generating systems. *Arzneimittelforschung Drug Res* 44(1): 608–611, 1994.

17. Sumiyoshi H, et al. Chronic toxicity test of garlic extracts in rats. *J Toxicol Sci* 9: 61–75, 1984.

18. Schulz V, et al. Rational phytotherapy. New York: Springer-Verlag, 1998.

19. Beck E, et al. *Allium sativum* in der Stufentherapie der Hyperlipidamie. *Med Welt* 44: 516–520, 1993. As cited in Schulz V, et al. Rational phytotherapy. New York: Springer-Verlag, 1998.

20. Heber D, et al. Cholesterol-lowering effects of a proprietary Chinese red yeast rice dietary supplement. *FASEB J* 12(4): A206, 1998.

21. Rippe J, et al. A multi-center, self-controlled study of Cholestin in subjects with elevated cholesterol. Results presented at the March, 1999 American Heart Association's 39th Annual Conference on Cardiovascular Disease Epidemiology and Prevention in Orlando, Florida.

22. Chang J, et al. Elderly patients with primary hyperlipidemia benefited from treatment with a *Monacus purpureus* rice preparation: A placebo-controlled, double-blind clinical trial. Results presented at the March, 1999 American Heart Association's 39th Annual Conference on Cardiovascular Disease Epidemiology and Prevention in Orlando, Florida.

23. Chang M. Cholestin: Health-care professional product guide. Simi Valley: Pharmanex, 1998: 1–6.

24. Illingworth DR, et al. Comparative effects of lovastatin and niacin in primary hypercholesterolemia. *Arch Intern Med* 154: 1586–1595, 1994.

25. Guyton JR, Goldberg AC, Kreisberg RA, et al. Effectiveness of once-nightly dosing of extended-release niacin alone and in combination for hypercholesterolemia. *Am J Cardiol* 82: 737–743, 1998.

26. Vega GL and Grundy SM. Lipoprotein responses to treatment with lovastatin, gemfibrozil, and nicotinic acid in normolipidemic patients with hypoalphalipoproteinemia. *Arch Intern Med* 154: 73–82, 1994.

27. Lal SM, et al. Effects of nicotinic acid and lovastatin in renal transplant patients: A prospective, randomized, open-label crossover trial. *Am J Kidney Dis* 25: 616–622, 1995.

28. Crouse JR III. New developments in the use of niacin for treatment of hyperlipidemia: new considerations in the use of an old drug. *Coron Artery Dis* 7: 321–326, 1996.

29. Head KA. Inositol hexaniacinate: a safer alternative to niacin. *Alt Med Rev* 1: 176–184, 1996.

30. Glore SR, et al. Soluble fiber and serum lipids: a literature review. *J Am Diet Assoc* 94: 425–436, 1994.

31. Anderson JW, Johnstone BM, and Cook-Newell ME. Meta-analysis of the effects of soy protein intake on serum lipids. *N Engl J Med* 333: 276–282, 1995.

32. Agarwal RC, et al. Clinical trial of gugulipid—a new hyperlipidemic agent of plant origin in primary hyperlipidemia. *Indian J Med Res* 84: 626–634, 1986.

33. Nityanand, S, et al. Clinical trials with gugulipid. A new hypolipidaemic agent. *J Assoc Physicians India* 37(5): 323–328, 1989.

34. Singh RB, et al. Hypolipidemic and antioxidant effects of *Commiphora mukul* as an adjunct to dietary therapy in patients with hypercholesterolemia. *Cardiovasc Drug Ther* 8(4): 659–664, 1994.

35. Gaddi A, et al. Controlled evaluation of pantethine, a natural hypolipidemic compound, in patients with different forms of hyperlipoproteinemia. *Atherosclerosis* 50(1): 73–83, 1984.

36. Rubba R, Postiglione A, DeSimone B, et al. Comparative evaluation of the lipid-lowering effects of fenofibrate and pantethine in type II hyperlipoproteinemia. *Curr Ther Res Clin Exp* 38: 719–727, 1985.

37. Angelico M, et al. Improvement in serum lipid profile in hyperlipoproteinaemic patients after treatment with pantethine: a crossover, double-blind trial versus placebo. *Curr Ther Res* 33: 1091, 1983.

38. Dacol PG, et al. Pantethine in the treatment of hypercholesterolemia: a randomized double-blind trial versus tiadenol. *Curr Ther Res* 36: 314–322, 1984.

39. Davini P, et al. Controlled study on L-carnitine therapeutic efficacy in post-infarction. *Drugs Exp Clin Res* 18(8): 355–365, 1992.

40. Vecchio F, Zanchin G, Maggioni F, et al. Mesoglycan in treatment of patients with cerebral ischemia: effects on hemorrheologic and hematochemical parameters. *Acta Neurol* (Napoli) 15(6): 449–456, 1993.

41. Saba P, Galeone F, Giuntoli F, et al. Hypolipidemic effect of mesoglycan in hyperlipidemic patients. *Curr Ther Res* 40: 761–768, 1986.

42. Postiglione A, De Simone B, Rubba P, et al. Effect of oral mesoglycan on plasma lipoprotein concentration and on lipoprotein lipase activity in primary hyperlipidemia. *Pharmacol Res Commun* 16(1): 1–8, 1984.

43. Mertz W. Chromium in human nutrition: a review. *J Nutr* 123: 626–633, 1993.

44. Bell L, et al. Cholesterol-lowering effects of calcium carbonate in patients with mild to moderate hypercholesterolemia. *Arch Intern Med* 152: 2441–2444, 1992.

45. Schwarz B, Bischof H, Kunze M. Coffee, tea, and lifestyle. *Prev Med* 23: 377–384, 1994.

## Colds and Flus

1. Dorn M. Milderung grippaler Effekte durch ein pflanzliches Immunstimulans. *Natur und Ganzheitsmedizin* 2: 314–319, 1989. As cited in Schulz V, et al. Rational phytotherapy. New York: Springer-Verlag, 1998: 277.

2. Braunig B, et al. *Echinacea purpurea* root for strengthening the immune response in flu-like infections. *Z Phytother* 13: 7–13, 1992.

3. Hoheisel O, et al. Echinagard treatment shortens the course of the common cold: a double-blind placebo-controlled clinical trial. *Eur J Clin Res* 9: 261–268, 1997.

4. Brinkeborn R, Shah D, Geissbuhler S, et al. Echinaforce in the treatment of acute colds. *Schweiz Zschr Gunsheits Medizin* 10: 26–29, 1998.

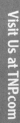

5. Dorn M, et al. Placebo-controlled double-blind study of *Echinacea pallidae radix* in upper respiratory tract infections. *Complement Ther Med* 3: 40–42, 1997.

6. Hoheisel O, et al. Echinagard treatment shortens the course of the common cold: a double-blind placebo-controlled clinical trial. *Eur J Clin Res* 9: 261–268, 1997.

7. Melchart MD, et al. Immunomodulation with echinacea—A sytematic review of controlled clinical trials. *Phytomedicine* 1: 245–254, 1994.

8. Melchart, MD, et al. Echinacea root extracts for the prevention of upper respiratory tract infections: a double-blind, placebo-controlled randomized trial. *Arch Fam Med* 7: 541–545, 1998.

9. Schoenberger D. The influence of immune-stimulating effects of pressed juice from *Echinacea purpurea* on the course and severity of colds. *Forum Immunol* 8: 2–12, 1992.

10. Carlo Calabrese N.D., Bastyr University. Unpublished communication.

11. Bauer R, et al. Echinacea species as potential immunostimulatory drugs. *Econ Med Plant Res* 5: 253–321, 1991.

12. Wagner V, et al. Immunostimulating polysaccharides (heteroglycans) of higher plants. *Arzneimittelforschung* 35: 1069–1075, 1985.

13. Stimpel M, et al. Macrophage activation and induction of macrophage cytotoxicity by purified polysaccharide fractions from the plant *Echinacea purpurea*. *Infect Immun* 46: 845–849, 1984.

14. Luettig B, et al. Macrophage activation by the polysaccharide arabinogalactan isolated from plant cell cultures of *Echinacea purpurea*. *J Natl Cancer Inst* 81: 669–675, 1989.

15. Mose J. Effect of echinacin on phagocytosis and natural killer cells. *Med Welt* 34: 1463–1467, 1983.

16. Vomel V. Influence of a non-specific immune stimulant on phagocytosis of erythrocytes and ink by the reticuloendothelial system of isolated perfused rat livers of different ages. *Arzneimittelforschung* 34: 691–695, 1984.

17. Hobbs C. The echinacea handbook. Portland, OR: Eclectic Medical Publications, 1989.

18. Schulz V, et al. Rational phytotherapy. New York: Springer-Verlag, 1998: 278.

19. Bergner P. Goldenseal and the common cold: the antibiotic myth. *Med Herbalism* 8(4): 1–10, 1997.

20. Schulz V, et al. Rational phytotherapy. New York: Springer-Verlag, 1998.

21. Mengs U, et al. Toxicity of *Echinacea purpurea* acute, subacute and genotoxicity studies. *Arzneimittelforschung Drug Res* 41(11): 1076–1081, 1991.

22. Parnham MJ. Benefit-risk assessment of the squeezed sap of the purple coneflower (*Echinacea purpurea*) for long-term oral immunostimulation. *Phytomedicine* 3(1): 99–102, 1996.

23. Parnham MJ. Benefit-risk assessment of the squeezed sap of the purple coneflower (*Echinacea purpurea*) for long-term oral immunostimulation. *Phytomedicine* 3(1): 99–102, 1996.

24. Melchior J, et al. Controlled clinical study of standardized *Andrographis paniculata* extract in common cold: a pilot trial. *Phytomedicine* 34: 314–318, 1996–1997.

25. Hancke J, et al. A double-blind study with a new monodrug Kan Jang: decrease of symptoms and improvements in the recovery from common colds. *Phytother Res* 9: 559–562, 1995.

26. Thamlikitkul V, et al. Efficacy of *Andrographis paniculata* (Nees) for pharyngotonsillitis in adults. *J Med Assoc Thai* 74(10): 437–442, 1991.

27. Hancke J, et al. A double-blind study with a new monodrug Kan Jang: decrease of symptoms and improvements in the recovery from common colds. *Phytother Res* 9: –559–562, 1995.

28. Akbarsha MA, et al. Antifertility effect of *Andrographis paniculata* (Nees) in male albino rat. *Indian J Exp Biol* 28(5): 421–426, 1990.

29. Burgos RA, et al. Testicular toxicity assessment of *Andrographis paniculata* dried extract in rats. *J Ethnopharmacol* 58(3): 219–224, 1997.

30. Zoha MS, et al. Antifertility effect of *Andrographis paniculata* in mice. *Bangladesh Med Res Counc Bull* 15(1): 34–37, 1989.

31. Chandra RK. Trace element regulation of immunity and infection. *J Am Coll Nutr* 4(1): 5–16, 1985.

32. Fraker PJ, et al. Interrelationships between zinc and immune function. *Fed Proc* 45(5): 1474–1479, 1986.

33. Werbach M. Nutritional influences on illness. CD-ROM. Tarzana, CA: Third Line Press, 1998: 630.

34. Girodon F, Lombard M, Galan P, et al. Effect of micronutrient supplementation on infection in institutionalized elderly subjects: a controlled trial. *Ann Nutr Metab* 41(2): 98–107, 1997.

35. Mossad SB, et al. Zinc gluconate lozenges for treating the common cold: a randomized, double-blind placebo-controlled study. *Ann Intern Med* 125: 142–144, 1996.

36. Petrus EJ, Lawson KA, and Bucci LR. Randomized, double-masked, placebo-controlled clinical study of the effectiveness of zinc acetate lozenges on common cold

symptoms in allergy-tested subjects. *Curr Ther Res* 59: 595–607, 1998.

37. Macknin ML, et al. Zinc gluconate lozenges for treating the common cold in children: a randomized controlled trial. *JAMA* 279(24): 1962–1967, 1998.

38. Marshall S. Zinc gluconate and the common cold: review of randomized controlled trials. *Can Fam Physician* 44: 1037–1042, 1998.

39. Eby GA. Zinc ion availability—the determinant of efficacy in zinc lozenge treatment of common colds. *Antimicrob Chemother* 40(4): 483–493, 1997.

40. Macknin ML, et al. Zinc gluconate lozenges for treating the common cold in children: a randomized controlled trial. *JAMA* 279(24): 1962–1967, 1998.

41. Hemilä H. Vitamin C and the common cold. *Br J Nutr* 67: 3–16, 1992.

42. Hemilä H. Does vitamin C alleviate symptoms of the common cold?—a review of current evidence. *Scand J Infect Dis* 26: 1–6, 1994.

43. Peters EM, Goetzsche JM, Grobbelaar B, et al. Vitamin C supplementation reduces the incidence of postrace symptoms of upper-respiratory-tract infection in ultramarathon runners. *Am J Clin Nutr* 57(2): 170–174, 1993.

44. Hemilä H. Vitamin C and common cold incidence: a review of studies with subjects under heavy physical stress. *Int J Sports Med* 17(5): 379–383, 1996.

45. Hemilä H. Vitamin C intake and susceptibility to the common cold. *Br J Nutr* 77: 1–14, 1997.

46. Scaglione F, et al. Efficacy and safety of the standardised ginseng extract G115 for potentiating vaccination against the influenza syndrome and protection against the common cold. *Drugs Exp Clin Res* 22(2): 65–72, 1996.

47. Ploss E. *Panax ginseng*. C. A. Meyer. Scientific report. Cologne: Kooperation Phytopharmaka, 1998.

48. Lawrence Review of Natural Products. Ginseng monograph. St. Louis, Missouri: Facts and Comparisons Division, J.B. Lipincott Company, March, 1990.

49. Tyler V. Herbs of choice. New York: Pharmaceutical Production Press, 1994.

50. Tyler V. Herbs of choice. New York: Pharmaceutical Production Press, 1994.

51. Schulz V, et al. Rational phytotherapy. New York: Springer-Verlag, 1998: 271, 273.

52. Meydani SM, et al. Vitamin E supplementation and in vivo immune response in healthy elderly subjects: a randomized controlled trial. *JAMA* 277: 1380–1386, 1997.

53. Zakay-Rones Z, et al. Inhibition of several strains of influenza virus and reduction of symptoms by an elderberry extract (*Sambucus nigra* L.) during an outbreak of influenza B Panama. *J Altern Complement Med* 1(4): 361–369, 1995.

## Congestive Heart Failure

1. Hofman-Bang C, et al. Coenzyme $Q_{10}$ as an adjunctive treatment of congestive heart failure. *J Am Coll Cardiol* 19: 216A, 1992.

2. Morisco C, et al. Effect of coenzyme $Q_{10}$ therapy in patients with congestive heart failure: a long-term multicenter randomized study. *Clin Invest* 71(Suppl. 8): S134–S136, 1993.

3. Lampetico M, et al. Italian multicenter study on the efficacy and safety of coenzyme $Q_{10}$ as adjuvant therapy in heart failure. *Clin Invest* 71(Suppl. 8): S129–S133, 1993.

4. Popping S, et al. Effect of a hawthorn extract on contraction and energy turnover of isolated rat cardiomyocytes. *Arzneimittelforschung Drug Res* 45: 1157–1161, 1995.

5. Joseph G. Pharmacologic action profile of crataegus extract in comparison to epinephrine, amirinone, milrinone and digoxin in the isolated perfused guinea pig heart. *Arzneimittelforschung* 45(12): 1261–1265, 1995.

6. Schulz V, et al., Rational phytotherapy. New York: Springer-Verlag, 1998.

7. Schulz V, et al., Rational phytotherapy. New York: Springer-Verlag, 1998: 91–94.

8. Schulz V, et al., Rational phytotherapy. New York: Springer-Verlag, 1998: 90–98.

9. Schulz V, et al., Rational phytotherapy. New York: Springer-Verlag, 1998: 95.

10. Azuma J, et al. Therapy of congestive heart failure with orally administered taurine. *Clin Ther* 5(4): 398–408, 1983.

11. Azuma J, et al. Double-blind randomized crossover trial of taurine in congestive heart failure. *Curr Ther Res* 34(4): 543–557, 1983.

12. Azuma J, Sawamura A, Awata N, et al. Therapeutic effect of taurine in congestive heart failure: a double-blind crossover trial. *Clin Cardiol* 8: 276–282, 1985.

13. Azuma J, Takihara K, Awata N, et al. Taurine and failing heart: experimental and clinical aspects. *Prog Clin Biol Res* 179: 195–213, 1985.

14. Takihara K, et al. Beneficial effect of taurine in rabbits with chronic congestive heart failure. *Am Heart J* 112: 1278, 1986.

15. Azuma J, et al. Beneficial effect of taurine on congestive heart failure induced by chronic aortic regurgitation in rabbits. *Res Comm Chem Pathol Pharmacol* 435: 261, 1984.

16. Azuma J, Sawamura A, and Awata N. Usefulness of taurine in chronic congestive heart failure and its prospective application. *Jpn Circ J* 56: 95–99, 1992.

17. Azuma J, Sawamura A, and Awata N. Usefulness of taurine in chronic congestive heart failure and its prospective application. *Jpn Circ J* 56: 95–99, 1992.

18. Caponnetto S, et al. Efficacy of L-propionylcarnitine treatment in patients with left ventricular dysfunction. *Eur Heart J* 15(9): 1267–1273, 1994.

19. Mancini M, et al. Controlled study on the therapeutic efficacy of propionyl- L-carnitine in patients with congestive heart failure. *Arzneimittelforschung* 42: 1101–1104, 1992.

20. Cacciatore L, et al. The therapeutic effect of L-carnitine in patients with exercise-induced stable angina: a controlled study. *Drugs Exp Clin Res* 17: 225–235, 1991.

21. Pucciarelli G, et al. The clinical and hemodynamic effects of propionyl-L-carnitine in patients with congestive heart failure. *Clin Ther* 141: 379–384, 1992.

## Cyclic Mastalgia

1. Horrobin DF, et al. Abnormalities in plasma essential fatty acid levels in women with premenstrual syndrome and with nonmalignant breast disease. *J Nutr Med* 2: 259–264, 1991.

2. Pye JK, et al. Clinical experience of drug treatment for mastalgia. *Lancet* ii: 373–377, 1985.

3. Pashby NL, et al. A clinical trial of evening primrose oil in mastalgia. *Br J Surg* 68: 801–824, 1981.

4. Mansel RE, et al. Effect and tolerability of n-6 essential fatty acid supplementation in patients with recurrent breast cysts—a randomized double-blind placebo-controlled trial. *J Nutr Med* 1: 195–200, 1990.

5. Mansel RE, et al. A randomized trial of dietary intervention with essential fatty acids in patients with categorized cysts. *Ann N Y Acad Sci* 586: 288–294, 1990.

6. Horrobin DF. Nutritional and medical importance of gamma-linolenic acid. *Prog Lipid Res* 31: 163–194, 1992.

7. Horrobin DF, et al. Gamma-linolenic acid: An intermediate in essential fatty acid metabolism with potential as an ethical pharmaceutical and as a food. *Rev Contemp Pharmacother* 1: 1–45, 1990.

8. Horrobin DF. Essential fatty acids in the management of impaired nerve function in diabetes. *Diabetes* 46(Suppl. 2): S90–S93, 1997.

9. Tamborini A, et al. Value of standardized *Ginkgo biloba* extract in the management of congestive symptoms of premenstrual syndrome. *Rev Fr Gynecol Obstet* 88(7–9): 447–457, 1993.

10. De Feudis FV. *Ginkgo biloba* extract: Pharmacological activity and clinical applications. Paris: Elsevier, 1991: 143–146.

11. Kleijnen J and Knipschild P. *Ginkgo biloba* for cerebral insufficiency. *Br J Clin Pharamcol* 34: 352–358, 1992.

12. De Feudis FV. *Ginkgo biloba* extract: Pharmacological activity and clinical applications. Paris: Elsevier, 1991: 143–146.

13. Dittmar FW, et al. Premenstrual syndrome: treatment with a phytopharmaceutical. *Therapie Gynakol* 5: 60–68, 1992.

14. Peteres-Welte C, et al. Menstrual abnormalities and PMS: *Vitex agnus-castus*. *Therapie Gynakol* 7: 49–52, 1994.

15. Coeugniet E, et al. Premenstrual syndrome (PMS) and its treatment. *Arztezeitschr Naturheilverf* 27: 619–622, 1986.

## Depression

1. Laakman G, et al. St. John's wort in mild to moderate depression: the relevance of hyperforin for the clinical efficacy. *Pharmacopsychiatry* 31(Suppl.): 54–59, 1998.

2. Linde K, et al. St. John's wort for depression—an overview and meta-analysis of randomized clinical trials. *BMJ* 313: 253–258, 1996.

3. Ernst E. St. John's wort, an antidepressant? A systematic, criteria-based review. *Phytomedicine* 2(1): 67–71, 1995.

4. Suzuki O, et al. Inhibition of monoamine oxidase by hypericin. *Planta Medica* 50: 2722–2724, 1984.

5. Bladt S, et al. Inhibition of MAO by fractions and constituents of hypericum extract. *J Geriatr Psychiatry Neurol* 7(Suppl. 1): S57–S59, 1994.

6. Thiede B, et al. Inhibition of MAO and COMT by hypericum extracts and hypericin. *J Geriatr Psychiatry Neurol* 7(Suppl. 1): 54–56, 1994.

7. Muller WEG, et al. Effects of hypericum extract on the expression of serotonin receptors. *J Geriatr Psychiatry Neurol* 7(Suppl. 1): S63–S64, 1994.

8. Muller WE, et al. Hypericum extract (LI160) as an herbal antidepressant. *Pharmacopsychiatry* 30(Suppl. 2): 71–134, 1997.

9. Laakman G, et al. St. John's wort in mild to moderate depression: the relevance of hyperforin for the clinical efficacy. *Pharmacopsychiatry* 31(Suppl.): 54–59, 1998.

10. Woelk H, et al. Benefits and risks of the hypericum extract LI 160: drug monitoring study with 3,250 patients. *J Geriatr Psychiatry Neurol* 7(Suppl 1): S34–S38, 1994.

11. Smet P and Nolen W. St. John's wort as an antidepressant. *BMJ* 3: 241–242, 1996.

12. Schulz V, et al. Rational phytotherapy. New York: Springer-Verlag, 1998: 56.

13. Seigers CP, et al. Phototoxicity caused by hypericum. *Nervenhielkunde* 12: 320–322, 1993.

14. Brockmoller J, et al. Hypericin and pseudohypericin: pharmacokinetics and effects on photosensitivity in humans. *Pharmacopsychiatry* 30(Suppl. 2): 94–101, 1997.

15. Roberts J. 1999 meeting of the American Society for Photobiology.

16. Suzuki O, et al. Inhibition of monoamine oxidase by hypericin. *Planta Medica* 50: 2722–2724, 1984.

17. Bladt S, et al. Inhibition of MAO by fractions and constituents of hypericum extract. *J Geriatr Psychiatry Neurol* 7(Suppl. 1): S57–S59, 1994.

18. Thiede B, et al. Inhibition of MAO and COMT by hypericum extracts and hypericin. *J Geriatr Psychiatry Neurol* 7(Suppl. 1): 54–56, 1994.

19. Demott K. St. John's wort tied to serotonin syndrome. *Clin Psychiatr News* 26: 28, 1998.

20. Gordon JB. SSRIs and St. John's wort: possible toxicity? *Am Fam Phys* 57: 950, 1998.

21. Baker RK, et al. Inhibition of human DNA topoisomerase IIalpha by the naphthodianthrone, hypericin. *Proc Am Assoc Cancer Res* 39: 422, 1998.

22. Nebel A, et al. Potential metabolic interaction between theophylline and St. John's wort. Submitted to *Ann Pharmacother* 1998.

23. Baker RK, et al. Catalytic inhibition of human DNA topoisomerase IIalpha by hypericin, a naphthodianthone from St. John's wort *(Hypericum perforatum)*. Manuscript in preparation.

24. Heller B. Pharmacological and clinical effects of D-phenylalanine in depression and Parkinson's disease. As cited in Mosnaim and Wolf, eds. Noncatecholic phenylethylamines, Part 1. New York: Marcel Dekker, 1978: 397–417.

25. Beckmann H, et al. DL-phenylalanine versus imipramine: a double-blind controlled study. *Arch Psychiat Nervenkr* 227: 49–58, 1979.

26. Beckmann H. Phenylalanine in affective disorders. *Adv Biol Psychiatry* 10: 137–147, 1983.

27. Werbach M. Nutritional influences on mental illness. Tarzana, CA: Third Line Press, 1991: 142.

28. Werbach M. Nutritional influences on mental illness. Tarzana, CA: Third Line Press, 1991: 141–142.

29. Simonson M. L-phenylalanine. Letter. *J Clin Psychiatry* 46(8): 355, 1985.

30. Richardson MA. Amino acids in psychiatric disease. Washington, DC: American Psychiatric Press, 1990.

31. Mosnik DM, Spring B, Rogers K, and Baruah SL. Tardive dyskinesia exacerbated after ingestion of phenylalanine by schizophrenic patients. *Neuropsychopharmacology* 16(2): 136–146, 1997.

32. Byerly WF, et al. 5-hydroxytryptophan: a review of its antidepressant efficacy and adverse effects. *J Clin Psychopharmacol* 7: 127–137, 1987.

33. Poldinger W, et al. A functional-dimensional approach to depression: serotonin deficiency as a target syndrome in a comparison of 5-hydroxytryptophan and fluvoxamine. *Psychopathology* 24: 53–81, 1991.

34. Eckmann F. Cerebral insufficiency treatment with *Ginkgo-biloba* extract: time of onset of effect in a double-blind study with 60 inpatients. *Fortschr Med* 108: 557–560, 1990.

35. Schubert H, et al. Depressive episode primarily unresponsive to therapy in elderly patients: efficacy of *Ginkgo-biloba* (EGb 761) in combination with antidepressants. *Geriatr Forsch* 3: 45–53, 1993.

36. Huguet F, et al. Decreased cerebral 5-HT receptors during aging: reversal by *Ginkgo-biloba* extract (EGb 761). *J Pharm Pharmacol* 46: 316–318, 1994.

37. Schulz V, et al. Rational phytotherapy. New York: Springer-Verlag, 1998: 41.

38. De Feudis FV. *Ginkgo biloba* extract (EGb 761): Pharmacological activity and clinical applications. Paris: Elsevier, 1991: 143–146.

39. Cenacchi T, et al. Cognitive decline in the elderly: a double-blind, placebo-controlled multicenter study on efficacy of phosphatidylserine administration. *Aging* 5: 123–133, 1993.

40. Benjamen J, et al. Inositol treatment in psychiatry. *Psychopharmacol Bull* 31(1): 167–175, 1995.

41. Bell I, et al. Complex vitamin patterns in geriatric and young adult inpatients with major depression. *J Am Geriatr Soc* 39: 252–257, 1991.

42. Zucker DK et al. $B_{12}$ deficiency and psychiatric disorders: case report and literature review. *Biol Psychiatry* 16: 197–205, 1981.

43. Alpert JE and Fava M. Nutrition and depression: the role of folate. *Nutr Rev* 55(5): 145–149, 1997

44. Passeri M, Cucinotta D, Abate G, et al. Oral 5'-methyltetrahydrofolic acid in senile organic mental

disorders with depression: results of a double-blind multicenter study. *Aging* (Milano) 5(1): 63–71, 1993.

45. Godfrey PS, Toone BK, Carney MW, et al. Enhancement of recovery from psychiatric illness by methylfolate. *Lancet* 336: 392–395, 1990.

46. Heseker H, Kubler W, Pudel V, and Westenhoffer J. Psychological disorders as early symptoms of a mild-moderate vitamin deficiency. *Ann N Y Acad Sci* 669: 352–357, 1992.

47. Crellin R, Bottiglierei T, and Reynolds EH. Folates and psychiatric disorders. Clinical potential. *Drugs* 45(5): 623–636, 1993.

48. Brattstrom LE, Hultberg BL, and Hardebo JE. Folic acid responsive postmenopausal homocysteinemia. *Metabolism* 34(11): 1073–1077, 1985.

49. Botez MI. Folate deficiency and neurological disorders in adults. *Med Hypothesis* 2: 135–140, 1976.

50. Coppen A, et al. Depression and tetrahydrobiopterin: the folate connection. *J Affect Disord* 16(2–3): 103–107, 1989.

51. Alpert JE and Fava M. Nutrition and depression: the role of folate. *Nutr Rev* 55(5): 145–149, 1997.

## Diabetes

1. Anderson RA, et al. Elevated intakes of supplemental chromium improve glucose and insulin variables in individuals with type II diabetes. *Diabetes* 46(11): 1786–1791, 1997.

2. Ravina A, et al. Chromium in the treatment of clinical diabetes mellitus. *Harefuah* 125(5–6): 142–145, 1993.

3. Rabinowitz MB, et al. Effect of chromium and yeast supplements on carbohydrate and lipid metabolism in diabetic men. *Diabetes Care* 6: 319–327, 1983.

4. Certulli J, et al. Chromium picolinate toxicity. *Ann Pharmacother* 32: 428–431, 1998.

5. Wasser WG, et al. Chronic renal failure after ingestion of over-the-counter chromium picolinate. *Ann Intern Med* 126(5): 410, 1997.

6. Sharma RD, Sarkar A, Hazra DK, et al. Use of fenugreek seed powder in the management of non-insulin-dependent diabetes mellitus. *Nutr Res* 16: 1331–1339, 1996.

7. Madar Z, et al. Glucose-lowering effect of fenugreek in non-insulin-dependent diabetics. *Eur J Clin Nutr* 42: 51–54, 1988.

8. Sharma RD, Raghuram TC, and Rao NS. Effect of fenugreek seeds on blood glucose and serum lipids in type I diabetes. *Eur J Clin Nutr* 44: 301–306, 1990.

9. Leung A, et al. Encyclopedia of common natural ingredients in food, drugs, and cosmetics. New York: John Wiley and Sons, 1996: 243–244.

10. Baskaran K, et al. Antidiabetic effect of a leaf extract from *Gymnema sylvestre* in non-insulin-dependent diabetes mellitus patients. *J Ethnopharmacol* 30: 295–305, 1990.

11. Shanmugasundaram ERB, et al. Use of *Gymnema sylvestre* leaf extract in the control of blood glucose in insulin-dependent diabetes mellitus. *J Ethnopharmacol* 30: 281–294, 1990.

12. Authors not noted. Flexible dose open trial of Vijayasar in cases of newly-diagnosed non-insulin-dependent diabetes mellitus. Indian Council of Medical Research (ICMR), Collaborating Centres, New Delhi. *Indian J Med Res* 108: 24–29, 1998.

13. Sotaneimi EA, et al. Ginseng therapy in non-insulin-dependent diabetic patients. *Diabetes Care* 18(10): 1373–1375, 1995.

14. Yaniv Z, Dafni A, Friedman J, et al. Plants used for the treatment of diabetes in Israel. *J Ethnopharmacol* 19(2): 145–151, 1987.

15. Teixeira CC, et al. The effect of *Syzygium cumini* (L.) skeels on post-prandial blood glucose levels in non-diabetic rats and rats with streptozotocin-induced diabetes mellitus. *J Ethnopharmacol* 56: 209–213, 1997.

16. Bever BO and Zahnd GR. Plants with oral hypoglycemic action. *Q J Crude Drug Res* 17: 139–196, 1979.

17. Mathew PT and Augusti KT. Hypoglycaemic effects of onion, *Allium cepa* Linn. on diabetes mellitus—a preliminary report. *Indian J Physiol Pharmacol* 19: 213–217, 1975.

18. Manickam M, Ramanathan M, Jahromi MA, et al. Antihyperglycemic activity of phenolics from *Pterocarpus marsupium*. *J Nat Prod* 60: 609–610, 1997.

19. Ahmad F, Khalid P, Khan MM, et al. Insulin-like activity in epicatechin. *Acta Diabetol Lat* 26: 291–300, 1989.

20. Stern E. Successful use of *Atriplex halimus* in the treatment of type 2 diabetic patients: a preliminary study. Zamenhoff Medical Center, Tel Aviv, 1989.

21. Earon G, Stern E, and Lavosky H. Successful use of *Atriplex hamilus* in the treatment of type 2 diabetic patients. Controlled clinical research report on the subject of Atriplex. Unpublished study conducted at the Hebrew University, Jerusalem, 1989.

22. Khan AK, Akhtar S, and Mahtab H. Treatment of diabetes mellitus with *Coccinia indica*. *BMJ* 280: 1044, 1980.

23. Welihinda J, et al. Effect of *Momordica charantia* on the glucose tolerance in maturity onset diabetes. *J Ethnopharmacol* 17: 277–282, 1986.

24. Akhtar MS. Trial of *Momordica charantia* Linn (Karela) powder in patients with maturity-onset diabetes. *J Pak Med Assoc* 32: 106–107, 1982.

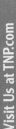

25. Leatherdale BA, Panesar RK, Singh G, et al. Improvement of glucose tolerance due to *Momordica charantia* (Karela). *BMJ [Clin Res Ed]* 282: 1823–1824, 1981.

26. Cignarella A, et al. Novel lipid-lowering properties of *Vaccinium myrtillus* L. leaves, a traditional antidiabetic treatment, in several models of rat dyslipidaemia: a comparison with ciprofibrate. *Thromb Res* 84: 311–322, 1996.

27. Paolisso G, D'Amore A, Galzerano D, et al. Daily vitamin E supplements improve metabolic control but not insulin secretion in elderly non-insulin-dependent diabetic patients. *Diabetes Care* 16: 1433–1437, 1993.

28. Paolisso G, D'Amore A, Giugliano D, et al. Pharmacologic doses of vitamin E improve insulin action in healthy subjects and non-insulin-dependent diabetic patients. *Am J Clin Nutr* 57: 650–656, 1993.

29. Pozzilli P, Visalli N, Signore A, et al. Double-blind trial of nicotinamide in recent-onset IDDM (the IMDIAB III study). *Diabetologia* 38: 848–852, 1995.

30. Kagan VE, et al. Dihydrolipoic acid—A universal antioxidant both in the membrane and in the aqueous phase. *Biochem Pharmacol* 44: 1637–1649, 1992.

31. Hounsom L, et al. A lipoic acid—gamma-linolenic acid conjugate is effective against multiple indices of experimental diabetic neuropathy. *Diabetologia* 41(7): 839-843,1998.

32. Cameron NE, et al. Effects of alpha-lipoic acid on neurovascular function in diabetic rats. Interaction with essential fatty acids. *Diabetologia* 41(4): 390 –399, 1998.

33. Packer L, Witt EH, and Tritschler HJ. Alpha-lipoic acid as a biological antioxidant. *Free Radical Biol Med* 19: 227–250, 1995.

34. Ziegler D, et al. Alpha-lipoic acid in the treatment of diabetic peripheral and cardiac autonomic neuropathy. *Diabetes* 46(Suppl. 2): S62–S66, 1997.

35. Kahler W, et al. Diabetes mellitus—A free radical–associated disease: results of adjuvant antioxidant supplementation. *Gesamte Inn Med* 48: 223–232, 1993.

36. Ziegler D, et al. Alpha-lipoic acid in the treatment of diabetic peripheral and cardiac autonomic neuropathy. *Diabetes* 46(Suppl. 2): S62–S66, 1997.

37. Stevens EJ, et al. Essential fatty acid treatment prevents nerve ischaemia and associated conduction anomalies in rats with experimental diabetes mellitus. *Diabetologia* 36(5): 397–401, 1993.

38. Reichert RG. Evening primrose oil and diabetic neuropathy. *Q Rev Natl Med*: 141–145, 1995.

39. Keen H, et al. Treatment of diabetic neuropathy with gamma-linolenic acid: the gamma-linolenic acid multicenter trial group. *Diabetes Care* 16(1): 8–15, 1993.

40. Horrobin DF. The use of gamma-linolenic acid in diabetic neuropathy. *Agents Actions* 37 (Suppl.): 120–144, 1992.

41. Horrobin DF. Nutritional and medical importance of gamma-linolenic acid. *Prog Lipid Res* 31: 163–194, 1992.

42. Horrobin DF, et al. Gamma-linolenic acid: an intermediate in essential fatty acid metabolism with potential as an ethical pharmaceutical and as a food. *Rev Contemp Pharmacother* 1: 1–45, 1990.

43. Horrobin DF. Essential fatty acids in the management of impaired nerve function in diabetes. *Diabetes* 46(Suppl. 2): S90–S93, 1997.

44. Vaddadi KS. The use of gamma-linolenic acid and linoleic acid to differentiate between temporal lobe epilepsy and schizophrenia. *Prostaglandins Med* 6: 375–379, 1981.

45. Horrobin DF. The regulation of prostaglandin biosynthesis by the manipulation of essential fatty acid metabolism. *Rev Pure Appl Pharmacol* 4: 339–383, 1983.

46. Salway JG, et al. Effect of myo-inositol on peripheral-nerve function in diabetes. *Lancet* ii: 1282–1284, 1978.

47. Gregersen G, et al. Oral supplementation of myo-inositol: effects on peripheral nerve function in human diabetics and on the concentration in plasma, erythrocytes, urine and muscle tissue in human diabetics and normals. *Acta Neurol Scand* 67: 164–172, 1983.

48. Bravetti G. Preventive medical treatment of senile cataract with vitamin E and anthocyanosides: clinical evaluation. *Ann Ottalmol Clin Ocul* 115: 109, 1989.

49. Scharrer A, et al. Anthocyanosides in the treatment of retinopathies. *Klin Monatsbl Augenheilkd* 178: 386–389, 1981.

50. Carson C, Lee S, De Paola C, et al. Antioxidant intake and cataract in the Melbourne Visual Impairment Project. *Am J Epidemiol* 139(11): S18, 1994.

51. Hankinson S, Stampfer M, Seddon J, et al. Nutrient intake and cataract extraction in women: a prospective study. *BMJ* 305: 335–339, 1992.

52. Will JC, et al. Does diabetes mellitus increase the requirement for vitamin C? *Nutr Rev* 54: 193–202, 1996.

53. Elamin A and Tuvemo T. Magnesium and insulin-dependent diabetes mellitus. *Diabetes Res Clin Pract* 10: 203–209, 1990.

54. Tosiello L. Hypomagnesemia and diabetes mellitus. *Arch Intern Med* 156: 1143–1148, 1996.

55. Schmidt LE, Arfken CL, and Heins JM. Evaluation of nutrient intake in subjects with non-insulin-dependent diabetes mellitus. *J Am Diet Assoc* 94(7): 773–774, 1994.

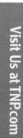

56. Blostein-Fujii A, DeSilvestro RA, Frid D, et al. Short-term zinc supplementation in women with non-insulin-dependent diabetes mellitus: effects on plasma 5'-nucleotidase activities, insulin-like growth factor I concentrations, and lipoprotein oxidation rates in vitro. *Am J Clin Nutr* 66: 639–642, 1997.

57. Sjogren A, Floren CH, and Nilsson A. Magnesium, potassium, and zinc deficiency in subjects with type II diabetes mellitus. *Acta Med Scand* 224: 461–466, 1988.

58. Cunningham J. Reduced mononuclear leukocyte ascorbic acid content in adults with insulin-dependent diabetes mellitus consuming adequate dietary vitamin C. *Metabolism* 40: 146–149, 1991.

59. Sinclair AJ, et al. Low plasma ascorbate levels in patients with type 2 diabetes mellitus consuming adequate dietary vitamin C. *Diabet Med* 11: 893–898, 1994.

60. Will JC, et al. Does diabetes mellitus increase the requirement for vitamin C? *Nutr Rev* 54: 193–202, 1996.

61. Singh RB, et al. Dietary intake and plasma levels of antioxidant vitamins in health and disease: a hospital-based case-control study. *J Nutr Environ Med* 5: 235–242, 1995.

62. Basu TK, et al. Serum vitamin A and retinol-binding protein in patients with insulin-dependent diabetes mellitus. *Am J Clin Nutr* 50: 329–331, 1989.

63. Wako Y, et al. Vitamin A transport in plasma of diabetic patients. *Tohoku J Exp Med* 149: 133–143, 1986.

64. Franconi F, Bennardini F, Mattana A, et al. Plasma and platelet taurine are reduced in subjects with insulin-dependent diabetes mellitus: effects of taurine supplementation. *Am J Clin Nutr* 61: 1115–1119, 1995.

65. Kosenko LG. *Klin Med* 42: 113, 1964. Cited in Werbach M. Nutritional influences on illness. CD ROM. Tarzana, CA: Third Line Press, 1998.

66. Elliott RB, Pilcher CC, Fergusson DM, et al. A population-based strategy to prevent insulin-dependent diabetes using nicotinamide. *J Pediatr Endocrinol Metab* 9: 501–509, 1996.

67. Lampeter EF, et al. The Deutsche Nicotinamide Intervention Study: an attempt to prevent type 1 diabetes. DENIS Group. *Diabetes* 47: 980–984, 1998.

### Dysmenorrhea

1. Harel Z, Biro FM, Kottenhahn RK, et al. Supplementation with omega-3 polyunsaturated fatty acids in the management of dysmenorrhea in adolescents. *Am J Obstet Gynecol* 174(4): 1335–1338, 1996.

2. Harel Z, Biro FM, Kottenhahn RK, et al. Supplementation with omega-3 polyunsaturated fatty acids in the management of dysmenorrhea in adolescents. *Am J Obstet Gynecol* 174(4): 1335–1338, 1996.

3. Harris WS. Dietary fish oil and blood lipids. *Curr Opin Lipidol* 7: 3–7, 1996.

4. Harris WS. Fish oils and plasma lipid and lipoprotein metabolism in humans: a critical review. J Lipid Res 30: 785–807, 1989.

5. Harris WS. N-3 fatty acids and serum lipoproteins: human studies. *Am J Clin Nutr* 65(Suppl.): 1645S–1654S, 1997.

6. Cobiac L, Clifton PM, and Abbey M. Lipid, lipoprotein, and hemostatic effects of fish vs fish-oil n-3 fatty acids in mildly hyperlipidemic males. *Am J Clin Nutr* 53: 1210–1216, 1991.

7. Harris WS. N-3 fatty acids and serum lipoproteins: human studies. *Am J Clin Nutr* 65(Suppl.): 1645S–1654S, 1997.

8. Fontana-Klaiber H, Hogg B. Therapeutic effects of magnesium in dysmenorrhea. *Schweiz Rundsch Med Prax* 79(16): 491–494, 1990.

9. Seifert B, et al. Magnesium—A new therapeutic alternative in primary dysmenorrhea. *Zentralbl Gynakol* 111(11): 755–760, 1989.

### Eczema

1. Morse PF, et al. Meta-analysis of placebo-controlled studies of the efficacy of Epogam in the treatment of atopic eczema: relationship between plasma essential fatty acid changes and clinical response. *Br J Dermatol* 121(1): 75–90, 1989.

2. Berth-Jones J and Graham-Brown RAC. Placebo-controlled trial of essential fatty acid supplementation in atopic dermatitis. *Lancet* 341: 1557–1560, 1993.

3. Hederos CA, et al. Epogam evening primrose oil treatment in atopic dermatitis and asthma. *Arch Dis Child* 75(6): 494–497, 1996.

4. Whitaker DK, et al. Evening primrose oil (Epogam) in the treatment of chronic hand dermatitis: disappointing therapeutic results. *Dermatology* 193: 115–120, 1996.

5. Bamford JT, et al. Atopic eczema unresponsive to evening primrose oil (linoleic and gamma-linolenic acids). *J Am Acad Dermatol* 13: 959–965, 1985.

6. Horrobin DF and Stewart C. Evening primrose oil in atopic eczema (letter). *Lancet* i: 864–865, 1990.

7. Wright S. Essential fatty acids in clinical dermatology. *J Nutr Med* 1: 301–313, 1990.

8. Biagi PL, et al. The effect of gamma-linolenic acid on clinical status, red cell fatty acid composition and membrane microviscosity in infants with atopic dermatitis. *Drugs Exp Clin Res* 20(2): 77–84, 1994.

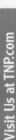

## Gallstones

1. Somerville KW, et al. Stones in the common bile duct: experience with medical dissolution therapy. *Postgrad Med J* 61: 313–316, 1985.

2. Nassauto G, et al. Effect of silibinin on biliary lipid composition: experimental and clinical study. *J Hepatol* 12: 290–295, 1991.

3. Schulz V, et al. Rational phytotherapy. New York: Springer-Verlag, 1998: 173–177.

## Gout

1. Lewis AS, et al. Inhibition of mammalian xanthine oxidase by folate compounds and amethopterin. *J Biol Chem* 259: 12–15, 1984.

2. Blouvier B and Duvulder B. Folic acid, xanthine oxidase, and uric acid (Letter). *Ann Intern Med* 88(2): 269, 1978.

3. Boss GR, et al. Failure of folic acid (pteroylglutamic acid) to affect hyperuricemia. *J Lab Clin Med* 96: 783, 1980.

4. ESCOP monographs. Fascicule 2: *Harpagophyti radix.* Exeter, UK: European Scientific Cooperative on Phytotherapy, 1997: 4.

5. Murray, M. Encyclopedia of natural medicine, 2nd ed. Rocklin, CA: Prima Publishing, 1997: 493–94.

6. Blau LW. Cherry diet control for gout and arthritis. *Texas Rep Biol Med* 8: 309–312, 1950.

## Hemorrhoids

1. Wijayanegara H, et al. A clinical trial of hydroxyethylrutosides in the treatment of hemorrhoids of pregnancy. *J Int Med Res* 20: 54–60, 1992.

2. Boisseau MR, et al. Fibrinolysis and hemorrheology in chronic venous insufficiency: a double-blind study of troxerutin efficiency. *J Cardiovasc Surg* 36: 369–374, 1995.

3. Wadworth AN, et al. Hydroxyethylrutosides: a review of its pharmacology and therapeutic efficacy in venous insufficiency and related disorders. *Drugs* 44: 1013–1032, 1992.

4. Saggloro A, et al. Treatment of hemorrhoidal syndrome with mesoglycan. *Minerva Diet Gastroenterol* 31: 311–315, 1985.

5. Annoni R, et al. Treatment of hemorrhoidal syndrome with mesoglycan. *Minerva Diet Gastroenterol* 31: 311–315, 1985.

## Hepatitis

1. Berenguer J, et al. Double-blind trial of silymarin vs. placebo in the treatment of chronic hepatitis. *Muench Med Wochenschr* 119: 240–260, 1977.

2. Buzzelli G, et al. A pilot study on the liver protective effect of silybin-phosphatidylcholine complex (IdB 1016) in chronic active hepatitis. *Int J Clin Pharm Ther Toxicol* 31(9): 456–460, 1993.

3. Liruss F, et al. Cytoprotection in the nineties: experience with ursodeoxycholic acid and silymarin in chronic liver disease. *Acta Physiol Hung* 80(1–4): 363–367, 1992.

4. Bode JC, et al. Silymarin for the treatment of acute viral hepatitis? Report of a controlled trial. *Med Klin* 72: 513–518, 1977.

5. Schulz V, et al. Rational phytotherapy. New York: Springer-Verlag, 1998: 216.

6. Hikino H, et al. Natural products for liver disease. As cited in Wagner H, et al. (eds.). Economic and medicinal plant research, Vol 2. New York: Academic Press, 1988: 39–72.

7. Muzes G, et al. Effects of silymarin (Legalon) therapy on the antioxidant defense mechanism and lipid peroxidation in alcoholic liver disease (double-blind protocol). *Orv Hetil* 131(16): 863–866, 1990.

8. Lorenz D, et al. Pharmacokinetic studies with silymarin in human serum and bile. *Methods Find Exp Clin Pharmacol* 6(10): 655–661, 1984.

9. Dehmlow C, et al. Inhibition of Kupffer cell functions as an explanation for the hepatoprotective properties of silibinin. *Hepatology* 23(4): 749–754, 1996.

10. Comoglio A, et al. Scavenging effect of silipide, a new silybin-phospholipid complex, on ethanol-derived free radicals. *Biochem Pharmacol* 50(8): 1313–1316, 1995.

11. Barzaghi N, et al. Pharmacokinetic studies on IdB 1016, a silybin-phosphatidylcholine complex in healthy human subjects. *Eur J Drug Metab Pharmacokinet* 15(4): 333–338, 1990.

12. Schandalik R, et al. Pharmacokinetics of silybin in bile following administration of silipide and silymarin in cholecystectomy patients. *Arnzneimittelforschung* 42(7): 964–968, 1992.

13. Awang D. Milk thistle. *Can Pharm J* 422: 403–404, 1983.

14. Albrecht M. Therapy of toxic liver pathologies with Legalon. *Z Klin Med* 47(2): 87–92, 1992.

15. Giannola C, et al. A two-center study on the effects of silymarin in pregnant women and adult patients with so-called minor hepatic insufficiency. *Clin Ther* 114(2): 129–135, 1985.

16. Kim DH, et al. Silymarin and its components are inhibitors of beta-glucuronidase. *Biol Pharm Bull* 17(3): 443–445, 1994.

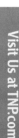

17. Arase Y, et al. The long-term efficacy of glycyrrhizin in chronic hepatitis C patients. *Cancer* 79: 1494–1500, 1997.

18. Okumura M, et al. A multicenter randomized controlled clinical trial of Sho-saiko-to in chronic active hepatitis. *Gastroenterol Jpn* 24: 715–719, 1989.

## Herpes

1. Wolbling RH, et al. Local therapy of herpes simplex with dried extract from *Melissa officinalis*. *Phytomedicine* 1: 25–31, 1994.

2. Wolbling RH, et al. Clinical therapy of herpes simplex. *Therapiewoche* 34: 1193–1200, 1984.

3. Wolbling RH, et al. Local therapy of herpes simplex with dried extract from *Melissa officinalis*. *Phytomedicine* 1: 25–31, 1994.

4. Flodin NW. The metabolic roles, pharmacology, and toxicology of lysine. *J Am Coll Nutr* 16(1): 7–21, 1997.

5. Griffith RS, Walsh DE, and Myrmel KH. Success of L-lysine therapy in frequently recurrent herpes simplex infection. Treatment and prophylaxis. *Dermatologica*, 175: 183–190, 1987.

6. McCune MA, Perry HO, Muller SA, et al. Treatment of recurrent herpes simplex infections with L-lysine monohydrochloride. *Cutis* 34: 366–373, 1984.

7. DiGiovanna JJ and Blank H. Failure of lysine in frequently recurrent herpes simplex infection: treatment and prophylaxis. *Arch Dermatol* 120: 48–51, 1984.

8. Kritchevsky D, et al. Gallstone formation in hamsters: influence of specific amino acids. *Nutr Rep Int* 29: 117, 1984.

9. Lexzczynski DE, et al. Excess dietary lysine induces hypercholesterolemia in chickens. *Experientia* 38: 266–267, 1982.

10. Hovi T, et al. Topical treatment of recurrent mucocutaneous herpes with ascorbic acid–containing solution. *Antiviral Res* 27(3): 263–270, 1995.

11. Terezhalmy GT, Bottomley WK, and Pelleu GB. The use of water-soluble bioflavonoid-ascorbic acid complex in the treatment of recurrent herpes labialis. *Oral Surg Oral Med Oral Pathol* 45(1): 56–62, 1978.

## Hypertension

1. Silagy CA, et al. A meta-analysis of the effect of garlic on blood pressure. *J Hypertens* 12: 463–468, 1994.

2. Auer W, et al. Hypertension and hyperlipidemia: garlic helps in mild cases. *Br J Clin Pract Symp Suppl* 69: 3–6, 1990.

3. Digiesi V, et al. Effect of coenzyme $Q_{10}$ on essential arterial hypertension. *Curr Ther Res* 47: 841–845, 1990.

4. Langsjoen P, et al. Treatment of essential hypertension with coenzyme $Q_{10}$. *Mol Aspects Med* 15(Suppl.): S265–S272, 1994.

5. Digiesi V, et al. Coenzyme $Q_{10}$ in essential hypertension. *Mol Aspects Med* 15(Suppl.): S257–S263, 1994.

6. Appel LJ, et al. Does supplementation of diet with "fish oil" reduce blood pressure? A meta-analysis of controlled clinical trials. *Arch Intern Med* 153(12): 1429–1438, 1993.

7. McCarron DA, et al. Dietary calcium and blood pressure: modifying factors in specific populations. *Am J Clin Nutr* 54: 215S–219S, 1991.

8. Bucher HC, Cook RJ, Guyatt GH, et al. Effects of dietary calcium supplementation on blood pressure. *JAMA* 275(13): 1016–1022, 1996.

9. Altura BM and Altura BT. Cardiovascular risk factors and magnesium: relationships to atherosclerosis, ischemic heart disease and hypertension. *Magnes Trace Elements* 10: 182–192, 1991.

10. Ma J, Folsom AR, Melnick SL, et al. Associations of serum and dietary magnesium with cardiovascular disease, hypertension, diabetes, insulin, and carotid artery wall thickness: the ARIC study. *J Clin Epidemiol* 48(7): 927–940, 1995.

11. Yamamoto ME, Applegate WB, Klag MJ, et al. Lack of blood pressure effect with calcium and magnesium supplementation in adults with high-normal blood pressure: Results from phase I of the trials of hypertension prevention (TOHP). *Ann Epidemiol* 5: 96–107, 1995.

12. Barri YM and Wingo CS. The effects of potassium depletion and supplementation on blood pressure: a clinical review. *Am J Med Sci* 314(1): 37–40, 1997.

13. Whelton PK, He J, Cutler JA, et al. Effects of oral potassium on blood pressure. Meta-analysis of randomized controlled clinical trials. *JAMA* 277(20): 1624–1632, 1997.

14. Preuss HG. Diet, genetics and hypertension. *J Am Coll Nutr* 16(4): 296–305, 1997.

15. Schulz V, et al. Rational phytotherapy. New York: Springer-Verlag, 1998: 97.

16. Feldman E, Gold S, Greene J, et al. Ascorbic acid supplements and blood pressure. *Ann N Y Acad Sci* 669: 342–344, 1992.

17. Feldman EB, Gold S, Greene J, et al. Vitamin C administration and blood pressure regulation (Abstract). *Am J Clin Nutr* 56: 760, 1992.

18. Koh ET. Effect of vitamin C on blood parameters of hypertensive subjects. *J Okla State Med Assoc* 77: 177–182, 1984.

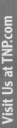

19. Ghosh S, Ekpo E, and Shah I. A double-blind, placebo-controlled parallel trial of vitamin C treatment in elderly patients with hypertension. *Gerontology* 40: 268–272, 1994.

20. Osilesi O, et al. Blood pressure and plasma lipids during ascorbic acid supplementation in borderline hypertensive and normotensive adults. *Nutr Res* 11: 405–412, 1991.

## Impotence

1. Sikora R, et al. *Ginkgo biloba* extract in the therapy of erectile dysfunction. *J Urol* 141: 188A, 1989.

2. Cohen AJ and Bartlik B. *Ginkgo biloba* for antidepressant-induced sexual dysfunction. *J Sex Marital Ther* 24: 139–143, 1988.

## Infertility in Men

1. Werbach, M. Nutritional influences on illness, 2nd ed. Tarzana, CA: Third Line Press, 1993: 628–629.

2. Kumamoto Y, et al. Clinical efficacy of mecobalamin in treatment of oligozoospermia: Results of double-blind comparative clinical study. *Acta Urol Jpn* 34: 1109–1132, 1988.

3. Sandler B, and Faragher B. Treatment of oligospermia with vitamin $B_{12}$. *Infertility* 7: 133–138, 1984.

4. Bedwal R, et al. Zinc, copper, and selenium in reproduction. *Experientia* 50: 626–640, 1994.

5. Netter A, et al. Effect of zinc administration on plasma testosterone, dihydrotestosterone, and sperm count. *Arch Androl* 7: 69–73, 1981.

6. Suleiman SA, Ali ME, Zaki ZM, et al. Lipid peroxidation and human sperm motility: protective role of vitamin E. *J Androl* 17(5): 530–537, 1996.

7. Dawson EB, et al. Effect of ascorbic acid on male fertility. *Ann N Y Acad Sci* 498: 312–323, 1987.

## Infertility in Women

1. Propping D, et al. Diagnosis and therapy of corpus luteum insufficiency in general practice. *Therapiewoche* 38: 2992–3001, 1988.

2. Czeizel A, Metnek J, and Dudas I. The effect of preconceptional multivitamin supplementation on fertility. *Int J Vitam Nutr Res* 66: 55–58, 1996.

## Insomnia

1. Schulz V, et al. Rational phytotherapy. New York: Springer-Verlag, 1998: 75–77, 81.

2. Hendriks H, et al. Central nervous depressant activity of valerenic acid in the mouse. *Planta Medica* 51: 28–31, 1985.

3. Krieglstein J, et al. Valepotriate, valenrensaure, valeranon und atherisches Ol sind jedoch unwirksam. Zentraldampfende Inhaltsstoffe im Baldrian. *Dtsch Apoth Ztg* 128: 2041–2046, 1988.

4. Leuschner J, et al. Characterization of the central nervous depressant activity of a commercially available valerian root extract. *Arzneimittelforschung* 43(6): 638–641, 1993.

5. Vorbach EU, et al. Therapie von Insomnien. Wirksamkeit und Vertraglichkeit eines Baldrianpraparats. *Psychopharmakotherapie* 3: 109–115, 1996. As cited in Schulz V, et al. Rational phytotherapy. New York: Springer-Verlag, 1998.

6. Leathwood PD, et al. Aqueous extract of valerian root (*Valeriana officinalis* L.) improves sleep quality in man. *Pharmacol Biochem Behav* 17(1): 65–71, 1982.

7. Leathwood PD, et al. Aqueous extract of valerian reduces latency to fall asleep in man. *Planta Medica* 51: 144–148, 1985.

8. Lindahl O, et al. Double-blind study of a valerian preparation. *Pharmacol Biochem Behav* 32(4): 1065–1066, 1989.

9. Kamm-Khol AV, et al. Moderne Baldriantherapie gegen nervose Storungen im Senium. *Med Welt* 35: 1450–1454, 1985. As cited in ESCOP monographs. Fascicule 4: *Valerianae radix* (valerian root). Exeter, UK: European Society Cooperative on Phytotherapy, 1997.

10. Andreatini R and Leite JR. Effect of valepotriates on the behavior of rats in the elevated plus-maze during diazepam withdrawal. *Eur J Pharmacol* 260(2–3): 233–235, 1994.

11. Holzl J, et al. Receptor binding studies with *Valeriana officinalis* on the benzodiazepine receptor. *Planta Medica* 55: 642, 1989.

12. Mennini T, et al. In vitro study on the interaction of extracts and pure compounds from *Valeriana officinalis* roots with GABA, benzodiazepine and barbiturate receptors in rat brain. *Fitoterapia* 54: 291–300, 1993.

13. Santos MS, et al. Synaptosomal GABA release as influenced by valerian root extract—involvement of the GABA carrier. *Arch Int Pharmacodyn* 327: 220–231, 1994.

14. Santos MS, et al. An aqueous extract of valerian influences the transport of GABA in synaptosomes. *Planta Medica* 60: 278–279, 1994.

15. Cavadas C, et al. In vitro study on the interaction of *Valeriana officinalis* L: Extracts and their amino acids on GABA receptor in rat brain. *Arzneimittelforschung* 45(7): 753–755, 1995.

**Notes**

**Visit Us at TNP.com**
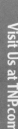

16. Santos MS, et al. The amount of GABA present in aqueous extracts of valerian is sufficient to account for [³H] GABA release in synaptosomes. *Planta Medica* 60: 475–476, 1994.

17. Schulz V, et al. Rational phytotherapy. New York: Springer-Verlag, 1998.

18. Dressing H, et al. Insomnia: Are valerian/balm combinations of equal value to benzodiazepine? *Therapiewoche* 42: 726-736, 1992.

19. Wiley LB, et al. Valerian overdose: a case report. *Vet Hum Toxicol* 37(4): 364–365, 1995.

20. Rosecrans JA, et al. Pharmacological investigation of certain *Valeriana officinalis* L. extracts. *J Pharm Sci* 50: 240–244, 1996.

21. Schulz V, et al. Rational phytotherapy. New York: Springer-Verlag, 1998.

22. Albrecht M, et al. Psychopharmaceuticals and safety in traffic. *Z Allg Med* 71: 1215–1221, 1995.

23. Gerhard U, et al. Vigilance-decreasing effects of 2 plant-derived sedatives. *Schweiz Rundsch Med Prax* 85(15): 473–481, 1996.

24. Sakamoto T, et al. Psychotropic effects of Japanese valerian root extract. *Chem Pharm Bull* (Tokyo) 40(3): 758–761, 1992.

25. Albrecht M, et al. Psychopharmaceuticals and safety in traffic. *Z Allg Med* 71: 1215–1221, 1995.

26. Lamberg L. Melatonin potentially useful but safety, efficacy remain uncertain. *JAMA* 276(13): 1011–1014, 1996.

27. Suhner A, et al. Optimal melatonin dosage form for the alleviation of jet lag. *Chronobiol Int* 14: 41, 1997.

28. Garfinkel D, et al. Improvement of sleep quality in elderly people by controlled-release melatonin. *Lancet* 346: 541–544, 1995.

29. Petrie K, et al. A double-blind trial of melatonin as a treatment for jet lag in international cabin crew. *Biol Psych* 33(7): 526–530, 1993.

30. Chase JE, et al. Melatonin: therapeutic use in sleep disorders. *Ann Pharmacother* 346(10): 1218–1226, 1997.

31. Spitzer RL, et al. Failure of melatonin to affect jet lag in a randomized double- blind trial. *Soc Light Treatment Biol Rhythms Abstr* 9: 1, 1997.

32. Arendt J, et al. Efficacy of melatonin in jet lag, shift work and blindness. *J Biol Rhythms* 12(6): 604–617, 1997.

33. Suhner A, et al. Optimal melatonin dosage form for the alleviation of jet lag. *Chronobiol Int* 14: 41, 1997.

34. Waterhouse J, et al. Jet lag. *Lancet* 350: 1611–1616, 1997.

## Intermittent Claudication

1.Schulz V, et al. Rational phytotherapy. New York: Springer-Verlag, 1998: 126.

2. Peters H, Kieser M, and Holscher U. Demonstration of the efficacy of *Ginkgo biloba* special extract EGb 761 on intermittent claudication—a placebo-controlled, double-blind multicenter trial. *Vasa* 27: 106–110, 1998.

3. Peters H, Kieser M, and Holscher U. Demonstration of the efficacy of *Ginkgo biloba* special extract EGb 761 on intermittent claudication—a placebo-controlled, double-blind multicenter trial. *Vasa* 27: 106–110, 1998.

4. Brevetti G, et al. Propionyl-L-carnitine in intermittent claudication: double-blind, placebo-controlled, dose titration, multicenter study. *J Am Coll Cardiol* 26(6): 1411–1416, 1995.

5. O'Hara J, Jolly PN, and Nicol CG. The therapeutic efficacy of inositol nicotinate (Hexopal) in intermittent claudication: a controlled trial. *Br J Clin Pract* 42(9): 377–383, 1988.

6. Kiff RS. Does inositol nicotinate (Hexopal) influence intermittent claudication? A controlled trial. *Br J Clin Pract* 42(4): 141–145, 1988.

7. Head A. Treatment of intermittent claudication with inositol nicotinate. *Practitioner* 230: 49–54, 1986.

8. O'Hara J. A double-blind placebo-controlled study of Hexopal in the treatment of intermittent claudication. *J Int Med Res* 13: 322–327, 1985.

9. Tyson VCH. Treatment of intermittent claudication. *Practitioner* 223: 121–126, 1979.

10. O'Hara J, Jolly PN, and Nicol CG. The therapeutic efficacy of inositol nicotinate (Hexopal) in intermittent claudication: a controlled trial. *Br J Clin Pract* 42(9): 377–383, 1988.

11. Maxwell A. Annual meeting of American College of Cardiology. 1999.

## Irritable Bowel Syndrome

1. Rees WDW, et al. Treating irritable bowel syndrome with peppermint oil. *BMJ* 2: 835–836, 1979.

2. Dew MJ, et al. Peppermint oil for the irritable bowel syndrome: A multicentre trial. *Br J Clin Pract* 34: 55–57, 1989.

3. Lawson MJ, et al. Failure of enteric-coated peppermint oil in the irritable bowel syndrome: A randomized double-blind crossover study. *J Gastroenterol Hepatol* 3: 235–238, 1988.

4. Nash P, et al. Peppermint oil does not relieve the pain of irritable bowel syndrome. *Br J Clin Pract* 40: 292–293, 1986.

5. ESCOP monographs. Fascicule 3: *Menthae piperitae aetheroleum* (peppermint oil). Exeter, UK: European Scientific Cooperative on Phytotherapy, 1997: 1–2.

6. Halpern GM, et al. Treatment of irritable bowel syndrome with lacteol fort: a randomized, double-blind, cross-over trial. *Am J Gastroenterol* 91: 1579–1585, 1996.

## Macular Degeneration

1. Mares-Perlman J, Klein R, Klein B, et al. Relationship between age-related maculopathy and intake of vitamin and mineral supplements (Abstract). *Invest Ophthalmol Vis Sci* 34: 1133, 1993.

2. Mares-Perlman JA, et al. Association of zinc and antioxidant nutrients with age- related maculopathy. *Arch Ophthalmol* 114: 991–997, 1996.

3. Age-Related Macular Degeneration Study Group. Multicenter ophthalmic and nutritional age-related macular degeneration study—Part 2: antioxidant intervention and conclusions. *J Am Optom Assoc* 67: 30–49, 1996.

4. Seddon JM, Ajani UA, Sperduto RD, et al. Dietary carotenoids, vitamins A, C, and E, and advanced age-related macular degeneration. *JAMA* 272: 1413–1420, 1994.

5. Mares-Perlman JA, Brady W, Klein R, et al. Serum antioxidants and age-related macular degeneration in a population-based case-control study. *Arch Ophthalmol* 113: 1518–1523, 1995.

6. Landrum JT, Bone RA, and Kilburn MD. The macular pigment: a possible role in protection from age-related macular degeneration. *Adv Pharmacol* 38: 537–555, 1997.

7. Snodderly DM. Evidence for protection against age-related macular degeneration by carotenoids and antioxidant vitamins. *Am J Clin Nutr* 62(14): 48S–61S, 1995.

8. Scharrer A, et al. Anthocyanosides in the treatment of retinopathies. *Klin Monatsbl Augenheilkd* 178: 386–389, 1981.

9. Lebuisson DA, et al. Treatment of senile macular degeneration with *Ginkgo biloba* extract: A preliminary double-blind, drug vs. placebo study. *Presse Med* 15: 1556–1558, 1986.

10. Caselli L. Clinical and electroretinographic study on activity of anthocyanosides. *Arch Med Int* 37: 29–35, 1985.

11. Watson V. Wine consumption decreases risk of age-related blindness. *Medical Tribune*, June 5, 1997.

12. Stur M, et al. Oral zinc and the second eye in age-related macular degeneration. *Invest Ophthalmol Visual Sci* 37(7): 1225–1235, 1996.

13. Mares-Perlman JA, et al. Association of zinc and antioxidant nutrients with age-related maculopathy. *Arch Ophthalmol* 114: 991–997, 1996.

14. Newsome DA, Swartz M, Leone NC, et al. Oral zinc in macular degeneration. *Arch Ophthalmol* 106(2): 192–198, 1988.

## Menopausal Symptoms

1. Stoll W. Phythopharmacon influences atrophic vaginal epithelium. Double-blind study: *Cimicifuga* vs. estrogenic substances. *Therapeuticum* 1: 23–28, 1987.

2. Stolze H. An alternative to treat menopausal complaints. *Gyne* 3: 14–16, 1982.

3. Warnecke G. Influencing menopausal symptoms with a phytotherapeutic agent. *Med Welt* 36: 871–874, 1985.

4. Stoll W. Phythopharmacon influences atrophic vaginal epithelium. Double-blind study: *Cimicifuga* vs. estrogenic substances. *Therapeuticum* 1: 23–28, 1987.

5. Stolze H. An alternative to treat menopausal complaints. *Gyne* 3: 14–16, 1982.

6. Warnecke G. Influencing menopausal symptoms with a phytotherapeutic agent. *Med Welt* 36: 871–874, 1985.

7. Jarry H, et al. The endocrine effects of constituents of *Cimicifuga racemosa*. 2. In vitro binding of constituents to estrogen receptors. *Planta Medica* 4: 316–319, 1985.

8. Jarry H, et al. Endocrine effects of constituents of *Cimicifuga racemosa*. 1. The effect on serum levels of pituitary hormones in ovariectomized rats. *Planta Medica* 1: 46–49, 1985.

9. Duker EM, et al. Effects of extracts from *Cimicifuga racemosa* on gonadotropin release in menopausal women and ovariectomized rats. *Planta Medica* 57(5): 420–424, 1991.

10. Liske P. Therapeutic efficacy and safety of *Cimicifuga racemosa* for gynecologic disorders. *Advances in Therapy* 15(1):45–53, 1998.

11. Einer-Jensen N, Zhao J, Andersen KP, et al. *Cimicifuga* and melbosia lack oestrogenic effects in mice and rats. *Maturitas* 25:149–153, 1996.

12. Jones TK, et al. Profound neonatal congestive heart failure caused by maternal consumption of blue cohosh herbal medication. *J Pediatrics* 132: 550–552, 1998.

13. Korn WD. Six-month oral toxicity study with Remifemin-granulate in rats followed by an 8-week recovery period. Hannover, Germany: International Bioresearch, 1991.

14. Nesselhut T, et al. Influence of *Cimicifuga racemosa* extracts with estrogen-like activity on the in vitro proliferation of mammalian carcinoma cells. *Arch Gynecol Obstet* 254: 817–818, 1993.

15. Newall C. Herbal medicines: a guide for the health-care professional. London: The Pharmaceutical Press, 1996: 80.

16. Albertazzi P, et al. The effect of dietary soy supplementation on hot flashes. *Obstet Gynecol* 91(1): 6–11, 1998.

17. Hughes C. Complementary medicine for the physician. 3(4): 26–27, 1998.

18. Messina M. To recommend or not to recommend soy foods. *J Am Diet Assoc* 94(11): 1253–1254.

19. Hirata JD, et al. Does dong quai have estrogenic effects in postmenopausal women? A double-blind placebo-controlled trial. *Fertil Steril* 68(6): 981–986, 1997.

## Migraine Headaches

1. Johnson ES, et al. Efficacy of feverfew as a prophylactic treatment of migraine. *BMJ* 291: 569–573, 1985.

2. Murphy JS, et al. Randomized, double-blind, placebo-controlled trial of feverfew in migraine prevention. *Lancet* 23: 189–192, 1988.

3. Palevitch DG, et al. Feverfew (*Tanacetum parthenium*) as a prophylactic treatment for migraine: A double-blind, placebo-controlled study. *Phytother Res* 11(7): 506–511, 1997.

4. De Weerdt C, et al. Herbal medicines in migraine prevention. Randomized double-blind placebo controlled crossover trial of a feverfew preparation. *Phytomedicine* 3(3): 225–230, 1996.

5. Bohlmann F, et al. Sesquiterpene lactones and other constituents from *Tanacetum parthenium*. *Phytochemistry* 21: 2543–2549, 1982.

6. Makheja AM, et al. The active principle in feverfew. *Lancet* ii: 1054, 1981.

7. Makheja AM, et al. A platelet phospholipase inhibitor from the medicinal herb feverfew (*Tanacetum parthenium*). *Prostaglandins Leukotriens Med* 8: 653–660, 1982.

8. Heptinstall S, et al. Extracts from feverfew inhibit granule secretion in blood platelets and polymorphonuclear leukocytes. *Lancet* 8437: 1071–1074, 1985.

9. Tyler V. Herbs of choice. New York: Pharmaceutical Products Press, 1994: 127.

10. Murphy JS, et al. Randomized, double-blind, placebo-controlled trial of feverfew in migraine prevention. *Lancet* 23: 189–192, 1988.

11. Johnson ES, et al. Efficacy of feverfew as a prophylactic treatment of migraine. *BMJ* 291: 569–573, 1985.

12. Johnson ES, et al. Efficacy of feverfew as a prophylactic treatment of migraine. *BMJ* 291: 569–573, 1985.

13. Newall C, et al. Herbal medicines: a guide for health-care professionals. London: The Pharmaceutical Press, 1996: 120.

14. Peikert A, et al. Prophylaxis of migraine with oral magnesium: results from a prospective, multicenter, placebo-controlled and double-blind randomized study. *Cephalalgia* 6(4): 257–263, 1996.

15. Taubert K. Magnesium in migraine: Results of a multicenter pilot study (in German). *Fortschr Med* 112(24): 328–330, 1994.

16. Facchinetti F, Sances G, Borella P, et al. Magnesium prophylaxis of menstrual migraine: effects on intracellular magnesium. *Headache* 31(5): 298–301, 1991.

17. Pfaffenrath V, et al. Magnesium in the prophylaxis of migraine—a double-blind, placebo-controlled study. *Cephalalgia* 16: 436–440, 1996.

18. Gaby AR. Research Review. *Nutrition & Healing*, March 1997.

19. Titus F, et al. 5-hydroxytryptophan versus methysergide in the prophylaxis of migraine: randomized clinical trial. *Eur Neurol* 25(5): 327–329, 1986.

20. De Benedittis G and Massei R. Serotonin precursors in chronic primary headache. A double-blind cross-over study with L-5-hydroxytryptophan vs. placebo. *J Neurosurg Sci* 29(3): 239–248, 1985.

21. Maissen CP and Ludin HP. Comparison of the effect of 5-hydroxytryptophan and propranolol in the interval treatment of migraine. *Schweiz Med Wochenschr* 121(43): 1585–1590, 1991.

22. Longo G, Rudoi I, Iannuccelli M, et al. Treatment of essential headache in developmental age with L-5-HTP (crossover double-blind study versus placebo). *Pediatr Med Chir* 6(2): 241–245, 1984.

23. Santucci M, et al. L-hydroxytryptophan versus placebo in childhood migraine prophylaxis: a double-blind crossover study. *Cephalalgia* 6: 155–157, 1986.

24. Glueck CJ, et al. Amelioration of severe migraine with omega-3 fatty acids: A double-blind, placebo-controlled clinical trial (Abstract). *Am J Clin Nutr* 43: 710, 1986.

25. Macaroon T, et al. Amelioration of severe migraine by fish oil (w-3) fatty acids (Abstract). *Am J Clin Nutr* 41: 874a, 1985.

26. Schoenen, J, Jacquy J, and Lenaerts M. Effectiveness of high-dose riboflavin in migraine prophylaxis. A randomized controlled trial. *Neurology* 50: 466–470, 1998.

27. Trotsky MB. Neurogenic vascular headaches, food and chemical triggers. *Ear Nose Throat J* 73(4): 228–230, 235–236, 1994.

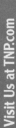

28. Vincent CA. A controlled trial of the treatment of migraine by acupuncture. *Clin J Pain* 5(4): 305–312, 1989.

## Nausea

1. Fischer-Rasmussen W, et al. Ginger treatment of hyperemesis gravidarum. *Eur J Obstet Gynecol Reprod Biol* 38: 19–24, 1990.

2. Mowrey DB. Motion sickness, ginger, and psychophysics. *Lancet* i: 655–657, 1982.

3. ESCOP monographs. Fascicule 1: *Zingiberis rhizoma* (ginger). Exeter, UK: European Scientific Cooperative on Phytotherapy, 1997: 2.

4. Grontved A, et al. Ginger root against seasickness: A controlled trial on the open sea. *Acta Otolaryngol* (Stockh) 105: 45–49, 1988.

5. Stott JRR, et al. A double-blind comparative trial of powdered ginger root, hyosine (sic) hydrobromide and cinnarizine in the prophylaxis of motion sickness induced by cross coupled stimulation. *Advisory Group for Aerospace Research and Development, Conference Proceedings* 372(39): 1–6, 1985.

6. Stewart JJ, et al. Effects of ginger on motion sickness susceptibility and gastric function. *Pharmacology* 42: 111–120, 1991.

7. Bone ME, Wilkinson DJ, Young JR, et al. Ginger root: a new anti-emetic. The effect of ginger root on postoperative nausea and vomiting after major gynecological surgery. *Anaesthesia* 45: 669–671, 1990.

8. Phillips S, et al. *Zingiber officinale* (ginger)—an anti-emetic for day case surgery. *Anaesthesia* 48: 715–717, 1993.

9. Arfeen Z, et al. A double-blind randomized controlled trial of ginger for the prevention of postoperative nausea and vomiting. *Anaesth Intensive Care* 23(4): 449–452, 1995.

10. Visalyaputra S, et al. The efficacy of ginger root in the prevention of postoperative nausea and vomiting after outpatient gynaecological laparoscopy. *Anaesthesia* 53: 506–510, 1998.

11. Srivastava KC. Isolation and effects of some ginger components on platelet aggregation and eicosanoid biosynthesis. *Prostaglandins Leukot Med* 25: 187–198, 1986.

12. Srivastava K. Effects of aqueous extracts of onion, garlic, and ginger on the platelet aggregation and metabolism of arachidonic acid in the blood vascular system: In vitro study. *Prostaglandins Leukot Med* 13: 227–235, 1984.

13. Srivastava KC. Effect of onion and ginger consumption on platelet thromboxane production in humans. *Prostaglandins Leukot Essent Fatty Acids* 35: 183–185, 1989.

14. Janssen PL, et al. Consumption of ginger (*Zingiber officinale* Roscoe) does not affect ex vivo platelet thromboxane production in humans. *Eur J Clin Nutr* 50(11): 772–774, 1996.

15. Bordia A, et al. Effect of ginger (*Zingiber officinale* Rosc.) and fenugreek (*Trigonella foenumgraecum* L.) on blood lipids, blood sugar and platelet aggregation in patients with coronary artery disease. *Prostaglandins Leukot Essent Fatty Acids* 56(5): 379–384, 1997.

16. Lumb AB. Effect of dried ginger on human platelet function. *Thromb Haemost* 71: 110–111, 1994.

17. Vutyananich T, Wongtra-ngan S, and Rung-aroon R. Pyridoxine for nausea and vomiting of pregnancy. A randomized, double-blind placebo-controlled trial. *Am J Obstet Gynecol* 173: 881–884, 1995.

18. Merkel RL. The use of menadione bisulfite and ascorbic acid in the treatment of nausea and vomiting of pregnancy. *Am J Obstet Gynecol* 78: 33–36, 1952.

19. Signorello LB, et al. Saturated fat intake and the risk of severe hyperemesis gravidarum. *Am J Epidemiol* 143(Suppl. 11): S25, 1996.

## Night Vision

1. Jayle GE, et al. Action des glucosides d'anthocyanes sur la vision scotopique et mesopique du sujet normal. *Therapie* 19: 171–185, 1964. As cited in Bone K, et al. *Mediherb Professional Review*. Queensland, Australia, 59, 1997.

2. Jayle GE, et al.. Title not stated. *Ann Ocul* 198: 556, 1965. As cited in Bone K, et al. *Mediherb Professional Review*. Queensland, Australia, 59, 1997.

3. Sala D, et al. Effect of anthocyanosides on visual performance at low illumination. *Minerva Oftalmol* 21: 283–285, 1979.

4. Gloria E, et al. Effect of anthocyanosides on the absolute visual threshold. *Ann Ottalmol Clin Ocul* 92: 595–607, 1966.

5. Caselli L. Clinical and electroretinographic study on activity of anthocyanosides. *Arch Med Int* 37: 29–35, 1985.

6. Wegmann R, et al. Effects of anthocyanosides on photoreceptors. Cyto-enzymatic aspects. *Ann Histochem* 14: 237–256, 1969.

7. Lietti A, et al. Studies on *Vaccinium myrtillus* anthocyanosides: vasoprotective and anti-inflammatory activity. *Arzneimittelforschung* 26: 829–832, 1976.

8. Lietti A, et al. Studies on *Vaccinium myrtillus* anthocyanosides: aspects of anthocyanin pharmacokinetics in the rat. *Arzneimittelforschung* 26: 832–835, 1976.

9. Eandi M. Unpublished results. As cited in Morazzoni P, et al., *Vaccinium myrtillus*. *Fitoterapia* 67(1): 3–29 1996.

10. Corbe C, et al. Light vision and chorioretinal circulation. Study of the effect of procyanidolic oligomers (Endotelon). *J Fr Ophtalmol* 11: 453–460, 1988.

11. Boissin JP, et al. Chorioretinal circulation and dazzling: Use of procyanidolic oligomers. *Bull Soc Ophtamol Fr* 88: 173–174, 177–179, 1988.

## Osteoarthritis

1. Brandt KD. Effects of nonsteroidal anti-inflammatory drugs on chondrocyte metabolism in vitro and in vivo. *Am J Med* 83 (Suppl. 5A): 29–34, 1987.

2. Brooks PM, et al. NSAID and osteoarthritis—help or hindrance. *J Rheumatol* 9: 3–5, 1982.

3. Shield MJ, Anti-inflammatory drugs and their effects on cartilage synthesis and renal function. *Eur J Rheumatol Inflam* 13: 7–16, 1993.

4. Palmoski MJ, et al. Effects of some nonsteroidal anti-inflammatory drugs on proteoglycan metabolism and organization in canine articular cartilage. *Arthritis Rheum* 23: 1010–1020, 1980.

5. Rahad S, et al. Effects of nonsteroidal anti-inflammatory drugs on the course of osteoarthritis. *Lancet* 2: 519–522, 1989.

6. Jimenez SA, et al. The effects of glucosamine on human chondrocyte gene expression. Madrid, Spain: The Ninth Eular Symposium, 1996: 8–10.

7. Hellio MP, et al. The effects of glucosamine on human chondrocyte gene expression. Madrid, Spain: The Ninth Eular Symposium, 1996: 11–12.

8. Setnikar I, et al. Anti-arthritic effects of glucosamine sulfate studied in animal models. *Arzneim Forsch* 41: 542–545, 1991.

9. Setnikar I. Antireactive properties of "chondroprotective" drugs. *Int J Tissue React* 14(5): 253–261, 1992.

10. Crolle G, et al. Glucosamine sulfate for the management of arthrosis: A controlled clinical investigation. *Current Medical Research and Opinion* 7(2): 104–109, 1980.

11. Qiu GX, et al. Efficacy and safety of glucosamine sulfate versus ibuprofen in patients with knee arthritis. *Arzneimittelforschung* 48: 469–474, 1998.

12. Karzel K, et al. Effect of hexosamine derivatives and uronic acid derivatives on glycosaminoglycan metabolism of fibroblast cultures. *Pharmacology* 5: 337–345, 1971.

13. Vidal y Plana, et al. Articular cartilage pharmacology: I. In vitro studies on glucosamine and nonsteroidal anti-inflammatory drugs. *Pharmacol Res Comm* 10: 557–569, 1978.

14. Noack W, et al. Glucosamine sulfate in osteoarthritis of the knee. *Osteoarthritis Cartilage* 2: 51–59, 1994.

15. Rovati, LC, et al. A large, randomized, placebo controlled, double-blind study of glucosamine sulfate vs. Piroxicam and vs. their association, on the kinetics of the symptomatic effect in knee osteoarthritis. *Osteoarthritis Cartilage* 2(Suppl. 1): 56, 1994.

16. Muller-Fassbender H, et al. Glucosamine sulfate compared to ibuprofen in osteoarthritis of the knee. *Osteoarthritis Cartilage* 2: 61–69, 1994.

17. Qiu GX, et al. Efficacy and safety of glucosamine sulfate versus ibuprofen in patients with knee arthritis. *Arzneimittelforschung* 48: 469–474, 1998.

18. Setnikar I, et al. Pharmacokinetics of glucosamine in man. *Arzneimittelforschung* 43(10): 1109–1113, 1993.

19. Tapadinhas MJ, et al. Oral glucosamine sulfate in the management of arthrosis: Report on multi-centre open investigation in Portugal. *Pharmatherapeutica* 3: 157–168, 1982.

20. Conte A, et al. Biochemical and pharmacokinetic aspects of oral treatment with chondroitin sulfate. *Arzneimittelforschung Drug Res* 45: 918–925, 1995.

21. Hungerford, DS. Treating osteoarthritis with chondroprotective agents. *Orthopedic Special Edition* 4(1): 39–42, 1998.

22. Busci L and Poór G. Efficacy and tolerability of oral chondroitin sulfate as a symptomatic slow-acting drug for osteoarthritis (SYSADOA) in the treatment of knee osteoarthritis. *Osteoarthritis and Cartilage* 6(Suppl. A): 31–36, 1998.

23. Bourgeois R, Chales G, Dehais J, et al. Efficacy and tolerability of CS 1,200 mg/day versus CS 3x400 mg/day versus placebo. *Osteoarthritis and Cartilage* 6(Suppl. A): 25–30, 1998.

24. Uebelhart D, et al. Effects of oral chondroitin sulfate on the progression of knee osteoarthritis: a pilot study. *Osteoarthritis Cartilage* 6(Suppl. A): 39–46, 1998.

25. Verbruggen G, Goemaere S, and Veys EM. Chondroitin sulfate: S/DMOAD (structure/disease modifying anti-osteoarthritis drug) in the treatment of finger joint OA. *Osteoarthritis Cartilage* 6(Suppl. A): 37–38, 1998.

26. Uebelhart D, et al. Protective effect of exogenous chondroitin 4,6-sulfate in the acute degradation of articular cartilage in the rabbit. *Osteoarthritis Cartilage* 6(Suppl. A): 6–13, 1998.

27. di Padova C. S-adenosylmethionine in the treatment of osteoarthritis: Review of the clinical studies. *Am J Med* 83(Suppl. 5A): 60–65, 1989.

28. Caruso I and Peitrogrande V. Italian double-blind multicenter study comparing S-adenosylmethionine, naproxen, and placebo in the treatment of degenerative joint disease. *Am J Med* 83(Suppl. 5A): 66–71, 1987.

29. Kalbhen DA, et al. Pharmakologische Untersuchungen zur antidegenerativen Wirkung von Ademetionin bei der tierexperimentellen Arthrose. *Arzneimittelforschung* 40(9): 1017–1021.

30. Barcelo HA, et al. Experimental osteoarthritis and its course when treated with S-adenyl-L-methionine. *Rev Clin Esp* 187(2): 74–78, 1990.

31. Cozens DD, et al. Reproductive toxicity studies of ademetionine. *Arzneimittelforschung* 38(11): 1625–1629, 1988.

32. Berger R, et al. A new medical approach to the treatment of osteoarthritis: Report of an open phase IV study with ademethionine (Gumbaral). *Am J Med* 83(Suppl 5A): 84–88, 1987.

33. Konig B. A long-term (two years) clinical trial with S-adenosylmethionine for the treatment of osteoarthritis. *Am J Med* 83(Suppl. 5A): 89–94, 1987.

34. Caruso I and Peitrogrande V. Italian double-blind multicenter study comparing S-adenosylmethionine, naproxen, and placebo in the treatment of degenerative joint disease. *Am J Med* 83(Suppl. 5A): 66–71, 1987.

35. di Padova C. S-adenosylmethionine in the treatment of osteoarthritis: Review of the clinical studies. *Am J Med* 83(Suppl. 5A): 60–65, 1989.

36. Carney MWP, et al. Switch and S-adenosylmethionine. *Ala J Med Sci* 25(3): 316–319, 1988.

37. Carney MWP, et al. The switch mechanism and the bipolar/unipolar dichotomy. *Br J Psych* 154: 48–51, 1989.

38. Reicks M, et al. Effects of methionine and other sulfur compounds on drug conjugations. *Pharmacol Ther* 37: 67–79, 1988.

39. Iruela LM, et al. Toxic interaction of S-adenosylmethionine and clomipramine. *Am J Psych* 150: 522, 1993.

40. Jonas WB, Rapoza CP, and Blair WF. The effect of niacinamide on osteoarthritis: a pilot study. *Inflamm Res* 45: 330–334, 1996.

41. ESCOP monographs. Fascicule 2: *Harpagophyti radix* (devil's claw). Exeter, UK: European Scientific Cooperative on Phytotherapy, 1997: 4.

42. ESCOP monographs. Fascicule 2: *Harpagophyti radix* (devil's claw). Exeter, UK: European Scientific Cooperative on Phytotherapy, 1997: 1–2.

43. ESCOP monographs. Fascicule 2: *Harpagophyti radix* (devil's claw). Exeter, UK: European Scientific Cooperative on Phytotherapy, 1997: 1–2.

44. McAlindon TE, et al. Do antioxidant micronutrients protect against the development and progression of knee OA? *Arth Rheum* 39: 648–656, 1996.

## Osteoporosis

1. Reid IR. The roles of calcium and vitamin D in the prevention of osteoporosis. *Endocrinol Metab Clin North Am* 27: 389–398, 1998.

2. Cumming RG. Calcium intake and bone mass: A qualitative review of the evidence. *Calcif Tissue Int* 47: 194–201, 1990.

3. Dawson-Hughes B, Dallal GE, Krall EA, et al. A controlled trial of the effect of calcium supplementation on bone density in postmenopausal women. *N Engl J Med* 323(13): 878–883, 1990.

4. Prince R. Diet and the prevention of osteoporotic fractures. *N Engl J Med* 337(10): 701–702, 1997.

5. Nieves JW, et al. Calcium potentiates the effect of estrogen and calcitonin on bone mass: review and analysis. *Am J Clin Nutr* 67(1): 18–24, 1998.

6. Aloia JF, et al. Calcium supplementation with and without hormone replacement therapy to prevent postmenopausal bone loss. *Annals Intern Med* 120: 97–103, 1994.

7. Lloyd T, Andon MB, and Rollings N. Calcium supplementation and bone mineral density in adolescent girls. *JAMA* 270(7): 841–844, 1993.

8. Saltman PD, et al. The role of trace minerals in osteoporosis. *J Am Coll Nutr* 12(4): 384–389, 1993.

9. Strause L, et al. Spinal bone loss in postmenopausal women supplemented with calcium and trace minerals. *J Nutr* 124: 1060–1064, 1994.

10. Kruger MC, et al. Calcium, gamma-linolenic acid (GLA) and eicosapentaenoic acid (EPA) supplementation in osteoporosis. *Osteoporosis Int* 6(Suppl. 1): 250, 1996.

11. van Papendorp DH, Coetzer H, and Kruger MC. Biochemical profile of osteoporotic patients on essential fatty acid supplementation. *Nutr Res* 15(3): 325–334, 1995.

12. NIH Consensus Development Panel on Optimal Calcium Intake. *Nutrition* 11: 409–417, 1994.

13. Curhan GC, Willett WC, Speizer FE, et al. Comparison of dietary calcium with supplemental calcium and other nutrients as factors affecting the risk for kidney stones in women. *Ann Intern Med* 126: 497–504, 1997.

14. Curhan GC, Willett WC, Rimm EB, et al. A prospective study of dietary calcium and other nutrients and the risk of symptomatic kidney stones. *N Engl J Med* 328: 833–838, 1993.

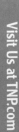

15. Agnusdei D, et al. A double-blind placebo-controlled trial of ipriflavone for prevention of postmenopausal spinal bone loss. *Calcif Tissue Int* 61: 142–147, 1997.

16. Genari C, Adami S, Agusei L, et al. Effect of chronic treatment with ipriflavone in postmenopausal women with low bone mass. *Calcif Tissue Int* 61: S19–S22, 1997.

17. Valente M, Bufalino L, et al. Effects of 1-year treatment with ipriflavone on bone in postmenopausal women with low bone mass. *Calcif Tissue Int* 54: 377–380, 1994.

18. Kovacs AB. Efficacy of ipriflavone in the prevention and treatment of postmenopausal osteoporosis. *Agents Actions* 41: 86–87, 1994.

19. Adami S, et al. Ipriflavone prevents radial bone loss in postmenopausal women with low bone mass over 2 years. *Osteoporos Int* 7(2): 119–125, 1997.

20. Agnusdei D, et al. Efficacy of ipriflavone in established osteoporosis and long-term safety. *Calcif Tissue Int* 61(1): S23–S27, 1997.

21. Agnusdei D, et al. A double-blind placebo-controlled trial of ipriflavone for prevention of postmenopausal spinal bone loss. *Calcif Tissue Int* 61: 142–147, 1997.

22. Agnusdei D, et al. Effects of ipriflavone on bone mass and bone remodeling in patients with established postmenopausal osteoporosis. *Curr Ther Res* 51(1): 82–91, 1992.

23. Gambacciani M, Cappagli B, Piaggesi M, et al. Ipriflavone prevents the loss of bone mass in pharmacological menopause produced by GnRH-agonists. *Calcif Tissue Int* 61: S15–S18, 1997.

24. Melis GB and Paoletti AM. Ipriflavone and low doses of estrogens in the prevention of bone mineral loss in climacterium. *Bone Mineral* 19: S49–S56, 1992.

25. Nozaki M, Hashimoto K, et al. Treatment of bone loss in oophorectomized women with a combination of ipriflavone and conjugated equine estrogen. *Int J Gyn Ob* 62: 69–75, 1998.

26. Agnusdei D and Bufalino L. Efficacy of ipriflavone in established osteoporosis and long-term safety. *Calcif Tissue Int* 61: S23–S27, 1997.

27. Melis G, Paoletti A, and Cagnacci A. Lack of any estrogenic effect of ipriflavone in postmenopausal women. *J Endrocrinol Invest* 15: 755–761, 1992.

28. Feskanich D, Weber P, Willett WC, et al. Vitamin K intake and hip fractures in women: a prospective study. *Am J Clin Nutr* 69: 74–79, 1999.

29. Kanai T, Takagi T, Masuhiro K, et al. Serum vitamin K level and bone mineral density in post-menopausal women. *Int J Gynecol Obstet* 56: 25–30, 1997.

30. Hart JP. Electrochemical detection of depressed circulating levels of vitamin K in osteoporosis. *J Clin Endocrinol Metab* 60: 1268–1269, 1985.

31. Hart JP, et al. Circulation vitamin K levels in patients with fractures. *J Bone Joint Surg* 70-B: 663, 1998.

32. Hodges SJ, Pilkington MJ, Stamp TCB, et al. Depressed levels of circulating menaquinones in patients with osteoporotic fractures of the spine and femoral neck. *Bone* 12: 387–389, 1991.

33. Jie K-SG, et al. Effects of vitamin K and oral anticoagulants on urinary calcium excretion. *Br J Haematol* 83: 100–104, 1993.

34. Knapen MHJ, et al. The effect of vitamin K supplementation on circulating osteocalcin (bone Gla protein) and urinary calcium excretion. *Ann Intern Med* 111: 1001–1005, 1989.

35. Tomita A. Postmenopausal osteoporosis 47 Ca study with vitamin $K_2$. *Clin Endocrinol* (Jpn) 19: 731–736, 1971.

36. Orimo H, Shiraki M, Fujita T, et al. Clinical evaluation of menatetrenone in the treatment of involutional osteoporosis—a double-blind multicenter comparative study with 1a hydroxy vitamin $D_3$. *J Bone Miner Res*(Suppl. 1) 7: S122, 1992.

37. Nielsen FH, et al. Effect of dietary boron on mineral, estrogen and testosterone metabolism in postmenopausal women. *FASEB J* 1: 394–397, 1987.

38. Naghii MR and Samman S. The effect of boron supplementation on its urinary excretion and selected cardiovascular risk factors in healthy male subjects. *Biol Trace Elem Res* 56(3): 273–286, 1997.

39. Nielsen FH, et al. Effect of dietary boron on mineral, estrogen and testosterone metabolism in postmenopausal women. *FASEB J* 1: 394–397, 1987.

40. Prior JC. Progesterone as a bone-trophic hormone. *Endocr Rev* 1: 386–398, 1986.

41. Leonetti HB, et al. Transdermal progesterone cream for vasomotor symptoms and postmenopausal bone loss. *Obstet Gynecol* 94: 225–228, 1999.

## Periodontal Disease

1. Hanoika T, et al. Effect of topical application of coenzyme $Q_{10}$ on adult periodontitis. *Mol Aspects Med* 15(Suppl.): S241–S248, 1994.

2. Iwamoto Y, Watanabe T, Okamoto H, et al. Clinical effect of coenzyme $Q_{10}$ on periodontal disease. As cited in Folkers K, Yamamura Y, eds. Biomedical & clinical aspects of coenzyme $Q_{10}$, Vol. 3. Amsterdam: Elsevier/North-Holland Biomedical Press, 1981: 109–119.

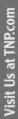

3. Folkers K and Yamamura Y. Biomedical and clinical aspects of coenzyme Q$_{10}$, Vol. 1. Amsterdam: Elsevier/North-Holland Biomedical Press, 1977: 294–311.

4. Wilkinson EG, Arnold RM, and Folkers K. Treatment of periodontal and other soft tissue diseases of the oral cavity with coenzyme Q$_{10}$. As cited in Folkers K, Yamamura Y, eds. Biomedical & clinical aspects of coenzyme Q$_{10}$, Vol. 1. Amsterdam: Elsevier/North-Holland Biomedical Press, 1977.

5. Wilkinson EG, Arnold RM, and Folkers K. Bioenergetics and clinical medicine. VI. Adjunctive treatment of periodontal disease with coenzyme Q$_{10}$. *Res Commun Chem Pathol Pharmacol* 14(4): 715–719, 1976.

6. Littarru G, et al. Deficiency of coenzyme Q$_{10}$ in gingival tissue from patients with periodontal disease. *Proc Natl Acad Sci USA* 68(10): 2332–2335, 1971.

7. Iwamoto Y, Watanabe T, Okamoto H, et al. Clinical effect of coenzyme Q$_{10}$ on periodontal disease. As cited in Folkers K, Yamamura Y, eds. Biomedical & clinical aspects of coenzyme Q$_{10}$, Vol. 3. Amsterdam: Elsevier/North-Holland Biomedical Press, 1981: 109–119.

8. Pack ARC. Folate mouthwash: Effects on established gingivitis in periodontal patients. *J Clin Periodontol* 11: 619–628, 1984.

9. Thomson ME and Pack ARC. Effects of extended systemic and topical folate supplementation on gingivitis of pregnancy. *J Clin Periodontol* 9(3): 275–280, 1982.

10. Pack ARC and Thomson ME. Effects of topical and systemic folic acid supplementation on gingivitis in pregnancy. *J Clin Periodontol* 7(5): 402–414, 1980.

11. Vogel RI, et al. The effect of topical application of folic acid on gingival health. *J Oral Med* 33(1): 20–22, 1978.

## PMS

1. Thys-Jacobs S, et al. Calcium carbonate and the premenstrual syndrome: Effects on premenstrual and menstrual symptoms. *Am J Ob Gyn* 179(2): 444–452, 1998.

2. Alvir JM and Thys-Jacobs S. Premenstrual and menstrual symptom clusters and response to calcium treatment. *Psychopharmacol Bull* 27(2): 145–148, 1991.

3. Thys-Jacobs S, Ceccarelli S, Bierman A, et al. Calcium supplementation in premenstrual syndrome: A randomized crossover trial. *J Gen Intern Med* 4(3): 183–189, 1989.

4. Milewicz A, et al. *Vitex agnus-castus* extract in the treatment of luteal phase defects due to latent hyperprolactinemia. Results of a randomized placebo-controlled double-blind study. *Arzneimittelforschung* 43(7): 752–756, 1993.

5. Jarry H, et al. In vitro prolactin but not LH and FSH release is inhibited by compounds in extracts of *Agnus-castus*: direct evidence for a dopaminergic principle by the dopamine receptor assay. *EYP Clin Endocrinol* 102: 448–454, 1994.

6. Sliutz G, et al. *Agnus-castus* extracts inhibit prolactin secretion of rat pituitary cells. *Horm Metab Res* 25(5): 253–255, 1993.

7. Schulz V, et al. Rational phytotherapy. New York: Springer-Verlag, 1998: 241–242.

8. Dittmar FW, et al. Premenstrual syndrome: Treatment with a phytopharmaceutical. *Therapiewoche Gynakol* 5: 60–68, 1992.

9. Peteres-Welte C, et al. Menstrual abnormalities and PMS: *Vitex agnus-castus*. *Therapiewoche Gynakol* 7: 49–52, 1994.

10. Coeugniet E, et al. Premenstrual syndrome (PMS) and its treatment. *Arztezeitschr Naturheilverf* 27: 619–622, 1986.

11. Lauritzen C, et al. Treatment of premenstrual tension syndrome with *Vitex agnus-castus*. Controlled, double-blind study vs. pyridoxine. *Phytomedicine* 4(3): 183–189, 1997.

12. Lauritzen C, et al. Treatment of premenstrual tension syndrome with *Vitex agnus-castus*. Controlled, double-blind study vs. pyridoxine. *Phytomedicine* 4(3): 183–189, 1997.

13. Schulz V, et al. Rational phytotherapy. New York: Springer-Verlag, 1998: 243.

14. Cahill DJ, et al. Multiple follicular development associated with herbal medicine. *Hum Reprod* 9(8): 1469–1470, 1994.

15. Propping D, et al. *Agnus-castus*: treatment of gynaecological syndromes. *Therapeutikon* 5(110): 581–585, 1991.

16. Diegoli MS, et al. A double-blind trial of four medications to treat severe premenstrual syndrome. *Int J Gynaecol Obstet* 62: 63–67, 1998.

17. Kleijnen J, Ter Riet G, and Knipschild P. Vitamin B$_6$ in the treatment of premenstrual syndrome—a review. *Br J Obstet Gynaecol* 97(9): 847–852, 1990.

18. London RS, et al. Efficacy of alpha-tocopherol in the treatment of the premenstrual syndrome. *J Reprod Med* 32(6): 400–404, 1987.

19. Facchinetti F, Bolrella P, Sances G, et al. Oral magnesium successfully relieves premenstrual mood changes. *Obstet Gynecol* 78(2): 177–181, 1991.

20. Facchinetti F, et al. Magnesium prophylaxis of menstrual migraine: effects on intracellular magnesium. *Headache* 31: 298–304, 1991.

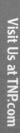

21. London RS, Bradley L, and Chiamori NY. Effect of a nutritional supplement on premenstrual symptomatology in women with premenstrual syndrome: a double-blind longitudinal study. *J Am Coll Nutr* 10(5): 494–499, 1991.

22. Reynolds MA and London RS. Efficacy of a multivitamin/mineral supplement in the treatment of the premenstrual syndrome (Abstract). *J Am Coll Nutr* 7(5): 416, 1988.

23. Stewart A. Clinical and biochemical effects of nutritional supplementation on the premenstrual syndrome. *J Reprod Med* 32(6): 435–441, 1987.

24. Chakmakjian ZH, Higgins CE, and Abraham GE. The effect of a nutritional supplement, Optivite for Women, on premenstrual tension syndromes: II. Effect on symptomatology, using a double-blind, cross-over design. *J Appl Nutr* 37(1): 12–17, 1985.

25. Puolakka J, et al. Biochemical and clinical effects of treating the premenstrual syndrome with prostaglandin synthesis precursors. *J Reprod Med* 30: 149–153, 1985.

26. Dittmar FW, et al. Premenstrual syndrome: Treatment with a phytopharmaceutical. *Therapiewoche Gynakol* 5: 60–68, 1992.

## Psoriasis

1. Bittiner SB, et al. A double-blind, randomised, placebo-controlled trial of fish oil in psoriasis. *Lancet* i: 378–380, 1988.

2. Soyland E, Funk J, Rajka G, et al. Effect of dietary supplementation with very-long-chain n-3 fatty acids in patients with psoriasis. *N Engl J Med* 328: 1812–1816, 1993.

3. Harris WS. Dietary fish oil and blood lipids. *Curr Opin Lipidol* 7: 3–7, 1996.

4. Harris WS. Fish oils and plasma lipid and lipoprotein metabolism in humans: a critical review. *J Lipid Res* 30: 785–807, 1989.

5. Harris WS. N-3 fatty acids and serum lipoproteins: human studies. *Am J Clin Nutr* 65(Suppl.): 1645S–1654S, 1997.

6. Cobiac L, Clifton PM, and Abbey M. Lipid, lipoprotein, and hemostatic effects of fish vs fish-oil n-3 fatty acids in mildly hyperlipidemic males. *Am J Clin Nutr* 53: 1210–1216, 1991.

7. Harris WS. N-3 fatty acids and serum lipoproteins: human studies. *Am J Clin Nutr* 65(Suppl.): 1645S–1654S, 1997.

8. Syed TA, Ahmad A, Holt AH, et al. Management of psoriasis with *Aloe vera* extract in a hydrophilic cream: a placebo-controlled, double-blind study. *Trop Med Internat Health* 1: 505–509, 1996.

## Raynaud's Phenomenon

1. Sunderland GT, Belch JJF, Sturrock RD, et al. A double-blind randomised placebo-controlled trial of Hexopal in primary Raynaud's disease. *Clin Rheumatol* 7(1): 46–49, 1988.

2. DiGiacomo RA, Kremer JM, and Shah DM. Fish-oil dietary supplementation in patients with Raynaud's phenomenon: a double-blind, controlled, prospective study. *Am J Med* 86: 158–164, 1989.

3. Ringer TV, et al. Fish oil blunts the pain response to cold pressor testing in normal males (Abstract). *J Am Coll Nutr* 8(5): 435, 1989.

4. Belch JJF, et al. Evening primrose oil (Efamol) as a treatment for cold-induced vasospasm (Raynaud's phenomenon). *Prog Lipid Res* 25: 335–340, 1986.

5. Belch JJF, et al. Evening primrose oil (Efamol) in the treatment of Raynaud's phenomenon: A double-blind study. *Thromb Haemost* 54(2): 490–494, 1985.

6. Jung F, et al. Effect of *Ginkgo biloba* on fluidity of blood and peripheral microcirculation in volunteers. *Arzneimittelforschung Drug Res* 40: 589–593, 1990.

## Rheumatoid Arthritis

1. James MJ, et al. Dietary n-3 fatty acids and therapy for rheumatoid arthritis. *Semin Arthritis Rheum* 27: 85–97, 1997.

2. Harris WS. Dietary fish oil and blood lipids. *Curr Opin Lipidol* 7: 3–7, 1996.

3. Harris WS. Fish oils and plasma lipid and lipoprotein metabolism in humans: a critical review. *J Lipid Res* 30: 785–807, 1989.

4. Cobiac L, Clifton PM, and Abbey M. Lipid, lipoprotein, and hemostatic effects of fish vs. fish-oil n-3 fatty acids in mildly hyperlipidemic males. *Am J Clin Nutr* 53: 1210–1216, 1991.

5. Harris WS. N-3 Fatty acids and serum lipoproteins: human studies. *Am J Clin Nutr* 65(Suppl.): 1645S–1654S, 1997.

6. Nordstrom DCE, et al. Alpha-linolenic acid in the treatment of rheumatoid arthritis. A double-blind placebo-controlled and randomized study: flaxseed vs. safflower oil. *Rheumatol Int* 14: 231–234, 1995.

7. Shapiro JA, Koepsell TD, Voight LF, et al. Diet and rheumatoid arthritis in women: a possible protective effect of fish consumption. *Epidemiology* 7: 256–263, 1996.

8. Singh GB and Atal CK. Pharmacology of an extract of salai guggal ex-*Boswellia serrata,* a new non-steroidal anti-inflammatory agent. *Agents Actions* 18: 407–412, 1986.

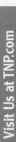

9. Wildfeuer A, Neu IS, Safayhi H, et al. Effects of boswellic acids extracted from an herbal medicine on the biosynthsis of leukotrienes and the course of experimental autoimmune encephalomyelitis. *Arzneimittelforschung* 48(6): 668–674, 1998.

10. Etzel R. Special extract of *Boswellia serrata* in the treatment of rheumatoid arthritis. *Phytomedicine* 3(1): 67–70, 1996.

11. Sander O, Herborn G, and Rau R. Is H15 (resin extract of *Boswellia serrata,* "incense") a useful supplement to established drug therapy of chronic polyarthritis? Results of a double-blind pilot study. English abstract only. *Z Rheumatol* 57(1): 11–16, 1998.

12. ESCOP monographs. Fascicule 2: *Harpagophyti radix* (devil's claw). Exeter, UK: European Scientific Cooperative on Phytotherapy, 1997: 5.

13. ESCOP monographs. Fascicule 2: *Harpagophyti radix* (devil's claw). Exeter, UK: European Scientific Cooperative on Phytotherapy, 1997: 4

14. ESCOP monographs. Fascicule 2: *Harpagophyti radix* (devil's claw). Exeter, UK: European Scientific Cooperative on Phytotherapy, 1997: 5.

15. ESCOP monographs. Fascicule 2: *Harpagophyti radix* (devil's claw). Exeter, UK: European Scientific Cooperative on Phytotherapy, 1997: 4.

16. Satoskar RR, et al. Evaluation of anti-inflammatory property of curcumin diferuloyl methane. *Ind J Med Res* 71: 632–634, 1980.

17. Deodhar SD, et al. Preliminary studies on antirheumatic activity of curcumin. *Ind J Med Res* 71: 632–634, 1980.

18. Schulz V, et al. Rational phytotherapy. New York: Springer-Verlag, 1998: 263.

19. Ammon HPT, et al. Pharmacology of *Curcuma longa. Planta Medica* 57: 1–7, 1991.

20. Bingham R, et al. Yucca plant saponin in the management of arthritis. *J Appl Nutr* 27: 45–50, 1975.

21. Zurier RB, Rossetti RG, Jacobson EW, et al. Gamma-linolenic acid treatment of rheumatoid arthritis. A randomized, placebo-controlled trial. *Arthritis Rheum* 39: 1808–1817, 1996.

22. Leventhal LJ, Boyce EG, and Zurier RB. Treatment of rheumatoid arthritis with black currant seed oil. *Br J Rheumatol* 33: 847–852, 1994.

23. Leventhal LJ, Boyce EG, and Zurier RB. Treatment of rheumatoid arthritis with gamma linolenic acid. *Ann Intern Med* 119: 867–873, 1993.

24. Rothman D, et al. Botanical lipids: Effects on inflammation, immune responses and rheumatoid arthritis. *Semin Arthritis Rheum* 25: 87–96, 1995.

25. Peretz A, et al. Zinc distribution in blood components, inflammatory status, and clinical indexes of disease activity during zinc supplementation in inflammatory rheumatic diseases. *Am J Clin Nutr* 57: 690–694, 1993.

26. Rasker JJ and Kardaun SH. Lack of beneficial effect of zinc sulphate in rheumatoid arthritis. *Scand J Rheumatol* 11: 168–170, 1982.

27. Simkin PA. Treatment of rheumatoid arthritis with oral zinc sulfate. *Agents Actions* 8(Suppl.): 587–596, 1981.

28. Tarp U. Selenium in rheumatoid arthritis. A review. *Analyst* 120: 877–881, 1995.

29. Darlington LG and Ramsey NW. Review of dietary therapy for rheumatoid arthritis. *Br J Rheumatol* 32(6): 507–514, 1993.

30. Kjeldsen-Kragh J. Controlled trial of fasting and one-year vegetarian diet in rheumatoid arthritis. *Lancet* 338(8772): 899–902, 1991.

31. Nenonen M, et al. Effects of uncooked vegan food "living food" on rheumatoid arthritis, a three-month controlled and randomised study (Abstract). *Am J Clin Nutr* 56: 762, 1992.

## Ulcers

1. Kassir ZA. Endoscopic controlled trial of four drug regimens in the treatment of chronic duodenal ulceration. *Irish Med J* 78: 153–156, 1985.

2. Morgan AG, et al. Comparison between cimetidine and Caved-S in the treatment of gastric ulceration and subsequent maintenance therapy. *Gut* 23: 545–551, 1982.

3. Morgan AG, et al. Maintenance therapy: A two-year comparison between Caved-S and cimetidine treatment in the prevention of symptomatic gastric ulcer. *Gut* 26: 599–602, 1985.

4. Murray M and Pizzorno J. Encyclopedia of natural medicine, 2nd ed. Rocklin, CA: Prima Publishing, 1997: 815.

5. Murray M and Pizzorno J. Encyclopedia of natural medicine, 2nd ed. Rocklin, CA: Prima Publishing, 1997: 816.

6. Beil W, et al. Effects of flavonoids on parietal cell acid secretion, gastric mucosal prostaglandin production and *Helicobacter pylori* growth. *Arzneimittelforschung Drug Res* 45: 697–700, 1995.

## Varicose Veins

1. Schulz V, et al. Rational phytotherapy. New York: Springer-Verlag, 1998: 131–134.

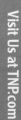

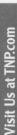

2. Neiss A, et al. Zum Wirksamkeitsnachweis von Rosskastaniensamenextrakt beim varikosen Symptomenkomplex. *Munch Med Wochenschr* 7: 213–216, 1976.

3. Diehm C, et al. Comparison of leg compression stocking and oral horse-chestnut seed extract therapy in patients with chronic venous insufficiency. *Lancet* 347: 292–294, 1996.

4. Kreysel HW, et al. A possible role of lysosomal enzymes in the pathogenesis of varicocosis and the reduction in their serum activity by Venostatin. *Vasa* 12: 377–382, 1983.

5. Bougelet C. Effect of aescine on hypoxia-induced neutrophil adherence to umbilical vein endothelium. *Eur J Pharmacol* 345(1): 89–95, 1998.

6. Schulz V, et al. Rational phytotherapy. New York: Springer-Verlag, 1998: 131.

7. Newall C, et al. Herbal medicines: a guide for healthcare professionals. London: Pharmaceutical Press, 1996: 166–167.

8. Grasso A and Corvaglia E. Two cases of suspected oxic tubulonephrosis due to escine. *Gazz Med Ital* 335: 581–584, 1976.

9. Schulz V, et al. Rational phytotherapy. New York: Springer-Verlag, 1998: 132.

10. Schwitters B, et al. OPC in practice: Bioflavanols and their applications. Rome: Alfa Omega, 1993.

11. Masquelier J, et al. Stabilization of collagen by procyanidolic oligomers. *Acta Ther* 7: 101–105, 1981.

12. Masquelier J. Procyanidolic oligomers. *J Parums Cosm Arom* 95: 89–97, 1990.

13. Tixier JM, et al. Evidence by in vivo and in vitro studies that binding of pycnogenols to elastin affects its rate of degradation by elastases. *Biochem Pharmacol* 33: 3933–3939, 1984.

14. Bombardelli E, et al. *Vitis vinifera* L. *Fitoterapia* 66: 291–317, 1995.

15. Henriet JP. Exemplary study for a phlebotropic substance, the EIVE study. On file with Primary Services International, Southport, CT.

16. Delacroix P, et al. Double-blind study of endotelon in chronic venous insufficiency. *La Revue de Medicine* 31: 27–28, 1793–1802, 1981.

17. Bombardelli E, et al. *Vitis vinifera* L. *Fitoterapia* 66: 291–317, 1995.

18. Schulz V, et al., Rational phytotherapy. New York: Springer-Verlag, 1998: 283.

19. Kartnig T. Clinical applications of *Centella asiatica* (L.) Urb. *Herbs Spices Med Plants* 3: 146–173, 1988.

20. Castellani C, et al. The *Centella asiatica. Boll Chim Farm* 120: 570–605, 1981.

21. Belcaro GV, et al. Capillary filtration and ankle edema in patients with venous hypertension treated with TTFCA. *Angiology* 41: 12–18, 1990.

22. Cesarone MR, et al. The microcirculatory activity of *Centella asiatica* in venous insufficiency: A double-blind study. *Minerva Cardioangiol* 42: 299–304, 1994.

23. Pointel JP, et al. Titrated extract of *Centella asiatica* (TECA) in the treatment of venous insufficiency of the lower limbs. *Angiology* 38: 46–50, 1987.

24. Cesarone MR, et al. Activity of *Centella asiatica* in venous insufficiency. *Minerva Cardioangiol* 42: 137–143, 1992.

25. Kartnig T. Clinical applications of *Centella asiatica* (L.) Urb. *Herbs Spices Med Plants* 3: 146–173, 1988.

26. Nalini K, et al. Effect of *Centella asiatica* fresh leaf aqueous extract on learning and memory and biogenic amine turnover in albino rats. *Fitoterapia* 63(3): 232–237, 1992.

27. Bosse JP, et al. Clinical study of a new antikeloid drug. *Ann Plast Surg* 3: 13–21, 1979.

28. Basellini A, et al. Varicose disease in pregnancy. *Ann Obstet Gyn Med Perinat* 106: 337–341, 1985.

29. Bone K. *Mediherb Professional Review* 59: 3, 1997.

30. Bone K. *Mediherb Professional Review* 59: 3, 1997.

31. Gabor M. Pharmacologic effects of flavonoids on blood vessels. *Angiologica* 9: 355–374, 1972.

32. Mian E, et al. Anthocyanosides and the walls of microvessels: Further aspects of the mechanism of action of their protective effect in syndromes due to abnormal capillary fragility. *Minerva Med* 68: 3565–3581, 1977.

33. Havsteen B. Flavonoids, a class of natural products of high pharmacological potency. *Biochem Pharmacol* 32: 1141–1148, 1983.

34. Lietti A, et al. Studies on *Vaccinium myrtillus* anthocyanosides. I. Vasoprotective and anti-inflammatory activity. *Arzneimittelforschung* 26: 829–832, 1976.

35. Eandi M. Unpublished results. As cited in Morazzoni P, et al. eds. *Vaccinium myrtillus. Fitoterapia* 67(1): 3–29, 1996.

36. Petruzezellis V, et al. Therapeutic action of oral doses of mesoglycan in the pharmacological treatment of varicose syndrome and its complications. *Minerva Med* 76: 543–548, 1985.

37. Sangrigoli V. Mesoglycan in acute and chronic venous insufficiency of the legs. *Clin Ther* 129(3): 207–209, 1989.

38. Oddone G, et al. Assessment of the effects of oral mesoglycan sulphate in patients with chronic venous

pathology of the lower extremities. *Gazzetta Medica Italiana* 146: 111–114, 1987.

## Acidophilus and Other Probiotics

1. Elmer GW, et al. Biotherapeutic agents. *JAMA* 275 (111): 870–876, 1996.

2. Halpern GM, et al. Treatment of irritable bowel syndrome with lacteol fort: a randomized, double-blind, cross-over trial. *Am J Gastroenterol* 91: 1579–1585, 1996.

3. Scarpignato C, et al. Prevention and treatment of traveler's diarrhea: a clinical pharmacological approach. *Chemotherapy* 41: 48–81, 1995.

4. Shornikova AV, Casas IA, Mykkanen H, et al. Bacteriotherapy with *Lactobacillus reuteri* in rotavirus gastroenteritis. *Pediatr Infect Dis J* 12: 1103–1107, 1997.

5. Shornikova AV, Casas IA, Isolauri E, et al. *Lactobacillus reuteri* as a therapeutic agent in acute diarrhea in young children. *J Pediatr Gastroenterol Nutr* 24(4): 399–404, 1997.

6. Elmer GW, et al. Biotherapeutic agents. *JAMA* 275 (111): 870–876, 1996.

7. Halpern GM, et al. Treatment of irritable bowel syndrome with lacteol fort: a randomized, double-blind, cross-over trial. *Am J Gastroenterol* 91: 1579–1585, 1996.

8. Scarpignato C, et al. Prevention and treatment of traveler's diarrhea: a clinical pharmacological approach. *Chemotherapy* 41: 48–81, 1995.

9. Shornikova AV, Casas IA, Mykkanen H, et al. Bacteriotherapy with *Lactobacillus reuteri* in rotavirus gastroenteritis. *Pediatr Infect Dis J* 12: 1103–1107, 1997.

10. Shornikova AV, Casas IA, Isolauri E, et al. *Lactobacillus reuteri* as a therapeutic agent in acute diarrhea in young children. *J Pediatr Gastroenterol Nutr* 24(4): 399–404, 1997.

## Aloe

1. Marshall HM. *Aloe vera* gel: What is the evidence? *Pharmacol J* 244: 360–362, 1990.

2. Chithra, P, et al. Influence of *Aloe vera* on collagen characteristics in healing dermal wounds in rats. *Mol Cell Biochem* 181(1&2) 71–76, 1998.

3. Schmidt JM, et al. *Aloe vera* dermal wound gel is associated with a delay in wound healing. *Obstet Gynecol* 78: 115–117, 1991.

4. Hart LA, et al. Effects of low molecular weight constituents from *Aloe vera* gel on oxidative metabolism and cytotoxic and bactericidal activities of human neutrophils. *Int J Immunol Pharmacol* 12: 427–434, 1990.

5. Sheets MA, et al. Studies of the effect of acemannan on retrovirus infections: Clinical stabilization of feline leukemia virus-infected cats. *Mol Biother* 3: 41–45, 1991.

6. Kemp MC, et al. In-vitro evaluation of the antiviral effects of acemannan on the replication and pathogenesis of HIV-1 and other enveloped viruses: Modification of the processing of glycoprotein precursors. *Antiviral Res* 13(Suppl. 1): 83, 1990.

7. Syed TA, Ahmad A, Holt AH, et al. Management of psoriasis with *Aloe vera* extract in a hydrophilic cream: a placebo-controlled, double-blind study. *Trop Med Internat Health* 1: 505–509, 1996.

8. Davis RH, et al. *Aloe vera* as a biologically active vehicle for hydrocortisone acetate. *J Am Pod Med Assoc* 81(1): 1–9, 1991.

## Andrographis

1. Hancke J, et al. A double-blind study with a new monodrug Kan Jang: Decrease of symptoms and improvements in the recovery from common colds. *Phytotherapy Res* 9: 559–562, 1995.

2. Melchior J, et al. Controlled clinical study of standardized *Andrographis paniculata* extract in common cold: A pilot trial. *Phytomedicine* 34: 314–318, 1996–1997.

3. Hancke J, et al. A double-blind study with a new monodrug Kan Jang: Decrease of symptoms and improvements in the recovery from common colds. *Phytotherapy Res* 9: 559–562, 1995.

4. Thamlikitkul V, et al. Efficacy of *Andrographis paniculata* (Nees) for pharyngotonsillitis in adults. *J Med Assoc Thai* 74(10): 437–442, 1991.

5. Hancke J, et al. A double-blind study with a new monodrug Kan Jang: Decrease of symptoms and improvements in the recovery from common colds. *Phytotherapy Res* 9: 559–562, 1995.

6. Akbarsha MA, et al. Antifertility effect of *Andrographis paniculata* (Nees) in male albino rat. *Indian J Exp Biol* 28(5): 421–426, 1990.

7. Burgos RA, et al. Testicular toxicity assessment of *Andrographis paniculata* dried extract in rats. *J Ethnopharmacol* 58(3): 219–224, 1997.

8. Zoha MS, et al. Antifertility effect of *Andrographis paniculata* in mice. *Bangladesh Med Res Counc Bull* 15(1): 34–37, 1989.

## Androstenedione

1. Yesalis CE, ed. Anabolic steroids in sport and exercise. Champaign, IL: Human Kinetics, 1993.

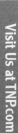

## Aortic Glycosaminoglycans

1. Laurora G, Cesarone MR, Belcaro G, et al. Control of the progress of arteriosclerosis in high risk subjects treated with mesoglycan. Measuring the intima media. *Minerva Cardioangiol* 46: 41–47, 1998.

2. Laurora G, Cesarone MR, De Sanctis MT, et al. Delayed arteriosclerosis progression in high risk subjects treated with mesoglycan. Evaluation of intima-media thickness. *J Cardiovasc Surg* (Torino) 34(4): 313–318, 1993.

3. Petruzzellis V and Velon A. Therapeutic action of oral mesoglycan in the pharmacologic treatment of the varicose syndrome and its complications. English abstract only. *Minerva Med* 76(12): 543–548, 1985.

4. Agrati AM, De Bartolo G and Palmieri G. Heparan sulfate: Efficacy and safety in patients with chronic venous insufficiency. English abstract only. *Minerva Cardioangiol* 39(10): 395–400, 1991.

5. Saggioro A, Chiozzini G, Pallini P, et al. Treatment of hemorrhoidal crisis with mesoglycan sulfate. English abstract only. *Minerva Dietol Gastroenterol* 31(2): 311–315, 1985.

6. Prandoni P, Cattelan AM, and Carta M. Long-term sequelae of deep venous thrombosis of the legs. *Ann Ital Med Int* 4: 378–385, 1989.

7. Laurora G, Cesarone MR, Belcaro G, et al. Control of the progress of arteriosclerosis in high risk subjects treated with mesoglycan. Measuring the intima media. *Minerva Cardioangiol* 46: 41–47, 1998.

8. Tanganelli P, Bianciardi G, Carducci A, et al. Updating on in-vivo and in-vitro effects of heparin and other glycosaminoglycans (mesoglycan) on arterial endothelium: a morphometrical study. *Int J Tissue React* 14(3): 149–153, 1992.

9. Morrison LM and Enrick L. Coronary heart disease: Reduction of death rate by chondroitin sulfate A. *Angiology* 24(5): 269–287, 1973.

10. Nakazawa K and Murata K. The therapeutic effect of chondroitin polysulphate in elderly atherosclerotic patients. *J Int Med Res* 6(3): 217–225, 1978.

11. Saba P, Galeone F, Giuntoli F, et al. Hypolipidemic effect of mesoglycan in hyperlipidemic patients. *Curr Ther Res* 40:761–768, 1986.

12. Agrati AM, De Bartolo G, and Palmieri G. Heparan sulfate: Efficacy and safety in patients with chronic venous insufficiency. English abstract only. *Minerva Cardioangiol* 39(10): 395–400, 1991.

13. Saggioro A, Chiozzini G, Pallini P, et al. Treatment of hemorrhoidal crisis with mesoglycan sulfate. English abstract only. *Minerva Dietol Gastroenterol* 31(2): 311–315, 1985.

14. Petruzzellis V and Velon A. Therapeutic action of oral mesoglycan in the pharmacologic treatment of the varicose syndrome and its complications. English abstract only. *Minerva Med*) 76(12): 543–548, 1985.

15. Prandoni P, Cattelan AM, and Carta M. Long-term sequelae of deep venous thrombosis of the legs. *Ann Ital Med Int* 4: 378–385, 1989.

## Arginine

1. Baligan M, Giardina A, Giovannini G, et al. L-arginina e immunita. Studio in soggetti pediatrici. *Minerva Pediatr* 49: 537–542, 1997.

2. Maxwell A. Annual meeting of American College of Cardiology. 1999.

3. Rector TS, et al. Randomized, double-blind, placebo-controlled study of supplemental oral L-arginine in patients with heart failure. *Circulation* 93: 2135–2141, 1996.

4. Koifman B, et al. Improvement of cardiac performance by intravenous infusion of L-arginine in patients with moderate congestive heart failure. *J Am Coll Cardiol* 26: 1251–1256, 1995.

5. de Aloysio D, Mantuano R, Mauloni M, and Nicoletti G. The clinical use of arginine aspartate in male infertility. *Acta Eur Fertil* 13: 133–167, 1982.

6. Tanimura J. Studies on arginine in human semen. Part II. The effects of medication with L-arginine-HCl on male infertility. *Bull Osaka Med School* 13: 84–89, 1967.

7. Schacter A, Goldman JA, and Zukerman Z. Treatment of oligospermia with the amino acid arginine. *J Urol* 110: 311–313, 1973.

8. Schacter A, et al. Treatment of oligospermia with the amino acid arginine. *Int J Gynaecol Obstet* 11: 206–209, 1973.

9. Mroueh A. Effect of arginine on oligospermia. *Fertil Steril* 21: 217–219, 1970.

10. Pryor JP, Blandy JP, Evans P, Chaput de Saintonge DM, and Usherwood M. Controlled clinical trial of arginine for infertile men with oligozoospermia. *Brit J Urol* 50: 47–50, 1978.

11. Baligan M, Giardina A, Giovannini G, et al. L-arginina e immunita. Studio in soggetti pediatrici. *Minerva Pediatr* 49: 537–542, 1997.

12. Maxwell A. Annual meeting of American College of Cardiology, 1999.

## Ashwaganda

1. Devi PU, et al. In vivo growth inhibitory effect of *Withania somnifera* (ashwaganda) on a transplantable mouse tumour, Sarcoma 180. *Indian J Exp Biol* 30: 169–172, 1992.

2. Al-Hindawi MK, et al. Anti-granuloma activity of Iraqi *Withania somnifera*. *J Ethnopharmacol* 37: 113–116, 1992.

3. Kuppurajan K, et al. Effect of ashwaganda (*Withania somnifera* Dunal) on the process of aging in human volunteers. *J Res Ayurveda Siddha* 1: 247–258, 1980.

4. Bone, K. MediHerb Professional Newsletter No. 30 Warwick, Australia, 1998.

## Astragalus

1. Benksy D and Gamble A. Chinese herbal medicine: Materia medica. Seattle, WA: Eastland Press, 1986: 457–459.

2. Hou Y, et al. Effect of *Radix Astragali Seu Hedysari* on the interferon system. *Chin Med J* 94: 35–40, 1981.

3. Sun Y, et al. Immune restoration and/or augmentation of local graft versus host reaction by traditional Chinese medicinal herbs. *Cancer* 52: 70–73, 1983.

4. Benksy D and Gamble A. Chinese herbal medicine: Materia medica. Seattle, WA: Eastland Press, 1986: 457–459.

5. Liang R, et al. Clinical study on braincalming tablets in treating 450 cases of atherosclerosis. *J North Chin Med* 1: 63–65, 1985.

6. Xiao S, et al. Hyperthyroidism treated with yiqiyangyin decoction. *J Trad Chin Med* 6(2): 79–82, 1986.

7. Zhang ND, et al. Effects on blood pressure and inflammation of astragalus saponin 1, a principle isolated from *Astragalus membranaceus* Bge. *Acta Pharm Suec* 19(5): 333–337, 1984.

8. Zhang H, et al. Treatment of adult diabetes with jiangtangjia tablets. *J Trad Chin Med* 7(4): 37–39, 1986.

9. Zhou MX, et al. Therapeutic effect of astragalus in treating chronic active hepatitis and the changes in immune function. *J Chin People's Liberation Army* 7(4): 242–244, 1982.

10. Benksy D and Gamble A. Chinese herbal medicine: Materia medica. Seattle, WA: Eastland Press, 1986: 457–459.

## BCAAs (Branched-Chain Amino Acids)

1. Cangiano C, et al. Effects of administration of oral branched-chain amino acids on anorexia and caloric intake in cancer patients. *J Natl Cancer Inst* 88: 550–551, 1996.

2. Plaitakis A, Mandeli J, et al. Pilot trial of branched-chain amino acids in amyotrophic lateral sclerosis. *Lancet*: 1: 1015–1018, 1988.

3. Kelly GS. Sports nutrition: A review of selected nutritional supplements for bodybuilders and strength athletes. *Alt Med Rev* 2: 184–201, 1997.

4. MacLean DA, Graham TE, and Saltin B. Stimulation of muscle ammonia production during exercise following branched-chain amino acid supplementation in humans. *J Physiol* (Lond) 15: 493, 1996.

5. Mendell JR, et al. Clinical investigation in Duchenne muscular dystrophy: IV. Double-blind controlled trial of leucine. *Muscle Nerve* 7: 535–541, 1984.

6. Cangiano C, et al. Effects of administration of oral branched-chain amino acids on anorexia and caloric intake in cancer patients. *J Natl Cancer Inst* 88: 550–551, 1996.

7. Plaitakis A, Mandeli J, et al. Pilot trial of branched-chain amino acids in amyotrophic lateral sclerosis. *Lancet*: 1: 1015–1018, 1988.

8. Mendell JR, et al. Clinical investigation in Duchenne muscular dystrophy: IV. Double-blind controlled trial of leucine. *Muscle Nerve* 7: 535–541, 1984.

## Beta-Carotene

1. Holt GA. Food and drug interactions. Chicago: Precept Press, 1998: 169, 179.

2. Steinmetz KA and Potter JD. Vegetables, fruit, and cancer prevention: a review. *J Am Diet Assoc* 96: 1027–1039, 1996.

3. Ziegler RG. A review of epidemiologic evidence that carotenoids reduce the risk of cancer. *J Nutr* 119: 116–122, 1989.

4. Flagg EW, Coates RJ, and Greenberg RS. Epidemiologic studies of antioxidants and cancer. *J Am Coll Nutr* 14: 419–427, 1995.

5. Vena JE, Graham S, Freudenheim J, et al. Diet in the epidemiology of bladder cancer in western New York. *Nutr Cancer* 18: 255–264, 1992.

6. Rock CL, Saxe GA, and Ruffin MT, et al. Carotenoids, vitamin A, and estrogen receptor status in breast cancer. *Nutr Cancer* 25: 281–296, 1996.

7. Zheng W, Sellers TA, Doyle TJ, et al. Retinol, antioxidant vitamins, and cancer of the upper digestive tract in a prospective cohort study of postmenopausal women. *Am J Epidemiol* 142: 955–960, 1995.

8. Kohlmeier L and Hastings SB. Epidemiologic evidence of a role of carotenoids in cardiovascular disease prevention. *Am J Clin Nutr* 62(suppl.): 1370S–1376S, 1995.

9. Albanes D, et al. Alpha-Tocopherol, Beta-Carotene Cancer Prevention Study Group. The effect of vitamin E and beta-carotene on the incidence of lung cancer and other cancers in male smokers. *N Engl J Med* 330: 1029–1035, 1994.

10. Rapola JM, Virtamo J, Ripatti S, et al. Randomized trial of alpha-tocopherol and beta-carotene supplements

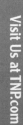

on incidence of major coronary events in men with previous myocardial infarction. *Lancet* 349: 1715–1720, 1997.

11. Rapola JM, Virtamo J, Haukka JK, et al. Effect of vitamin E and beta-carotene on the incidence of angina pectoris. *JAMA* 275(9): 693–698, 1996.

12. White WS, et al. Pharmacokinetics of beta-carotene and canthaxanthin after individual and combined doses by human subjects. *J Am Coll Nutr* 13: 665–671, 1994.

13. Omenn GS, et al. The beta-carotene and retinol efficacy trial (CARET) for chemoprevention of lung cancer in high risk populations: Smokers and asbestos-exposed workers. *Cancer Research* 54(Suppl.): 2038S–2043S, 1996.

14. Carson C, Lee S, De Paola C, et al. Antioxidant intake and cataract in the Melbourne Visual Impairment Project. *Am J Epidemiol* 139: S18, 1994.

15. Vitale S, West S, Hallfrish H, et al. Plasma antioxidants and risk of cortical and nuclear cataract. *Epidemiology* 4: 195–203, 1993.

16. Teikari JM, Rautalahti M, Haukka J, et al. Incidence of cataract operations in Finnish male smokers unaffected by alpha-tocopherol or beta-carotene supplements. *J Epidemiol Community Health* 52: 468–472, 1998.

17. Seddon JM, Ajani UA, Sperduto RD, et al. Dietary carotenoids, vitamins A, C, and E, and advanced age-related macular degeneration. *JAMA* 272: 1413–1420, 1994.

18. Goldberg J, et al. Factors associated with age-related macular degeneration. An analysis of data from the First National Health and Nutrition Examination Survey. *Am J Epidemiol* 128: 700–710, 1988.

19. McAlindon, TE, et al. Do antioxidant micronutrients protect against the development and progression of knee OA. *Arth Rheum.* 39: 648–656; 1996.

20. Krook G and Haeger-Aronsen B. Beta-carotene in the treatment of erythropoietic protoporphyria. A short review. *Acta Derm Venereol Suppl* (Stockh) 100: 125–129, 1982.

21. Suhonen R and Plosila M. The effect of beta-carotene in combination with canthaxanthin, Ro 8–8427 (Phenoro), in treatment of polymorphous light eruptions. *Dermatologica* 163: 172–176, 1981.

22. Corbett MF, Hawk JL, Herxheimer A, and Magnus IA. Controlled therapeutic trials in polymorphic light eruption. *Br J Dermatol* 107: 571–581, 1982.

23. Corbett MF, Herxheimer A, Magnus IA, et al. The long term treatment with beta-carotene in erythropoietic protoporphyria: a controlled trial. *Br J Dermatol* 97: 655–662, 1977.

24. Steinmetz KA and Potter JD. Vegetables, fruit, and cancer prevention: a review. *J Am Diet Assoc* 96: 1027–1039, 1996.

25. Ziegler RG. A review of epidemiologic evidence that carotenoids reduce the risk of cancer. *J Nutr* 119: 116–122, 1989.

26. Flagg EW, Coates RJ, and Greenberg RS. Epidemiologic studies of antioxidants and cancer. *J Am Coll Nutr* 14: 419–427, 1995.

27. Vena JE, Graham S, Freudenheim J, et al. Diet in the epidemiology of bladder cancer in western New York. *Nutr Cancer* 18: 255–264, 1992.

28. Rock CL, Saxe GA, and Ruffin MT, et al. Carotenoids, vitamin A, and estrogen receptor status in breast cancer. *Nutr Cancer* 25: 281–296, 1996.

29. Zheng W, Sellers TA, Doyle TJ, et al. Retinol, antioxidant vitamins, and cancer of the upper digestive tract in a prospective cohort study of postmenopausal women. *Am J Epidemiol* 142: 955–960, 1995.

30. Zheng W, Sellers TA, Doyle TJ, et al. Retinol, antioxidant vitamins, and cancer of the upper digestive tract in a prospective cohort study of postmenopausal women. *Am J Epidemiol* 142: 955–960, 1995.

31. Albanes D, Heinonen OP, Huttunen JK, et al. Effects of alpha-tocopherol and beta-carotene supplements on cancer incidence in the Alpha-Tocopherol Beta-Carotene Cancer Prevention Study. *Am J Clin Nutr* 62(suppl.): 1427S–1430S, 1995.

32. Omenn GS, et al. The beta-carotene and retinol efficacy trial (CARET) for chemoprevention of lung cancer in high risk populations: Smokers and asbestos-exposed workers. *Cancer Research* 54(Suppl.): 2038S–2043S, 1996.

33. Hennekens CH, Buring JE, Manson JAE, et al. Lack of effect of long-term supplementation with beta-carotene on the incidence of malignant neoplasms and cardiovascular disease. *N Engl J Med* 334: 1145–1149, 1996.

34. White WS, et al. Pharmacokinetics of beta-carotene and canthaxanthin after individual and combined doses by human subjects. *J Am Coll Nutr* 13: 665–671, 1994.

35. Kohlmeier L and Hastings SB. Epidemiologic evidence of a role of carotenoids in cardiovascular disease prevention. *Am J Clin Nutr* 62(suppl.): 1370S–1376S, 1995.

36. Albanes D, et al. Alpha-Tocopherol, Beta-Carotene Cancer Prevention Study Group. The effect of vitamin E and beta-carotene on the incidence of lung cancer and other cancers in male smokers. *N Engl J Med* 330: 1029–1035, 1994.

37. Rapola JM, Virtamo J, Ripatti S, et al. Randomized trial of alpha-tocopherol and beta-carotene supplements on incidence of major coronary events in men with previous myocardial infarction. *Lancet* 349: 1715–1720, 1997.

38. Rapola JM, Virtamo J, Haukka JK, et al. Effect of vitamin E and beta-carotene on the incidence of angina pectoris. *JAMA* 275(9): 693–698, 1996.

39. McAlindon, TE, et al. Do antioxidant micronutrients protect against the development and progression of knee OA. *Arth. Rheum.* 39: 648–656; 1996.

40. McAlindon, TE, et al. Do antioxidant micronutrients protect against the development and progression of knee OA. *Arth. Rheum.* 39: 648–656; 1996.

## Bilberry

1. Monboisse JC, et al. Non-enzymatic degradation of acid-soluble calf skin collagen by superoxide ion: Protective effect of flavonoids. *Biochem Pharmacol* 32: 53–58, 1983.

2. Havsteen B. Flavonoids, a class of natural products of high pharmacological potency. *Biochem Pharmacol* 32: 1141–1148, 1983.

3. Gabor M. Pharmacologic effects of flavonoids on blood vessels. *Angiologica* 9: 355–374, 1972.

4. Mian E, et al. Anthocyanosides and the walls of microvessels: Further aspects of the mechanism of action of their protective effect in syndromes due to abnormal capillary fragility. *Minerva Med* 68: 3565–3581, 1977.

5. Puilleiro G, et al. Ex vivo study of the inhibitory effects of *Vaccinium myrtillus* anthocyanosides on human platelet aggregation. *Fitoterapia* 60: 69–75, 1989.

6. Wegmann R, et al. Effects of anthocyanosides on photo receptors. Cyto-enzymatic aspects. *Ann Histochim* 14: 237–256, 1969.

7. Jayle GE and Aubert L. Action des glucosides d'anthocyanes sur la vision scotopique et mesopique du sujet normal. *Therapie* 19: 171–185, 1964.

8. Jayle GE, et al. Etude concernant l'action sur la vision nocturne. *Ann Ocul* (Paris) 198: 556-562, 1965.

9. Bone K, et al. *Mediherb Professional Review.* 59(3): 1997.

10. Sala D, et al. Effect of anthocyanosides on visual performance at low illumination. *Minerva Oftalmol* 21: 283–285, 1979.

11. Gloria E, et al. Effect of anthocyanosides on the absolute visual threshold. *Ann Ottalmol Clin Ocul* 92: 595–607, 1966.

12. Caselli L. Clinical and electroretinographic study on activity of anthocyanosides. *Arch Intern Med* 37: 29–35, 1985.

13. Bone K, et al. *Mediherb Professional Review.* 59(3): 1997.

14. Bone K, et al. *Mediherb Professional Review.* 59(3): 1997.

15. Scharrer A, et al. Anthocyanosides in the treatment of retinopathies. *Klin Monatsbl Augenheilkd* 178: 386–389, 1981.

16. Bravetti G. Preventive medical treatment of senile cataract with vitamin E and anthocyanosides: Clinical evaluation. *Ann Ottalmol Clin Ocul* 115: 109, 1989.

17. Bone K, et al. *Mediherb Professional Review.* 59(3): 1997.

18. Bone K, et al. *Mediherb Professional Review.* 59(3): 1997.

19. Ghiringhelli C, et al. Capillarotropic activity of anthocyanosides in high doses in phlebopathic stasis. *Minerva Cardioangiol* 26: 255–276, 1978.

20. Grismond GL. Treatment of pregnancy-induced phlebopathies. *Minerva Ginecol* 33: 221–230, 1981.

21. Lietti A, et al. Studies on *Vaccinium myrtillus* anthocyanosides. I. Vasoprotective and anti-inflammatory activity. *Arzneimittelforschung* 26: 829–832, 1976.

22. Lietti A, et al. Studies on *Vaccinium myrtillus* anthocyanosides. II. Aspects of anthocyanin pharmacokinetics in the rat. *Arzneimittelforschung* 26: 832–835, 1976.

23. Eandi M. Unpublished results as cited in Morazzoni P, et al. *Vaccinium myrtillus. Fitoterapia* 67(1): 3–29, 1996.

24. Grismond GL. Treatment of pregnancy-induced phlebopathies. *Minerva Ginecol* 33: 221–230, 1981.

25. Scharrer A, et al. Anthocyanosides in the treatment of retinopathies. *Klin Monatsbl Augenheilkd* 178: 386–389, 1981.

## Biotin

1. Maebashi M, Makino Y, Furukawa Y, et al. Therapeutic evaluation of the effect of biotin on hyperglycemia in patients with non-insulin-dependent diabetes mellitus. *J Clin Biochem Nutr* 14: 211–218, 1993.

2. Coggeshall JC, et al. Biotin status and glucose in diabetics. *Ann N Y Acad Sci* 447: 389–392, 1985.

3. Koutsikos D, Agroyannis B, and Tzanatos-Exarchou H. Biotin for diabetic peripheral neuropathy. *Biomed Pharmacother* 44: 511–514, 1990.

4. Floersheim GL. Behandlung bruchiger Fingernagel mit Biotin. *Z Hautkr* 64: 41–48, 1989.

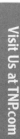

## Bitter Melon

1. Srivastava Y, et al. Antidiabetic and adaptogenic properties of *Momordica charantia* extract: An experimental and clinical evaluation. *Phytother Res* 7: 285–289, 1993.

2. Welihinda J, et al. The insulin-releasing activity of the tropical plant *Momordica charantia*. *Acta Biol Med Germ* 41: 1229–1240, 1982.

3. Murray M. The healing power of herbs. Rocklin, CA: Prima Publishing, 1995: 358.

4. Leatherdale BA, et al. Improvement in glucose tolerance due to *Momordica charantia* (karela) *BMJ* 282: 1823–1824, 1981.

5. Welhinda J, et al. Effect of *Momordica charantia* on the glucose tolerance in maturity onset diabetes. *J Ethnopharm* 17: 277–282, 1986.

6. Aslam M, et al. Interaction between curry ingredient (karela) and drug (chlorporamine). *Lancet:* 607, March 17, 1979.

## Black Cohosh

1. Jarry H, et al. II. Endocrine effects of constituents of *Cimicifuga racemosa*. 1. The effect on serum levels of pituitary hormones in ovariectomized rats. *Planta Med* 1: 46–49, 1985.

2. Jarry H, et al. The endocrine effects of constituents of *Cimicifuga racemosa*. 2. In vitro binding of constituents to estrogen receptors. *Planta Med* 4: 316–319, 1985.

3. Duker EM, et al. Effects of extracts from *Cimicifuga racemosa* on gonadotropin release in menopausal women and ovariectomized rats. *Planta Med* 57(5): 420–424, 1991.

4. Stolze H. An alternative to treat menopausal complaints. *Gyne* 3: 14–16, 1982.

5. Schulz V, et al. Rational phytotherapy. New York: Springer-Verlag, 1998: 246.

6. Warnecke G. Influencing menopausal symptoms with a phytotherapeutic agent. *Med Welt* 36: 871–874, 1985.

7. Stoll W. Phytopharmacon influences atrophic vaginal epithelium. Double-blind study: *Cimicifuga* vs. estrogenic substances. *Therapeuticum* 1: 23–31: 1987.

8. Liske P. Therapeutic efficacy and safety of *Cimicifuga racemosa* for gynecologic disorders. *Advances in Therapy* 15(1): 45–53, 1998.

9. Einer-Jensen N, Zhao J, Andersen KP, et al. *Cimicifuga* and melbosia lack oestrogenic effects in mice and rats. *Maturitas*; 25:149–153, 1996.

10. Jones TK, et al. Profound neonatal congestive heart failure caused by maternal consumption of blue cohosh herbal medication. *J Pediatr* 132: 550–552, 1998.

11. Korn WD. Six-month oral toxicity study with Remifemin-granulate in rats followed by an 8-week recovery period. Hannover, Germany: International Bioresearch, 1991.

12. Nesselhut T, et al. Influence of *Cimicifuga racemosa* extracts with estrogen-like activity on the in vitro proliferation of mammalian carcinoma cells. *Arch Gynecol Obstet* 254: 817–818, 1993.

13. Newall C. Herbal medicines: A guide for health-care professionals. London: Pharmaceutical Press, 1996: 80.

## Bloodroot

1. Godowski KC. Antimicrobial action of sanguinarine. *J Clin Dentistry* 1: 96–101, 1989.

2. Lawrence Review of Natural Products. Bloodroot monograph. St. Louis, MO: Facts and Comparisons Division, J. B. Lipincott Company, 1992.

3. Newall C, et al. Herbal medicines: A guide for health-care professionals. London: Pharmaceutical Press, 1996: 42–43.

4. Newall C, et al. Herbal medicines: A guide for health-care professionals. London: Pharmaceutical Press, 1996: 42–43.

## Boron

1. de Fabio A. Treatment and prevention of osteoarthritis. *Townsend Letter for Doctors:* 143–148, February–March 1990.

2. Travers RL, Rennie GC, and Newnham RE. Boron and arthritis: the results of a double-blind pilot study. *J Nutr Med* 1: 127–132, 1990.

3. Travers RL and Rennie GC. Clinical trial—boron and arthritis. The results of a double-blind pilot study. *Townsend Letter for Doctors:* 360–362, June 1990.

4. Nielsen FH, Hunt CD, Mullen LM, and Hunt JR. Effect of dietary boron on mineral, estrogen, and testosterone metabolism in postmenopausal women. *FASEB J* 1: 394–397, 1987.

5. de Fabio A. Treatment and prevention of osteoarthritis. *Townsend Letter for Doctors:* 143–148, February–March 1990.

6. Travers RL, Rennie GC, and Newnham RE. Boron and arthritis: the results of a double-blind pilot study. *J Nutr Med* 1: 127–132, 1990.

7. Travers RL and Rennie GC. Clinical trial—boron and arthritis. The results of a double-blind pilot study. *Townsend Letter for Doctors:* 360–362, June 1990.

8. Nielsen FH, Hunt CD, Mullen LM, and Hunt JR. Effect of dietary boron on mineral, estrogen, and testos-

terone metabolism in postmenopausal women. *FASEB J* 1: 394–397, 1987.

9. Beattie, JH, et al. The influence of a low boron diet and boron supplementation on bone, major mineral and sex steroid metabolism in postmenopausal women. *Br J Nutr* 69: 871–884, 1993.

10. Nielsen FH, Hunt CD, Mullen LM and Hunt JR. Effect of dietary boron on mineral, estrogen, and testosterone metabolism in postmenopausal women. *FASEB J* 1: 394–397, 1987.

11. Naghii and Samman S. The effect of boron supplementation on its urinary excretion and selected cardiovascular risk factors in healthy male subjects. *Biol Trace Elem Res* 56(3): 273–286, 1997.

## Boswellia

1. Safyhi H, et al. 5-lipoxygenase inhibition by acetyl-11-keto-b-boswellic acid. *Phytomedicine* 3: 71–72, 1996.

2. Singh G, et al. Pharmacology of an extract of salai guggal ex-*Boswellia serrata*, a new non-steroidal anti-inflammatory agent. *Agents Actions* 18: 407–412, 1986.

3. Reddy CK, et al. Studies on the metabolism of glycosaminoglycans under the influence of new herbal anti-inflammatory agents. *Biochem Pharmacol* 20: 3527–3534, 1989.

4. Etzel R. Special extract of *Boswellia serrata* in the treatment of rheumatoid arthritis. *Phytomed* 3(1): 67–70, 1996.

5. Sander O, Herborn G, and Rau R. Is H15 resin extract of *Boswellia serrata* "incense" a useful supplement to established drug therapy of chronic polyarthritis? Results of a double-blind pilot study. English abstract only. *Z Rheumatol* 57(1): 11–16, 1998.

## Bromelain

1. Taussig S, et al. Bromelain, a proteolytic enzyme and its clinical application. A review. *Hiroshima J Med Sci* 24: 185–193, 1975.

2. Taussig S, et al. Bromelain, the enzyme complex of pineapple (*Ananas comosus*) and its clinical application. An update. *J Ethnopharmacol* 22: 191–203, 1988.

3. Schulz V, et al. Rational phytotherapy. New York: Springer-Verlag, 1998: 263.

4. Schulz V, et al. Rational phytotherapy. New York: Springer-Verlag, 1998: 263.

5. Izaka K, et al. Gastrointestinal absorption and anti-inflammatory effect of bromelain. *Jpn J Pharmacol* 22: 519–534, 1972.

6. Seligman B. Bromelain: An anti-inflammatory agent. *Angiology* 13: 508–510, 1962.

7. Pirotta F, et al. Bromelain—A deeper pharmacological study. Note I. Anti-inflammatory and serum fibrinolytic activity after oral administration in the rat. *Drugs Exp Clin Res* 4: 1–20, 1978.

8. Schulz V, et al. Rational phytotherapy. New York: Springer-Verlag, 1998: 263.

9. Seligman B. Bromelain: An anti-inflammatory agent. *Angiology* 13: 508–510, 1962.

10. Blonstein J. Control of swelling in boxing injuries. *Practitioner* 203: 206, 1960.

11. Blumenthal M, et al. The complete German Commission E monographs. Boston: Integrative Medicine Communications, 1998: 94.

## Burdock

1. Newall C, et al. Herbal medicines: A guide for healthcare professionals. London: Pharmaceutical Press, 1996: 52–53.

2. Brinker F. Herb contraindications and drug interactions, 2nd ed. Sandy, Oregon: Eclectic Medical Publications, 1998: 45.

## Butcher's Broom

1. Bouskela E, et al. Effects of Ruscus extract on the internal diameter of arterioles and venules of the hamster cheek pouch microcirculation. *J Cardiovasc Pharmacol* 22: 221–224, 1993.

2. Bouskela E, et al. Inhibitory effect of the Ruscus extract and of the flavonoid heperidine methylchalcone on increased microvascular permeability induced by various agents in the hamster cheek pouch. *J Cardiovasc Pharmacol* 22: 225–230, 1993.

## Calcium

1. McCarron DA and Hatton D. Dietary calcium and lower blood pressure. We can all benefit. Editorial. *JAMA* 275(14): 1128–1129, 1996.

2. Bourgoin B and Evans D. Lead content in 70 brands of dietary calcium supplements. *Amer J Pub Health* 83(8): 1155–1160, 1993.

3. Dawson-Hughes B. A controlled trial of calcium supplementation on bone density in postmenopausal women. *N Engl J Med* 323(13): 878–883, 1990.

4. Sheikh MS. Gastrointestinal absorption of calcium from milk and calcium salts. *N Engl J Med* 317(9): 532–536, 1987.

5. Miller J, Smith DL, Flora L, and Slemenda C. Calcium absorption from calcium carbonate and a new form of calcium (CCM) in healthy male and female adolescents. *Am J Clin Nutr* 48: 1291–1294, 1988.

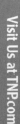

6. Werbach M. Foundations of nutritional medicine. Tarzana, CA: Third Line Press, 1997: 179.

7. Seaborn C and Stoecker B. Effects of antacid or ascorbic acid on tissue accumulation and urinary excretion of chromium. *Nutr Res* 10: 1401–1417, 1990.

8. Freeland-Graves JH. Manganese: An essential nutrient for humans. *Nutr Today* 23: 10–13, 1989.

9. Holt, GA. Food and drug interactions. Chicago: Precept Press. 1998.

10. Hallberg L. Does calcium interfere with iron absorption? *Am J Cl Nutr* 68: 3–4, 1998.

11. Minihane AM and Fairweather-Tait, SJ. Effect of calcium supplementation on daily nonheme-iron absorption and long-term iron status. *Am J Cl Nutr* 68: 96–102, 1998.

12. Cumming RG. Calcium intake and bone mass: a qualitative review of the evidence. *Calcif Tissue Int* 47: 194–201, 1990.

13. Dawson-Hughes B, Dallal GE, Krall EA, et al. A controlled trial of the effect of calcium supplementation on bone density in postmenopausal women. *N Engl J Med* 323(13): 878–883, 1990.

14. Prince R. Diet and the prevention of osteoporotic fractures. *N Engl J Med* 337: 10, 701–702, 1997.

15. Nieves JW, Komar L, Cosman F, Lindsay R. Calcium potentiates the effect of estrogen and calcitonin on bone mass: review and analysis. *Am J Clin Nutr* 67: 1, 18–24, 1998.

16. Aloia JF, et al. Calcium supplementation with and without hormone replacement therapy to prevent postmenopausal bone loss. *Annals Intern Med* 120: 97–103, 1994.

17. Lloyd T, Andon MB, and Rollings N. Calcium supplementation and bone mineral density in adolescent girls. *JAMA* 270(7): 841–844, 1993.

18. Thys-Jacobs S, et al. Calcium carbonate and the premenstrual syndrome: Effects on premenstrual and menstrual symptoms. *Am J Obst Gyn* 179(2): 444–452, 1998.

19. Thys-Jacobs S, et al. Reduced bone mass in women with premenstrual syndrome. *J Women's Health* 4: 161–168, 1995.

20. Lee SJ and Kanis JA. An association between osteoporosis and premenstrual and postmenstrual symptoms. *Bone Miner* 24: 127–134, 1994.

21. Baron JA, Beach M, and Mandel JS. Calcium supplements for the prevention of colorectal adenomas. *New Engl J Med* 340: 101–107, 1999.

22. Cappuccio F, Elliot P, Allender P, et al. Epidemiologic association between dietary calcium intake and blood pressure: a meta-analysis of published data. *Am J Epidemiol* 142(9): 935–945, 1995.

23. Van Leer EM, Seidell JC, and Kromhout D. Dietary calcium, potassium, magnesium and blood pressure in the Netherlands. *Int J Epidemiol* 24(6): 1117–1123, 1995.

24. Bell L, et al. Cholesterol-lowering effects of calcium carbonate in patients with mild to moderate hypercholesterolemia. *Arch Intern Med* 152: 2441–2444, 1992.

25. Levine RJ, Hauth JC, Curet LB, et al. Trial of calcium to prevent preeclampsia. *N Engl J Med* 337(2): 69–76, 1997.

26. Cumming RG. Calcium intake and bone mass: a qualitative review of the evidence. *Calcif Tissue Int* 47: 194–201, 1990.

27. Dawson-Hughes B, Dallal GE, Krall EA, et al. A controlled trial of the effect of calcium supplementation on bone density in postmenopausal women. *N Engl J Med* 323(13): 878–883, 1990.

28. Prince R. Diet and the prevention of osteoporotic fractures. *N Engl J Med* 337: 10, 701–702, 1997.

29. Nieves JW, Komar L, Cosman F, Lindsay R. Calcium potentiates the effect of estrogen and calcitonin on bone mass: review and analysis. *Am J Clin Nutr* 67: 1, 18–24, 1998.

30. Aloia JF, et al. Calcium supplementation with and without hormone replacement therapy to prevent postmenopausal bone loss. *Annals Intern Med* 120: 97–103, 1994.

31. Lloyd T, Andon MB, and Rollings N. Calcium supplementation and bone mineral density in adolescent girls. *JAMA* 270(7): 841–844, 1993.

32. Thys-Jacobs S, et al. Calcium carbonate and the premenstrual syndrome: Effects on premenstrual and menstrual symptoms. *Am J Obst Gyn* 179(2): 444–452, 1998.

33. Thys-Jacobs S, et al. Calcium supplementation in premenstrual syndrome: a randomized crossover trial. *J Gen Intern Med* 4: 183–189, 1989.

34. Penland JG and Johnson PE. Dietary calcium and manganese effects on menstrual cycle symptoms. *Am J Obst Gynecol* 168: 1417–1423, 1993.

35. Baron JA, Beach M, and Mandel JS. Calcium supplements for the prevention of colorectal adenomas. *New Engl J Med* 340: 101–107, 1999.

36. Hyman J, Baron JA, Dain BJ, et al. Dietary and supplemental calcium and the recurrence of colorectal adenomas. *Cancer Epidemiol Biomarkers Prev* 7:291–295, 1998.

37. NIH Consensus Development Panel on Optimal Calcium Intake. *Nutrition* 11: 409–417, 1994.

38. Curhan GC, Willett WC, Speizer FE, et al. Comparison of dietary calcium with supplemental calcium and other nutrients as factors affecting the risk for kidney stones in women. *Ann Intern Med* 126: 497–504, 1997.

39. Curhan GC, Willett WC, Rimm EB, et al. A prospective study of dietary calcium and other nutrients and the risk of symptomatic kidney stones. *N Engl J Med* 328: 833–838, 1993.

## Calendula

1. Schulz V, et al. Rational phytotherapy. New York: Springer-Verlag, 1998: 259.

2. Lawrence Review of Natural Products. Calendula monograph. St. Louis, MO: Facts and Comparisons Division, J. B. Lipincott Company, 1995.

3. Schulz V, et al. Rational phytotherapy. New York: Springer-Verlag, 1998: 259.

4. Brinker F. Herb contraindications and drug interactions, 2nd ed. Sandy, Oregon: Eclectic Medical Publications, 1998: 46.

## Carnitine

1. Hug C, McGraw CA, Bates SR, et al. Reduction of serum carnitine concentrations during anticonvulsant therapy with phenobarbital, valproic acid, phenytoin, and carbamazepine in children. *J Pediatr* 119: 799–802, 1991.

2. Chung S, Choi J, Hyun T, et al. Alterations in the carnitine metabolism in epileptic children treated with valproic acid. *J Korean Med Sci* 12: 553–558, 1997.

3. Melegh B and Trombitas K. Valproate treatment induces lipid globule accumulation with ultrastructual abnormalities of mitochondria in skeletal muscle. *Neuropediatrics* 28: 257–261, 1997.

4. Cacciatore L, et al. The therapeutic effect of L-carnitine in patients with exercise-induced stable angina: A controlled study. *Drugs Exp Clin Res* 17: 225–235, 1991.

5. Bartels GL, et al. Effects of L-propionylcarnitine on ischemia-induced myocardial dysfunction in men with angina pectoris. *Am J Cardiol* 74: 125–130, 1994.

6. Bartels GL, et al. Additional anti-ischemic effects of long-term L-propionylcarnitine in anginal patients treated with conventional antianginal therapy. *Cardiovasc Drugs Ther* 9: 749–753, 1995.

7. Bartels GL, et al. Anti-ischemic efficacy of L-propionyl-carnitine—a promising novel metabolic approach to ischaemia? *Eur Heart J* 17: 414–420, 1996.

8. Cherchi A, et al. Effects of L-carnitine on exercise tolerance in chronic, stable angina: A multicenter, double-blind, randomized, placebo controlled crossover study. *Int J Clin Pharmacol Ther Toxicol*, 23: 569–572, 1985.

9. Lagioia R, et al. Propionyl-L-carnitine: A new compound in the metabolic approach to the treatment of effort angina. *Int J Cardiol* 34: 167–172,1992.

10. Davini P, Bigalli A, Lamanna F, and Boem A. Controlled study on L-carnitine therapeutic efficacy in post-infarction. *Drugs Exp Clin Res* 18(8): 355–365, 1992.

11. Iliceto S, et al. Effect of L-carnitine administration on left ventricular remodeling after acute anterior myocardial infarction: the L-Carnitine Echocardiografia Digitalizzata Infarto Miocardico (CEDIM) trial. *J Am Coll Cardiol*, 26: 380–387, 1995.

12. Brevetti G, et al. Propionyl-L-carnitine in intermittent claudication: Double-blind, placebo-controlled, dose titration, multicenter study. *J Am Coll Cardiol* 26(6): 1411–1416, 1995.

13. Bolognesi M, Amodio P, Merkel C, et al. Effect of 8-day therapy with propionyl-L-carnitine on muscular and subcutaneous blood flow of the lower limbs in patients with peripheral arterial disease. *Clin Physiol* 15(5): 417–423, 1995.

14. Brevetti G, Perna S, Sabba C, et al. Superiority of L-propionylcarnitine vs L-carnitine in improving walking capacity in patients with peripheral vascular disease: an acute, intravenous, double-blind, cross-over study. *Eur Heart J* 13(2): 251–255, 1992.

15. Greco AV, Mingrone G, Bianchi M, and Ghirlanda G. Effect of propionyl-L-carnitine in the treatment of diabetic angiopathy: controlled double-blind trial versus placebo. *Drugs Exp Clin Res* 18(2): 69–80, 1992.

16. Brevetti G, Chiariello M, Ferulano G, et al. Increases in walking distance in patients with peripheral vascular disease treated with L-carnitine: A double-blind, cross-over study. *Circulation* 77(4): 767–773, 1988.

17. Deckert J. Propionyl-L-carnitine for intermittent claudication. *J Fam Pract* 44(6): 533–534, 1997.

18. Sabba C, Berardi E, Antonica G, et al. Comparison between the effect of L-propionylcarnitine, L-carnitine and nitroglycerin in chronic peripheral arterial disease: a haemodynamic double-blind echo-doppler study. *Eur Heart J* 15: 1348–1352, 1994.

19. Pepine CJ. The therapeutic potential of carnitine in cardiovascular disorders. *Clin Ther* 13(1): 2–21, 1991.

20. Brevetti G, et al. Effect of L-carnitine on the reactive hyperemia in patients affected by peripheral vascular disease: a double-blind, crossover study. *Angiology* 40(10): 857–862, 1989.

21. Caponetto S, et al. Efficacy of L-propionylcarnitine treatment in patients with left ventricular dysfunction. *Eur Heart J* 15: 1267–1273, 1994.

Notes

Visit Us at TNP.com

22. Mancini M, et al. Controlled study on the therapeutic efficacy of propionyl-L-carnitine in patients with congestive heart failure. *Arzneimittelforschung* 42: 1101–1104, 1992.

23. Pucciarelli G, et al. The clinical and hemodynamic effects of propionyl-L-carnitine in patients with congestive heart failure. *Clin Ther* 141: 379–384, 1992.

24. Cacciatore L, et al. The therapeutic effect of L-carnitine in patients with exercise-induced stable angina: A controlled study. *Drugs Exp Clin Res* 17: 225–235, 1991.

25. Winter S, Jue K, Prochazka J, et al. The role of L-carnitine in pediatric cardiomyopathy. *J Child Neurol* (Canada) 10(Suppl. 2): 2S45–2S51, 1995.

26. Pepine CJ. The therapeutic potential of carnitine in cardiovascular disorders. *Clin Ther* 13(1): 2–21, 1991.

27. Passeri M, et al. Acetyl-L-carnitine in the treatment of mildly demented elderly patients. *Int J Clin Pharmacol Res* 10: 75–79, 1990.

28. Calvani M, et al. Action of acetyl-L-carnitine in neurodegeneration and Alzheimer's disease. *Ann N Y Acad Sci* 663: 483–486, 1992.

29. Sano M, et al. Double-blind parallel design pilot study of acetyl-levocarnitine in patients with Alzheimer's disease. *Arch Neurol* 49: 1137–1141, 1992.

30. Spagnoli A, et al. Long-term acetyl-L-carnitine treatment in Alzheimer's disease. *Neurology* 41: 1726–1732, 1991.

31. Campi N, et al. Seleginine versus L-acetylcarnitine in the treatment of Alzheimer-type dementia. *Clin Ther* 12: 306–314, 1990.

32. Vecchi GP, et al. Methodology of a controlled clinical study for cerebral aging evaluation. *Int J Clin Pharmacol Res* 10: 145–152, 1990.

33. Garzya G, et al. Evaluation of the effects of L-acetylcarnitine on senile patients suffering from depression. *Drugs Exp Clin Res* 16: 101–106, 1990.

34. Bonavita E. Study of the efficacy and tolerability of L-acetylcarnitine therapy in the senile brain. *Int J Clin Pharmacol Ther Toxicol* 24: 511–516, 1986.

35. Bella R, Biondi R, Raffaele R, and Pennisi G. Effect of acetyl-L-carnitine on geriatric patients suffering from dysthymic disorders. *Int J Clin Pharmacol Res* 10: 355–360, 1990.

36. Thal LJ, Carta A, Clarke WR, et al. A 1-year multi-center placebo-controlled study of acetyl-L-carnitine in patients with Alzheimer's disease. *Neurology* 47: 705–711, 1996.

37. Davini P, Bigalli A, Lamanna F, and Boem A. Controlled study on L-carnitine therapeutic efficacy in post-infarction. *Drugs Exp Clin Res* 18(8): 355–365, 1992.

38. Heinonen OJ. Carnitine and physical exercise. *Sports Med* 22(2): 109–132, 1996.

39. Cacciatore L, et al. The therapeutic effect of L-carnitine in patients with exercise-induced stable angina: A controlled study. *Drugs Exp Clin Res* 17: 225–235, 1991.

40. Cherchi A, et al. Effects of L-carnitine on exercise tolerance in chronic, stable angina: A multicenter, double-blind, randomized, placebo-controlled crossover study. *Int J Clin Pharmacol Ther Toxicol*, 23: 569–572, 1985.

41. Bartels GL, et al. Effects of L-propionylcarnitine on ischemia-induced myocardial dysfunction in men with angina pectoris. *Am J Cardiol* 74: 125–130, 1994.

42. Bartels GL, et al. Additional anti-ischemic effects of long-term L-propionylcarnitine in anginal patients treated with conventional antianginal therapy. *Cardiovasc Drugs Ther* 9: 749–753, 1995.

43. Bartels GL, et al. Anti-ischemic efficacy of L-propionyl-carnitine—a promising novel metabolic approach to ischaemia? *Eur Heart J* 17: 414–420, 1996.

44. Lagioia R, et al. Propionyl-L-carnitine: A new compound in the metabolic approach to the treatment of effort angina. *Int J Cardiol* 34: 167–172,1992.

45. Brevetti G, et al. Propionyl-L-carnitine in intermittent claudication: Double-blind, placebo-controlled, dose titration, multicenter study. *J Am Coll Cardiol* 26(6): 1411–1416, 1995.

46. Bolognesi M, Amodio P, Merkel C, et al. Effect of 8-day therapy with propionyl-L-carnitine on muscular and subcutaneous blood flow of the lower limbs in patients with peripheral arterial disease. *Clin Physiol* 15(5): 417–423, 1995.

47. Brevetti G, Perna S, Sabba C, et al. Superiority of L-propionylcarnitine vs L-carnitine in improving walking capacity in patients with peripheral vascular disease: an acute, intravenous, double-blind, cross-over study. *Eur Heart J* 13(2): 251–255, 1992.

48. Greco AV, Mingrone G, Bianchi M, and Ghirlanda G. Effect of propionyl-L-carnitine in the treatment of diabetic angiopathy: controlled double-blind trial versus placebo. *Drugs Exp Clin Res* 18(2): 69–80, 1992.

49. Brevetti G, Chiariello M, Ferulano G, et al. Increases in walking distance in patients with peripheral vascular disease treated with L-carnitine: A double-blind, cross-over study. *Circulation* 77(4): 767–773, 1988.

50. Deckert J. Propionyl-L-carnitine for intermittent claudication. *J Fam Pract* 44(6): 533–534, 1997.

51. Sabba C, Berardi E, Antonica G, et al. Comparison between the effect of L-propionylcarnitine, L-carnitine

and nitroglycerin in chronic peripheral arterial disease: a haemodynamic double-blind echo-doppler study. *Eur Heart J* 15: 1348–1352, 1994.

52. Pepine CJ. The therapeutic potential of carnitine in cardiovascular disorders. *Clin Ther* 13(1): 2–21, 1991.

53. Brevetti G, et al. Effect of L-carnitine on the reactive hyperemia in patients affected by peripheral vascular disease: a double-blind, crossover study. *Angiology* 40(10): 857–862, 1989.

54. Caponetto S, et al. Efficacy of L-propionylcarnitine treatment in patients with left ventricular dysfunction. *Eur Heart J* 15: 1267–1273, 1994.

55. Mancini M, et al. Controlled study on the therapeutic efficacy of propionyl-L-carnitine in patients with congestive heart failure. *Arzneimittelforschung* 42: 1101–1104, 1992.

56. Pucciarelli G, et al. The clinical and hemodynamic effects of propionyl-L-carnitine in patients with congestive heart failure. *Clin Ther* 141: 379–384, 1992.

57. Cacciatore L, et al. The therapeutic effect of L-carnitine in patients with exercise-induced stable angina: A controlled study. *Drugs Exp Clin Res* 17: 225–35, 1991.

58. Davini P, Bigalli A, Lamanna F, and Boem A. Controlled study on L-carnitine therapeutic efficacy in postinfarction. *Drugs Exp Clin Res* 18(8): 355–365, 1992.

59. Iliceto S, et al. Effect of L-carnitine administration on left ventricular remodeling after acute anterior myocardial infarction: the L-Carnitine Echocardiografia Digitalizzata Infarto Miocardico (CEDIM) trial. *J Am Coll Cardiol* 26: 380–387, 1995.

60. Calvani M, et al. Action of acetyl-L-carnitine in neurodegeneration and Alzheimer's disease. *Ann N Y Acad Sci* 663: 483–486, 1992.

61. Cipolli C, et al. Effects of L-acetylcarnitine on mental deterioration in the aged: Initial results. *Clin Ther* 132: 479–510, 1990.

62. Garzya G, et al. Evaluation of the effects of L-acetylcarnitine on senile patients suffering from depression. *Drugs Exp Clin Res* 16: 101–106, 1990.

63. Passeri M, et al. Acetyl-L-carnitine in the treatment of mildly demented elderly patients. *Int J Clin Pharmacol Res* 10: 75–79, 1990.

64. Salvioli G and Neri M. L-acetylcarnitine treatment of mental decline in the elderly. *Drugs Exp Clin Res* 20: 169–176, 1994.

65. Spagnoli A, et al. Long-term acetyl-L-carnitine treatment in Alzheimer's disease. *Neurology* 41: 1726–1732, 1991.

66. Vecchi GP, et al. Acetyl-L-carnitine treatment of mental impairment in the elderly: Evidence from a multicenter study. *Arch Gerontol Geriatr* 2(Suppl): 159–168, 1991.

67. Thal LJ, et al. A 1-year multicenter placebo-controlled study of acetyl-L-carnitine in patients with Alzheimer's disease. *Neurology* 47(3): 705–711, 1996.

68. Sano M, et al. Double-blind parallel design pilot study of acetyl-levocarnitine in patients with Alzheimer's disease. *Arch Neurol* 49: 1137–1141, 1992.

69. Campi N, et al. Selegiline versus l-acetylcarnitine in the treatment of Alzheimer-type dementia. *Clin Ther* 12: 306–314, 1990.

70. Rai G, et al. Double-blind, placebo-controlled study of acetyl-l-carnitine in patients with Alzheimer's dementia. *Curr Med Res Opin* 11(10): 638–647.

71. Bonavita E. Study of the efficacy and tolerability of L-acetylcarnitine therapy in the senile brain. *Int J Clin Pharmacol Ther Toxicol* 24: 511–516, 1986.

72. Spagnoli A, et al. Long-term acetyl-L-carnitine treatment in Alzheimer's disease. *Neurology* 41: 1726–1732, 1991.

73. Thal LJ, Carta A, Clarke WR, et al. A 1-year multicenter placebo-controlled study of acetyl-L-carnitine in patients with Alzheimer's disease. *Neurology* 47: 705–711, 1996.

74. Heinonen OJ. Carnitine and physical exercise. *Sports Med* 22(2): 109–132, 1996.

## Cartilage

1. Dupont E, et al. Antiangiogenic properties of a novel shark cartilage extract: Potential role in the treatment of psoriasis. *J Cutan Med Surg* 2: 146–152, 1998.

2. Sheu JR, et al. Effect of U-995, a potent shark cartilage-derived angiogenesis and anti-tumor activities. *Anticancer Res* 18: 4435–4441, 1998.

3. Davis PF, et al. Inhibition of angiogenesis by oral ingestion of powdered shark cartilage in a rat model. *Microvasc Res* 54: 178–182, 1997.

## Cat's Claw

1. Jones K. Cat's claw. *Herbs for Health* September/October: 42–46, 1996.

2. Lininger S, et al. The natural pharmacy. Rocklin, CA: Prima Publishing, 1998: 246.

## Cayenne

1. Yeoh KG, et al. Chili protects against aspirin-induced gastroduodenal mucosal injury in humans. *Dig Dis Sci* 40(3): 580–583, 1995.

2. Graham DY, et al. Spicy food and the stomach: Evaluation by videoendoscopy. *JAMA* 260(23): 3473–3475, 1988.

Notes

Visit Us at TNP.com

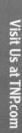

3. Brinker F. Herb contraindications and drug interactions, 2nd ed. Sandy, Oregon: Eclectic Medical Publications, 1998: 51.

## Chamomile

1. Brinker F. Herb contraindications and drug interactions, 2nd ed. Sandy, Oregon: Eclectic Medical Publications, 1998: 53.

2. Hormann HP, et al. Evidence for the efficacy and safety of topical herbal drugs in dermatology: Part 1. Anti-inflammatory agents. *Phytomedicine* 1: 161–167, 1994.

3. Schulz V, et al. Rational phytotherapy. New York: Springer-Verlag, 1998: 254–256.

4. Schulz V, et al. Rational phytotherapy. New York: Springer-Verlag, 1998: 256.

## Chasteberry

1. Milewicz A, et al. *Vitex agnus-castus* extract in the treatment of luteal phase defects due to latent hyperprolactinemia. Results of a randomized placebo-controlled double-blind study. *Arzneimittelforschung* 43(7): 752–756, 1993.

2. Jarry H, et al. In vitro prolactin but not LH and FSH release is inhibited by compounds in extracts of *Agnus castus:* Direct evidence for a dopaminergic principle by the dopamine receptor assay. *EYP Clin Endocrinol* 102: 448–454, 1994.

3. Sliutz G, et al. *Agnus castus* extracts inhibit prolactin secretion of rat pituitary cells. *Horm Metab Res* 25(5): 253–255, 1993.

4. Schulz V, et al. Rational phytotherapy. New York: Springer-Verlag, 1998: 241–242.

5. Propping D, et al. Diagnosis and therapy of corpus luteum insufficiency in general practice. *Therapiewoche* 38: 2992–3001, 1988.

6. Dittmar FW, et al. Premenstrual syndrome: Treatment with a phytopharmaceutical. *Therapiewoche Gynakol* 5: 60–68, 1992.

7. Peteres-Welte C, et al. Menstrual abnormalities and PMS: *Vitex agnus-castus. Therapiewoche Gynakol* 7: 49–52, 1994.

8. Lauritzen C, et al. Treatment of premenstrual tension syndrome with *Vitex agnus-castus*. Controlled, double-blind study vs. pyridoxine. *Phytomedicine* 4(3): 183–189, 1997.

9. Lauritzen C, et al. Treatment of premenstrual tension syndrome with *Vitex agnus-castus*. Controlled, double-blind study vs. pyridoxine. *Phytomedicine* 4(3): 183–189, 1997.

10. Kleijnen J, et al. Vitamin $B_6$ in the treatment of PMS—A review. *Br J Obstet Gynaecol* 97: 847–852, 1990.

11. Milewicz A, et al. *Vitex agnus-castus* extract in the treatment of luteal phase defects due to latent hyperprolactinemia. Results of a randomized placebo-controlled double-blind study. *Arzneimittelforschung* 43(7): 752–756, 1993.

12. Schulz V, et al. Rational phytotherapy. New York: Springer-Verlag, 1998: 243.

13. Cahill DJ, et al. Multiple follicular development associated with herbal medicine. *Hum Reprod* 9(8): 1469–1470, 1994.

## Chondroitin

1. Brandt KD. Effects of nonsteroidal anti-inflammatory drugs on chondrocyte metabolism in vitro and in vivo. *Am J Med* 83 (Suppl. 5A): 29–34, 1987.

2. Brooks PM, et al. NSAID and osteoarthritis—help or hindrance. *J Rheumatol* 9: 3–5, 1982.

3. Shield MJ Anti-inflammatory drugs and their effects on cartilage synthesis and renal function. *Eur J Rheumatol Inflam* 13: 7–16, 1993.

4. Palmoski MJ, et al. Effects of some nonsteroidal anti-inflammatory drugs on proteoglycan metabolism and organization in canine articular cartilage. *Arthritic Rheum* 23: 1010–1020, 1980.

5. Rahad S, et al. Effect of nonsteroidal anti-inflammatory drugs on the course of osteoarthritis. *Lancet* 2: 519–522, 1989.

6. Bucsi L and Poör G. Efficacy and tolerability of oral chondroitin sulfate as a symptomatic slow-acting drug for osteoarthritis (SYSADOA) in the treatment of knee osteoarthritis. *Osteoarthritis Cartilage* 6 (Suppl. A): 31–36, 1998.

7. Bourgeois R, Chales G, Dehais J, et al. Efficacy and tolerability of CS 1200 mg/day vs CS 3x400 mg/day vs. placebo. *Osteoarthritis Cartilage* 6(Suppl. A): 25–30, 1998.

8. Uebelhart D, et al. Effects of oral chondroitin sulfate on the progression of knee osteoarthritis: a pilot study. *Osteoarthritis Cartilage* 6(Suppl. A): 39–46, 1998.

9. Bourgeois R, Chales G, Dehais J, et al. Efficacy and tolerability of CS 1200 mg/day vs CS 3x400 mg/day vs. placebo. *Osteoarthritis Cartilage* 6(Suppl. A): 25–30, 1998.

10. Verbruggen G, Goemaere S, and Veys EM. Chondroitin sulfate: S/DMOAD (structure/disease modifying anti-osteoarthritis drug) in the treatment of finger joint OA. *Osteoarthritis Cartilage* 6(Suppl. A): 37–38, 1998.

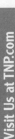

11. Uebelhart D, et al. Effects of oral chondroitin sulfate on the progression of knee osteoarthritis: a pilot study. *Osteoarthritis Cartilage* 6(Suppl. A): 39–46, 1998.

12. Uebelhart D, Thonar EJMA, Zhang J, and Williams JM. Protective effect of exogenous chondroitin 4, 6-sulfate in the acute degradation of articular cartilage in the rabbit. *Osteoarthritis Cartilage* 6(Suppl. A): 6–13, 1998.

13. Nakazawa K. Effect of chondroitin sulfates on atherosclerosis. I. Long-term oral administration of chondroitin sulfates to atherosclerotic subjects. *Nippon Naika Gakkai Zasshi* 59: 1084–1092, 1970.

14. Nakazawa K and Murata K. Comparative study of the effects of chondroitin sulfate isomers on atherosclerotic subjects. *ZFA* 34: 153–159, 1979.

15. Conte A, Volpi N, Palmieri L, Bahous I, and Ronca G. Biochemical and pharmacokinetic aspects of oral treatment with chondroitin sulfate. *Arzneimittelforschung Drug Res* 45: 918–925, 1995.

16. Bucsi L and Poör G. Efficacy and tolerability of oral chondroitin sulfate as a symptomatic slow-acting drug for osteoarthritis (SYSADOA) in the treatment of knee osteoarthritis. *Osteoarthritis Cartilage* 6 (Suppl. A): 31–36, 1998.

17. Bourgeois R, Chales G, Dehais J, et al. Efficacy and tolerability of CS 1200 mg/day vs CS 3x400 mg/day vs. placebo. *Osteoarthritis Cartilage* 6(Suppl. A): 25–30, 1998.

18. Uebelhart D, et al. Effects of oral chondroitin sulfate on the progression of knee osteoarthritis: a pilot study. *Osteoarthritis Cartilage* 6(Suppl. A): 39–46, 1998.

19. Conrozier T. Anti-arthrosis treatments: efficacy and tolerance of chondroitin sulfates (CS 4 & 6). English abstract only. *Presse Med* 27(36): 1862–1865, 1998.

20. Mazieres B, Loyau G, Menkes CJ, et al. Chondroitin sulfate in the treatment of gonarthrosis and coxarthrosis. Five months result of a multicenter double-blind controlled prospective study using placebo. English abstract only. *Rev Rhum Mal Osteoartic* 59(7–8): 466–472, 1992.

21. L'Hirondel JL. Klinische Doppelblind-studie mit oral verbreichtem chondroitinsulfat gegen placebo bei der tibio-femoralengonarthrose. English abstract only. *Litera Rheumatol* 14: 77–84, 1992.

22. Morreale P, Monopulo R, Galati M, et al. Comparison of the anti-inflammatory efficacy of chondroitin sulfate and diclofenac sodium in patients with knee arthritis. *J Rheum* 23(8): 1385–1391, 1996.

23. Verbruggen G, Goemaere S, and Veys EM. Chondroitin sulfate: S/DMOAD (structure/disease modifying anti-osteoarthritis drug) in the treatment of finger joint OA. *Osteoarthritis Cartilage* 6(Suppl. A): 37–38, 1998.

24. Uebelhart D, Thonar EJMA, Zhang J, and Williams JM. Protective effect of exogenous chondroitin 4, 6-sulfate in the acute degradation of articular cartilage in the rabbit. *Osteoarthritis Cartilage* 6(Suppl. A): 6–13, 1998.

25. Uebelhart D, Thonar EJMA, Zhang J, and Williams JM. Protective effect of exogenous chondroitin 4, 6-sulfate in the acute degradation of articular cartilage in the rabbit. *Osteoarthritis Cartilage* 6(Suppl. A): 6–13, 1998.

26. Ronca F, Palmieri L, Panicucci P, and Ronca G. Anti-inflammatory activity of chondroitin sulfate. *Osteoarthritis Cartilage* 6(Suppl. A): 14–21, 1998.

27. Hungerford, DS. Treating osteoarthritis with chondroprotective agents. *Orthopedic Special Edition* 4(1): 39–42, 1998.

28. Ronca F, Palmieri L, Panicucci P, and Ronca G. Anti-inflammatory activity of chondroitin sulfate. *Osteoarthritis Cartilage* 6(Suppl. A): 14–21, 1998.

## Chromium

1. Mertz W. Chromium in human nutrition: A review. *J Nutr* 123: 626–633, 1993.

2. Mertz W. Chromium in human nutrition: A review. *J Nutr* 123: 626–633, 1993.

3. Seaborn C and Stoecker B. Effects of antacid or ascorbic acid on tissue accumulation and urinary excretion of chromium. *Nutr Res* 10: 1401–1417, 1990.

4. Anderson RA, Cheng N, Bryden NA, et al. Elevated intakes of supplemental chromium improve glucose and insulin variables in individuals with type 2 diabetes. *Diabetes* 46: 1786–1791, 1997.

5. Ravina A, et al. Chromium in the treatment of clinical diabetes mellitus. *Harefuah* 125: 142–145, 1993.

6. Anderson RA, et al. Chromium supplementation of human subjects: effects on glucose, insulin and lipid parameters. *Metabolism* 32: 894–899, 1983.

7. Anderson RA, et al. Supplemental-chromium effects on glucose, insulin, glucagon, and urinary chromium losses in subjects consuming controlled low-chromium diets. *Am J Clin Nut* 54: 909–916, 1991.

8. Kaats G, et al. A randomized, double-masked, placebo-controlled study of the effects of chromium picolinate supplementation on body composition: a replication and extension of a previous study *Curr Ther Res* 59: 379–388, 1998.

9. Mertz W. Chromium in human nutrition: A review. *J Nutr* 123: 626–633, 1993.

10. Anderson RA, Cheng N, Bryden NA, et al. Elevated intakes of supplemental chromium improve glucose and insulin variables in individuals with type 2 diabetes. *Diabetes* 46: 1786–1791, 1997.

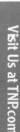

11. Ravina A, et al. Chromium in the treatment of clinical diabetes mellitus. *Harefuah* 125: 142–145, 1993.

12. Wilson BE, et al. Effects of chromium supplementation on fasting insulin levels and lipid parameters in healthy, non-obese young subjects. *Diabetes Res Clin Pract* 28:179–184, 1995.

13. Anderson RA, et al. Chromium supplementation of human subjects: effects on glucose, insulin and lipid parameters. *Metabolism* 32: 894–899, 1983.

14. Rabinowitz MB, et al. Effect of chromium and yeast supplements on carbohydrate and lipid metabolism in diabetic men. *Diabetes Care* 6: 319–327, 1983.

15. Anderson RA, et al. Chromium supplementation of human subjects: effects on glucose, insulin and lipid parameters. *Metabolism* 32: 894–899, 1983.

16. Wilson BE, et al. Effects of chromium supplementation on fasting insulin levels and lipid parameters in healthy, non-obese young subjects. *Diabetes Res Clin Pract* 28:179–184, 1995.

17. Anderson RA, et al. Supplemental-chromium effects on glucose, insulin, glucagon, and urinary chromium losses in subjects consuming controlled low-chromium diets. *Am J Clin Nut* 54: 909–916, 1991.

18. Uusitupa MI. Chromium supplementation in impaired glucose tolerance of elderly: effects on blood glucose, plasma insulin, c-peptide and lipid levels. *Br J Nutr* 68(1): 209–216, 1992.

19. Kaats G, et al. A randomized, double-masked, placebo-controlled study of the effects of chromium picolinate supplementation on body composition: a replication and extension of a previous study *Curr Ther Res* 59: 379–388, 1998.

20. Anderson RA, et al. Lack of toxicity of chromium chloride and chromium picolinate in rats. *J Am Coll Nutr* 163: 273–279, 1997.

21. Certulli J, et al. Chromium picolinate toxicity. *Ann Pharmacother* 32: 428–431, 1998.

22. Wasser WG, et al. Chronic renal failure after ingestion of over-the-counter chromium picolinate. *Ann Intern Med* 126(5): 410, 1997.

23. Reading SA. Chromium picolinate. *J Fla Med Assoc* 83(1): 29–31, 1996.

## Coenzyme Q10

1. Weiss M. Bioavailability of four oral coenzyme $Q_{10}$ formulations in healthy volunteers. *Mol Aspects Med* 15(Suppl.): S273–S280, 1994.

2. Morisco C, et al. Effect of coenzyme $Q_{10}$ therapy in patients with congestive heart failure: A long-term multicenter randomized study. *Clin Invest* 71(Suppl. 8): S134–S136, 1993.

3. Hashiba K, Kuramoto K, Ishimi Z, et al. *Heart* (in Japanese) 4:1579–1589, 1972. As cited in Werbach M. Nutritional influences on illness. CD-ROM. Tarzana, CA: Third Line Press, 1998.

4. Hofman-Bang C, et al. Coenzyme $Q_{10}$ as an adjunctive treatment of congestive heart failure. *J Am Coll Cardiol* 19: 216A, 1992.

5. Sinatra ST. Refractory congestive heart failure successfully managed with high-dose coenzyme $Q_{10}$ administration. *Mol Aspects Med* 18(Suppl.): S299–S305, 1997.

6. Langsjoen H, Langsjoen P, Langsjoen P, et al. Usefulness of coenzyme $Q_{10}$ in clinical cardiology: a long-term study. *Mol Aspects Med* 15(Suppl. PS): 165–175, 1994.

7. Langsjoen PH, et al. Response of patients in classes III and IV of cardiomyopathy to therapy in a blind and crossover trial with coenzyme $Q_{10}$. *Proc Natl Acad Sci* 82: 4240, 1985.

8. Pogessi L, Galanti G, Comeglio M, et al. Effect of coenzyme $Q_{10}$ on left ventricular function in patients with dilative cardiomyopathy. *Curr Ther Res* 49: 878–886, 1991.

9. Digiesi V, et al. Effect of coenzyme $Q_{10}$ on essential arterial hypertension. *Curr Ther Res* 47: 841–845, 1990.

10. Langsjoen P, et al. Treatment of essential hypertension with coenzyme $Q_{10}$. *Mol Aspects Med* 15(Suppl.): S265–S272, 1994.

11. Digiesi V, et al. Coenzyme $Q_{10}$ in essential hypertension. *Mol Aspects Med* 15(Suppl.): S257–S263, 1994.

12. Werbach M. Nutritional influences on illness. CD-ROM. Tarzana, CA: Third Line Press, 1998.

13. Bargossi AM, et al. Exogenous $CoQ_{10}$ supplementation prevents plasma ubiquinone reduction induced by HMG-CoA reductase inhibitors. *Mol Aspects Med* 15(Suppl.): S187–S193, 1994.

14. Ghirlanda G, et al. Evidence of plasma $CoQ_{10}$-lowering effect by HMG-CoA reductase inhibitors: a double-blind, placebo-controlled study. *J Clin Pharmacol* 33(3): 226–229, 1993.

15. Mortensen SA, et al. Dose-related decrease of serum coenzyme $Q_{10}$ during treatment with HMG-CoA reductase inhibitors. *Mol Aspects Med* 18(Suppl.): S137–S144, 1997.

16. Kishi T, et al. Bioenergetics in clinical medicine. XI. Studies on CoQ and diabetes mellitus. *J Med* 7(3–4): 307–321, 1976.

17. Kishi H, et al. Bioenergetics in clinical medicine. III. Inhibition of coenzyme $Q_{10}$-enzymes by clinically used

anti-hypertensive drugs. *Res Commun Chem Pathol Pharmacol* 12(3): 533–540, 1975.

18. Kishi T, et al. Bioenergetics in clinical medicine XV. Inhibition of coenzyme $Q_{10}$ enzymes by clinically used adrenergic blockers of beta receptors. *Res Commun Chem Pathol Pharmacol* 17(1): 157–164, 1977.

19. Folkers K. Basic chemical research on coeznyme $Q_{10}$ and integrated clinical research on therapy of diseases. As cited in G Lenaz, ed. Coenzyme Q. New York: John Wiley and Sons, 1985.

20. Kishi T, et al. In Y Yamamura K Folkers, and Y Ito, eds. Biochemical and clinical aspects of coenzyme Q, Vol. 2. Amsterdam: Elsevier/North-Holland Biomedical Press, 1980: 139–157.

21. Werbach M. Nutritional influences on illness. CD-ROM. Tarzana, CA: Third Line Press, 1998.

22. Morisco C, et al. Effect of coenzyme $Q_{10}$ therapy in patients with congestive heart failure: A long-term multicenter randomized study. *Clin Invest* 71(Suppl. 8): S134–S136, 1993.

23. Hashiba K, Kuramoto K, Ishimi Z, et al. *Heart* (in Japanese) 4:1579–1589, 1972. As cited in Werbach M. Nutritional influences on illness. CD-ROM. Tarzana, CA: Third Line Press, 1998.

24. Hofman-Bang C, et al. Coenzyme $Q_{10}$ as an adjunctive treatment of congestive heart failure. *J Am Coll Cardiol* 19: 216A, 1992.

25. Sinatra ST. Refractory congestive heart failure successfully managed with high-dose coenzyme $Q_{10}$ administration. *Mol Aspects Med* 18(Suppl.): S299–S305, 1997.

26. Langsjoen H, Langsjoen P, Langsjoen P, et al. Usefulness of coenzyme Q10 in clinical cardiology: a long-term study. *Mol Aspects Med* 15(Suppl. PS): 165–175, 1994.

27. Langsjoen PH, et al. Response of patients in classes III and IV of cardiomyopathy to therapy in a blind and crossover trial with coenzyme $Q_{10}$. *Proc Natl Acad Sci* 82: 4240, 1985.

28. Pogessi L, Galanti G, Comeglio M, et al. Effect of coenzyme $Q_{10}$ on left ventricular function in patients with dilative cardiomyopathy. *Curr Ther Res* 49: 878–886, 1991.

29. Digiesi V, et al. Effect of coenzyme $Q_{10}$ on essential arterial hypertension. *Curr Ther Res* 47: 841–845, 1990.

30. Langsjoen P, et al. Treatment of essential hypertension with coenzyme $Q_{10}$. *Mol Aspects Med* 15(Suppl.): S265–S272, 1994.

31. Digiesi V, et al. Coenzyme $Q_{10}$ in essential hypertension. *Mol Aspects Med* 15(Suppl.): S257–S263, 1994.

32. Werbach M. Nutritional influences on illness. CD-ROM. Tarzana, CA: Third Line Press, 1998.

33. Lampetico M, et al. Italian multicenter study on the efficacy and safety of coenzyme $Q_{10}$ as adjuvant therapy in heart failure. *Clin Invest* 71(Suppl. 8): S129–S133, 1993.

## *Coleus forskohlii*

1. Seamon KB and Daly JW. Forskolin: A unique diterpene activator of cAMP-generating systems. *J Cyclic Nucleotide Res* 7: 201–224, 1981.

2. Laurenza A, Sutkowski EM, and Seamon KB. Forskolin: A specific stimulator of adenylyl cyclase or a diterpene with multiple sites of action? *Trends Pharmacol Sci* 10: 442–447, 1989.

3. Marone G, et al. Forskolin inhibits the release of histamine from human basophils and mast cells. *Agents Actions* 18: 96–99, 1986.

4. Ammon HPT, et al. Forskolin: From Ayurvedic remedy to a modern agent. *Planta Med* 51: 473–477, 1985.

5. DeSouza NJ. Industrial development of traditional drugs: The forskolin example. A mini-review. *J Ethnopharmacol* 38: 1177–1180, 1993.

6. Kreutner W, et al. Bronchodilatory and antiallergy activity of forskolin. *Eur J Pharmacol* 11: 1–8, 1985.

7. Schlepper M, et al. Cardiovascular effects of forskolin and phosphodiesterase-III inhibitors. *Basic Res Cardiol* 84(Suppl. 1): 197–212, 1989.

8. Dubey MP, et al. Pharmacological studies on coleonol, a hypotensive diterpene from *Coleus forskohlii*. *J Ethnopharmacol* 3: 1–13, 1981.

9. Bauer K, et al. Pharmacodynamic effects of inhaled dry powder formulations of fenoterol and colforsin in asthma. *Clin Pharmacol Ther* 53: 76–83, 1993.

10. Meyer BH, et al. The effects of forskolin eye drops on intraocular pressure. *S Afr Med* J 71(9): 570–571, 1987.

## Colostrum

1. Okhuysen PC, Chappell CL, and Crabb J. Prophylactic effect of bovine anti-cryptosporidium hyperimmune colostrum immunoglobulin in healthy volunteers challenged with *Cryptosporidium parvum*. *Clin Infect Dis* 26: 1324–1329, 1998.

2. Greenberg PD and Cello JP. Treatment of severe diarrhea caused by *Cryptosporidium parvum* with oral bovine immunoglobulin concentrate in patients with AIDS. *J Acquir Immune Defic Syndr Hum Retrovirol* 13: 348–354, 1996.

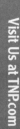

Notes

3. Plettenberg A, Stoehr A, Stellbrink HJ, et al. A preparation from bovine colostrum in the treatment of HIV-positive patients with chronic diarrhea. *Clin Invest* 71: 42–45, 1993.

4. Casswall TH, Sarker SA, Albert MJ, Fuchs GJ, et al. Treatment of *Helicobacter pylori* infection in infants in rural Bangladesh with oral immunoglobulins from hyperimmune bovine colostrum. *Aliment Pharmacol Ther* 2: 563–568, 1998.

5. Ylitalo S, Uhari M, Rasi S, et al. Rotaviral antibodies in the treatment of acute rotaviral gastroenteritis. *Acta Paediatr* 87: 264–267, 1998.

6. Tacket CO, Binion SB, and Bostwick E. Efficacy of bovine milk immunoglobulin concentrate in preventing illness after *Shigella flexneri* challenge. *Am J Trop Med Hyg* 47: 276–283, 1992.

7. Okhuysen PC, Chappell CL, and Crabb J. Prophylactic effect of bovine anti-cryptosporidium hyperimmune colostrum immunoglobulin in healthy volunteers challenged with *Cryptosporidium parvum*. *Clin Infect Dis* 26: 1324–1329, 1998.

8. Greenberg PD and Cello JP. Treatment of severe diarrhea caused by *Cryptosporidium parvum* with oral bovine immunoglobulin concentrate in patients with AIDS. *J Acquir Immune Defic Syndr Hum Retrovirol* 13: 348–354, 1996.

9. Plettenberg A, Stoehr A, Stellbrink HJ, et al. A preparation from bovine colostrum in the treatment of HIV-positive patients with chronic diarrhea. *Clin Invest* 71: 42–45, 1993.

10. Tacket CO, Binion SB, and Bostwick E. Efficacy of bovine milk immunoglobulin concentrate in preventing illness after *Shigella flexneri* challenge. *Am J Trop Med Hyg* 47: 276–283, 1992.

11. Casswall TH, Sarker SA, Albert MJ, Fuchs GJ, et al. Treatment of *Helicobacter pylori* infection in infants in rural Bangladesh with oral immunoglobulins from hyperimmune bovine colostrum. *Aliment Pharmacol Ther* 2: 563–568, 1998.

12. Ylitalo S, Uhari M, Rasi S, et al. Rotaviral antibodies in the treatment of acute rotaviral gastroenteritis. *Acta Paediatr* 87: 264–267, 1998.

## Conjugated Linolenic Acid

1. Erling T. A pilot study with the aim of studying the efficacy and tolerability of CLA (Tonalin) on the body composition in humans. Medstat Research Ltd., Liilestrom, Norway, 1997.

2. West D. Reduced body fat with conjugated linoleic acid feeding in the mouse. *FASEB J* 11: A599, 1997.

## Copper

1. Werbach M. Foundations of nutritional medicine. Tarzana, CA: Third Line Press, 1997: 54.

2. Werbach M. Foundations of nutritional medicine. Tarzana, CA: Third Line Press, 1997: 170–171.

3. Saltman PD, et al. The role of trace minerals in osteoporosis. *J Am Coll Nutr* 12(4): 384–389, 1993.

4. Strause L, et al. Spinal bone loss in postmenopausal women supplemented with calcium and trace minerals. *J Nutr* 124: 1060–1064, 1994.

5. Jones AA, DiSilvestro RA, Coleman M, and Wagner TL. Copper supplementation of adult men: effects on blood copper enzyme activities and indicators of cardiovascular disease risk. *Metabolism* 46: 1380–1383, 1997.

6. Werbach M. Foundations of nutritional medicine. Tarzana, CA: Third Line Press, 1997: 169–171, 206.

## Cranberry

1. Sobota AE. Inhibition of bacterial adherence by cranberry juice: Potential use for the treatment of urinary tract infections. *J Urol* 131: 1013–1016, 1984.

2. Schmidt DR, et al. An examination of the anti-adherence activity of cranberry juice on urinary and nonurinary bacterial isolates. *Microbios* 55: 173–181, 224–225, 1988.

3. Zafriri D, et al. Inhibitory activity of cranberry juice on adherence of type 1 and type P fimbriated *Escherichia coli* to eucaryotic cells. *Antimicrob Agents Chemother* 33(1): 92–98, 1989.

4. Avorn J, et al. Reduction of bacteriuria and pyuria after ingestion of cranberry juice. *JAMA* 271: 751–754, 1994.

5. Schaefer AJ. Recurrent urinary tract infections in the female patient. *Urology* 32(Suppl.): 12–15, 1988.

## Creatine

1. Williams MH, et al. Creatine supplementation and exercise performance: An update. *J Am Coll Nutr* 17: 216–234, 1998.

2. Williams MH, et al. Creatine supplementation and exercise performance: An update. *J Am Coll Nutr* 17: 216–234, 1998.

3. Balsom PD, Eckblom B, Soderlund K, et al. Creatine supplementation and dynamic high-intensity intermittent exercise. *Scand J Med Sci Sports* 3: 143–149, 1993.

4. Mujika I, et al. Creatine supplementation as an ergogenic acid for sports performance in highly trained athletes: a critical review. *Int J Sports Med* 18: 491–496, 1997.

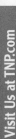

5. Williams MH, et al. Creatine supplementation and exercise performance: An update. *J Am Coll Nutr* 17: 216–234, 1998.

6. Williams MH, et al. Creatine supplementation and exercise performance: An update. *J Am Coll Nutr* 17: 216–234, 1998.

7. Balsom PD, Ekblom B, Soderlund K, et. al. Creatine supplementation and dynamic high-intensity intermittent exercise. *Scand J Med Sci Sport* 3: 143–149, 1993.

8. Mujika I, et al. Creatine supplementation as an ergogenic acid for sports performance in highly trained athletes: a critical review. *Int J Sports Med* 18: 491–496, 1997.

9. Williams MH, et al. Creatine supplementation and exercise performance: An update. *J Am Coll Nutr* 17: 216–234, 1998.

10. Balsom PD, Eckblom K, Soderlund K, et al. Creatine supplementation and dynamic high-intensity intermittent exercise. *Scand J Med Sci Sports* 3: 143–149, 1993.

11. Williams MH, et al. Creatine supplementation and exercise performance: An update. *J Am Coll Nutr* 17: 216–234, 1998.

12. Balsom PD, Harridge SDR, Soderlund K, et al. Creatine supplementation per se does not enhance endurance exercise performance. *Acta Physiol Scand* 149: 521–523, 1993.

13. Burke LM, et al. Effect of oral creatine supplementation on single-effort sprint performance in elite swimmers. *Int J Sport Nutr* 6: 222–233, 1966.

14. Mujika I, et al. Creatine supplementation does not improve sprint performance in competitive swimmers. *Med Sci Sports Exerc* 30:1435–1441, 1996.

15. Creatine is innocent; FDA rejects creatine role in deaths. Associated Press: April 30, 1998.

16. Williams MH, et al. Creatine supplementation and exercise performance: An update. *J Am Coll Nutr* 17: 216–234, 1998.

## Damiana

1. Willard T. The wild rose scientific herbal. Calgary, Canada: Wild Rose College of Natural Healing, Ltd., 1991: 104–105.

2. Duke JA. CRC handbook of medicinal herbs. Boca Raton, FL: CRC Press, 1985: 492.

3. Newall C, et al. Herbal medicines: A guide for healthcare professionals. London: Pharmaceutical Press, 1996: 94.

## Dandelion

1. Leung A and Foster S. Encyclopedia of common natural ingredients used in food, drugs, and cosmetics, 2nd edition. New York: John Wiley and Sons, 1996: 205–206.

2. Murray M. The healing power of herbs, 2nd ed. Rocklin, CA: Prima Publishing, 1995.

3. Susnik F. Present state of knowledge of the medicinal plant *Taraxacum officinale* Weber. *Med Razgledi* 21: 323–328, 1982.

4. ESCOP monographs. Fascicule 2: *Taraxaci radix* (dandelion). Exeter, UK: European Scientific Commission on Phytotherapy, 1996: 2.

5. Bohm K. Studies on the choleretic action of some drugs. *Arzneimittelforschung* 9: 376–378, 1959.

6. Racz-Kotilla, et al. The action of *Taraxacum officinale* extracts on the body weight and diureses of laboratory animals. *Planta Med* 26: 212–217, 1974.

7. Newall C, et al. Herbal medicines: A guide for healthcare professionals. London: Pharmaceutical Press, 1996: 96.

8. ESCOP monographs. Fascicule 2: *Taraxaci radix* (dandelion). Exeter, UK: European Scientific Commission on Phytotherapy, 1996: 2.

9. Review of natural products, dandelion. St. Louis, MO: Facts and Comparisons Division, J.B. Lipincott Company, August 1998.

10. Hirono I, et al. *J Environ Pathol Toxicol* 1: 71, 1978.

11. Blumenthal M, et al., eds. The complete German Commission E monographs. Boston: Integrative Medicine Communications, 119–120, 1998.

12. McGuffin M, et al., eds. Botanical safety handbook. New York: CRC Press, 1997: 114.

## Devil's Claw

1. Lecomte A, et al. *Harpagophytum* dans l'arthrose: Etude en double insu contre placebo. *Le Magazine* 15: 27–30, 1992.

2. ESCOP monograph. Fascicule 2: *Harpagophyti radix* (devil's claw). Exeter, UK: European Scientific Cooperative on Phytotherapy, 1997.

3. Chrubasik S, et al. Effectiveness of *Harpagophytum procumbens* in treatment of acute low back pain. *Phytomedicine* 3(1): 1–10, 1996.

4. Schulz V, et al. Rational phytotherapy. New York: Springer-Verlag, 1998: 263.

5. ESCOP monograph. Fascicule 2: *Harpagophyti radix* (devil's claw). Exeter, UK: European Scientific Cooperative on Phytotherapy, 1997.

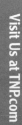

6. Moussard C, et al. A drug used in traditional medicine, *Harpagophytum procumbens*: No evidence for NSAID-like effect on whole blood eicosonoid production in humans. *Prostaglandins Leukot Essent Fatty Acids* 46: 283–286, 1992.

7. ESCOP monograph. Fascicule 2: *Harpagophyti radix* (devil's claw). Exeter, UK: European Scientific Cooperative on Phytotherapy, 1997.

## DHEA

1. van Vollenhoven RF, Morabito LM, Engleman EG, and McGuire JL. Treatment of systemic lupus erythematosus with dehydroepiandrosterone: 50 patients treated up to 12 months. *J Rheumatol* 25: 285–289, 1998.

2. Labrie F, et al. Effect of 12-month dehydroepiandrosterone replacement therapy on bone, vagina and endometrium in postmenopausal women. *J Clin End Met* 82: 3498–3505, 1997.

3. Wolf OT, Neumann O, Hellhammer DH, et al. Effects of a two-week physiological dehydroepiandrosterone substitution on cognitive performance and well-being in healthy elderly women. *J Clin Endocrinol Metab* 82(7): 2363–2367, 1997.

4. van Vollenhoven RF, Morabito LM, Engleman EG, and McGuire JL. Treatment of systemic lupus erythematosus with dehydroepiandrosterone: 50 patients treated up to 12 months. *J Rheumatol* 25: 285–289, 1998.

5. van Vollenhoven RF, Morabito LM, Engleman EG, and McGuire JL. Treatment of systemic lupus erythematosus with dehydroepiandrosterone: 50 patients treated up to 12 months. *J Rheumatol* 25: 285–289, 1998.

6. van Vollenhoven RF, Engleman EG, and McGuire JL. Dehydroepiandrosterone in systemic lupus erythematosus. Results of a double-blind, placebo-controlled, randomized clinical trial. *Arthritis Rheum* 38(12): 1826–1831, 1995.

7. Gatto V, Aragno M, Gallo M, et al. Dehydroepiandrosterone inhibits the growth of DMBA-induced rat mammary carcinoma via the androgen receptor. *Oncol Rep* 5: 241–243, 1998.

8. Orner GA, Mathews C, Hendricks JD, et al. Dehydroepiandrosterone is a complete hepatocarcinogen and potent tumor promoter in the absence of peroxisome proliferation in rainbow trout. *Carcinogenesis* 16: 2893–2898, 1995.

9. Shibata M, Hasegawa R, Imaida K, et al. Chemoprevention by dehydroepiandrosterone and indomethacin in a rat multiorgan carcinogenesis model. *Cancer Res* 55: 4870–4874, 1995.

10. Simile M, Pascale RM, De Miglio MR, et al. Inhibition by dehydroepiandrosterone of growth and progression of persistent liver nodules in experimental rat liver carcinogenesis. *Int J Cancer* 62: 210–215, 1995.

## Dong Quai

1. Chang HM, et al. Pharmacology and application of Chinese materia medica. Singapore: World Scientific, 1983.

2. Igarashi M. Proceedings of the satellite symposium on Sino-Japanese traditional medicine (Kampo). 16th World International Congress on Pharmacology. Excerpta Medica, 1987: 141–143.

3. Bensky D and Gamble A. Chinese herbal medicine: Materia medica. Seattle, WA: Eastland Press, 1986.

4. Hsu HY, et al. Oriental materia medica: A concise guide. Long Beach, CA: Oriental Healing Arts Institute, 1986: 540–542.

5. Zhu D. Dong quai. *Am J Chin Med* 90(3–4): 117–125, 1987.

6. Hirata JD, et al. Does dong quai have estrogenic effects in postmenopausal women? A double-blind placebo-controlled trial. *Fertil Steril* 68(6): 981–986, 1997.

7. Chang HM, et al. Pharmacology and application of Chinese materia medica. Singapore: World Scientific, 1983.

8. Igarashi M. Proceedings of the satellite symposium on Sino-Japanese traditional medicine (Kampo). 16th World International Congress on Pharmacology. Excerpta Medica, 1987: 141–143.

9. Bensky D and Baronet R. Chinese herbal medicine formulas and strategies. Seattle, WA: Eastland Press, 1990.

10. Chang HM, et al. Pharmacology and application of Chinese materia medica. Singapore: World Scientific, 1983.

11. Bensky D and Baronet R. Chinese herbal medicine formulas and strategies. Seattle, WA: Eastland Press, 1990.

12. Zhu D. Dong quai. *Am J Chin Med* 90(3–4): 117–125, 1987.

## Echinacea

1. Dorn M. Milderung grippaler Effekte durch ein pflanzliches Immunstimulans. *Natur und Ganzheitsmedizin* 2: 314–319, 1989. As cited in Schulz V, et al. Rational phytotherapy. New York: Springer-Verlag, 1998: 277.

2. Braunig B, et al. *Echinacea purpurea* root for strengthening the immune response in flu-like infections. *Z Phytother* 13: 7–13, 1992.

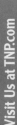

3. Brinkeborn R, Shah D, Geissbuhler S, et al. Echinaforce in the treatment of acute colds. *Schweiz Zschr Gunsheits Medizin* 10: 26–29, 1998.

4. Dorn M, et al. Placebo-controlled double-blind study of *Echinacea pallidae radix* in upper respiratory tract infections. *Complement Ther Med* 3: 40–42, 1997.

5. Hoheisel O, et al. Echinagard treatment shortens the course of the common cold: A double-blind placebo-controlled clinical trial. *Eur J Clin Res* 9: 261–268, 1997.

6. Melchart MD, et al. Echinacea root extracts for the prevention of upper respiratory tract infections. A double-blind placebo-controlled randomized trial. *Arch Fam Med* 7: 541–545, 1998.

7. Carlo Calabrese, N.D., Bastyr University. Unpublished communication.

8. Melchart D, et al. Immunomodulation with echinacea—A systematic review of controlled clinical trials. *Phytomedicine* 1: 245–254, 1994.

9. Bauer R, et al. Echinacea species as potential immunostimulatory drugs. *Econ Med Plant Res* 5: 253–321, 1991.

10. Wagner V, et al. Immunostimulating polysaccharides (heteroglycans) of higher plants. *Arzneimittelforschung* 35: 1069–1075, 1985.

11. Stimpel M, et al. Macrophage activation and induction of macrophage cytotoxicity by purified polysaccharide fractions from the plant *Echinacea purpurea*. *Infect Immun* 46: 845–849, 1984.

12. Luettig B, et al. Macrophage activation by the polysaccharide arabinogalactan isolated from plant cell cultures of *Echinacea purpurea*. *J Natl Cancer Inst* 81: 669–675, 1989.

13. Mose J. Effect of echinacin on phagocytosis and natural killer cells. *Med Welt* 34: 1463–1467, 1983.

14. Vomel V. Influence of a non-specific immune stimulant on phagocytosis of erythrocytes and ink by the reticuloendothelial system of isolated perfused rat livers of different ages. *Arzneimittelforschung* 34: 691–695, 1984.

15. Hobbs C. The echinacea handbook. Portland, OR: Eclectic Medical Publications, 1989.

16. Schulz V, et al. Rational phytotherapy. New York: Springer-Verlag, 1998: 278.

17. Bergner P. Goldenseal and the common cold: The antibiotic myth. *Med Herbalism* 8(4): 1–10, 1997.

18. Schulz V, et al. Rational phytotherapy. New York: Springer-Verlag, 1998: 276.

19. Mengs U, et al. Toxicity of *Echinacea purpurea* acute, subacute, and genotoxicity studies. *Arzneimittelforschung Drug Res* 41(11): 1076–1081, 1991.

20. Parnham MJ. Benefit-risk assessment of the squeezed sap of the purple coneflower (*Echinacea purpurea*) for long-term oral immunostimulation. *Phytomedicine* 3(1): 99–102, 1996.

21. Parnham MJ. Benefit-risk assessment of the squeezed sap of the purple coneflower (*Echinacea purpurea*) for long-term oral immunostimulation. *Phytomedicine* 3(1): 99–102, 1996.

## Elderberry

1. Zakay-Rones Z, et al. Inhibition of several strains of influenza virus and reduction of symptoms by an elderberry extract (*Sambucus nigra* L.) during an outbreak of influenza B Panama. *J Altern Complement Med* 1(4): 361–369, 1995.

2. Shapira-Nahor B, et al. The effect of Sambucol on HIV infection in vitro. Annual Israel Congress of Microbiology, February 6–7, 1995.

3. Morag A, et al. Inhibition of sensitive and acyclovir-resistant HSV-1 strains by an elderberry extract in vitro. Xth International Congress of Virology, Abstract 18–23 (Jerusalem, 1996).

## Elecampane

1. Reiter M, et al. Relaxant effects on tracheal and ileal smooth muscles of the guinea pig. *Arzneimittelforschung* 35: 408–414, 1985.

2. Newall C, et al. Herbal medicines: A guide for health-care professionals. London: Pharmaceutical Press, 1996: 106.

## Ephedra

1. Blumenthal M. A review of the botany, chemistry, medicinal uses, safety concerns, and legal status of ephedra and its alkaloids. *Herbal Gram* 34: 22–57, 1995.

2. Physicians' desk reference for herbal medicines. Montvale, NJ: Medical Economics Company, Inc., 1998: 827.

## Eyebright

1. Lawrence Review of Natural Products. Eyebright monograph. St. Louis, MO: Facts and Comparisons Division, J.B. Lipincott Company, 1996.

2. Duke JA. CRC handbook of medicinal herbs. Boca Raton, FL: CRC Press, 1985: 141.

## Fenugreek

1. Sharma RD, et al. Use of fenugreek seed powder in the management of non-insulin-dependent diabetes mellitus. *Nutr Res* 16:1331–1339, 1996.

2. Madar Z, et al. Glucose-lowering effect of fenugreek in non-insulin dependent diabetics. *Eur J Clin Nutr* 42: 51–54, 1988.

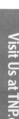

3. Sharma RD, Raghuram TC, and Rao NS. Effect of fenugreek seeds on blood glucose and serum lipids in type I diabetes. *Eur J Clin Nutr* 44: 301–306, 1990.

4. Leung A, et al. Encyclopedia of common natural ingredients used in food, drugs, and cosmetics. New York: John Wiley and Sons, 1996: 243–244.

## Feverfew

1. Castleman, M. The healing herbs. Emmaus, PA: Rodale Press, 1991: 173–176.

2. Johnson ES, et al. Efficacy of feverfew as a prophylactic treatment of migraine. *BMJ* 291: 569–573, 1985.

3. Bohlmann F, et al. Sesquiterpene lactones and other constituents from *Tanacetum parthenium*. *Phytochemistry* 21: 2543–2549, 1982.

4. Makheja AM, et al. The active principle in feverfew. *Lancet* ii: 1054, 1981.

5. Makheja AM, et al. A platelet phospholipase inhibitor from the medicinal herb feverfew (*Tanacetum parthenium*). *Prostaglandins Leukot Med* 8: 653–660, 1982.

6. Heptinstall S, et al. Extracts from feverfew inhibit granule secretion in blood platelets and polymorphonuclear leukocytes. *Lancet* 8437: 1071–1074, 1985.

7. Tyler V. Herbs of choice. New York: Pharmaceutical Products Press, 1994: 127.

8. De Weerdt CJ, et al. Herbal medicines in migraine prevention. Randomized double-blind placebo controlled crossover trial of a feverfew preparation. *Phytomedicine* 3(3): 225–230, 1996.

9. Murphy JS, et al. Randomized, double-blind, placebo-controlled trial of feverfew in migraine prevention. *Lancet* 23: 189–192, 1988.

10. Palevitch DG, et al. Feverfew (*Tanacetum parthenium*) as a prophylactic treatment for migraine: A double-blind, placebo-controlled study. *Phytomed Res* 11(7): 506–511, 1997.

11. De Weerdt CJ, et al. Herbal medicines in migraine prevention. Randomized double-blind placebo-controlled crossover trial of a feverfew preparation. *Phytomedicine* 3(3): 225–230, 1996.

12. Newall C. Herbal medicines: A guide for health-care professionals. London: Pharmaceutical Press, 1996: 120.

13. Murphy JS, et al. Randomized, double-blind, placebo-controlled trial of feverfew in migraine prevention. *Lancet* 23: 189–192, 1988.

14. Johnson ES, et al. Efficacy of feverfew as a prophylactic treatment of migraine. *BMJ* 291: 569–573, 1985.

15. Johnson ES, et al. Efficacy of feverfew as a prophylactic treatment of migraine. *BMJ* 291: 569–573, 1985.

16. ESCOP monographs. Fascicule 2: *Tanaceti parthenii herba/folium* (feverfew). Exeter UK: European Scientific Cooperative on Phytotherapy, 1996.

## Fish Oil

1. Harris WS. N-3 fatty acids and serum lipoproteins: human studies. *Am J Clin Nutr* 65(suppl.): 1645S–1654S, 1997.

2. Shekelle RB, et al. Diet, serum cholesterol, and death from coronary heart disease. The Western Electric Study. *N Engl J Med* 304: 65, 1981.

3. Kromhout D, Arntzenius AC, Kempen-Voogd N, et al. The inverse relation between fish consumption and twenty year mortality from coronary heart disease. *N Engl J Med* 312: 1205, 1985.

4. Harris WS. N-3 fatty acids and serum lipoproteins: human studies. *Am J Clin Nutr* 65(suppl.): 1645S–1654S, 1997.

5. Cobiac L, Clifton PM, and Abbey M. Lipid, lipoprotein, and hemostatic effects of fish vs fish-oil n-3 fatty acids in mildly hyperlipidemic males. *Am J Clin Nutr* 53: 1210–1216, 1991.

6. Dyerberg, J. N-3 fatty Acids and coronary artery disease. Potentials and problems. *Omega-3, Lipoproteins, and Atherosclerosis* 27: 251–258, 1996.

7. Lungershausen YK, Abbey M, Nestel PJ, and Howe PR. Reduction of blood pressure and plasma triglycerides by omega-3 fatty acids in treated hypertensives. *J Hypertens* 12: 1041–1045, 1994.

8. Radack K, Deck C, and Huster G. The effects of low doses of n-3 fatty acid supplementation on blood pressure in hypertensive subjects. A randomized controlled trial. *Arch Intern Med* 151: 1173–1180, 1991.

9. Singer P, et al. Lipid and blood-pressure lowering effect of mackerel diet in man. *Atherosclerosis* 49: 99, 1983.

10. Singer P, Melzer S, Goschel M, and Augustin S. Fish oil amplifies the effect of propranolol in mild essential hypertension. *Hypertension* 16: 682–691, 1990.

11. Whelton PK, Kumanyika SK, and Cook NR. Efficacy of nonpharmacologic interventions in adults with high-normal blood pressure: results from phase 1 of the Trials of Hypertension Prevention. Trials of Hypertension Prevention Collaborative Research Group. *Am J Clin Nutr* 65: 652S–660S, 1997.

12. James MJ and Cleland LG. Dietary n-3 fatty acids and therapy for rheumatoid arthritis. *Semin Arthritis Rheum* 27: 85–97, 1997.

13. Harel Z, Biro FM, Kottenhahn RK, et al. Supplementation with omega-3 polyunsaturated fatty acids in

the management of dysmenorrhea in adolescents. *Am J Obstet Gynecol* 174: 1335–1338, 1996.

14. Stoll AL, et al. Omega 3 fatty acids in bipolar disorder: a preliminary double-blind, placebo-controlled trial. *Arch Gen Psychiatry* 56(5): 407–412, 1999.

15. DiGiacomo RA, Kremer JM, and Shah DM. Fish-oil dietary supplementation in patients with Raynaud's phenomenon: a double-blind, controlled, prospective study. *Am J Med* 86: 158–164, 1989.

16. Ringer TV, et al. Fish oil blunts the pain response to cold pressor testing in normal males. Abstract. *J Am Coll Nutr* 8: 435, 1989.

17. Kruger MC, et al. Calcium, gamma-linolenic acid (GLA) and eicosapentaenoic acid (EPA) supplementation in osteoporosis. *Osteoporosis Int* 6(suppl. 1): 250, 1996.

18. van Papendorp DH, Coetzer H, and Kruger MC. Biochemical profile of osteoporotic patients on essential fatty acid supplementation. *Nutr Res* 15: 325–334, 1995.

19. Walton AJ, Snaith ML, and Locniskar M. Dietary fish oil and the severity of symptoms in patients with systemic lupus erythematosus. *Ann Rheum Dis* 50: 463–466, 1991.

20. Bittiner SB, Tucker WF, and Cartwright I. A double-blind, randomised, placebo-controlled trial of fish oil in psoriasis. *Lancet* 1: 378–380, 1988.

21. Soyland E, Funk J, Rajka G, et al. Effect of dietary supplementation with very-long-chain n-3 fatty acids in patients with psoriasis. *N Engl J Med* 328: 1812–1816, 1993.

22. Thien FC, et al. Fish oils and asthma—a fishy story? *Med J Australia* 164: 135–136, 1996.

23. Arm JP, Thien FC, and Lee TH. Leukotrienes, fish-oil and asthma. *Allergy Proc* 15: 129–134, 1994.

24. Shekelle RB, et al. Diet, serum cholesterol, and death from coronary heart disease. The Western Electric Study. *N Engl J Med* 304: 65, 1981.

25. Kromhout D, Arntzenius AC, Kempen-Voogd N, et al. The inverse relation between fish consumption and twenty year mortality from coronary heart disease. *N Engl J Med* 312: 1205, 1985.

26. Harris WS. N-3 fatty acids and serum lipoproteins: human studies. *Am J Clin Nutr* 65(suppl.): 1645S–1654S, 1997.

27. Cobiac L, Clifton PM, and Abbey M. Lipid, lipoprotein, and hemostatic effects of fish vs fish-oil n-3 fatty acids in mildly hyperlipidemic males. *Am J Clin Nutr* 53: 1210–1216, 1991.

28. Harris WS. N-3 fatty acids and serum lipoproteins: human studies. *Am J Clin Nutr* 65(suppl.): 1645S–1654S, 1997.

29. Dyerberg, J. N-3 fatty Acids and coronary artery disease. Potentials and problems. *Omega-3, Lipoproteins, and Atherosclerosis* 27: 251–258, 1996.

30. Lungershausen YK, Abbey M, Nestel PJ, and Howe PR. Reduction of blood pressure and plasma triglycerides by omega-3 fatty acids in treated hypertensives. *J Hypertens* 12: 1041–1045, 1994.

31. Radack K, Deck C, and Huster G. The effects of low doses of n-3 fatty acid supplementation on blood pressure in hypertensive subjects. A randomized controlled trial. *Arch Intern Med* 151: 1173–1180, 1991.

32. Singer P, et al. Lipid and blood-pressure lowering effect of mackerel diet in man. *Atherosclerosis* 49: 99, 1983.

33. Singer P, Melzer S, Goschel M, and Augustin S. Fish oil amplifies the effect of propranolol in mild essential hypertension. *Hypertension* 16: 682–691, 1990.

34. Appel LJ, Miller ER, Seidler AJ, et al. Does supplementation of diet with "fish oil" reduce blood pressure? A meta-analysis of controlled clinical trials. *Arch Intern Med* 153: 1429–1438, 1993.

35. Whelton PK, Kumanyika SK, and Cook NR. Efficacy of nonpharmacologic interventions in adults with high-normal blood pressure: results from phase 1 of the Trials of Hypertension Prevention. Trials of Hypertension Prevention Collaborative Research Group. *Am J Clin Nutr* 65: 652S–660S, 1997.

36. James MJ and Cleland LG. Dietary n-3 fatty acids and therapy for rheumatoid arthritis. *Semin Arthritis Rheum* 27: 85–97, 1997.

37. Harel Z, Biro FM, Kottenhahn RK, et al. Supplementation with omega-3 polyunsaturated fatty acids in the management of dysmenorrhea in adolescents. *Am J Obstet Gynecol* 174: 1335–1338, 1996.

38. Stoll AL, et al. Omega 3 fatty acids in bipolar disorder: a preliminary double-blind, placebo-controlled trial. *Arch Gen Psychiatry* 56(5): 407–412, 1999.

39. DiGiacomo RA, Kremer JM, and Shah DM. Fish-oil dietary supplementation in patients with Raynaud's phenomenon: a double-blind, controlled, prospective study. *Am J Med* 86: 158–164, 1989.

40. Ringer TV, et al. Fish oil blunts the pain response to cold pressor testing in normal males. Abstract. *J Am Coll Nutr* 8: 435, 1989.

41. Kruger MC, et al. Calcium, gamma-linolenic acid (GLA) and eicosapentaenoic acid (EPA) supplementation in osteoporosis. *Osteoporosis Int* 6(suppl. 1): 250, 1996.

42. van Papendorp DH, Coetzer H, and Kruger MC. Biochemical profile of osteoporotic patients on essential fatty acid supplementation. *Nutr Res* 15: 325–334, 1995.

43. Walton AJ, Snaith ML, and Locniskar M. Dietary fish oil and the severity of symptoms in patients with systemic lupus erythematosus. *Ann Rheum Dis* 50: 463–466, 1991.

44. Harris WS. Dietary fish oil and blood lipids. *Curr Opin Lipidol* 7: 3–7, 1996.

45. Harris WS. Fish oils and plasma lipid and lipoprotein metabolism in humans: a critical review. *J Lipid Res* 30: 785–807, 1989.

46. Harris WS. N-3 fatty acids and serum lipoproteins: human studies. *Am J Clin Nutr* 65(suppl.): 1645S–1654S, 1997.

47. Cobiac L, Clifton PM, and Abbey M. Lipid, lipoprotein, and hemostatic effects of fish vs fish-oil n-3 fatty acids in mildly hyperlipidemic males. *Am J Clin Nutr* 53: 1210–1216, 1991.

48. Harris WS. N-3 fatty acids and serum lipoproteins: human studies. *Am J Clin Nutr* 65(suppl.): 1645S–1654S, 1997.

## 5-HTP

1. Byerly WF, et al. 5-hydroxytryptophan: a review of its antidepressant efficacy and adverse effects. *J Clin Psychopharmacol* 7: 127–137, 1987.

2. Poldinger W, et al. A functional-dimensional approach to depression: serotonin deficiency as a target syndrome in a comparison of 5-hydroxytryptophan and fluvoxamine. *Psychopathology* 24: 53–81, 1991.

3. Titus F, et al. 5-hydroxytryptophan versus methysergide in the prophylaxis of migraine. Randomized clinical trial. *Eur Neurol* 25: 327–329, 1986.

4. Bono G, et al. Serotonin precursors in migraine prophylaxis. *Adv Neurol* 33: 357–363, 1982.

5. Maissen CP and Ludin HP. Comparison of the effect of 5-hydroxytryptophan and propranolol in the interval treatment of migraine. *Schweiz Med Wochenschr* 121: 1585–1590, 1991.

6. De Giorgis G, et al. Headache in association with sleep disorders in children: A psychodiagnostic evaluation. *Drugs Exp Clin Res* 13: 425–433, 1987.

7. Longo G, et al. Treatment of essential headache in developmental age with L-5-HTP (cross over double-blind study versus placebo). *Pediatr Med Chir* 6: 241–245, 1984.

8. Santucci M, et al. L-hydroxytryptophan versus placebo in childhood migraine prophylaxis: a double-blind crossover study. *Cephalalgia* 6: 155–157, 1986.

9. De Benedittis G and Massei R. Serotonin precursors in chronic primary headache. A double-blind cross-over study with L-5-hydroxytryptophan vs. placebo. *J Neurosurg Sci* 29: 239–248, 1985.

10. Caruso I, et al. Double-blind study of 5-hydroxytryptophan versus placebo in the treatment of primary fibromyalgia syndrome. *J Int Med Res* 18: 201–209, 1990.

11. Ceci F, et al. The effects of 5-hydroxytryptophan administration on feeding behavior in obese adult female subjects. *J Neural Transm* 76: 109–117, 1989.

12. Cangiano C, Ceci F, Cairella M, et al. Effects of 5-hydroxytryptophan on eating behavior and adherence to dietary prescriptions in obese adult subjects. *Adv Exp Med Biol* 294: 591–593, 1991.

13. Cangiano C, Ceci F, Cascino A, et al . Eating behavior and adherence to dietary prescriptions in obese adult subjects treated with 5-hydroxytryptophan. *Am J Clin Nutr* 56: 863–867, 1992.

14. Byerly WF, et al. 5-hydroxytryptophan: a review of its antidepressant efficacy and adverse effects. *J Clin Psychopharmacol* 7: 127–137, 1987.

15. Poldinger W, et al. A functional-dimensional approach to depression: serotonin deficiency as a target syndrome in a comparison of 5-hydroxytryptophan and fluvoxamine. *Psychopathology* 24: 53–81, 1991.

16. Titus F, et al. 5-hydroxytryptophan versus methysergide in the prophylaxis of migraine. Randomized clinical trial. *Eur Neurol* 25: 327–329, 1986.

17. Bono G, et al. Serotonin precursors in migraine prophylaxis. *Adv Neurol* 33: 357–363, 1982.

18. Maissen CP and Ludin HP. Comparison of the effect of 5-hydroxytryptophan and propranolol in the interval treatment of migraine. *Schweiz Med Wochenschr* 121: 1585–1590, 1991.

19. De Giorgis G, et al. Headache in association with sleep disorders in children: A psychodiagnostic evaluation. *Drugs Exp Clin Res* 13: 425–433, 1987.

20. Longo G, et al. Treatment of essential headache in developmental age with L-5-HTP (cross over double-blind study versus placebo). *Pediatr Med Chir* 6: 241–245, 1984.

21. Santucci M, et al. L-hydroxytryptophan versus placebo in childhood migraine prophylaxis: a double-blind crossover study. *Cephalalgia* 6: 155–157, 1986.

22. De Benedittis G and Massei R. Serotonin precursors in chronic primary headache. A double-blind cross-over study with L-5-hydroxytryptophan vs. placebo. *J Neurosurg Sci* 29: 239–248, 1985.

23. Ceci F, et al. The effects of 5-hydroxytryptophan administration on feeding behavior in obese adult female subjects. *J Neural Transm* 76: 109–117, 1989.

24. Cangiano C, Ceci F, Cairella M, et al. Effects of 5-hydroxytryptophan on eating behavior and adherence to

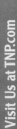

dietary prescriptions in obese adult subjects. *Adv Exp Med Biol* 294: 591–593, 1991.

25. Cangiano C, Ceci F, Cascino A, et al . Eating behavior and adherence to dietary prescriptions in obese adult subjects treated with 5-hydroxytryptophan. *Am J Clin Nutr* 56: 863–867, 1992.

26. Caruso I, et al. Double-blind study of 5-hydroxytryptophan versus placebo in the treatment of primary fibromyalgia syndrome. *J Int Med Res* 18: 201–209, 1990.

27. Sternberg EM, et al. Development of a scleroderma-like illness during therapy with L-5-hydroxytryptophan and carbidopa. *New Engl J Med* 303: 782–787, 1980.

28. Joly P, et al. Develoment of pseudobullous morphea and scleroderma-like illness during therapy with L-5-hydroxytryptophan and carbidopa. *J Am Acad Dermatol* 25: 332–333, 1991.

29. Auffranc JC, et al. Sclerodermiform and poikilodermal syndrome observed during treatment with carbidopa and 5-hydroxytryptophan. *Ann Dermatol Venereol* 112: 691–692, 1985.

## Flaxseed Oil

1. Siguel EN. Essential and trans fatty acid metabolism in health and disease. *Compr Ther* 20: 500–510, 1994.

2. Prasad K. Dietary flax seed in prevention of hypercholesterolemic atherosclerosis. *Atherosclerosis* 132: 69–76, 1997.

3. Arjmandi BH, et al. Whole flaxseed consumption lowers serum LDL-cholesterol and lipoprotein (a) concentrations in postmenopausal women. *Nutr Res* 18: 1203–1214, 1998.

4. Singer P, et al. Effects of dietary oleic, linoleic, and alpha-linolenic acids on blood pressure, serum lipids, lipoproteins and the formation of eicosanoid precursors in patients with mild essential hypertension. *J Human Hypertension* 4: 227–233, 1990.

5. deLorgeril M, et al. Mediterranean alpha-linolenic acid–rich diet in secondary prevention of coronary heart disease. *Lancet* 343: 1454–1459, 1994.

6. Rice RD. Mediterranean diet. *Lancet* 344: 893–894, 1994.

7. Nordstrom DCE, et al. Alpha-linolenic acid in the treatment of rheumatoid arthritis. A double-blind placebo-controlled and randomized study: flaxseed vs. safflower oil. *Rheumatol Int* 14: 231–234, 1995.

8. Serraino M and Thompson LU. The effect of flaxseed supplementation on the initiation and promotional stages of mammary tumorigenesis. *Nutr Cancer* 17: 153–159, 1992.

9. Bougnoix P, et al. Alpha-linolenic acid content of adipose breast tissue: A host determinant of the risk of early metastasis in breast cancer. *Br J Cancer* 70: 330–334, 1994.

10. Rose DP. Dietary fatty acids and cancer. *Am J Clin Nutr* 66(suppl.): 998S–1003S, 1997.

## Folic Acid

1. Oakley GP Jr, Adams MJ, and Dickinson CM . More folic acid for everyone, now. *J Nutr* 126(3): 751S–755S, 1996.

2. Werbach, M. Foundations of nutritional medicine. Tarzana, CA: Third Line Press, 1997: 55–57.

3. Werbach, M. Foundations of nutritional medicine. Tarzana, CA: Third Line Press, 1997: 205–247.

4. Holt GA. Food and drug interactions. Chicago: Precept Press, 1998.

5. Russell RM, et al. Impairment of folic acid absorption by oral pancreatic extracts. *Dig Dis Sci* 25: 369–373, 1980.

6. Werler MM, Shapiro S, and Mitchell AA. Periconceptional folic acid exposure and risk of occurrent neural tube defects. *JAMA* 269: 1257–1261, 1993.

7. Milunsky A, et al. Multivitamin/folic acid supplementation in early pregnancy reduces the prevalence of neural tube defects. *JAMA* 262: 2847–2852, 1989.

8. Rimm EB, et al. Folate and vitamin $B_6$ from diet and supplements in relation to risk of coronary heart disease among women. *JAMA* 279: 359–364, 1998.

9. Moghadasian MH, et al. Homocysteine and coronary artery disease. *Arch Intern Med* 157: 2299–2308, 1997.

10. Ubbink JB, et al. Hyperhomocysteinemia and the response to vitamin supplementation. *Clin Invest* 71: 993–998, 1993.

11. den Heijer M, Brouwer IA, and Bos GM. Vitamin supplementation reduces blood homocysteine levels: a controlled trial in patients with venous thrombosis and healthy volunteers. *Arterioscler Thromb Vasc Biol* 18: 356–361, 1998.

12. Ward M, McNulty H, and McPartlin J. Plasma homocysteine, a risk factor for cardiovascular disease, is lowered by physiological doses of folic acid. *QJM* 90: 519–524, 1997.

13. Graham IM, et al. Plasma homocysteine as a risk factor for vascular disease. The European Concerted Action Project. *JAMA* 277: 1775–1781, 1997.

14. Oakley GP Jr, Adams MJ, and Dickinson CM . More folic acid for everyone, now. *J Nutr* 126(3): 751S–755S, 1996.

15. Butterworth CE Jr. Effect of folate on cervical cancer. Synergism among risk factors. *Ann N Y Acad Sci* 669: 293–299, 1992.

16. Kim Y-I, Mason JB, et al. Folate, epithelial dysplasia and colon cancer. *Proc Assoc Am Physicians* 107: 218–227, 1995.

17. Heimberger DC. Localized deficiencies of folic acid in aerodigestive tissues. *Ann N Y Acad Sci* 669: 87–96, 1992.

18. Heimberger DC. Localized deficiencies of folic acid in aerodigestive tissues. *Ann N Y Acad Sci* 669: 87–96, 1992.

19. Butterworth CE Jr. Effect of folate on cervical cancer. Synergism among risk factors. *Ann N Y Acad Sci* 669: 293–299, 1992.

20. Zarcone R, Bellini P, Carfora E, et al. Folic acid and cervix dysplasia. *Minerva Ginecol* 48: 397–400, 1996.

21. Childers JM, Chu J, Voigt LF, et al. Chemoprevention of cervical cancer with folic acid: a phase III Southwest Oncology Group Intergroup study. *Cancer Epidemiol Biomarkers Prev* 4: 155–159, 1995.

22. Oster KA. Evaluation of serum cholesterol reduction and xanthine oxidase inhibition in the treatment of atherosclerosis. *Recent Adv Stud Cardiac Struct Metab* 3: 73–80, 1973.

23. Boss GR, et al. Failure of folic acid (pteroylglutamic acid) to affect hyperuricemia. *J Lab Clin Med* 96: 783, 1980.

24. Blouvier B and Duvulder B. Folic acid, xanthine oxidase, and uric acid. Letter. *Ann Intern Med* 88(2): 269, 1978.

25. Boss GR, et al. Failure of folic acid (pteroylglutamic acid) to affect hyperuricemia. *J Lab Clin Med* 96: 783, 1980.

26. Alpert JE and Fava M. Nutrition and depression: the role of folate. *Nutr Rev* 55(5): 145–149, 1997.

27. Passeri M, Cucinotta D, Abate G, et al. Oral 5'-methyltetrahydrofolic acid in senile organic mental disorders with depression: results of a double-blind multicenter study. *Aging* (Milano) 5(1): 63–71, 1993.

28. Godfrey PS, Toone BK, Carney MW, et al. Enhancement of recovery from psychiatric illness by methylfolate. *Lancet* 336: 392–395, 1990.

29. Heseker H, Kubler W, Pudel V, and Westenhoffer J. Psychological disorders as early symptoms of a mild-moderate vitamin deficiency. *Ann N Y Acad Sci* 669: 352–357, 1992.

30. Crellin R, Bottiglierei T, and Reynolds EH. Folates and psychiatric disorders. Clinical potential. *Drugs* 45(5): 623–636, 1993.

31. Brattstrom LE, Hultberg BL, and Hardebo JE. Folic acid responsive postmenopausal homocysteinemia. *Metabolism* 34(11): 1073–1077, 1985.

32. Botez MI. Folate deficiency and neurological disorders in adults. *Med Hypothesis* 2: 135–140, 1976.

33. Coppen A, et al. Depression and tetrahydrobiopterin: the folate connection. *J Affect Disord* 16(2–3): 103–107, 1989.

34. Flynn MA, Irvin W, and Krause G. The effect of folate and cobalamin on osteoarthritic hands. *J Am Coll Nutr* 13(4): 351–356, 1994.

35. Kremer JM and Bigaouette J. Nutrient intake of patients with rheumatoid arthritis is deficient in pyridoxine, zinc, copper, and magnesium. *J Rheumatol* 23(6): 990–994, 1996.

36. Montes LF, Diaz ML, Lajous J, and Garcia NJ. Folic acid and vitamin $B_{12}$ in vitiligo: a nutritional approach. *Cutis* 50: 39–42, 1992.

37. Werler MM, Shapiro S, and Mitchell AA. Periconceptional folic acid exposure and risk of occurrent neural tube defects. *JAMA* 269: 1257–1261, 1993.

38. Milunsky A, et al. Multivitamin/folic acid supplementation in early pregnancy reduces the prevalence of neural tube defects. *JAMA* 262: 2847–2852, 1989.

39. Rimm EB, et al. Folate and vitamin $B_6$ from diet and supplements in relation to risk of coronary heart disease among women. *JAMA* 279: 359–364, 1998.

40. Graham IM, et al. Plasma homocysteine as a risk factor for vascular disease. The European Concerted Action Project. *JAMA* 277: 1775–1781, 1997.

41. Moghadasian MH, et al. Homocysteine and coronary artery disease. *Arch Intern Med* 157: 2299–2308, 1997.

42. Ubbink JB, et al. Hyperhomocysteinemia and the response to vitamin supplementation. *Clin Invest* 71: 993–998, 1993.

43. den Heijer M, Brouwer IA, and Bos GM. Vitamin supplementation reduces blood homocysteine levels: a controlled trial in patients with venous thrombosis and healthy volunteers. *Arterioscler Thromb Vasc Biol* 18: 356–361, 1998.

44. Ward M, McNulty H, and McPartlin J. Plasma homocysteine, a risk factor for cardiovascular disease, is lowered by physiological doses of folic acid. *QJM* 90: 519–524, 1997.

45. Butterworth, CE Jr and Tamura T. Folic acid safety and toxicity. A brief review. *Am J Clin Nutr* 50: 353–358, 1989.

46. Holt GA. Food and drug interactions. Chicago: Precept Press, 1998: 207, 215.

47. Morgan SL, et al. Supplementation with folic acid during methotrexate therapy for rheumatoid arthritis: a double-blind, placebo-controlled trial. *Ann Intern Med* 121: 833–841, 1994.

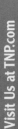

48. Duhra P. Treatment of gastrointestinal symptoms associated with methotrexate therapy for psoriasis. *J Acad Dermatol* 28: 466–469, 1993.

## Gamma Oryzanol

1. Murase Y and Iishima H. Clinical studies of oral administration of gamma-oryzanol on climacteric complaints and its syndrome. *Obstet Gynecol Prac* 12: 147–149, 1963.

2. Rong N, Ausman LM, and Nicolosi RJ. Oryzanol decreases cholesterol absorption and aortic fatty streaks in hamsters. *Lipids* 32: 303–309, 1997.

3. Sasaki J, Takada Y, Handa K, et al. Effects of gamma-oryzanol on serum lipids and apolipoproteins in dyslipidemic schizophrenics receiving major tranquilizers. *Clin Ther* 12: 263–268, 1990.

4. Rosenbloom C, Millard-Stafford M, and Lathrop J. Contemporary ergogenic aids used by strength/power athletes. *J Am Diet Assoc* 92(10): 1264–1265, 1992.

5. Murase Y and Iishima H. Clinical studies of oral administration of gamma-oryzanol on climacteric complaints and its syndrome. *Obstet Gynecol Prac* 12: 147–149, 1963.

6. Schulz V, et al. Rational phytotherapy. New York: Springer-Verlag, 1998: 246.

7. Rong N, Ausman LM, and Nicolosi RJ. Oryzanol decreases cholesterol absorption and aortic fatty streaks in hamsters. *Lipids* 32: 303–309, 1997.

8. Sasaki J, Takada Y, Handa K, et al. Effects of gamma-oryzanol on serum lipids and apolipoproteins in dyslipidemic schizophrenics receiving major tranquilizers. *Clin Ther* 12: 263–268, 1990.

## Garlic

1. Efendi JL, et al. The effect of the aged garlic extract, "kyolic," on the development of experimental atherosclerosis. *Atherosclerosis* 132(1): 37–42, 1997.

2. Schulz V, et al. Rational phytotherapy. New York: Springer-Verlag, 1998: 112.

3. Quereshi AA, et al. Inhibition of cholesterol and fatty acid biosynthesis in liver enzymes and chicken hepatocytes by polar fractions of garlic. *Lipids* 18: 343–348, 1983.

4. Gebhardt R. Multiple inhibitory effects of garlic extracts on cholesterol biosynthesis in hepatocytes. *Lipids* 28(6): 613–619, 1993.

5. Gebhardt R, et al. Inhibition of cholesterol biosynthesis by allicin and ajoene in rat hepatocytes and HepG2 cells. *Biochem Biophys Acta* 1213: 57–62, 1994.

6. Schulz V, et al. Rational phytotherapy. New York: Springer-Verlag, 1998: 113.

7. Agarwal KC, et al. Therapeutic actions of garlic constituents. *Med Res Rev* 16(1): 111–124, 1996.

8. Legnani C, et al. Effects of dried garlic preparation on fibrinolysis and platelet aggregation in healthy subjects. *Arzneimittelforschung* 43: 119–121, 1993.

9. Chutani SK, et al. The effect of dried vs. raw garlic on fibrinolytic activity in man. *Atherosclerosis* 38: 417–421, 1981.

10. Kiesewetter H, et al. Effect of garlic on thrombocyte aggregation, microcirculation, and other risk factors. *Int J Clin Pharmacol Ther Toxicol* 29: 151–155, 1991.

11. Reuter HD, et al. *Allium sativum* and *Allium ursinum:* Chemistry, pharmacology, and medical applications. *Econ Med Plant Res* 6: 56–108, 1994.

12. Popov I, et al. Antioxidant effects of aqueous garlic extract, 1st communication: Direct detection using photochemoluminescence. *Arzneimittelforschung Drug Res* 44(1): 602–604, 1994.

13. Torok B, et al. Effectiveness of garlic on radical activity in radical generating systems. *Arzneimittelforschung Drug Res* 44(1): 608–611, 1994.

14. Silagy CA, et al. A meta-analysis of the effect of garlic on blood pressure. *J Hypertens* 12(4): 463–468, 1994.

15. Warshafsky S, et al. Effect of garlic on total serum cholesterol. A meta-analysis. *Ann Intern Med* 119(7) Part 1: 599–605.

16. Mader FH. Treatment of hyperlipidaemia with garlic-powder tablets. Evidence from the German Association of General Practitioners' multicentric placebo-controlled double-blind study. *Arzneimittelforschung* 40(10): 1111–1116, 1990.

17. Steiner M, et al. A double-blind crossover study in moderately hypercholesterolemic men that compared the effect of aged garlic extract and placebo administration on blood lipids. *Am J Clin Nutr* 64(6): 866–870, 1996.

18. Holzgartner H, et al. Comparison of the efficacy and tolerance of a garlic preparation vs. bezafibrate. *Arzneimittelforschung* 42(12): 1473–1477, 1992.

19. Neil HA, et al. Garlic powder in the treatment of moderate hyperlipidaemia: A controlled trial and meta-analysis. *J R Coll Physicians Lond* 30(4): 329–334, 1996.

20. Simons LA, et al. On the effect of garlic on plasma lipids and lipoproteins in mild hypercholesterolaemia. *Atherosclerosis* 113(2): 219–225, 1995.

21. Santos OS de A, et al. Effects of garlic powder and garlic oil preparations on blood lipids, blood pressure and well being. *Br J Clin Res* 6: 91–100, 1995.

22. Silagy CA, et al. A meta-analysis of the effect of garlic on blood pressure. *J Hypertens* 12(4): 463–468, 1994.

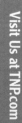

23. Schulz V, et al. Rational phytotherapy. New York: Springer-Verlag, 1998: 119.

24. Auer W, et al. Hypertension and hyperlipidemia: Garlic helps in mild cases. *Br J Clin Pract Symp* 69 (Suppl.): 3–6, 1990.

25. Santos OS de A, et al. Effects of garlic powder and garlic oil preparations on blood lipids, blood pressure and well being. *Br J Clin Res* 6: 91–100, 1995.

26. Breithaupt-Grogler K, et al. Protective effect of chronic garlic intake on the elastic properties of the aorta in the elderly. *Circulation* 96(7): 2649–2655, 1997.

27. Bordia A. Knoblauch und koronare Herzkrankheit: Wirkungen einer Dreijahrigen Behandlung mit Knoblauchextrakt auf die Reinfarkt-und Mortalitatsrate. *Dtsch Apoth Ztg* 129(Suppl. 15): 16–17. As reported in the ESCOP monographs. Fascicule 3: *Allii sativi bulbus* (garlic). Exeter, UK: European Scientific Cooperative on Phytotherapy, 1997: 4.

28. Steinmetz KA, et al. Vegetables, fruit, and colon cancer in the Iowa Women's Health Study. *Am J Epidemiol* 139(1): 1–13, 1994.

29. Ernst E. Can allium vegetables prevent cancer? *Phytomedicine* 4(1): 79–83, 1997.

30. Agarwal KC, et al. Therapeutic actions of garlic constituents. *Med Res Rev* 16(1): 111–124, 1996.

31. Nagai K. Experimental studies on the preventive effect of garlic extract against infection with influenza virus. *Jpn J Infect Dis* 47: 321, 1973.

32. Chowdhury AK, et al. Efficacy of aqueous extract of garlic and allicin in experimental shigellosis in rabbits. *Indian J Med Res* 93: 33–36, 1991.

33. Sharma VD, et al. Antibacterial property of *Allium sativum* Linn.: In vivo and in vitro studies. *Indian J Exp Biol* 15(6): 466–468, 1977.

34. Hunan Hospital. Garlic in cryptococcal meningitis. A preliminary report of 21 cases. *Chin Med J* 93: 123–126, 1980.

35. Caporaso N, et al. Antifungal activity in human urine and serum after ingestion of garlic (*Allium sativum*). *Antimicrob Agents Chemother* 23(5): 700–702, 1983.

36. Sumiyoshi H, et al. Chronic toxicity test of garlic extracts in rats. *J Toxicol Sci* 9: 61–75, 1984.

37. Schulz V, et al. Rational phytotherapy. New York: Springer-Verlag, 1998: 121.

38. Schulz V, et al. Rational phytotherapy. New York: Springer-Verlag, 1998: 121.

## Gentian

1. Lininger S, et al. The natural pharmacy. Rocklin, CA: Prima Publishing, 1998: 267.

2. Newall C, et al. Herbal medicines: A guide for healthcare professionals. London: Pharmaceutical Press, 1996: 134.

## Ginger

1. Tyler V. Herbs of choice. New York: Haworth Press, 1994: 42.

2. Holtman S, et al. The anti-motion sickness mechanism of ginger. *Acta Otolaryngol* 108: 168–174, 1989.

3. Mowrey DB. Motion sickness, ginger, and psychophysics. *Lancet* i: 655–657, 1982.

4. ESCOP monographs. Fascicule 1: *Zingiberis rhizoma* (ginger). Exeter, UK: European Scientific Cooperative on Phytotherapy, 1997.

5. Grontved A, et al. Ginger root against seasickness. A controlled trial on the open sea. *Acta Otolaryngol* (Stockh) 105: 45–49, 1988.

6. Stott JRR, et al. A double-blind comparative trial of powdered ginger root, hyosine (sic) hydrobromide and cinnarizine in the prophylaxis of motion sickness induced by cross coupled stimulation. Advisory Group for Aerospace Research and Development, Conference Proceedings 372 (39):1–6, 1985.

7. Stewart JJ, et al. Effects of ginger on motion sickness susceptibility and gastric function. *Pharmacology* 42: 111–120, 1991.

8. Wood CD, et al. Comparison of efficacy of ginger with various antimotion sickness drugs. *Clin Res Pract Drug Reg Aff* 6:129–136, 1988.

9. Fischer-Rasmussen W, et al. Ginger treatment of hyperemesis gravidarum. *Eur J Obstet Gynecol Reprod Biol* 38: 19–24, 1990.

10. Bone ME, et al. Ginger root: A new anti-emetic. The effect of ginger root on postoperative nausea and vomiting after major gynecological surgery. *Anaesthesia* 45: 669–671, 1990.

11. Phillips S, et al. *Zingiber officinale* (ginger)—An anti-emetic for day case surgery. *Anaesthesia* 48: 715–717, 1993.

12. Arfeen Z, et al. A double-blind randomized controlled trial of ginger for the prevention of postoperative nausea and vomiting. *Anaesth Intensive Care* 23(4): 449–452, 1995.

13. Visalyaputra S, et al. The efficacy of ginger root in the prevention of postoperative nausea and vomiting after outpatient gynaecological laparoscopy. *Anaesthesia* 53: 506–510, 1998.

14. Srivastava KC. Isolation and effects of some ginger components on platelet aggregation and eicosanoid biosynthesis. *Prostaglandins Leukot Med* 25: 187–198, 1986.

15. Srivastava K. Effects of aqueous extracts of onion, garlic, and ginger on the platelet aggregation and metabolism of arachidonic acid in the blood vascular system: In vitro study. *Prostaglandins Leukot Med* 13: 227–235, 1984.

16. Srivastava KC. Effect of onion and ginger consumption on platelet thromboxane production in humans. *Prostaglandiins Leukot Essent Fatty Acids* 35: 183–185, 1989.

17. Janssen PL, et al. Consumption of ginger (*Zingiber officinale* Roscoe) does not affect ex vivo platelet thromboxane production in humans. *Eur J Clin Nutr* 50(11): 772–774, 1996.

18. Bordia A, et al. Effect of ginger (*Zingiber officinale* Rosc.) and fenugreek (*Trigonella foenumgraecum* L.) on blood lipids, blood sugar and platelet aggregation in patients with coronary artery disease. *Prostaglandins Leukot Essent Fatty Acids* 56(5): 379–384, 1997.

19. Lumb AB. Effect of dried ginger on human platelet function. *Thromb Haemost* 71: 110–111, 1994.

## Ginkgo

1. Schulz V, et al. Rational phytotherapy. New York: Springer-Verlag, 1998: 288–292.

2. Tamborini A, et al. Value of standardized *Ginkgo biloba* extract (EGb 761) in the management of congestive symptoms of premenstrual syndrome. *Rev Fr Gynecol Obstet* 88: 447–457, 1993.

3. Schulz V, et al. Rational phytotherapy. New York: Springer-Verlag, 1998: 41.

4. Jung F, et al. Effect of *Ginkgo biloba* on fluidity of blood and peripheral microcirculation in volunteers. *Arzneimittelforschung Drug Res* 40: 589–593, 1990.

5. De Feudis FV. *Ginkgo biloba* extract (EGb 761): Pharmacological activities and clinical applications. Paris: Elsevier, 1991: 143–146.

6. Kleijnen J and Knipschild P. *Ginkgo biloba*. *Lancet* 340: 1136–1139, 1992.

7. Schulz V, et al. Rational phytotherapy. New York: Springer-Verlag, 1998: 41.

8. Kleijnen J and Knipschild P. *Ginkgo biloba*. *Lancet* 340: 1136–1139, 1992

9. Kanowski S, et al. Proof of efficacy of the *Ginkgo biloba* special extract EGb 761 in outpatients suffering from mild to moderate primary degenerative dementia of the Alzheimer type or multi-infarct dementia. *Pharmacopsychiatry* 29: 47–56, 1996.

10. Hofferberth B. The efficacy of EGb 761 in patients with senile dementia of the Alzheimer type, a double-blind, placebo-controlled study on different levels of investigation. *Hum Psychopharmacol* 9: 215–222, 1994.

11. Schulz V, et al. Rational phytotherapy. New York: Springer-Verlag, 1998: 46.

12. LeBars PL, et al. A placebo-controlled, double-blind, randomized trial of an extract of *Ginkgo biloba* for dementia. *JAMA* 278: 1327–1332, 1997.

13. Winther K, Randlov C, Rein E, et al. Effect of *Ginkgo biloba* extract on cognitive function and blood pressure in elderly subjects. *Current Ther Res* 59: 881–888, 1998.

14. Schulz V, et al. Rational phytotherapy. New York: Springer-Verlag, 1998: 126.

15. Peters H, Kieser M, and Holscher U. Demonstration of the efficacy of *Ginkgo biloba* special extract EGb 761 on intermittent claudication—A placebo-controlled double-blind multicenter trial. *Vasa* 27: 106–110, 1998.

16. Tamborini A, et al. Value of standardized *Ginkgo biloba* extract (EGb 761) in the management of congestive symptoms of premenstrual syndrome. *Rev Fr Gynecol Obstet* 88: 447–457, 1993.

17. Lebuisson DA, et al. Treatment of senile macular degeneration with *Ginkgo biloba* extract: A preliminary double-blind, drug vs. placebo study. *Presse Med* 15: 1556–1558, 1986.

18. Cohen A, et al. Treatment of sexual dysfunction with *Ginkgo biloba* extract. Scientific Reports—Paper session from the proceedings of the APA annual meeting. 1997.

19. De Feudis FV. *Ginkgo biloba* extract (EGb 761): Pharmacological activities and clinical applications. Paris: Elsevier, 1991: 143–146

20. De Feudis FV. *Ginkgo biloba* extract (EGb 761): Pharmacological activities and clinical applications. Paris: Elsevier, 1991: 143–146

21. Schulz V, et al. Rational phytotherapy. New York: Springer-Verlag, 1998: 247.

22. Rosenblatt M and Mindel J. Spontaneous hyphema associated with ingestion of *Ginkgo biloba* extract. *N Engl J Med* 336(15): 1108, 1997.

23. Rowin J and Lewis SL. Spontaneous bilateral subdural hematomas associated with chronic *Ginkgo biloba* ingestion. *Neurology* 46: 1775–1776, 1996.

## Ginseng

1. Yoshimura H, Kumura N, and Sugiura K. Preventive effects of various ginseng saponins on the development of copulatory disorder induced by prolonged individual housing in male mice. *Methods Find Exp Clin Pharmcol* 20(1): 59–64, 1998.

2. Yun TK and Choi SY. Non-organ specific cancer prevention of ginseng: A prospective study in Korea. *Int J Epidemiol* 27: 359–364, 1998.

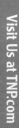

3. Takahashi M and Takuyama S. Pharmacological and physiological effects of ginseng on actions induced by opioids and psychostimulants. *Methods Find Exp Clin Pharmacol* 20(1): 77–84, 1998.

4. Schulz V, et al. Rational phytotherapy. New York: Springer-Verlag, 1998: 271, 273.

5. Brekhman II. *Eleutheroccoccus*: 20 years of research and clinical application. Presented at the 1st International symposium on *eleutherococcus*, Hamburg, Germany, 1980. In Brown D. Herbal prescriptions for better health. Rocklin, CA: Prima Publishing, 1997.

6. Brekhman II. *Eleutherococcus*: Clinical data. USSR Foreign Trade Publication. Medexport, 1970. In Brown D. Herbal prescriptions for better health. Rocklin, CA: Prima Publishing 1997.

7. Sonnenborn U, et al. Ginseng (*Panax ginseng* C.A. Meyer). *Z Phytother* 11: 35–49, 1990.

8. Schulz V, et al. Rational phytotherapy. New York: Springer-Verlag, 1998: 271, 273.

9. Scaglione F, et al. Efficacy and safety of the standardised ginseng extract G115 for potentiating vaccination against the influenza syndrome and protection against the common cold. *Drugs Exp Clin Res* 22(2): 65–72, 1996.

10. Sotaneimi EA, et al. Ginseng therapy in non-insulin–dependent diabetic patients. *Diabetes Care* 18(10): 1373–1375, 1995.

11. Sorenson H, et al. A double-masked study of the effects of ginseng on cognitive functions. *Curr Ther Res Clin Exp* 57(12): 959–968, 1996.

12. Dowling EA, et al. Effect of *Eleutherococcus senticosus* on submaximal and maximal exercise performance. *Med Sci Sports Exerc* 28(4): 482–489, 1996.

13. Enles HJ and Wirth JC. No ergogenic effects of ginseng (*Panax ginseng*, C.A. Meyer) during graded maximal aerobic exercise. *J Am Diet Assoc* 97: 1110–1115, 1997.

14. Yun TK and Choi SY. Non-organ specific cancer prevention of ginseng: A prospective study in Korea. *Int J Epidemiol* 27: 359–364, 1998.

15. Awang, DVC. Maternal use of ginseng and neonatal andiogenization. *JAMA* 266: 363, 1991.

16. Ploss E. *Panax ginseng*. C. A. Meyer. Scientific report. Cologne: Kooperation Phytopharmaka, 1988.

17. Lawrence Review of Natural Products. Ginseng monograph. St. Louis, Missouri: Facts and Comparisons Division, J.B. Lipincott Company, 1990.

18. Tyler V. Herbs of choice. New York: Haworth Press, 1994.

19. Siegel RK. *JAMA* 241: 1614–1615, 1979.

20. Tyler V. Herbs of choice. New York: Haworth Press, 1994.

21. Schulz V, et al. Rational phytotherapy. New York: Springer-Verlag, 1998.

22. Kroll D, University of Colorado School of Pharmacy. Unpublished communication. 1998.

23. Jones BD, et al. Interaction of ginseng with phenelzine. *J Clin Psychopharmacol* 7: 201–202, 1987.

24. McCrae S. Elevated serum digoxin levels in a patient taking digoxin and Siberian ginseng. *Can Med Assoc J* 155(3): 293–295, 1996.

25. Janetzky K and Morreale AP. Probable interaction between warfarin and ginseng. *Am J Health Syst Pharm* 54: 692–693, 1997.

## GLA (Gamma-Linolenic Acid)

1. Horrobin DF. Nutritional and medical importance of gamma-linolenic acid. *Prog Lipid Res* 31: 163–194, 1992.

2. Horrobin DF. The use of gamma-linolenic acid in diabetic neuropathy. *Agents Actions* 37(Suppl.): 120–144, 1992.

3. Horrobin DF, et al. Evening primrose oil in atopic eczema. Letter. *Lancet* 1: 864–865, 1990.

4. Horrobin DF, et al. Abnormalities in plasma essential fatty acid levels in women with premenstrual syndrome and with nonmalignant breast disease. *J Nutr Med* 2: 259–264, 1991.

5. Jenkins DK, et al. Effects of different sources of gamma-linolenic acid on the formation of essential fatty acids and prostanoid metabolism. *Med Sci Res* 16: 525–526, 1988.

6. Manku MS. Essential fatty acids in the plasma phospholipids of patients with atopic eczema. *Br J Dermatol* 110: 643–648, 1984.

7. Pye JK, Mansel RE, and Hughes LE. Clinical experience of drug treatments for mastalgia. *Lancet* 2: 373–377, 1985.

8. Pashby NL, Mansel RE, Hughes LE, Hanslip J, and Preece PE. A clinical trial of evening primrose oil in mastalgia. *Br J Surg* 68: 801, 1981.

9. Mansel RE, et al. Effect and tolerability of n-6 essential fatty acid supplementation in patients with recurrent breast cysts—a randomized double-blind placebo-controlled trial. *J Nutr Med* 1: 195–200, 1990.

10. Mansel RE, et al. A randomized trial of dietary intervention with essential fatty acids in patients with categorized cysts. *Ann N Y Acad Sci* 586: 288–294, 1990.

11. Drug evaluations subscription, vol. 2. Endocrine Drugs 6: 6. Chicago, Illinois: American Medical Association, 1991.

12. Budeiri D, et al. Is evening primrose oil of value in the treatment of premenstrual syndrome? *Control Clin Trials* 17: 60–68, 1996.

13. Keen H, Payan J, Allawi J, et al. Treatment of diabetic neuropathy with gamma-linolenic acid. The Gamma-Linolenic Acid Multicenter Trial Group. *Diabet Care* 16: 8–15 1993.

14. Jamal GA and Carmichael H. The effect of gamma-linolenic acid on human diabetic peripheral neuropathy: a double-blind placebo-controlled trial. *Diabet Med* 7: 319–323, 1990.

15. Morse PF, et al. Meta-analysis of placebo-controlled studies of the efficacy of Epogam in the treatment of atopic eczema. Relationship between plasma essential fatty acid changes and clinical response. *Br J Dermatol* 121: 75–90, 1989.

16. Sharpe GR, et al. Evening primrose oil and eczema. *Lancet* 335: 1283, 1990.

17. Hederos CA, et al. Epogam evening primrose oil treatment in atopic dermatitis and asthma. *Arch Dis Child* 75: 494–497, 1996.

18. Zurier RB, Rossetti RG, Jacobson EW, et al. Gamma-linolenic acid treatment of rheumatoid arthritis. A randomized, placebo-controlled trial. *Arthritis Rheum* 39: 1808–1817, 1996.

19. Leventhal LJ, Boyce EG, and Zurier RB. Treatment of rheumatoid arthritis with black currant seed oil. *Br J Rheumatol* 33: 847–852, 1994.

20. Leventhal LJ, Boyce EG, and Zurier RB. Treatment of rheumatoid arthritis with gamma linolenic acid. *Ann Intern Med* 119: 867–873, 1993.

21. Rothman D, et al. Botanical lipids: Effects on inflammation, immune responses and rheumatoid arthritis. *Sem Arthritis Rheum* 25: 87–96, 1995.

22. Belch JJF, et al. Evening primrose oil (Efamol) as a treatment for cold-induced vasospasm (Raynaud's phenomenon). *Prog Lipid Res* 25: 335–340, 1986.

23. Belch JJF, et al. Evening primrose oil (Efamol) in the treatment of Raynaud's phenomenon: A double-blind study. *Thromb Haemost* 54: 490–494, 1985.

24. Kruger MC, et al. Calcium, gamma-linolenic acid (GLA) and eicosapentaenoic acid (EPA) supplementation in osteoporosis. *Osteopor Int* 6(suppl. 1): 250, 1996.

25. van Papendorp DH, Coetzer H, Kruger MC. Biochemical profile of osteoporotic patients on essential fatty acid supplementation. *Nutr Res* 15: 325–334, 1995.

26. Horrobin DF, et al. Abnormalities in plasma essential fatty acid levels in women with premenstrual syndrome and with nonmalignant breast disease. *J Nutr Med* 2: 259–264, 1991.

27. Horrobin DF, et al. Abnormalities in plasma essential fatty acid levels in women with premenstrual syndrome and with nonmalignant breast disease. *J Nutr Med* 2: 259–264, 1991.

28. Pye JK, Mansel RE, and Hughes LE. Clinical experience of drug treatments for mastalgia. *Lancet* 2: 373–377, 1985.

29. Pashby NL, Mansel RE, Hughes LE, Hanslip J, and Preece PE. A clinical trial of evening primrose oil in mastalgia. *Br J Surg* 68: 801, 1981.

30. Mansel RE, et al. Effect and tolerability of n-6 essential fatty acid supplementation in patients with recurrent breast cysts—a randomized double-blind placebo-controlled trial. *J Nutr Med* 1: 195–200, 1990.

31. Mansel RE, et al. A randomized trial of dietary intervention with essential fatty acids in patients with categorized cysts. *Ann N Y Acad Sci* 586: 288–294, 1990.

32. Budeiri D, et al. Is evening primrose oil of value in the treatment of premenstrual syndrome? *Control Clin Trials* 17: 60–68, 1996.

33. Keen H, Payan J, Allawi J, et al. Treatment of diabetic neuropathy with gamma-linolenic acid. The Gamma-Linolenic Acid Multicenter Trial Group. *Diabet Care* 16: 8–15 1993.

34. Jamal GA and Carmichael H. The effect of gamma-linolenic acid on human diabetic peripheral neuropathy: a double-blind placebo-controlled trial. *Diabet Med* 7: 319–323, 1990.

35. Stevens EJ, et al. Essential fatty acid treatment prevents nerve ischaemia and associated conduction anomalies in rats with experimental diabetes mellitus. *Diabetologia* 36(5): 397–401, 1993.

36. Reichert RG. Evening primrose oil and diabetic neuropathy. *Q Rev Natl Med* Summer: 141–145, 1995.

37. Hounsom L, et al. A lipoic acid—gamma-linolenic acid conjugate is effective against multiple indices of experimental diabetic neuropathy. *Diabetologia* 41(7): 839–843, 1998.

38. Cameron NE, et al. Effects of alpha-lipoic acid on neurovascular function in diabetic rats. Interaction with essential fatty acids. *Diabetologia* 41(4): 390–399, 1998.

39. Morse PF, et al. Meta-analysis of placebo-controlled studies of the efficacy of Epogam in the treatment of atopic eczema. Relationship between plasma essential fatty acid changes and clinical response. *Br J Dermatol* 121: 75–90, 1989.

40. Sharpe GR, et al. Evening primrose oil and eczema. *Lancet* 335: 1283, 1990.

41. Biagi PL, Bordoni A, Hrelia S, et al. The effect of gamma-linolenic acid on clinical status, red cell fatty acid composition and membrane microviscosity in infants with atopic dermatitis. *Drugs Exp Clin Res* 20(Suppl. 2): 77–84, 1994.

42. Hederos CA, et al. Epogam evening primrose oil treatment in atopic dermatitis and asthma. *Arch Dis Child* 75: 494–497, 1996.

43. Horrobin DF, et al. Evening primrose oil in atopic eczema. Letter. *Lancet* 1: 864–865, 1990.

44. Zurier RB, Rossetti RG, Jacobson EW, et al. Gamma-linolenic acid treatment of rheumatoid arthritis. A randomized, placebo-controlled trial. *Arthritis Rheum* 39: 1808–1817, 1996.

45. Leventhal LJ, Boyce EG, and Zurier RB. Treatment of rheumatoid arthritis with black currant seed oil. *Br J Rheumatol* 33: 847–852, 1994.

46. Leventhal LJ, Boyce EG, and Zurier RB. Treatment of rheumatoid arthritis with gamma linolenic acid. *Ann Intern Med* 119: 867–873, 1993.

47. Rothman D, et al. Botanical lipids: Effects on inflammation, immune responses and rheumatoid arthritis. *Sem Arthritis Rheum* 25: 87–96, 1995.

48. Belch JJF, et al. Evening primrose oil (Efamol) as a treatment for cold-induced vasospasm (Raynaud's phenomenon). *Prog Lipid Res* 25: 335–340, 1986.

49. Belch JJF, et al. Evening primrose oil (Efamol) in the treatment of Raynaud's phenomenon: A double-blind study. *Thromb Haemost* 54: 490–494, 1985.

50. Kruger MC, et al. Calcium, gamma-linolenic acid (GLA) and eicosapentaenoic acid (EPA) supplementation in osteoporosis. *Osteopor Int* 6(suppl. 1): 250, 1996.

51. van Papendorp DH, Coetzer H, Kruger MC. Biochemical profile of osteoporotic patients on essential fatty acid supplementation. *Nutr Res* 15: 325–334, 1995.

52. Horrobin DF. Nutritional and medical importance of gamma-linolenic acid. *Prog Lipid Res* 31: 163–194, 1992.

53. Horrobin DF, et al. Gamma-linolenic acid: An intermediate in essential fatty acid metabolism with potential as an ethical pharmaceutical and as a food. *Rev Contemp Pharmacother* 1: 1–45, 1990.

54. Horrobin DF. Essential fatty acids in the management of impaired nerve function in diabetes. *Diabetes* 46(Suppl. 2): S90–S93, 1997.

55. Vaddad KS. The use of gamma-linolenic acid and linoleic acid to differentiate between temporal lobe epilepsy and schizophrenia. *Prostaglandins Med* 6: 375–379, 1981.

56. Horrobin DF. The regulation of prostaglandin biosynthesis by the manipulation of essential fatty acid metabolism. *Rev Pure Appl Pharmacol* 4: 339–383, 1983.

## Glucosamine

1. Brandt KD. Effects of nonsteroidal anti-inflammatory drugs on chondrocyte metabolism in vitro and in vivo. *Am J Med* 83 (Suppl. 5A): 29–34, 1987.

2. Brooks PM, et al. NSAID and osteoarthritis—help or hindrance. *J Rheumatol* 9: 3–5, 1982.

3. Shield MJ, Anti-inflammatory drugs and their effects on cartilage synthesis and renal function. *Eur J Rheumatol Inflam* 13: 7–16, 1993.

4. Palmoski MJ, et al. Effects of some nonsteroidal anti-inflammatory drugs on proteoglycan metabolism and organization in canine articular cartilage. *Arthritis Rheum* 23: 1010–1020, 1980.

5. Rahad S, et al. Effect of non-steroidal anti-inflammatory drugs on the course of osteoarthritis. *Lancet* 2: 519–522, 1989.

6. Noack W, et al. Glucosamine sulfate in osteoarthritis of the knee. *Osteoarthritis Cartilage* 2: 51–59, 1994.

7. Rovati LC, et al. A large, randomized, placebo-controlled, double-blind study of glucosamine sulfate vs. piroxicam and vs. their association, on the kinetics of the symptomatic effect in knee osteoarthritis. *Osteoarthritis Cartilage* 2(Suppl.1): 56, 1994.

8. Rovati LC. The practical clinical development of a selective drug for osteoarthritis: glucosamine sulfate. Madrid, Spain: The Ninth Eular Symposium, 1996: 4–7.

9. Qiu GX, et al. Efficacy and safety of glucosamine sulfate versus ibuprofen in patients with knee osteoarthritis. *Arzneimittelforschung* 48: 469–474, 1998.

10. Muller-Fassbender H, et al. Glucosamine sulfate compared to ibuprofen in osteoarthritis of the knee. *Osteoarthritis Cartilage* 2: 61–69, 1994.

11. Noack W, et al. Glucosamine sulfate in osteoarthritis of the knee. *Osteoarthritis Cartilage* 2: 51–59, 1994.

12. Rovati LC, et al. A large, randomized, placebo controlled, double-blind study of glucosamine sulfate vs. piroxicam and vs. their association, on the kinetics of the symptomatic effect in knee osteoarthritis. *Osteoarthritis Cartilage* 2(Suppl.1): 56, 1994.

13. Rovati LC. The practical clinical development of a selective drug for osteoarthritis: glucosamine sulfate. Madrid, Spain: The Ninth Eular Symposium, 1996: 4–7.

14. Qiu GX, et al. Efficacy and safety of glucosamine sulfate versus ibuprofen in patients with knee osteoarthritis. *Arzneimittelforschung* 48: 469–474, 1998.

15. Muller-Fassbender H, et al. Glucosamine sulfate compared to ibuprofen in osteoarthritis of the knee. *Osteoarthritis Cartilage* 2: 61–69, 1994.

16. Jimenez SA, et al. The effects of glucosamine on human chondrocyte gene expression, Madrid, Spain: The Ninth Eular Symposium, 8–10, 1996.

17. Hellio MP, et al. The effects of glucosamine on human osteoarthritic chondrocytes. In vitro investigations. Madrid, Spain: The Ninth Eular Symposium, 11–12, 1996.

18. Setnikar I, et al. Anti-arthritic effects of glucosamine sulfate studied in animal models. *Arzneimittelforschung* 41: 542–545, 1991.

19. Setnikar I. Antireactive properties of "chondroprotective" drugs. *Int J Tissue React* 14 (5): 253–261, 1992.

20. Crolle G and D'Este E. Glucosamine sulfate for the management of arthritis: A controlled clinical investigation. *Curr Med Res Opin* 7(2): 104–109, 1980.

21. Qiu GX, et al. Efficacy and safety of glucosamine sulfate versus ibuprofen in patients with knee osteoarthritis. *Arzneimittelforschung* 48: 469–474, 1998.

## Glutamine

1. Griffiths RD, Jones C, Palmer TE. Six-month outcome of critically ill patients given glutamine-supplemented parenteral nutrition. *Nutrition* 13: 295–302, 1997.

2. Van Der Hulst, RRJ, et al. Glutamine and the preservation of gut integrity. *Lancet* 341: 1363–1365, 1993.

3. Zoli G, et al. Effect of oral glutamine on intestinal permeability and nutritional status in Crohn's disease (Abstract). *Gastroenterology* 106: A766, 1995.

4. Griffiths RD, Jones C, Palmer TE. Six-month outcome of critically ill patients given glutamine-supplemented parenteral nutrition. *Nutrition* 13: 295–302, 1997.

## Goldenrod

1. Tyler V. Herbs of choice. New York: Haworth Press, 1994: 74–75.

2. ESCOP monographs. Fascicule 2: *Solidaginis virgaureae herba* (goldenrod). Exeter, UK: European Scientific Cooperative on Phytotherapy, 1996: 1–3.

3. ESCOP monographs. Fascicule 2: *Solidaginis virgaureae herba* (goldenrod). Exeter, UK: European Scientific Cooperative on Phytotherapy, 1996: 2.

4. ESCOP monographs. Fascicule 2: *Solidaginis virgaureae herba* (goldenrod). Exeter, UK: European Scientific Cooperative on Phytotherapy, 1996: 2.

## Goldenseal

1. Hahn FE, et al. Berberine. *Antibiotics* 3: 577–588, 1976.

2. Amin AH, et al. Berberine sulfate: Antimicrobial activity, bioassay, and mode of action. *Can J Microbiol* 15: 1067–1076, 1969.

3. Bensky D and Gamble H. Chinese herbal medicine: Materia medica. Seattle, WA: Eastland Press, 1986.

4. Bergner P. The healing power of echinacea and goldenseal. Rocklin, CA: Prima Publishing, 1997.

5. Bergner P. The healing power of echinacea and goldenseal. Rocklin, CA: Prima Publishing, 1997.

6. Foster S. Botanical Series No. 309: Goldenseal. Austin, TX: American Botanical Council, 1991: 5–6.

7. DeSmet PAGM, et al., eds. Adverse effects of herbal drugs. Berlin: Springer-Verlag, 1992: 97–104.

## Gotu Kola

1. Kartnig T. Clinical applications of *Centella asiatica* (L.) Urb. *Herbs Spices Med Plants* 3: 146–173, 1988.

2. Nalini K, et al. Effect of *Centella asiatica* fresh leaf aqueous extract on learning and memory and biogenic amine turnover in albino rats. *Fitoterapia* 63(3): 232–237, 1992.

3. Belcaro GV, et al. Capillary filtration and ankle edema in patients with venous hypertension treated with TTFCA. *Angiology* 41: 12–18, 1990.

4. Cesarone MR, et al. The microcirculatory activity of *Centella asiatica* in venous insufficiency: A double-blind study. *Minerva Cardioangiol* 42: 299–304, 1994.

5. Pointel JP, et al. Titrated extract of *Centella asiatica* (TECA) in the treatment of venous insufficiency of the lower limbs. *Angiology* 38: 46–50, 1987.

6. Cesarone MR, et al. Activity of *Centella asiatica* in venous insufficiency. *Minerva Cardioangiol* 42: 137–143, 1992.

7. Murray M. The healing power of herbs. Rocklin, CA: Prima Publishing, 1995: 177.

8. Bosse JP, et al. Clinical study of a new antikeloid drug. *Ann Plast Surg* 3: 13–21, 1979.

9. Kartnig T. Clinical applications of *Centella asiatica* (L.) Urb. *Herbs Spices Med Plants* 3: 146–173, 1988.

10. Laerum OD, et al. Reticuloses and epidermal tumors in hairless mice after topical skin applications of cantharidin and asiaticoside. *Cancer Res* 32: 1463–1469, 1972.

11. Bosse JP, et al. Clinical study of a new antikeloid drug. *Ann Plast Surg* 3: 13–21, 1979.

12. Basellini A, et al. Varicose disease in pregnancy. *Ann Obstet Gyn Med Perinat* 106: 337–341, 1985.

## Green Tea

1. Snow J. Herbal monograph: *Camellia sinensi* (L.) Kuntze (Theaceae) protocol. *J Botanical Medicine* Autumn: 47–51, 1995.

2. Imai K, et al. Cancer-preventive effects of drinking green tea among a Japanese population. *Prev Med* 26(6): 769–775, 1997.

3. Kohlmeier L, et al. Tea and cancer prevention: An evaluation of the epidemiologic literature. *Nutr Cancer* 27(1): 1–13, 1997.

## Guggul

1. Satyavati GV. Gum guggul (*Commiphor mukul*)—The success story of an ancient insight leading to a modern discovery. *Indian J Med Res* 87: 327–335, 1988.

2. Nityanand S, et al. Clinical trials with gugulipid. A new hypolipidaemic agent. *J Assoc Physicians India* 37(5): 323–328, 1989.

3. Agarwal RC, et al. Clinical trial of gugulipid—a new hyperlipidemic agent of plant origin in primary hyperlipidemia. *Indian J Med Res* 84: 626–634, 1986.

4. Nityanand S, et al. Clinical trials with gugulipid. A new hypolipidaemic agent. *J Assoc Physicians India* 37(5): 323–328, 1989.

5. Agarwal RC, et al. Clinical trial of gugulipid—a new hyperlipidemic agent of plant origin in primary hyperlipidemia. *Indian J Med Res* 84: 626–634, 1986.

6. Satyavati GV. Gum guggul (*Commiphor mukul*)—The success story of an ancient insight leading to a modern discovery. *Indian J Med Res* 87: 327–335, 1988.

7. Newall C, et al. Herbal medicines: A guide for healthcare professionals. London: Pharmaceutical Press, 1996: 200.

## Gymnema

1. Lininger S, et al. The natural pharmacy. Rocklin, CA: Prima Publishing, 1998: 276

2. Lawrence Review of Natural Products. Gymnema monograph. St. Louis, MO: Facts and Comparisons Division, J.B. Lipincott Company, 1993.

3. Shanmugasundaram ERB, et al. Use of *Gymnema sylvestre* leaf extract in the control of blood glucose in insulin-dependent diabetes mellitus. *J Ethnopharmacol* 30: 281–294, 1990.

4. Baskaran K, et al. Antidiabetic effect of a leaf extract from *Gymnema sylvestre* in non-insulin–dependent diabetes mellitus patients. *J Ethnopharmacol* 30: 295–305, 1990.

## Hawthorn

1. Popping S, et al. Effect of a hawthorn extract on contraction and energy turnover of isolated rat cardiomyocytes. *Arzneimittelforschung Drug Res* 45: 1157–1161, 1995.

2. Joseph G. Pharmacologic action profile of crataegus extract in comparison to epinephrine, amirinone, milrinone and digoxin in the isolated perfused guinea pig heart. *Arzneimittelforschung* 45(12): 1261–1265, 1995.

3. Schulz V, et al. Rational phytotherapy. New York: Springer-Verlag, 1998: 91–94.

4. Schulz V, et al. Rational phytotherapy. New York: Springer-Verlag, 1998: 91–95.

5. Ammon HTP, et al. Crataegus, toxicology, and pharmacology. *Planta Med* 43: 105–120, 209–239, 313–322, 1981.

6. Schulz V, et al. Rational phytotherapy. New York: Springer-Verlag, 1998: 97.

7. Tauchert M, et al. Crataegi folium cum flore bei herzinsuffizienz. As cited in Loew D, Tietbrock N, eds. Phytopharmaka in Forschung und klinischer Anwendung. Darmstadt: Steinkopff Verlag, 1995: 37–44.

8. Schulz V, et al. Rational phytotherapy. New York: Springer-Verlag, 1998: 90–98.

9. Tauchert M, et al. Weissdorn Extrakt als pflanzliches Cardiacum (Vorwort). Neubewertung der therapeutischen Wirksamkeit. *Munch Med Wschr* 136(Suppl. 1): 3–5, 1994.

10. Schulz V, et al. Rational phytotherapy. New York: Springer-Verlag, 1998: 95.

## He Shou Wu

1. Chang HM. Pharmacology and applications of Chinese materia medica. World Scientific I: 620–624, 1986.

## Histidine

1. Gerber DA, et al. Free serum histidine levels in patients with rheumatoid arthritis and control subjects following an oral load of free L-histidine. *J Clin Invest* 55: 1164, 1975.

2. Gerber DA and Gerber MG. Specificity of a low free serum histidine concentration for rheumatoid arthritis. *J Chronic Dis* 30: 115–127, 1977.

3. Pinals RS, Harris ED, Burnett JB, and Gerber DA. Treatment of rheumatoid arthritis with L-histidine: a randomized, placebo-controlled, double-blind trial. *J Rheumatol* 4: 414–419, 1997.

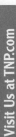

## HMB (Hydroxymethyl Butyrate)

1. Ostaszewski P, et al. The effect of leucine metabolite beta-hydroxy-beta-methylbutyrate (HMB) on muscle protein synthesis and protein breakdown in chick and rat muscle (Abstract). *J Anim Sci* 1996.

2. Nissen S, et al. Effect of leucine metabolite beta-hydroxy-beta-methylbutyrate on muscle metabolism during resistance training. *J App Phys* 81: 2095–2104, 1996.

3. Nissen S, et al. Effects of feeding beta-hydroxy beta-methylbutyrate (HMB) on body composition in women. *FASEB J* 11(3): A290, 1997.

4. Passwater R and Fuller, J. Building muscle mass, performance and health with HMB. New Canaan, CT: Keats Publishing, 1997.

5. Ostaszewski P, et al. The effect of leucine metabolite beta-hydroxy-beta-methylbutyrate (HMB) on muscle protein synthesis and protein breakdown in chick and rat muscle (Abstract). *J Anim Sci* 1996.

6. Nissen S, et al. Effect of leucine metabolite beta-hydroxy-beta-methylbutyrate on muscle metabolism during resistance training. *J App Phys* 81: 2095–2104, 1996.

7. Abumrad N and Flakoll P. The efficacy and safety of CaHMB (beta-hydroxy-beta-methylbutyrate) in humans. Annual Report. Vanderbilt University Medical Center: MTI, 1991.

## Hops

1. Schulz V, et al. Rational phytotherapy. New York: Springer-Verlag, 1998: 82–83.

2. Schulz V, et al. Rational phytotherapy. New York: Springer-Verlag, 1998: 83.

3. Duncan KL, et al. Malignant hyperthermia-like reaction secondary to ingestion of hops in five dogs. *J Am Vet Med Assoc* 210: 51–54, 1997.

4. Lee KM, et al. Effects of *Humulus lupulus* extract on the central nervous system in mice. *Planta Med* 59(Suppl.): A691, 1993.

## Horse Chestnut

1. Newall C, et al. Herbal medicines: A guide for healthcare professionals. London: Pharmaceutical Press, 1996: 166.

2. Kreysel HW, et al. A possible role of lysosomal enzymes in the pathogenesis of varicosis and the reduction in their serum activity by Venostatin. *Vasa* 12: 377–382, 1983.

3. Bougelet C. Effect of aescine on hypoxia induced neutrophil adherence to umbilical vein endothelium. *Eur J Pharmacol* 345(1): 89–95, 1998.

4. Schulz V, et al. Rational phytotherapy. New York: Springer-Verlag, 1998: 131–134.

5. Neiss A, et al. Zum Wirksamkeitsnachweis von Rosskastaniensamenextrakt beim varikosen Symptomenkomplex. *Munch Med Wschr* 7: 213–216.

6. Diehm C, et al. Comparison of leg compression stocking and oral horse-chestnut seed extract therapy in patients with chronic venous insufficiency. *Lancet* 347: 292–294, 1996.

7. Schulz V, et al. Rational phytotherapy. New York: Springer-Verlag, 1998: 131.

8. Schulz V, et al. Rational phytotherapy. New York: Springer-Verlag, 1998: 131.

9. Newall C, et al. Herbal medicines: A guide for healthcare professionals. London: Pharmaceutical Press, 1996: 166–167.

10. Grasso A and Corvaglia E. Two cases of suspected oxic tubulonephrosis due to escine. *Gazz Med Ital* 335: 581–584, 1976.

11. Brinker F. Herb contraindications and drug interactions, 2nd ed. Sandy, Oregon: Eclectic Medical Publications, 1998: 84.

12. Schulz V, et al. Rational phytotherapy. New York: Springer-Verlag, 1998: 132.

## Horsetail

1. Duke JA. CRC handbook of medicinal herbs. Boca Raton, FL: CRC Press, 1985: 492.

2. Fessenden RJ, et al. The biological properties of silicon compounds. *Adv Drug Res* 4: 95, 1987.

3. Weiss, R. Herbal medicine abstract arcanum. Gothenburg, Sweden: 1998: 238–239.

4. Fabre B, et al. Thiaminase activity in *Equisetum arvense* and its extracts. *Planta Med Phytother* 26: 190–197, 1993.

5. Leung A, Foster S. Encyclopedia of common natural ingredients used in food, drugs, and cosmetics. New York: John Wiley and Sons, 1996: 307.

6. Brinker F. Herb contraindications and drug interactions, 2nd ed. Sandy, Oregon: Eclectic Medical Publications, 1998: 85.

## Hydroxycitric Acid

1. Greenwood MR, Cleary MP, Gruen R, et al. Effect of (-)-hydroxycitrate on development of obesity in the Zucker obese rat. *Am J Physiol* 240: E72–78, 1981.

2. Sullivan AC and Triscari J. Metabolic regulation as a control for lipid disorders. *Am J Clin Nutr* 30: 767–776, 1977.

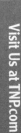

Notes

Visit Us at TNP.com

3. Sullivan AC, Triscari J, Hamilton JG, et al. Effect of (-)-hydroxycitrate upon the accumulation of lipid in the rat. I. Lipogenesis. *Lipids* 9: 121–128, 1974.

4. Sullivan AC, Triscari J, Hamilton JG, et al. Effect of (-)-hydroxycitrate upon the accumulation of lipid in the rat. II. Appetite. *Lipids* 9(2): 129–134, 1974.

5. Sergio W. A natural food, malabar tamarind, may be effective in the treatment of obesity. *Medical Hyp* 27: 40, 1988.

6. Lowenstein JM. Effect of (-)-hydroxycitrate on fatty acid synthesis by rat liver in vivo. *J Biol Chem* 246(3): 629–632, 1971.

7. Triscari J and Sullivan AC. Comparative effects of (-)-hydroxycitrate and (+)-allohydroxycitrate on acetyl CoA carboxylase and fatty acid and cholesterol synthesis in vivo. *Lipids* 12(4): 357–363, 1977.

8. Cheema-Dhadli S, Harlperin ML, and Leznoff CC. Inhibition of enzymes which interact with citrate by (-)hydroxycitrate and 1,2,3,-tricarboxybenzene. *Eur J Biochem* 38: 98–102, 1973.

9. Sullivan AC, Hamilton JG, Miller ON, et al. Inhibition of enzymes which interact with citrate by (-)hydroxy-citrate. *Arch Biochem Biophys* 150: 183–190, 1972.

## Inosine

1. Kipshidze NN, Korotkov AA, Chapidze GE, et al. Indications for the use of inosine in myocardial infarct (a clinical and experimental study). *Kardiologiia* 18: 18–28, 1978.

2. Starling RD, Trappe TA, Short KR, et al. Effect of inosine supplementation on aerobic and anaerobic cycling performance. *Med Sci Sports Exerc* 28: 1193–1198, 1996.

3. Dragan I, Baroga M, Eremia N, and Georgescu E. Studies regarding some effects of inosine in elite weightlifters. *Rom J Physiol* 30: 47–50, 1993.

4. Williams MH, Kreider RB, Hunter DW, et al. Effect of inosine supplementation on 3-mile treadmill run performance and VO2 peak. *Med Sci Sports Exerc* 22: 517–522, 1990.

5. Rosenbloom D, et al. Contemporary ergogenic aids used by strength/power athletes. *J Am Diet Assoc* 92: 10, 1264–1266, 1992.

6. Cheng Y and Jiang DH. Therapeutic effect of inosine in Tourette's syndrome and its possible mechanism of action. *Chung Hua Shen Ching Ching Shen Ko Tsa Chih* 23: 90–93, 126–127, 1990.

## Inositol

1. Levine J, Barak Y, Kofman O, and Belmaker RH. Follow-up and relapse analysis of an inositol study of depression. *Isr J Psychiatry Relat Sci* 32(1): 14–21, 1995.

2. Levine J. Controlled trials of inositol in psychiatry. *Eur Neuropsychopharmacol* 7: 147–155, 1997.

3. Benjamin J, Agam G, Levine J, et al. Inositol treatment in psychiatry. *Psychopharmacol Bull* 31(1): 167–175, 1995.

4. Benjamin J, Levine J, Fux M, et al. Double-blind, placebo-controlled, crossover trial of inositol treatment for panic disorder. *Am J Psychiatry* 152: 1084–1086, 1995.

5. Levine J. Controlled trials of inositol in psychiatry. *Eur Neuropsychopharmacol* 7: 147–155, 1997.

6. Fux M, Levine J, Aviv A, and Belmaker RH. Inositol treatment of obsessive-compulsive disorder. *Am J Psychiatry* 153: 1219–1221, 1996.

7. Levine J. Controlled trials of inositol in psychiatry. *Eur Neuropsychopharmacol* 7: 147–155, 1997.

8. Salway JG, et al. Effect of myo-inositol on peripheral-nerve function in diabetes. *Lancet* 2: 1282–1284, 1978.

9. Gregersen G, et al. Oral supplementation of myoinositol: effects on peripheral nerve function in human diabetics and on the concentration in plasma, erythrocytes, urine and muscle tissue in human diabetics and normals. *Acta Neurol Scand* 67: 164–172, 1983.

10. Levine J, Barak Y, Kofman O, and Belmaker RH. Follow-up and relapse analysis of an inositol study of depression. *Isr J Psychiatry Relat Sci* 32(1): 14–21, 1995.

11. Levine J. Controlled trials of inositol in psychiatry. *Eur Neuropsychopharmacol* 7: 147–155, 1997.

12. Benjamin J, Agam G, Levine J, et al. Inositol treatment in psychiatry. *Psychopharmacol Bull* 31(1): 167–175, 1995.

13. Benjamin J, Levine J, Fux M, et al. Double-blind, placebo-controlled, crossover trial of inositol treatment for panic disorder. *Am J Psychiatry* 152: 1084–1086, 1995.

## Iodine

1. Ghent WR, Eskin BA, Low DA, and Hill LP. Iodine replacement in fibrocystic disease of the breast. *Can J Surg* 36: 453–460, 1993.

2. Ghent WR, Eskin BA, Low DA, and Hill LP. Iodine replacement in fibrocystic disease of the breast. *Can J Surg* 36: 453–460, 1993.

## Iron

1. Werbach M. Foundations of nutritional medicine. Tarzana, CA: Third Line Press, 1997: 57.

2. Werbach M. Foundations of nutritional medicine. Tarzana, CA: Third Line Press, 1997: 57–59.

3. Holt GA. Food and drug interactions. Chicago: Precept Press, 1998.

4. Taymor ML, et al. The etiological role of chronic iron deficiency in production of menorrhagia. *JAMA* 187: 323–327, 1964.

5. Taymor ML, et al. The etiological role of chronic iron deficiency in production of menorrhagia. *JAMA* 187: 323–327, 1964.

6. Hallberg L, et al. Phytates and the inhibitory effects of bran on iron absorption in man. *Am J Clin Nutr* 45: 988–996, 1987.

7. Sandstrom B, et al. Oral iron, dietary ligands and zinc absorption. *J Nutr* 115(3): 411–414, 1985.

8. Werbach M. Foundations of nutritional medicine. Tarzana, CA: Third Line Press, 1997: 169–171.

9. Freeland-Graves JH. Manganese: An essential nutrient for humans. *Nutr Today* 23: 10–13, 1989.

10. Holt, GA. Food and drug interactions. Chicago: Precept Press. 1998.

## Isoflavones

1. Potter SM, Baum JA, Teng H, et al. Soy protein and isoflavones: their effects on blood lipids and bone density in postmenopausal women. *Am J Clin Nutr* 68(6 Suppl.): 1375S–1379S, 1998.

2. Anderson JW, et al. 1995. Meta-analysis of effects of soy protein on serum lipids in humans. *N Eng J Med* 333: 276–282, 1995.

3. Messina MJ, Persky V, and Setchell KD. Soy intake and cancer risk: a review of the in vitro and in vivo data. *Nutr Cancer* 21: 113–131, 1994.

4. Murkies A and Lombard C. Dietary flour supplementation decreases post-menopausal hot flushes: effect of soy and wheat. *Maturitas* 21(3): 189–195, 1995.

5. Genari C, Adami S, Agusei L, et al. Effect of chronic treatment with ipriflavone in postmenopausal women with low bone mass. *Calcif Tissue Int* 61: S19–S22, 1997.

6. Valente M, Bufalino L, et al. Effects of 1-year treatment with ipriflavone on bone in postmenopausal women with low bone mass. *Calcif Tissue Int* 54: 377–380, 1994.

7. Kovacs AB. Efficacy of ipriflavone in the prevention and treatment of postmenopausal osteoporosis. *Agents Actions* 41: 86–87, 1994.

8. Adami S, et al. Ipriflavone prevents radial bone loss in postmenopausal women with low bone mass over 2 years. *Osteoporos Int* 7(2): 119–125, 1997.

9. Agnusdei D, et al. Efficacy of ipriflavone in established osteoporosis and long-term safety. *Calcif Tissue Int* 61(1):S23–S27, 1997.

10. Agnusdei D, Crepaldi G, Isaia G, Mazzuoli S, et al. A double-blind placebo-controlled trial of ipriflavone for prevention of postmenopausal spinal bone loss. *Calcif Tissue Int* 61: 142–147, 1997.

11. Agnusdei D, Camporeale F, et al. 1992. Effects of ipriflavone on bone mass and bone remodeling in patients with established postmenopausal osteoporosis. *Curr Ther Res* 51: 82–91, 1992.

12. Gambacciani M, Cappagli B, Piaggesi M, et al. Ipriflavone prevents the loss of bone mass in pharmacological menopause induced by GnRH-agonists. *Calcif Tissue Int* 61: S15–S18, 1997.

13. Melis GB and Paoletti AM. Ipriflavone and low doses of estrogens in the prevention of bone mineral loss in climacterium. *Bone and Mineral* 19: S49–S56, 1992.

14. Nozaki M, Hashimoto K, et al. Treatment of bone loss in oophorectomized women with a combination of ipriflavone and conjugated equine estrogen. *Int J Gyn Ob* 62: 69–75, 1998.

15. Potter SM, Baum JA, Teng H, et al. Soy protein and isoflavones: their effects on blood lipids and bone density in postmenopausal women. *Am J Clin Nutr* 68(6 Suppl.): 1375S–1379S, 1998.

16. Harrison E, et al. The effect of soybean protein on bone loss in a rat model of postmenopausal osteoporosis. *J Nutr Sci Vitaminol* 44(2): 257–268, 1998.

17. Fanti O, et al. Systematic administration of genistein partially prevents bone loss in ovariectomized rats in a nonestrogen-like mechanism (Abstract). *Am J Clin Nutr*: 68(Suppl.): 1517, 1998.

18. Arjmandi BH, et al. Dietary soybean protein prevents bone loss in an ovariectomized rat model of osteoporosis. *J Nutr* 126: 161–167, 1996.

19. Arjmandi BH, et al. Role of soy protein with normal or reduced isoflavone content in reversing bone loss induced by ovarian hormone deficient rats is related to its isoflavone content. *Am J Clin Nutr* 68(Suppl.): 1364–1368, 1998.

20. Fanti P, et al. The phytoestrogen genistein reduces bone loss in short-term ovariectomized rats. *Osteoporos Int* 8: 274–281, 1998.

21. Anderson JJ, et al. Biphaic effects of genistein on bone tissue in the ovariectomized, lactating rat model. *Proc Soc Exp Biol Med* 217: 345–350, 1998.

22. Lees CJ and Ginn TA. Soy protein isolate diet does not prevent increased cortical bone turnover in ovariectomized macaques. *Calcif Tissue Int* 62: 557, 558, 1998.

23. Agnusdei D, Crepaldi G, Isaia G, Mazzuoli S., et al. A double-blind placebo-controlled trial of ipriflavone for

prevention of postmenopausal spinal bone loss. *Calcif Tissue Int* 61: 142–147, 1997.

## Juniper Berry

1. Newall C, et al. Herbal medicines: A guide for healthcare professionals. London: Pharmaceutical Press, 1996: 176.

2. Mascolo N, et al. Biological screening of Italian medicinal plants for anti-inflammatory activity. *Phytother Res* 1: 28–31, 1987.

3. Markkanen T, et al. Antiherpetic agent from juniper tree (*Juniperus cummunis*), its purification, identification, and testing in primary human amnion cell cultures. *Drugs Exp Clin Res* 7: 691–697, 1981.

4. Agarwal OP, et al. Antifertility effects of fruits of *Juniperus communis*. *Planta Med* 40(Suppl.): 98–101, 1980.

5. Newall C, et al. Herbal medicines: A guide for healthcare professionals. London: Pharmaceutical Press, 1990: 176.

## Kava

1. Meyer HJ, et al. Kawa-Pyrone-eine neuartige Substanzgruppe zentraler Muskelrelaxantien vom Typ des Mephenesins. *Klin Wschr* 44: 902–903, 1966.

2. Klohs MW, et al. A chemical and pharmacological investigation of *Piper methysticum* Forst. *J Med Pharm Chem* 1: 95–103, 1959.

3. Bruggenmann F, et al. Die analgetische Wirkung der Kawa-Inhaltsstoffe Dihydrokawain und Dihydromethysticin. *Arzneimittelforschung* 13: 407–409, 1963.

4. Meyer HJ. Pharmakologie der Wirksamen Prinzipien des Kawa-Rhizoms (*Piper methysticum* Forst). *Arch Intern Pharmacodyn* 138: 505–535, 1962.

5. Meyer HJ. Lokalanaesthetische Eigenschaften naturlicher Kawa-Pyrone. *Arzneimittelforschung* 42: 407, 1964.

6. Meyer HJ, et al. Kawa-Pyrone-eine neuartige Substanzgruppe zentraler Muskelrelaxantien vom Typ des Mephenesins. *Klin Wschr* 44: 902–903, 1966.

7. Singh YN. Effects of kava on neuromuscular transmission and muscle contractility. *J Ethnopharmacol* 7: 267–276, 1983.

8. Davies LP, et al. Kava pyrones and resin: Studies on GABA-A, GABA-B, and benzodiazepine binding sites in rodent brain. *Pharmacol Toxicol* 71(2): 120–126, 1992.

9. Jussofie A, Schmiz A, and Hiemke C. Kavapyrone enriched extract from *Piper methysticum* as modulator of the GABA binding site in different regions of rat brain. *Psychopharmacology* 116: 469–474, 1994.

10. Munte TF, et al. Effects of oxazepam and an extract of kava roots (*Piper methysticum*) on event-related potentials in a word recognition task. *Neuropsychobiology* 27(1): 46–53, 1993.

11. Heinze HJ, et al. Pharmacopsychological effects of oxazepam and kava extract in a visual search paradigm assessed with event-related potentials. *Pharmacopsychiatry* 27(6): 224–230, 1994.

12. Emser W and Bartylla K. Effect of kava extract WS 1490 on the sleep pattern in healthy subjects. *Neurol Psychiatr* 5: 636–642, 1991.

13. Holm E, et al. Studies on the profile of the neurophysiological effects of D,L-kavain. Cerebral sites of action and sleep-wakefulness-rhythm in animals. *Arzneimittelforschung* 41: 673–683, 1991.

14. Volz HP, et al. Kava-kava extract WS 1490 versus placebo in anxiety disorders—a randomized placebo-controlled 25 week outpatient trial. *Pharmacopsychiatry* 30(1): 1–5, 1997.

15. Kinzler E, et al. Effect of a special kava extract in patients with anxiety, tension, and excitation states of nonpsychotic genesis. Double-blind study with placebos over 4 weeks. *Arzneimittelforschung* 41(6): 584–588, 1991.

16. Warnecke G, et al. Wirksamkeit von Kawa-Kawa-Extract beim klimakterischen Syndrom. *Z Phytother* 11: 81–86, 1990.

17. Warnecke G. Psychosomatic dysfunctions in the female climacteric. Clinical effectiveness and tolerance of kava extract WS 1490. *Fortschr Med* 109(4): 119–122, 1991.

18. Woelk H, et al. Behandlung von Angst-Patienten. *Z Allg Med* 69: 271–277, 1993.

19. Schulz V, et al. Rational phytotherapy. New York: Springer-Verlag, 1998: 68.

20. Schulz V, et al. Rational phytotherapy. New York: Springer-Verlag, 1998: 71.

21. Schulz V, et al. Rational phytotherapy. New York: Springer-Verlag, 1998: 71.

22. Norton SA, et al. Kava dermopathy. *Am Acad Dermatol* 31(1): 89–97, 1994.

23. Munte TF, et al. Effects of oxazepam and an extract of kava roots (*Piper methysticum*) on event-related potentials in a word recognition task. *Neuropsychobiology* 27(1): 46–53, 1993.

24 Heinze HJ, et al. Pharmacopsychological effects of oxazepam and kava extract in a visual search paradigm assessed with event-related potentials. *Pharmacopsychiatry* 27(6): 224–230, 1994.

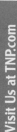

25. Herberg KW. Effect of kava special extract WS 1490 combined with ethyl alcohol on safety-relevant performance parameters. *Blutalkohol* 30(2): 96–105, 1993.

26. Munte TF, et al. Effects of oxazepam and an extract of kava roots (*Piper methysticum*) on event-related potentials in a word recognition task. *Neuropsychobiology* 27(1): 46–53, 1993.

27. Heinze HJ, et al. Pharmacopsychological effects of oxazepam and kava extract in a visual search paradigm assessed with event-related potentials. *Pharmacopsychiatry* 27(6): 224–230, 1994.

28. Schulz V, et al. Rational phytotherapy. New York: Springer-Verlag, 1998: 72.

29. Duffield PH and Jamieson D. Development of tolerance to kava in mice. *Clin Exp Pharmacol Physiol* 18: 571–578, 1991.

30. Almeida JC and Grimsley EW. Coma from the health food store: Interaction between kava and alprazolam. *Ann Intern Med* 125(11): 940–941, 1996.

31. Schelosky L, et al. Kava and dopamine antagonism. *J Neurol Neurosurg Psych* 58(5): 639–640, 1995.

## Kudzu

1. Keung WM, et al. Daidzin and daidzein suppress free choice ethanol intake by Syrian golden hamsters. *Proc Natl Acad Sci* 90: 10008–10012, 1993.

2. Overstreet DH. Suppression of alcohol intake after administration of the Chinese herbal medicine NPI-028 and its derivatives. *Alcohol Clin Exp Res* 20(2): 221–227, 1996.

## Lapacho

1. Li CJ, et al. Beta-lapachone, a novel DNA topoisomerase I inhibitor with a mode of action different from camptothecin. *J Biol Chem* 268: 22463–22468, 1993.

2. Guiraud P, et al. Comparison of antibacterial and antifungal activities of lapachol and beta-lapachone. *Planta Med* 60: 373–374, 1994.

3. Oswald EH. Lapacho. *Br J Phytother* 4(3): 112–117, 1993.

## Lecithin

1. Brook JG, et al. Dietary soya lecithin decreases plasma triglyceride levels and inhibits collagen- and ADP-induced platelet aggregation. *Biochem Med Metab Biol* 35: 31–39, 1986.

2. Wojcicki J, et al. Clinical evaluation of lecithin as a lipid-lowering agent. *Phytotherapy Res* 9: 597–599, 1995.

3. Oosthuizen W, et al. Lecithin has no effect on serum lipoprotein, plasma fibrinogen and macro molecular protein complex levels in hyperlipidaemic men in a double-blind controlled study. *Eur J Clin Nutr* 52(6): 419–424, 1998.

4. *Essentiale forté*. Cologne, Germany: Natterman International GMBH, 1989.

5. Buchman AL, Dubin M, Jenden D, et al. Lecithin increases plasma free choline and decreases hepatic steatosis in long-term total parenteral nutrition patients. *Gastroenterology* 102: 1363–1370, 1992.

6. Guan R, Ho KY, Kang JY, et al. The effect of polyunsaturated phosphatidylcholine in the treatment of acute viral hepatitis. *Ailment Pharmacol Ther* 9: 699–703, 1995.

7. Lieber CS, Robins SJ, Li J, et al. Phosphatidylcholine protects against fibrosis and cirrhosis in the baboon. *Gastroenterology* 106: 152–159, 1994.

8. Lieber CS, DeCarli LM, and Mak KM. Attenuation of alcohol-induced hepatic fibrosis by polyunsaturated lecithin. *Hepatology* 12: 1390–1398, 1990.

9. Lieber CS, et al. Choline fails to prevent liver fibrosis in ethanol-fed baboons but causes toxicity. *Hepatology* 5(4): 561–572, 1985.

10. Lieber CS and Rubin E. Alcoholic fatty liver. *N Engl J Med* 280(13): 705–708, 1969.

11. Schòller Perez A and González SMF. Controlled study using multiply-unsaturated phosphatidylcholine in comparison with placebo in the case of alcoholic liver steatosis. (In German.) *Med Welt* 36: 517–521, 1985.

12. Knuechel F. Double blind study in patients with alcohol-toxic fatty liver. (In German.) *Med Welt* 30: 411–416, 1979.

13. Jenkins PJ, et al. Use of polyunsaturated phosphatidylcholine in HBsAg negative chronic active hepatitis: Results of prospective double-blind controlled trial. *Liver* 2: 77–81, 1982.

14. Stoll AL, Sachs GS, Cohen BM, et al. Choline in the treatment of rapid-cycling bipolar disorder: clinical and neurochemical findings in lithium-treated patients. *Biol Psychiatry* 40: 382–388, 1996.

15. Cohen BM, Lipinski JF and Altesman RI. Lecithin in the treatment of mania: Double-blind placebo-controlled trials. *Am J Psychiatry* 139: 1162–1164, 1982.

16. Polinsky RJ, Ebert MH, Caine ED, et al. Cholinergic treatment in the Tourette syndrome. Letter. *N Engl J Med* 302: 1310, 1980.

17. Gelenberg AJ, et al. A crossover study of lecithin treatment of tardive dyskinesia. *J Clin Psychiatry* 51(4): 149–153, 1990.

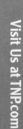

18. Domino EF, et al. Lack of clinically significant improvement of patients with tardive dyskinesia following phosphatidylcholine therapy. *Biol Psychiatry* 20(11): 1189–1196, 1985.

19. Weintraub S, et al. Lecithin in the treatment of Alzheimer's disease. *Arch Neurol* 40: 527, 1983.

20. Cohen BM, Miller AL, Lipinski JF, and Pope HG. Lecithin in mania: a preliminary report. *Am J Psychiatry* 137: 242–243, 1980.

21. Cohen BM, Lipinski JF and Altesman RI. Lecithin in the treatment of mania: Double-blind placebo-controlled trials. *Am J Psychiatry* 139: 1162–1164, 1982.

## Licorice

1. Newall C, et al. Herbal medicines: A guide for healthcare professionals. London: Pharmaceutical Press, 1996: 183–184.

2. van Marle J, et al. Deglycyrrhizinised liquorice (DGL) and the renewal of rat stomach epithelium. *Eur J Pharmacol* 72: 219–25, 1981.

3. Johnson B and McIssac R. Effect of some anti-ulcer agents on mucosal blood flow. *Br J Pharmacol* 1: 308, 1981.

4. Schulz V, et al. Rational phytotherapy. New York: Springer-Verlag, 1998: 185.

5. Brinker F. Herb contraindications and drug interactions, 2nd ed. Sandy, Oregon: Eclectic Medical Publications, 1998: 92.

6. Morgan AG, et al. Comparison between cimetidine and Caved-S in the treatment of gastric ulceration and subsequent maintenance therapy. *Gut* 23: 545–551, 1982.

7. Morgan AG, et al. Maintenance therapy: A two-year comparison between Caved-S and cimetidine treatment in the prevention of symptomatic gastric ulcer. *Gut* 26: 599–602, 1985.

8. Kassir ZA. Endoscopic controlled trial of four drug regimens in the treatment of chronic duodenal ulceration. *Ir Med J* 78: 153–156, 1985.

9. Brinker F. Herb contraindications and drug interactions, 2nd ed. Sandy, Oregon: Eclectic Medical Publications, 1998: 92.

## Lipoic Acid

1. Kagan VE, et al. Dihydrolipoic acid—A universal antioxidant both in the membrane and in the aqueous phase. *Biochem Pharmacol* 44: 1637–1649, 1992.

2. Matsugo S, et al. Elucidation of antioxidant activity of alpha-lipoic acid toward hydroxyl radical. *Biochem Biophys Res Commun* 208: 161–167, 1995.

3. Packer L, Witt EH, and Tritschler HJ. Alpha lipoic acid as a biological antioxidant. *Free Radical Biol Med* 19: 227–250, 1995.

4. Podda M, Tritschler HJ, Ulrich H, and Packer L. Alpha lipoic acid supplementation prevents symptoms of vitamin E deficiency. *Biochem Biophys Res Commun* 204: 98–104, 1994.

5. Ziegler D, et al. The ALADIN study group: Treatment of symptomatic diabetic peripheral neuropathy with the antioxidant alpha-lipoic acid: a 3 week randomized controlled trial (ALADIN study). *Diabetologia* 38: 1425–1433, 1995.

6. Ziegler D, et al. Alpha-lipoic acid in the treatment of diabetic peripheral and cardiac autonomic neuropathy. *Diabetes* 46(Suppl. 2): S62–S66, 1997.

7. Kahler W, et al. Diabetes mellitus—a free radical–associated disease: Results of adjuvant antioxidant supplementation. *Gesamte Inn Med* 48: 223–232, 1993.

8. Ziegler D, et al. Alpha-lipoic acid in the treatment of diabetic peripheral and cardiac autonomic neuropathy. *Diabetes* 46(Suppl. 2): S62–S66, 1997.

9. Jacob S, et al. Enhancement of glucose disposal in patients with type 2 diabetes by alpha lipoic acid. *Arzneimittelforschung* 45: 872–874, 1995.

10. Kawabata T, et al. Alpha-lipoate can protect against glycation of serum albumin, but not low density lipoprotein. *Biochem Biophys Res Commun* 203: 99–104, 1994.

11. Nagamatsu M, et al. Lipoic acid improves nerve blood flow, reduces oxidative stress and improves distal nerve conduction in experimental diabetic neuropathy. *Diabetes Care* 18: 1160–1167, 1995.

12. Suzuki, et al. Lipoate prevents glucose-induced protein modifications. *Free Radic Res Commun* 17: 211–217, 1992.

13. Ziegler D, et al. The ALADIN study group: Treatment of symptomatic diabetic peripheral neuropathy with the antioxidant alpha-lipoic acid: a 3 week randomized controlled trial (ALADIN study). *Diabetologia* 38: 1425–1433, 1995.

14. Ziegler D, et al. Alpha-lipoic acid in the treatment of diabetic peripheral and cardiac autonomic neuropathy. *Diabetes* 46(Suppl. 2): S62–S66, 1997.

15. Kahler W, et al. Diabetes mellitus—a free radical–associated disease: Results of adjuvant antioxidant supplementation. *Gesamte Inn Med* 48: 223–232, 1993.

16. Hounsom L, et al. A lipoic acid—gamma-linolenic acid conjugate is effective against multiple indices of experimental diabetic neuropathy. *Diabetologia* 41(7): 839–843, 1998.

17. Cameron NE, et al. Effects of alpha-lipoic acid on neurovascular function in diabetic rats. Interaction with essential fatty acids. *Diabetologia* 41(4): 390–399, 1998.

18. Ziegler D, et al. Alpha-lipoic acid in the treatment of diabetic peripheral and cardiac autonomic neuropathy. *Diabetes* 46(Suppl. 2): S62–S66, 1997.

19. Ziegler D, et al. Alpha-lipoic acid in the treatment of diabetic peripheral and cardiac autonomic neuropathy. *Diabetes* 46(Suppl. 2): S62–S66, 1997.

## Lutein

1. Mares-Perlman JA, Brady WE, Klein BE, et al. Diet and nuclear lens opacities. *Am J Epidemiol* 141: 322–334, 1995.

2. Hankinson S, Stampfer M, Seddon J, et al. Nutrient intake and cataract extraction in women: A prospective study. *BMJ* 305: 335–339, 1992.

3. Landrum JT, Bone RA, and Kilburn MD. The macular pigment: a possible role in protection from age-related macular degeneration. *Adv Pharmacol* 38: 537–555, 1997.

4. Hammond BR Jr, Wooten BR, and Snodderly DM. Density of the human crystalline lens is related to the macular pigment carotenoids, lutein and zeaxanthin. *Optom Vis Sci* 74: 499–504, 1997.

5. Dwyer J. Presentation. Federation of American Societies for Experimental Biology. Annual meeting. 1999.

## Lycopene

1. Weisburger JH. Evaluation of the evidence on the role of tomato products in disease prevention. *Proc Soc Exp Biol Med* 8: 140–143, 1998.

2. Sies H and Stahl W. Lycopene: antioxidant and biological effects and its bioavailability in the human. *Proc Soc Exp Biol Med* 218: 121–124, 1998.

3. Rao AV and Agarwal S. Bioavailability and in vivo antioxidant properties of lycopene from tomato products and their possible role in the prevention of cancer. *Nutr Cancer* 31: 199–203, 1998.

4. Giovannucci E, Ascherio A, Rimm EB, et al. Intake of carotenoids and retinol in relation to risk of prostate cancer. *J Natl Cancer Inst* 87: 1767–1776, 1995.

5. Paetau I, Khachik F, Brown ED, et al. Chronic ingestion of lycopene-rich tomato juice or lycopene supplements significantly increases plasma concentrations of lycopene and related tomato carotenoids in humans. *Am J Clin Nutr* 68: 1187–1195, 1998.

6. Giovannucci E, Ascherio A, Rimm EB, et al. Intake of carotenoids and retinol in relation to risk of prostate cancer. *J Natl Cancer Inst* 87: 1767–1776, 1995.

7. Giovannucci E and Clinton SK. Tomatoes, lycopene, and prostate cancer. *Proc Soc Exp Biol* 218: 129–139, 1998.

8. Franceschi S, et al. Tomatoes and risk of digestive-tract cancers. *Int J Cancer* 59: 181–184, 1994.

9. Kim DJ, Takasuka N and Kim JM. Chemoprevention by lycopene of mouse lung neoplasia after combined initiation treatment with DEN, MNU and DMH. *Cancer Lett* 120: 15–22, 1997.

10. Okajima E, Tsutsumi M, and Ozono S. Inhibitory effect of tomato juice on rat urinary bladder carcinogenesis after N-butyl-N-(4-hydroxybutyl)nitrosamine initiation. *Jpn J Cancer Res* 89: 22–26, 1998.

11. Mares-Perlman JA, Brady W, Klein R, et al. Serum antioxidants and age-related macular degeneration in a population-based case-control study. *Arch Ophthalmol* 113: 1518–1523, 1995.

12. Giovannucci E, Ascherio A, Rimm EB, et al. Intake of carotenoids and retinol in relation to risk of prostate cancer. *J Natl Cancer Inst* 87: 1767–1776, 1995.

13. Giovannucci E and Clinton SK. Tomatoes, lycopene, and prostate cancer. *Proc Soc Exp Biol* 218: 129–139, 1998.

14. Franceschi S, et al. Tomatoes and risk of digestive-tract cancers. *Int J Cancer* 59: 181–184, 1994.

15. Kim DJ, Takasuka N and Kim JM. Chemoprevention by lycopene of mouse lung neoplasia after combined initiation treatment with DEN, MNU and DMH. *Cancer Lett* 120: 15–22, 1997.

16. Okajima E, Tsutsumi M, and Ozono S. Inhibitory effect of tomato juice on rat urinary bladder carcinogenesis after N-butyl-N-(4-hydroxybutyl)nitrosamine initiation. *Jpn J Cancer Res* 89: 22–26, 1998.

17. Key TJ, Silcocks PB, Davey GK, et al. A case-control study of diet and prostate cancer. *Br J Cancer* 76: 678–687, 1997.

18. Nomura AM, Stemmermann GN, Lee J, and Craft NE. Serum micronutrients and prostate cancer in Japanese Americans in Hawaii. *Cancer Epidemiol Biomarkers* 6: 487–491, 1997.

## Lysine

1. Flodin NW. The metabolic roles, pharmacology, and toxicology of lysine. *J Am Coll Nutr* 16: 7–21, 1997.

2. Griffith RS, Walsh DE, and Myrmel KH. Success of L-lysine therapy in frequently recurrent herpes simplex infection. Treatment and prophylaxis. *Dermatologica* 175: 183–190, 1987.

3. McCune MA, Perry HO, Muller SA, and O'Fallon WM. Treatment of recurrent herpes simplex infections

with L-lysine monohydrochloride. *Cutis* 34: 366–373, 1984.

4. Simon CA, Van Melle GD, and Ramelet AA. Failure of lysine in frequently recurrent herpes simplex infection (letter). *Arch Dermatol* 121: 167–168, 1985.

5. DiGiovanna JJ and Blank H. Failure of lysine in frequently recurrent herpes simplex infection. Treatment and prophylaxis. *Arch Dermatol* 120: 48–51, 1984.

6. Griffith R, DeLong D and Nelson J. Relation of arginine-lysine antagonism to herpes simplex growth in tissue culture. *Chemotherapy* 27: 209–213, 1981.

7. Flodin NW. The metabolic roles, pharmacology, and toxicology of lysine. *J Am Coll Nutr* 16: 7–21, 1997.

8. Griffith RS, Walsh DE, and Myrmel KH. Success of L-lysine therapy in frequently recurrent herpes simplex infection. Treatment and prophylaxis. *Dermatologica* 175: 183–190, 1987.

9. McCune MA, Perry HO, Muller SA, and O'Fallon WM. Treatment of recurrent herpes simplex infections with L-lysine monohydrochloride. *Cutis* 34: 366–373, 1984.

10. Simon CA, Van Melle GD, and Ramelet AA. Failure of lysine in frequently recurrent herpes simplex infection (letter). *Arch Dermatol* 121: 167–168, 1985.

11. DiGiovanna JJ and Blank H. Failure of lysine in frequently recurrent herpes simplex infection. Treatment and prophylaxis. *Arch Dermatol* 120: 48–51, 1984.

12. Kritchevsky D, et al. Gallstone formation in hamsters: Influence of specific amino acids. *Nutr Rep Internat* 29: 117, 1984.

13. Lexzczynski DE, et al. Excess dietary lysine induces hypercholesterolemia in chickens. *Experientia* 38: 266–267, 1982.

## Magnesium

1. National Center for Health Statistics. Dietary intake of vitamins, minerals and fiber of persons age 2 months and over in the U.S. Advance data No. 258, Nov. 14, 1994.

2. Wester PO Magnesium. *Am J Clin Nutr* 45(5 suppl.): 1305–1312, 1987.

3. Holt, GA, Food and drug interactions. Chicago: Precept Press, 1998.

4. Spencer H, Norris C, and Williams D. Inhibitory effects of zinc on magnesium balance and magnesium adsorption in man. *J Am Coll Nutr* 13(5): 479–484, 1994.

5. Werbach M. Foundations of nutritional medicine. Tarzana, CA: Third Line Press, 1997: 180, 186.

6. Peikert A, et al. Prophylaxis of migraine with oral magnesium: results from a prospective, multi-center, placebo-controlled and double-blind randomized study. *Cephalalgia* 16: 257–263, 1996.

7. Taubert K. Magnesium in migraine. Results of a multicenter pilot study. *Fortschr Med* 112: 328–330, 1994.

8. Facchinetti F, Sances G, Borella P, et al. Magnesium prophylaxis of menstrual migraine: effects on intracellular magnesium. *Headache* 31: 298–301, 1991.

9. Attias J, et al. Oral magnesium intake reduces permanent hearing loss induced by noise exposure. *Am J Otolaryngol* 15: 26–32, 1994.

10. Johansson G, Backman U, Danielson B, et al. Biochemical and clinical effects of the prophylactic treatment of renal calcium stones with magnesium hydroxide. *J Urol* 124: 770–774, 1980.

11. Sanjuliani AF, et al. Effects of magnesium on blood pressure and intracellular ion levels of Brazilian hypertensive patients. *Int J Cardiol* 56: 177–183, 1996.

12. Witteman JCM, Grobbee DE, Derkx FHM, et al. Reduction of blood pressure with oral magnesium supplementation in women with mild to moderate hypertension. *Am J Clin Nutr* 60: 129–135, 1994.

13. Dyckner T and Wester PO. Effect of magnesium on blood pressure. *BMJ [Clin Res]* 286: 1847–1849, 1983.

14. Facchinetti F, Borella P, Sances G, et al. Oral magnesium successfully relieves premenstrual mood changes. *Obstet Gynecol* 78: 177–181, 1991.

15. Facchinetti F, Sances G, Borella P, et al. Magnesium prophylaxis of menstrual migraine: effects on intracellular magnesium. *Headache* 31: 298–301, 1991.

16. Fontana-Klaiber H and Hogg B. Therapeutic effects of magnesium in dysmenorrhea. *Schweiz Rundsch Med Prax* 79: 491–494, 1990.

17. Seifert B, et al. Magnesium—a new therapeutic alternative in primary dysmenorrhea. *Zentralbl Gynakol* 111: 755–760, 1989.

18. Elamin A and Tuvemo T. Magnesium and insulin-dependent diabetes mellitus. *Diabetes Res Clin Pract* 10: 203–209, 1990.

19. Tosiello L. Hypomagnesemia and diabetes mellitus. *Arch Intern Med* 156: 1143–1148, 1996.

20. Eibel NL, Kopp HP, Nowak HR, et al. Hypomagnesemia in type II diabetes: effect of a 3-month replacement therapy. *Diabetes Care* 18: 188–192, 1995.

21. Bernstein WK, Khastgir T, and Khastgir A. Lack of effectiveness of magnesium in chronic stable asthma. A prospective, randomized, double-blind, placebo-controlled, crossover trial in normal subjects and in patients

with chronic stable asthma. *Arch Intern Med* 155: 271–276, 1995.

22. Peikert A, et al. Prophylaxis of migraine with oral magnesium: results from a prospective, multi-center, placebo-controlled and double-blind randomized study. *Cephalalgia* 16: 257–263, 1996.

23. Taubert K. Magnesium in migraine. Results of a multicenter pilot study. *Fortschr Med* 112: 328–330, 1994.

24. Facchinetti F, Sances G, Borella P, et al. Magnesium prophylaxis of menstrual migraine: effects on intracellular magnesium. *Headache* 31: 298–301, 1991.

25. Pfaffenrath V, et al. Magnesium in the prophylaxis of migraine—a double-blind, placebo-controlled study. *Cephalalgia* 16: 436–440, 1996.

26. Gaby AR. Research Review. *Nutrition & Healing:* March 1997.

27. Attias J, et al. Oral magnesium intake reduces permanent hearing loss induced by noise exposure. *Am J Otolaryngol* 15: 26–32, 1994.

28. Johansson G, Backman U, Danielson B, et al. Biochemical and clinical effects of the prophylactic treatment of renal calcium stones with magnesium hydroxide. *J Urol* 124: 770–774, 1980.

29. Sanjuliani AF, et al. Effects of magnesium on blood pressure and intracellular ion levels of Brazilian hypertensive patients. *Int J Cardiol* 56: 177–183, 1996.

30. Witteman JCM, Grobbee DE, Derkx FHM, et al. Reduction of blood pressure with oral magnesium supplementation in women with mild to moderate hypertension. *Am J Clin Nutr* 60: 129–135, 1994.

31. Dyckner T and Wester PO. Effect of magnesium on blood pressure. *BMJ [Clin Res]* 286: 1847–1849, 1983.

32. Henderson DG, et al. Effect of magnesium supplementation on blood pressure and electrolyte concentrations in hypertensive patients receiving long term diuretic treatment. *BMJ[Clin Res]* 293: 664, 1986.

33. Holt, GA, Food and drug interactions. Chicago: Precept Press, 1998: 255, 275, 284.

34. Drug evaluations subscription, vol. 2 (section 10, chapter 3). Chicago: American Medical Association, Winter 1994.

## Maitake

1. Yamada Y, et al. Antitumor effect of orally administered extracts from fruit body of *Grifola frondosa* (maitake). *Chemotherapy* 38: 790–796, 1990.

2. Nanba H. Immunostimulant activity in vivo and anti-HIV activity in vitro of 3 branched b-1-6-glucans extracted from maitake mushrooms (*Grifola frondosa*).

Amsterdam: VIII International Conference on AIDS, 1992 (Abstract).

## Manganese

1. Freeland-Graves JH. Manganese: An essential nutrient for humans. *Nutr Today* 23: 10–13, 1989.

2. Holt, GA. Food and drug interactions. Chicago: Precept Press. 1998: 197.

3. Strause L, Saltman P, Smith KT, et al. Spinal bone loss in postmenopausal women supplemented with calcium and trace minerals. *J Nutr* 124: 1060–1064, 1994.

4. Penland JG and Johnson PE. Dietary calcium and manganese effects on menstrual cycle symptoms. *Am J Obstet Gynecol* 168: 1417–1423, 1993.

5. Akram M, Sullivan C, Mack G, and Buchanan N. What is the clinical significance of reduced manganese and zinc levels in treated epileptic patients? *Med J Aust* 151: 113, 1989.

6. Kosenko LG. *Klin Med 42*: 113, 1964. Cited in Werbach M. Nutritional influences on illness. CD ROM. Tarzana, CA: Third Line Press, 1998.

7. Strause L, Saltman P, Smith KT, et al. Spinal bone loss in postmenopausal women supplemented with calcium and trace minerals. *J Nutr* 124: 1060–1064, 1994.

8. Penland JG and Johnson PE. Dietary calcium and manganese effects on menstrual cycle symptoms. *Am J Obstet Gynecol* 168: 1417–1423, 1993.

## Marshmallow

1. Newall C, et al. Herbal medicines: A guide for healthcare professionals. London: Pharmaceutical Press, 1996: 188.

2. Tomodo M, et al. Hypoglycemic activity of twenty plant mucilages and three modified products. *Planta Med* 53: 8–12, 1987.

## Medium-Chain Triglycerides

1. Craig GB, Darnell BE, and Weinsier RL. Decreased fat and nitrogen losses in patients with AIDS receiving medium-chain-triglyceride-containing formulas. *J Am Diet Assoc* 97: 605–611, 1997.

2. Wanke CA, Pleskow D and Degirolami PC. A medium-chain triglyceride-based diet in patients with HIV and chronic diarrhea reduces diarrhea and malabsorption: a prospective, controlled trial. *Nutrition* 12: 766–771, 1996.

3. Caliari S, Benini L, and Sembenini C. Medium-chain triglyceride absorption in patients with pancreatic insufficiency. *Scand J Gastroenterol* 31: 90–94, 1996.

4. Bach, AC and Babayan VK. Medium triglycerides: a review. *Am J Clin Nutr* 36: 950, 1982.

5. Jeukendrup AE. Oxidation of orally ingested medium chain triglyceride (MCT) during prolonged exercise. *Med & Sci in Sport & Exer* 27 (Supplement): S101, 1995.

6. Anderson O. Putting medium-chain triglycerides in your sports drink can increase your endurance. *Running Res News:* 6, Sept–Oct 1994.

7. Signore JM. Ketogenic diet containing medium-chain triglycerides. *J Am Diet Assoc* 62: 285–290, 1973.

8. Craig GB, Darnell BE, and Weinsier RL. Decreased fat and nitrogen losses in patients with AIDS receiving medium-chain-triglyceride-containing formulas. *J Am Diet Assoc* 97: 605–611, 1997.

9. Wanke CA, Pleskow D and Degirolami PC. A medium chain triglyceride-based diet in patients with HIV and chronic diarrhea reduces diarrhea and malabsorption: a prospective, controlled trial. *Nutrition* 12: 766–771, 1996.

10. Caliari S, Benini L, and Sembenini C. Medium-chain triglyceride absorption in patients with pancreatic insufficiency. *Scand J Gastroenterol* 31: 90–94, 1996.

11. Bach, AC and Babayan VK. Medium triglycerides: a review. *Am J Clin Nutr* 36: 950, 1982.

12. Anderson O. Putting medium-chain triglycerides in your sports drink can increase your endurance. *Running Res News:* 6, Sept–Oct 1994.

13. Jeukendrup AE. Oxidation of orally ingested medium chain triglyceride (MCT) during prolonged exercise. *Med & Sci in Sport & Exer* 27 (Supplement): S101, 1995.

14. Jeukendrup AE, et al. Effect of medium-chain triacylglycerol and carbohydrate ingestion during exercise on substrate utilization and subsequent cycling performance. *Am J Clin Nutr* 67: 397–404, 1998.

## Melatonin

1. Suhner A, et al. Optimal melatonin dosage form for the alleviation of jet lag. *Chronobiol Int* 14: 41, 1997.

2. Suhner A, et al. Optimal melatonin dosage form for the alleviation of jet lag. *Chronobiol Int* 14: 41, 1997.

3. Arendt J, et al. Efficacy of melatonin in jet lag, shift work and blindness. *J Bio Rhythms* 12: 604–617, 1997.

4. Lissoni P, Meregalli S, Nosetto L, et al. Increased survival time in brain glioblastomas by a radioneuroendocrine strategy with radiotherapy plus melatonin compared to radiotherapy alone. *Oncology* 53: 43–46, 1996.

5. Lissoni P, Paolorossi F, Ardizzoia A, et al. A randomized study of chemotherapy with cisplatin plus etoposide versus chemoendocrine therapy with cisplatin, etoposide and the pineal hormone melatonin as a first-line treatment of advanced non-small cell lung cancer patients in a poor clinical state. *J Pineal Res* 23: 15–19, 1997.

6. Neri B, de Leonardis V, Gemelli MT. Melatonin as biological response modifier in cancer patients. *Anticancer Res* 18: 1329–1332, 1998.

7. Lissoni P, Tancini G, and Barni S. Treatment of cancer chemotherapy-induced toxicity with the pineal hormone melatonin. *Support Care Cancer* 5: 126–129, 1997.

8. Suhner A, et al. Optimal melatonin dosage form for the alleviation of jet lag. *Chronobiol Int* 14: 41, 1997.

9. Attenburrow ME, Cowen PJ, and Sharpley AL. Low dose melatonin improves sleep in healthy middle-aged subjects. *Psychopharmacology* (Berl) 126: 179–181, 1996.

10. Garfinkel D, et al. Improvement of sleep quality in elderly people by controlled-release melatonin. *Lancet* 346: 541–544, 1995.

11. Petrie K, et al. A double-blind trial of melatonin as a treatment for jet lag in international cabin crew. *Bio Psych* 33: 526–530, 1993.

12. Chase JE, et al. Melatonin: therapeutic use in sleep disorders. *Ann Pharmacother* 346: 1218–1226, 1997.

13. Arendt J, et al. Efficacy of melatonin in jet lag, shift work and blindness. *J Bio Rhythms* 12: 604–617, 1997.

14. Spitzer RL, et al. Failure of melatonin to affect jet lag in a randomized double blind trial. *Soc Light Treatment Biol Rhythms Abstr* 9: 1, 1997.

15. Lissoni P, Meregalli S, Nosetto L, et al. Increased survival time in brain glioblastomas by a radioneuroendocrine strategy with radiotherapy plus melatonin compared to radiotherapy alone. *Oncology* 53: 43–46, 1996.

16. Lissoni P, Paolorossi F, Ardizzoia A, et al. A randomized study of chemotherapy with cisplatin plus etoposide versus chemoendocrine therapy with cisplatin, etoposide and the pineal hormone melatonin as a first-line treatment of advanced non-small cell lung cancer patients in a poor clinical state. *J Pineal Res* 23: 15–19, 1997.

17. Lissoni P, Tancini G, and Barni S. Treatment of cancer chemotherapy-induced toxicity with the pineal hormone melatonin. *Support Care Cancer* 5: 126–129, 1997.

18. Neri B, de Leonardis V, Gemelli MT. Melatonin as biological response modifier in cancer patients. *Anticancer Res* 18: 1329–1332, 1998.

19. Waterhouse J, et al. Jet lag. *Lancet* 350: 1611–1616, 1997.

## Melissa

1. Wolbling RH, ct al. Clinical therapy of herpes simplex. *Therapiewoche* 34: 1193–1200, 1984.

2. Wolbling RH, et al. Local therapy of herpes simplex with dried extract from *Melissa officinalis*. *Phytomedicine* 1: 25–31, 1994.

3. Dimitrova Z, et al. Antiherpes effect of *Melissa officinalis* L. extracts. *Acta Microbiol Bulg* 29: 65–72, 1993.

4. May S, et al. Antivirale Wirkung wassriger Pflanzenextrakte in Gewebekulturen. *Arzneimittelforschung Drug Res* 28: 1–7, 1978.

5. Wolbling RH, et al. Local therapy of herpes simplex with dried extract from *Melissa officinalis*. *Phytomedicine* 1: 25–31, 1994.

6. Wolbling RH, et al. Clinical therapy of herpes simplex. *Therapiewoche* 34: 1193–1200, 1984.

7. Wolbling RH, et al. Local therapy of herpes simplex with dried extract from *Melissa officinalis*. *Phytomedicine* 1: 25–31, 1994.

8. Wolbling RH, et al. Clinical therapy of herpes simplex. *Therapiewoche* 34: 1193–1200, 1984.

9. Wolbling RH, et al. Local therapy of herpes simplex with dried extract from *Melissa officinalis*. *Phytomedicine* 1: 25–31, 1994.

10. Wolbling RH, et al. Local therapy of herpes simplex with dried extract from *Melissa officinalis*. *Phytomedicine* 1: 25–31, 1994.

11. Isselbacher K, et al., eds. Harrison's principles of internal medicine, 13th ed. New York: McGraw Hill, 1994: 779.

12. Soulimani R, et al. Neurotropic action of the hydroalcoholic extract of *Melissa officinalis* in the mouse. *Planta Med* 57: 105–109, 1991.

13. Dressing H, et al. Insomnia: Are valerian/balm combinations of equal value to benzodiazepine? *Therapiewoche* 42: 726–736, 1992.

14. Wolbling RH, et al. Local therapy of herpes simplex with dried extract from *Melissa officinalis*. *Phytomedicine* 1: 25–31, 1994.

## Methionine

1. Funfstuck R, Straube E, Schildbach O, and Tietz U. Prevention of reinfection by L-methionine in patients with recurrent urinary tract infection. *Med Klin* 92: 574–581: 1997.

2. Funfstuck R, Straube E, Schildbach O, and Tietz U. Prevention of reinfection by L-methionine in patients with recurrent urinary tract infection. *Med Klin* 92: 574–581: 1997.

3. Neuvonen PJ, Tokola O, Toivonen ML, and Simell O. Methionine in paracetamol tablets, a tool to reduce paracetamol toxicity. *Int J Clin Pharmacol Ther Toxicol* 23: 497–500, 1985.

4. Funfstuck R, Straube E, Schildbach O, and Tietz U. Prevention of reinfection by L-methionine in patients with recurrent urinary tract infection. *Med Klin* 92: 574–581: 1997.

5. Toborek M and Mennig B. Is methionine an atherogenic amino acid? *J Opt Nutr* 3: 80–83, 1994.

## Milk Thistle

1. Schulz V, et al. Rational phytotherapy. New York: Springer-Verlag, 1998: 215.

2. Muriel P, et al. Silymarin protects against paracetamol-induced lipid peroxidation and liver damage. *J Appl Toxicol* 12: 6439–6442, 1992.

3. Paulova J, et al. Verification of the hepatoprotective and therapeutic effect of silymarin in experimental liver injury with tetrachloromethane in dogs. *Vet Med* (Praha) 35(10): 629–635, 1990.

4. Skakun NP, et al. Clinical pharmacology of Fegalon (review of the literature). *Vrach Delo* 5: 5–10, 1988.

5. Tuchweber B, et al. Prevention of silybin of phalloidin-induced acute hepatotoxicity. *Toxicol Appl Pharmacol* 51(2): 265–275, 1979.

6. Boari C, et al. Toxic occupational liver diseases. Therapeutic effects of silymarin. *Minerva Med* 72(40): 2679–2688, 1981.

7. Szilard S. Protective effect of Legalon in workers exposed to organic solvents. *Acta Med Hung* 45(2): 249–256, 1988.

8. Rui YC. Advances in pharmacological studies of silymarin. *Mem Inst Oswaldo Cruz* 86(Suppl. 2): 79–85, 1991.

9. Schulz V, et al. Rational phytotherapy. New York: Springer-Verlag, 1998: 216.

10. Hikino H, et al. Natural products for liver disease. As cited in Wagner H, et al. Economic and medicinal plant research, Vol 2. New York: Academic Press, 1988: 39–72.

11. Muzes G, et al. Effects of silymarin (Legalon) therapy on the antioxidant defense mechanism and lipid peroxidation in alcoholic liver disease (double-blind protocol). *Orv Hetil* 131(16): 863–866, 1990.

12. Giannola C, et al. A two-center study on the effects of silymarin in pregnant women and adult patients with so-called minor hepatic insufficiency. *Clin Ther* 114(2): 129–135, 1985.

13. Schulz V, et al. Rational phytotherapy. New York: Springer-Verlag, 1998: 218.

14. Berenguer J, et al. Double-blind trial of silymarin vs. placebo in the treatment of chronic hepatitis. *Munch Med Wochenschr* 119: 240–260, 1977.

15. Buzzelli G, et al. A pilot study on the liver protective effect of silybin-phosphatidylcholine complex (IdB 1016) in chronic active hepatitis. *Int J Clin Pharmacol Ther Toxicol* 31(9): 456–460, 1993.

16. Liruss F, et al. Cytoprotection in the nineties: Experience with ursodeoxycholic acid and silymarin in chronic liver disease. *Acta Physiol Hung* 80(1–4): 363–367, 1992.

17. Magliulo E, et al. Results of a double blind study on the effect of silymarin in the treatment of acute viral hepatitis, carried out at two medical centers. *Med Klin* 73: 28–29, 1060–1065, 1978.

18. Bode JC, et al. Silymarin for the treatment of acute viral hepatitis? Report of a controlled trial. *Med Klin* 72(12): 513–518, 1977.

19. Salmi H, et al. Effect of silymarin on chemical, functional and morphological alterations of the liver. *Scand J Gastroenterol* 17: 517–521, 1982.

20. Feher J. Liver protective action of silymarin therapy in chronic alcoholic liver diseases. *Orv Hetil* 130(51): 2723–2727, 1989.

21. Trinchet JC. Treatment of alcoholic hepatitis with silymarin. A double-blind comparative study in 116 patients. *Gastroenterol Clin Biol* 13(2): 120–124, 1989.

22. Bunout D, et al. Controlled study of the effect of silymarin on alcoholic liver disease. *Rev Med Chil* 120(12): 1370–1375, 1992.

23. Ferenci P, et al. Randomized controlled trial of silymarin treatment in patients with cirrhosis of the liver. *J Hepatol* 9: 105–113, 1989.

24. Pares A, et al. Effects of silymarin in alcoholic patients with cirrhosis of the liver: Results of a controlled, double-blind, randomized and multicenter trial. *J Hepatology* 28: 615–621, 1998.

25. Brinker F. Herb contraindications and drug interactions, 2nd ed. Sandy, Oregon: Eclectic Medical Publications, 1998: 103.

26. Schandalik R, et al. Pharmacokinetics of silybin in bile following administration of silipide and silymarin in cholecsytectomy patients. *Arzneimittelforschung* 42(7): 964–968, 1992.

27. Barzaghi N, et al. Pharmacokinetic studies on IdB 1016, a silybin-phosphatidylcholine complex in healthy human subjects. *Eur J Drug Metab Pharmacokinet* 15(4): 333–338, 1990.

28. Awang D. Milk thistle. *Can Pharm J* 422: 403–404, 1983.

29. Albrecht M. Therapy of toxic liver pathologies with Legalon. *Z Klin Med* 47(2): 87–92, 1992.

30. Giannola C, et al. A two-center study on the effects of silymarin in pregnant women and adult patients with so-called minor hepatic insufficiency. *Clin Ther* 114(2): 129–135, 1985.

31. Kim DH, et al. Silymarin and its components are inhibitors of beta-glucuronidase. *Biol Pharm Bull* 17(3): 443–445, 1994.

## Mullein

1. Tyler V. The honest herbal, 3rd ed. Binghamton, New York: Pharmaceutical Products Press, 1993: 219–220.

## N-Acetyl Cysteine

1. Pizzulli L, Hagendorff A, and Zirbes M. N-acetylcysteine attenuates nitroglycerin tolerance in patients with angina pectoris and normal left ventricular function. *Am J Cardiol* 79: 28–33, 1997.

2. Ardissino D, Merlini PA, Savonitto S, et al. Effect of transdermal nitroglycerin or N-acetylcysteine, or both, in the long-term treatment of unstable angina pectoris. *J Am Coll Cardiol* 29: 941–947, 1997.

3. Bernard GR, Wheeler AP, Arons MM, et al. A trial of antioxidants N-acetylcysteine and procysteine in ARDS. The Antioxidant in ARDS Study Group. *Chest* 112: 164–172, 1997.

4. Ardissino D, Merlini PA, Savonitto S, et al. Effect of transdermal nitroglycerin or N-acetylcysteine, or both, in the long-term treatment of unstable angina pectoris. *J Am Coll Cardiol* 29: 941–947, 1997.

5. Pizzulli L, Hagendorff A, and Zirbes M. N-acetylcysteine attenuates nitroglycerin tolerance in patients with angina pectoris and normal left ventricular function. *Am J Cardiol* 79: 28–33, 1997.

6. Bernard GR, Wheeler AP, Arons MM, et al. A trial of antioxidants N-acetylcysteine and procysteine in ARDS. The Antioxidant in ARDS Study Group. *Chest* 112: 164–172, 1997.

7. Badawy AH, Abdel Aal SF, and Samour SA. Liver injury associated with N-acetylcysteine administration. *J Egypt Soc Parasitol* 19: 563–571, 1989.

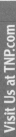

## NADH

1. Birkmayer JG, Vrecko C, Volc D, and Birkmayer W. Nicotinamideadenine dinucleotide (NADH)—a new therapeutic approach to Parkinson's disease. Comparison of oral and parenteral application. *Acta Neurol Scand* 146: 32–35, 1993.

2. Birkmayer W and Birkmayer JGD. The coenzyme nicotinamide adenine dinucleotide (NADH) as biological antidepressive agent. *New Trends in Neuropharmacology* 5: 19–25, 1991.

3. Birkmayer JGD. Coenzyme nicotinamide adenine dinucleotide: new therapeutic approach for improving dementia of the Alzheimer type. *Ann Clin Lab Sci* 26:1–9, 1996.


## Neem

1. Charles V, et al. Village pharmacy. The neem tree yields products from pesticides to soap. *Sci Am* 44(1–2): 132, 1992.

2. Neem Foundation: www.neemfoundation.org

3. Awasthy KS, Charuasia OP, Sinha SP. Prolonged murine genotoxic effects of crude extracted from neem. *Phytother Res* 13: 81–83, 1999.


## Nettle

1. Hryb DJ, et al. The effect of extracts of the roots of the stinging nettle (*Urtica dioica*) on the interaction of SHBG with its receptor on human prostatic membranes. *Planta Med* 61: 31–32, 1995.

2. Wagner H, et al. Search for the antiprostatic principle of stinging nettle (*Urtica dioica*) roots. *Phytomedicine* 1: 213–224, 1994.

3. Schulz V, et al. Rational phytotherapy. New York: Springer-Verlag, 1998: 229.

4. ESCOP monographs. Fascicule 2: *Urticae radix*. Exeter, UK: European Scientific Cooperative on Phytotherapy, 1996: 2–4.

5. ESCOP monographs. Fascicule 2: *Urticae radix*. Exeter, UK: European Scientific Cooperative on Phytotherapy, 1996: 4–5.

6. Dathe G, et al. Phytotherpie der beignen Prostatahyperplasie (BPH). *Urologe B* 27: 223–226, 1987.

7. ESCOP monographs. Fascicule 2: *Urticae radix*. Exeter, UK: 1996: European Scientific Cooperative on Phytotherapy, 4.

8. ESCOP monographs. Fascicule 2: *Urticae radix*. Exeter, UK: 1996: European Scientific Cooperative on Phytotherapy, 4.

9. Mittman P. Randomized, double-blind study of freeze-dried *Urtica dioica* in the treatment of allergic rhinitis. *Planta Med* 56: 44–47, 1990.

10. ESCOP monographs. Fascicule 2: *Urticae radix*. Exeter, UK: European Scientific Cooperative on Phytotherapy, 1996: 5.


## OPCs

1. Schwitters B, et al. OPC in practice. Bioflavanols and their applications. Rome, Italy: Alfa Omega, 1993.

2. Masquelier J, et al. Stabilization of collagen by procyanidolic oligomers. *Acta Ther* 7: 101–105, 1981.

3. Masquelier J. Procyanidolic oligomers. *J Parums Cosm Arom* 95: 89–97, 1990.

4. Tixier JM, et al. Evidence by in vivo and in vitro studies that binding of pycnogenols to elastin affects its rate of degradation by elastases. *Biochem Pharmacol* 33: 3933–3939, 1984.

5. Facino RM, et al. Free radical scavenging action and anti-enzyme activities of procyanidines from *Vitis vinifera*. A mechanism for their capillary protective action. *Arzneimittelforschung* 44: 592–601, 1994.

6. Kuttan R, et al. Collagen treated with catechin becomes resistant to the action of mammalian collagenase. *Experientia* 37: 221–223, 1981.

7. Masquelier J, et al. Stabilization of collagen by procyanidolic oligomers. *Acta Ther* 7: 101–105, 1981.

8. Thebaut JF, et al. Study of endotelon in functional manifestations of peripheral venous insufficiency. *Gazette Medicale* 92: 12, 1985.

9. Henriet JP. Exemplary study for a phlebotropic substance, the EIVE study. On file with Primary Services International, Southport, Connecticut.

10. Delacroix P, et al. Double-blind study of endotelon in chronic venous insufficiency. *La Revue de Medecine* 31: 27–28, 1793–1802, 1981.

11. Pecking A, et al. Oligomeric proanthocyanidins (endotelon) in the treatment of post therapeutic lymphedema in the upper limbs. Association de Lymphologie de Lange Française, Hôpital Saint-Louis, 75010, Paris, France: 69-73, 1989.

12. Baruch J. Effect of endotelon in post-surgical edemas. *Ann Chir Plast Esthet* 29(4): 393–395, 1984.

13. Parienti JJ, et al. Post traumatic edemas in sports: a controlled test of endotelon. *Gaz Med France* 90: 231–236, 1983.

14. Facino RM, et al. Free radical scavenging action and anti-enzyme activities of procyanidines from *vitis*

*vinifera.* A mechanism for their capillary protective action. *Arzneimittelforschung* 44: 592–601, 1994.

15. Kuttan R, et al. Collagen treated with catechin becomes resistant to the action of mammalian collagenase. *Experientia* 37: 221–223, 1981.

16. Masquelier J. Procyanidolic oligomers. *J Parums Cosm Arom* 95: 89–97, 1990.

17. Masquelier J, et al. Stabilization of collagen by procyanidolic oligomers. *Acta Therap* 7: 101–105, 1981.

18. Schwitters B, et al. OPC in practice. Bioflavanols and their applications. *Alfa Omega.* Rome, Italy, 1993.

19. Tixier JM, et al. Evidence by in vivo and in vitro studies that binding of pycnogenols to elastin affects its rate of degradation by elastases. *Biochem Pharmacol* 33: 3933–3939, 1984.

20. Bagchi D, Garg A, Krohn RL, et al. Oxygen free radical scavenging abilities of vitamins C and E, and a grape seed proanthocyanidin extract in vitro. *Res Commun Mol Pathol Pharmacol* 95: 179–189, 1997.

21. Thebaut JF, et al. Study of endotelon in functional manifestations of peripheral venous insufficiency. *Gazette Medicale* 92: 12, 1985.

22. Henriet, JP. Exemplary study for a phleboteropic substance, the EIVE study. On file with Primary Services International, Southport, CT.

23. Delacroix P, et al. Double-blind study of Endotelon in chronic venous insufficiency. English abstract only. *La Revue de Medecine* 31: 27–28, 1793–1802, 1981.

24. Pecking A, et al. Oligomeric proanthocyanidins (Endotelons) in the treatment of post-therapeutic lymphedema in the upper limbs. English abstract only. Association de Lymphologie de Lange Française, Hôpital Saint-Louis, 75010, Paris, France: 69–73, 1989.

25. Baruch J. Effect of Endotelon in post-surgical edemas. English abstract only. *Ann Chir Plast Esthet* 29 (4): 393–395, 1984.

26. Parienti JJ, et al. Post-traumatic edemas in sports: A controlled test of Endotelon. English abstract only. *Gaz Med France* 90 (3): 231–236.

27. Corbe C, et al. Light vision and chorioretinal circulation. Study of the effect of procyanidolic oligomers (Endotelon). *J Fr Ophtalmol* 11: 453–460, 1988.

28. Boissin JP, et al. Chorioretinal circulation and dazzling: Use of procyanidol oligomers. *Bull Soc Ophtamol Fr* 88: 173–174, 177–179, 1988.

29. Schwitters B, et al. OPC in practice. Bioflavanols and their applications. Rome, Italy: Alfa Omega, 1993.

30. Wegrowski J, et al. The effect of procyanidolic oligomers on the composition of normal and hypercholesterolemic rabbit aortas. *Biochem Pharmacol* 33: 3491–3497, 1984.

31. Uchida S, et al. Condensed tannins scavenge active free radicals. *Med Sci Res* 15: 831–832, 1987.

32. Gendre P. Effet protecteur des oligomeres procyandiloques sur le lathyrisme experimental chez le rat. *Ann Pharm Fr* 43(1): 61–71, 1985.

33. Schulz V, et al. Rational phytotherapy, 283. New York: Springer Verlag, 1998: 283.

## Ornithine Alpha-Ketoglutarate

1. Jeevanandam M, Holaday NJ, and Petersen SR. Ornithine-alpha-ketoglutarate (OKG) supplementation is more effective than its component salts in traumatized rats. *J Nutr* 126: 2141–2150, 1996.

2. Le Bricon T, Cynober L, and Baracos VE. Ornithine alpha-ketoglutarate limits muscle protein breakdown without stimulating tumor growth in rats bearing Yoshida ascites hepatoma. *Met Clin Exp* 43: 899–905, 1994.

## Osha

1. Bensky D and Gamble A. Chinese herbal medicine: Materia medica. Seattle, WA: Eastland Press, 1986: 383–384.

2. Moore M. Medicinal plants of the mountain west. Santa Fe, NM: Museum of New Mexico Press, 1979: 119.

## PABA (Para-Aminobenzoic Acid)

1. Zarafonetis CJ, Dabich L, and Skovronski JJ. Retrospective studies in scleroderma: skin response to potassium para-aminobenzoate therapy. *Clin Exp Rheumatol* 6: 261–268, 1988.

2. Zarafonetis CJ, Dabich L, Negri D et al. Retrospective studies in scleroderma: effect of potassium para-aminobenzoate on survival. *J Clin Epidemiol* 41: 193–205, 1988.

3. Clegg DO, Reading JC, and Mayes MD. Comparison of aminobenzoate potassium and placebo in the treatment of scleroderma. *J Rheumatol* 21: 105–110, 1994.

4. Hasche-Klunder R. Treatment of Peyronie's disease with para-aminobenzoacidic potassium (POTOBA). *Urologe* [A] 17: 224–247, 1978.

5. Carson CC. Potassium para-aminobenzoate for the treatment of Peyronie's disease: is it effective? *Tech Urol* 3: 135–139, 1997.

6. Ludwig G. Evaluation of conservative therapeutic approaches to Peyronie's disease (fibrotic induration of the penis). *Urol Int* 47: 236–239, 1991.

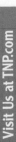

7. Sieve BF. The clinical effects of a new B complex factor, para-aminobenzoic acid, on pigmentation and fertility. *South Med Surg* 104: 135–139, 1942.

8. Physicians' desk reference. Montvale, NJ: Medical Economics Co., Inc., 1989.

9. Kantor GR and Ratz JL. Liver toxicity from potassium para-aminobenzoate. Letter. *J Am Acad Dermatol* 13: 671–672, 1985.

10. Hughes CG. Oral PABA and vitiligo. *J Am Acad Dermatol* 9: 770, 1983.

11. Drug evaluations subscription, vol. 2 (section 13, chapter 7). Chicago: American Medical Association, Spring 1993.

## Pantothenic Acid and Pantethine

1. Gaddi A, et al. Controlled evaluation of pantethine, a natural hypolipidemic compound, in patients with different forms of hyperlipoproteinemia. *Atherosclerosis* 50: 73–83, 1984.

2. Angelico M, et al. Improvement in serum lipid profile in hyper-lipoproteinaemic patients after treatment with pantethine: a crossover, double-blind trial versus placebo. *Curr Ther Res* 33: 1091, 1983.

3. Bertolini S, Donati C, Elicio N, Daga A, et al. Lipoprotein changes induced by pantethine in hyper-lipoproteinemic patients: adults and children. *Int J Clin Pharmacol Ther Toxicol* 24: 630–637, 1986.

4. Arsenio L, Caronna S, Lateana M, et al. Hyperlipidemia, diabetes and atherosclerosis: efficacy of treatment with pantethine. *Acta Biomed Ateneo Parmense* 55: 25–42, 1984.

5. Donati C, Barbi G, Cairo G, et al. Pantethine improves the lipid abnormalities of chronic hemodialysis patients: results of a multicenter clinical trial. *Clin Nephrol* 25: 70–74, 1986.

6. Donati C, Bertieri RS, and Barbi G. Pantethine, diabetes mellitus and atherosclerosis. Clinical study of 1045 patients. *Clin Ther* 128: 411–422, 1989.

7. Coronel F, Tornero F, Torrente J, et al. Treatment of hyperlipidemia in diabetic patients on dialysis with a physiological substance. *Am J Nephrol* 11: 32–36, 1991.

8. General Practitioner Research Group. Calcium pantothenate in arthritic conditions. *Practitioner* 224: 208–211, 1980.

9. Barton-Wright EC and Elliott WA. The pantothenic acid metabolism of rheumatoid arthritis. *Lancet* 2: 862–863, 1963.

10. Gaddi A, et al. Controlled evaluation of pantethine, a natural hypolipidemic compound, in patients with differ-

ent forms of hyperlipoproteinemia. *Atherosclerosis* 50: 73–83, 1984.

11. Angelico M, et al. Improvement in serum lipid profile in hyper-lipoproteinaemic patients after treatment with pantethine: a crossover, double-blind trial versus placebo. *Curr Ther Res* 33: 1091, 1983.

12. Bertolini S, Donati C, Elicio N, Daga A, et al. Lipoprotein changes induced by pantethine in hyperlipoproteinemic patients: adults and children. *Int J Clin Pharmacol Ther Toxicol* 24: 630–637, 1986.

13. Gaddi A, et al. Controlled evaluation of pantethine, a natural hypolipidemic compound, in patients with different forms of hyperlipoproteinemia. *Atherosclerosis* 50: 73–83, 1984.

14. Rubba R, Postiglione A, DeSimone B, et al. Comparative evaluation of the lipid-lowering effects of fenofibrate and pantethine in type II hyperlipoproteinemia. *Curr Ther Res Clin Exp* 38: 719–727, 1985.

15. Dacol PG, et al. Pantethine in the treatment of hypercholesterolemia: a randomized double-blind trial versus tiadenol. *Curr Ther Res* 36: 314–322, 1984.

16. Arsenio L, Caronna S, Lateana M, et al. Hyperlipidemia, diabetes and atherosclerosis: efficacy of treatment with pantethine. *Acta Biomed Ateneo Parmense* 55: 25–42, 1984.

17. Donati C, Barbi G, Cairo G, et al. Pantethine improves the lipid abnormalities of chronic hemodialysis patients: results of a multicenter clinical trial. *Clin Nephrol* 25: 70–74, 1986.

18. Donati C, Bertieri RS, and Barbi G. Pantethine, diabetes mellitus and atherosclerosis. Clinical study of 1045 patients. *Clin Ter* 128: 411–422, 1989.

19. Coronel F, Tornero F, Torrente J, et al. Treatment of hyperlipidemia in diabetic patients on dialysis with a physiological substance. *Am J Nephrol* 11: 32–36, 1991.

20. Carrara P, Matturri L, Galbussera M, et al. Pantethine reduces plasma cholesterol and the severity of arterial lesions in experimental hypercholesterolemic rabbits. *Atherosclerosis* 53: 255–264, 1984.

21. Barton-Wright EC and Elliott WA. The pantothenic acid metabolism of rheumatoid arthritis. *Lancet* 2: 862–863, 1963.

22. General Practitioner Research Group. Calcium pantothenate in arthritic conditions. *Practitioner* 224: 208–211, 1980.

## Passionflower

1. Schulz V, et al. Rational phytotherapy. New York: Springer-Verlag, 1998: 84.

2. Newall C, et al. Herbal medicines: A guide for healthcare professionals. London: Pharmaceutical Press, 1996: 206.

3. Brinker F. Herb contraindications and drug interactions, 2nd ed. Sandy, Oregon: Eclectic Medical Publications, 1998: 110.

## Peppermint

1. Somerville KW, et al. Stones in the common bile duct: experience with medical dissolution therapy. *Postgrad Med J* 61: 313–316, 1985.

2. Gunn JWC. The carminative action of volatile oils. *J Pharmacol Exp Ther* 16: 93–143, 1920.

3. Taylor BA, et al. Inhibitory effect of peppermint on gastrointestinal smooth muscle. *Gut* 24: 992, 1983.

4. Hawthorn M, et al. The actions of peppermint oil and menthol on calcium channel dependent processes in intestinal, neuronal and cardiac preparations. *Aliment Pharmcol Ther* 2: 101–118, 1988.

5. Rees WDW, et al. Treating irritable bowel syndrome with peppermint oil. *BMJ* ii: 835–836, 1979.

6. Dew MJ, et al. Peppermint oil for the irritable bowel syndrome: A multicentre trial. *Br J Clin Pract* 34: 55–57, 1989.

7. Nash P, et al. Peppermint oil does not relieve the pain of irritable bowel syndrome. *Br J Clin Pract* 40: 292–293, 1986.

8. Lawson MJ, et al. Failure of enteric-coated peppermint oil in the irritable bowel syndrome: A randomized double-blind crossover study. *J Gastroenterol Hepatol* 3: 235–238, 1988.

9. Carling L, et al. Short-term treatment of the irritable bowel syndrome: A placebo controlled trial of peppermint oil against hyoscyaminme. *Opuscula Medica* 34: 55–57, 1989.

10. Spindler P, et al. Subchronic toxicity study of peppermint oil in rats. *Toxicol Lett* 62: 215–220, 1992.

11. ESCOP monographs. Fascicule 3: *Menthae Piperitae Aetheroleum* (peppermint oil). Exeter, UK: European Scientific Cooperative on Phytotherapy, 1997: 1–6.

12. ESCOP monographs. Fascicule 3: *Menthae Piperitae Aetheroleum* (peppermint oil). Exeter, UK: European Scientific Cooperative on Phytotherapy, 1997: 5.

## Phenylalanine

1. Werbach M. Nutritional influences on mental illness. Tarzana, CA: Third Line Press, 1991: 142.

2. Werbach M. Nutritional influences on mental illness. Tarzana, CA: Third Line Press, 1991: 141–142.

3. Heller B. 1978. Pharmacological and clinical effects of D-phenylalanine in depression and Parkinson's disease. As cited in Werbach M, 1991, 141.

4. Beckmann H, et al. DL-phenylalanine versus imipramine: A double-blind controlled study. *Arch Psychiat Nervenkr* 227: 49–58, 1979.

5. Balagot RC, et al. Analgesia in mice and humans by D-phenylalanine: Relation to inhibition of enkephalin degradation and enkephalin levels. *Adv Pain Res Ther* 5: 289–292, 1983.

6. Walsh NE, et al. Letter. *Pain:* 409–410, 1986.

7. Budd K. Use of D-phenylalanine, an enkephalinase inhibitor, in the treatment of intractable pain. *Adv Pain Res Ther* 5: 305–308, 1983.

8. Walsh NE, et al. Analgesic effectiveness of D-phenylalanine in chronic pain patients. *Arch Phys Med Rehabil* 67: 436–439, 1986.

9. Siddiqui AH, Stolk LM, Bhaggoe R, et al. L-phenylalanine and UVA irradiation in the treatment of vitiligo. *Dermatology* 188: 215–218, 1994.

10. Zametkin AJ, et al. Treatment of hyperactive children with D-phenylalanine. *Am J Psychiatry* 144(6): 792–794, 1987.

11. Wood DR, et al. Treatment of attention deficit disorder with DL-phenylalanine. *Am J Psychiatry Res* 16: 21–26, 1985.

12. Heller B. 1978. Pharmacological and clinical effects of D-phenylalanine in depression and Parkinson's disease. As cited in Werbach M, 1991, 141.

13. Beckmann H, et al. DL-phenylalanine versus imipramine: A double-blind controlled study. *Arch Psychiat Nervenkr* 227: 49–58, 1979.

14. Sabelli HC, et al. Clinical studies on the phenylethylamine hypothesis of affective disorder: Urine and blood phenylacetic acid and phenylalanine dietary supplements. *J Clin Psychiatry* 47(2): 66–70, 1986.

15. Kravitz HM, Sabelli HC, and Fawcett J. Dietary supplements of phenylalanine and other amino acid precursors of brain neuroamines in the treatment of depressive disorders. *J Am Osteopathic Assoc* 84(Suppl.): 119–123, 1984.

16. Balagot RC, et al. Analgesia in mice and humans by D-phenylalanine: Relation to inhibition of enkephalin degradation and enkephalin levels. *Adv Pain Res Ther* 5: 289–292, 1983.

17. Walsh NE, et al. Letter. *Pain:* 409–410, 1986.

18. Budd K. Use of D-phenylalanine, an enkephalinase inhibitor, in the treatment of intractable pain. *Adv Pain Res Ther* 5: 305–308, 1983.

19. Walsh NE, et al. Letter. *Pain:* 409–410, 1986.

20. Walsh NE, et al. Analgesic effectiveness of D-phenylalanine in chronic pain patients. *Arch Phys Med Rehabil* 67: 436–439, 1986.

21. Simonson M. L-phenylalanine. Letter. *J Clin Psychiatry* 46(8): 355, 1985.

22. Richardson MA. Amino acids in psychiatric disease. Washington, DC: American Psychiatric Press, 1990.

23. Mosnik DM, Spring B, Rogers K, and Baruah SL. Tardive dyskinesia exacerbated after ingestion of phenylalanine by schizophrenic patients. *Neuropsychopharmacology* 16(2): 136–146, 1997.

## Phosphatidylserine

1. Toffano G, et al. Effect of brain cortex phospholipids on catechol-amine content of mouse brain. *Pharmacol Res Commun* 8(6): 581–590. 1976.

2. LaBrake C, et al. Phospholipid vesicles promote human hemoglobin oxidation. *J Biol Chem* 267:16703–16711, 1992.

3. Orlando P, et al. The fate of double-labeled brain phospholipids administered to mice. *Il Farmaco (Edizione Practica)* 30(9): 451–458, 1975.

4. Gindin J, et al. The effect of plant phosphatidylserine on age-associated memory impairment and mood in the functioning elderly. Rehovot, Israel. Geriatric Institute for Education and Research and Dept. of Geriatrics, Kaplan Hospital, 1995.

5. Crook T. The memory cure. New York: Pocket Books, 1998: 71, 72.

6. Gaby AR. Don't believe everything you read. Editorial. *Townsend Letter for Doctors and Patients.* May 1997: 122–123.

7. Gindin J, et al. The effect of plant phosphatidylserine on age-associated memory impairment and mood in the functioning elderly. Rehovot, Israel. Geriatric Institute for Education and Research and Dept. of Geriatrics, Kaplan Hospital, 1995.

8. Amaducci L, et al. Phosphatidylserine in the treatment of Alzheimer's disease: results of a multicenter study. *Psychopharmacol Bull* 24 (1): 130–134, 1988.

9. Crook T, et al. Effects of phosphatidylserine in age-associated memory impairment. *Neurology* 41: 644–649, 1991.

10. Crook T, et al. Effects of phosphatidylserine in Alzheimer's disease. *Psychopharmacol Bull* 28: 61–66, 1992.

11. Delwaide PJ, et al. Double-blind randomized controlled study of phosphatidylserine in senile demented patients. *Acta Neurol Scand* 73: 136–140, 1986.

12. Engel RR, et al. Double-blind cross-over study of phosphatidylserine vs. placebo in patients with early dementia of the Alzheimer type. *Eur Neuropsychopharmacol* 2: 149–155, 1992.

13. Funfgeld E, et al. Double-blind study with phosphatidylserine (PS) in Parkinsonian patients with senile dementia of Alzheimer's type (SDAT). *Prog Clin Biol Res* 317: 1235–1246, 1989.

14. Nerozzi D, et al. Phosphatidylserine and memory disorders in the aged (in Italian). *Clin Ther* 120: 399–404, 1987.

15. Palmieri G, et al. Double-blind controlled trial of phosphatidylserine in subjects with senile mental deterioration. *Clin Trials J* 24: 73–83, 1987.

16. Villardita C, et al. Multicentre clinical trial of brain phosphatidylserine in elderly subjects with mental deterioration. *Clin Trials J* 24: 84–93, 1987.

17. Cenacchi T, et al. Cognitive decline in the elderly: A double-blind, placebo-controlled multicenter study on efficacy of phosphatidylserine administration. *Aging* 5: 123–133, 1993.

18. Crook T, et al. Effects of phosphatidylserine in age-associated memory impairment. *Neurology* 41: 644–649, 1991.

19. Cenacchi T, et al. Cognitive decline in the elderly: A double-blind, placebo-controlled multicenter study on efficacy of phosphatidylserine administration. *Aging* 5: 123–133, 1993.

20. Maggioni M, Picotti GB, Bondiolotti GP et al. Effects of phosphatidylserine therapy in geriatric patients with depressive disorders. *Acta Psychiatr Scand* 81: 265–270, 1990.

21. Brambilla F, Maggioni M, Panerai, AE, et al. Beta-endorphin concentration in peripheral blood mononuclear cells of elderly depressed patients—effects of phosphatidylserine therapy. *Neuropsychobiology* 34: 18–21, 1996.

22. Fahey TD and Pearl M. Hormonal effects of phosphatidylserine during 2 weeks of intense training. Abstract submitted to national meeting of the American College of Sports Medicine, June 1998.

23. Monteleone P, Maj M, Beinat L, Natale M, and Kemali D. Blunting by chronic phosphatidylserine administration of the stress-induced activation of the hypothalamo-pituitary-adrenal axis in healthy men. *Eur J Clin Pharm* 43: 385–388, 1992.

24. Cenacchi T, et al. Cognitive decline in the elderly: A double-blind, placebo-controlled multicenter study on efficacy of phosphatidylserine administration. *Aging* 5: 123–133, 1993.

25. Amaducci L, et al. Phosphatidylserine in the treatment of Alzheimer's disease: results of a multicenter study. *Psychopharmacol Bull* 24 (1): 130–134, 1988.

26. Crook T, et al. Effects of phosphatidylserine in Alzheimer's disease. *Psychopharmacol Bull* 28: 61–66, 1992.

27. Delwaide PJ, et al. Double-blind randomized controlled study of phosphatidylserine in senile demented patients. *Acta Neurol Scand* 73: 136–140, 1986.

28. Engel RR, et al. Double-blind cross-over study of phosphatidylserine vs. placebo in patients with early dementia of the Alzheimer type. *Eur Neuropsychopharmacol* 2: 149–155, 1992.

29. Funfgeld E, et al. Double-blind study with phosphatidylserine (PS) in Parkinsonian patients with senile dementia of Alzheimer's type (SDAT). *Prog Clin Biol Res* 317: 1235–1246, 1989.

30. Nerozzi D, et al. Phosphatidylserine and memory disorders in the aged (in Italian). *Clin Ther* 120: 399–404, 1987.

31. Palmieri G, et al. Double-blind controlled trial of phosphatidylserine in subjects with senile mental deterioration. *Clin Trials J* 24: 73–83, 1987.

32. Villardita C, et al. Multicentre clinical trial of brain phosphatidylserine in elderly subjects with mental deterioration. *Clin Trials J* 24: 84–93, 1987.

33. Crook T, et al. Effects of phosphatidylserine in age-associated memory impairment. *Neurology* 41: 644–649, 1991.

34. Fahey TD and Pearl M. Hormonal effects of phosphatidylserine during 2 weeks of intense training. Abstract submitted to national meeting of the American College of Sports Medicine, June 1998.

35. Fahey TD and Pearl M. Hormonal effects of phosphatidylserine during 2 weeks of intense training. Abstract submitted to national meeting of the American College of Sports Medicine, June 1998.

36. Monteleone P, Maj M, Beinat L, Natale M, and Kemali D. Blunting by chronic phosphatidylserine administration of the stress-induced activation of the hypothalamo-pituitary-adrenal axis in healthy men. *Eur J Clin Pharm* 43: 385–388, 1992.

37. Cenacchi T, et al. Cognitive decline in the elderly: A double-blind, placebo- controlled multicenter study on efficacy of phosphatidylserine administration. *Aging* 5: 123–133, 1993.

38. Van den Besselaar AM. Phosphatidylethanolamine and phosphatidylserine synergistically promote heparin's anticoagulant effect. *Blood Coagul Fibrinolysis* 6: 239–244, 1995.

## Potassium

1. Overlack A, Maus B, Ruppert M, et al. Potassium citrate versus potassium chloride in essential hypertension. Effects on hemodynamic, hormonal and metabolic parameters. *Dtsch Med Wochenschr* 120: 631–635, 1995.

2. Werbach M. Foundations of nutritional medicine. Tarzana, CA: Third Line Press, 1997: 186.

3. Drug evaluation subscription, vol. 3 (section 19, chapter 5). Chicago: American Medical Association, Spring 1993.

4. Whelton PK, He J, Cutler JA, et al. Effects of oral potassium on blood pressure. Meta-analysis of randomized controlled clinical trials. *JAMA* 277(20): 1624–1632, 1997.

5. Whelton PK, Buring J, Borhani NO, et al. The effect of potassium supplementation in persons with a high-normal blood pressure. Results from phase I of the Trials of Hypertension Prevention (TOHP). *Ann Epidemiol* 5: 85–95, 1995.

6. Barcelo P, Wuhl O, Servitge E, et al. Randomized double-blind study of potassium citrate in idiopathic hypocitraturic calcium nephrolithiasis. *J Urol* 150: 1761–1764, 1993.

7. Ettinger B, Pak CY, Citron JT, et al. Potassium-magnesium citrate is an effective prophylaxis against recurrent calcium oxalate nephrolithiasis. *J Urol* 158: 2069–2073, 1997.

8. Whelton PK, He J, Cutler JA, et al. Effects of oral potassium on blood pressure. Meta-analysis of randomized controlled clinical trials. *JAMA* 277(20): 1624–1632, 1997.

9. Whelton PK, Buring J, Borhani NO, et al. The effect of potassium supplementation in persons with a high-normal blood pressure. Results from phase I of the Trials of Hypertension Prevention (TOHP). *Ann Epidemiol* 5: 85–95, 1995.

10. Davis BR, Oberman A, Blaufox MD, et al. Lack of effectiveness of a low-sodium/high-potassium diet in reducing antihypertensive medication requirements in overweight persons with mild hypertension. TAIM Research Group. Trial of Antihypertensive Interventions and Management. *Am J Hypertens* 7: 926–932, 1994.

11. Whelton PK, Buring J, Borhani NO, et al. The effect of potassium supplementation in persons with a high-normal blood pressure. Results from phase I of the Trials of Hypertension Prevention (TOHP). *Ann Epidemiol* 5: 85–95, 1995.

## Pregnenolone

1. Meldrum DR, Davidson BJ, Tataryn IV, and Judd HL. Changes in circulating steroids with aging in postmenopausal women. *Obstet Gynecol* 57: 624–628, 1981.

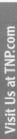

2. Flood JF, Morley JE, and Roberts E. Pregnenolone sulfate enhances post-training memory processes when injected in very low doses into limbic system structures: the amygdala is by far the most sensitive. *Proc Natl Acad Sci USA* 92: 10806–10810, 1995.

3. Flood JF, Morley JE, and Roberts E. Memory-enhancing effects in male mice of pregnenolone and steroids metabolically derived from it. *Proc Natl Acad Sci USA* 89: 1567–1571, 1992.

## Proteolytic Enzymes

1. Zuschlag JM. Double-blind clinical study using certain proteolytic enzyme mixtures in karate fighters. Working paper. *Mucos Pharma GmbH* (Germany): 1–5, 1988.

2. Rathgerber WF. The use of proteolytic enzymes (Chymoral) in sporting injuries. *S Afr Med J* 45: 181–183, 1971.

3. Schulz V, et al. Rational phytotherapy. New York: Springer-Verlag, 1998: 263.

4. Billigmann P. Enzymtherapie—eine Alternative bei der Behandlung des Zoster. Eine kontrollierte Studie an 192 Patienten. *Fortschr Med* 113: 43–48, 1995.

5. Zuschlag JM. Double-blind clinical study using certain proteolytic enzyme mixtures in karate fighters. Working paper. *Mucos Pharma GmbH* (Germany): 1–5, 1988.

6. Rathgerber WF. The use of proteolytic enzymes (Chymoral) in sporting injuries. *S Afr Med J* 45: 181–183, 1971.

7. Russell RM, et al. Impairment of folic acid absorption by oral pancreatic extracts. *Dig Dis Sci* 25: 369–373, 1980.

## Pygeum

1. Schulz V, et al. Rational phytotherapy. New York: Springer-Verlag, 1998: 232.

2. Schulz V, et al. Rational phytotherapy. New York: Springer-Verlag, 1998: 233.

3. Duvia R, et al. Advances in the phytotherapy of prostatic hypertrophy. *Med Pr* 4: 143–148, 1983.

4. Schulz V, et al. Rational phytotherapy. New York: Springer-Verlag, 1998: 233.

## Pyruvate

1. Stanko RT, Reynolds HR, Hoyson R, et al. Pyruvate supplementation of a low- cholesterol, low-fat diet: effects on plasma lipid concentrations and body composition in hyperlipidemic patients. *Am J Clin Nutr* 59: 423–427, 1994.

2. Stanko RT and Arch JE. Inhibition of regain in body weight and fat with addition of 3-carbon compound to the diet with hyperenergetic refeeding after weight reduction. *Int J Obes Relat Metab Disord* 20: 925–930, 1996.

3. Stanko RT, Tietze DL, and Arch JE. Body composition, energy utilization, and nitrogen metabolism with a severely restricted diet supplemented with dihydroxyacetone and pyruvate. *Am J Clin Nutr* 55: 771–772, 1992.

4. Stanko RT, Robertson RJ, Galbreath RW, et al. Enhanced leg exercise endurance with a high-carbohydrate diet and dihydroxyacetone and pyruvate. *J Appl Physiol* 69: 1651–1656, 1990.

5. Stanko RT, Robertson RJ, Spina RJ, et al. Enhancement of arm exercise endurance capacity with dihydroxyacetone and pyruvate. *J Appl Physiol* 68: 119–124, 1990.

6. Stanko RT, Reynolds HR, Hoyson R, et al. Pyruvate supplementation of a low-cholesterol, low-fat diet: effects on plasma lipid concentrations and body composition in hyperlipidemic patients. *Am J Clin Nutr* 59: 423–427, 1994.

7. Stanko RT and Arch JE. Inhibition of regain in body weight and fat with addition of 3-carbon compound to the diet with hyperenergetic refeeding after weight reduction. *Int J Obes Relat Metab Disord* 20: 925–930, 1996.

8. Stanko RT, Tietze DL, and Arch JE. Body composition, energy utilization, and nitrogen metabolism with a severely restricted diet supplemented with dihydroxyacetone and pyruvate. *Am J Clin Nutr* 55: 771–772, 1992.

## Quercetin

1. Ogasawara H and Middleton E Jr. Effect of selected flavonoids on histamine release (HR) and hydrogen peroxide ($H_2O_2$) generation by human leukocytes. *J Allergy Clin Immunol* 75: 184, 1985.

2. Yoshimoto T, et al. Flavonoids: Potent inhibitors of arachidonate 5-lipoxygenase. *Biochem Biophys Res Commun* 116: 612–618, 1983.

3. Constant J. Alcohol, ischemic heart disease, and the French paradox. *Coron Artery Dis* 8: 645–649, 1997.

4. Hayek T, Fuhrman B, and Vaya J. Reduced progression of atherosclerosis in apolipoprotein E-deficient mice following consumption of red wine, or its polyphenols quercetin or catechin, is associated with reduced susceptibility of LDL to oxidation and aggregation. *Arterioscler Thromb Vasc Biol* 17: 2744–2752, 1997.

5. Frankel EN, Waterhouse AL, and Kinsella JE. Inhibition of human LDL oxidation by resveratrol. Letter. *Lancet* 341: 1103–1104, 1993.

6. Alliangana DM. Effects of beta-carotene, flavonoid quercetin and quinacrine on cell proliferation and lipid peroxidation breakdown products in BHK-21 cells. *East Afr Med J* 73: 752–757, 1996.

7. Keli SO, et al. Dietary flavonoids, antioxidant vitamins, and incidence of stroke: the Zupthen study. *Arch Intern Med* 147: 637–642, 1996.

8. Balasubramanian S and Govindasamy S. Inhibitory effect of dietary quercetin on 7,12-dimethyl-benz(a)anthracene-induced hamster buccal pouch carcinogenesis. *Carcinogenesis* 17: 877–879, 1996.

9. Cross JH, et al. Effect of quercetin on the genotoxic potential of cisplatin. *Int J Cancer* 66: 404–409, 1996.

10. Hoffman R, et al. Enhanced anti-proliferative action of busulphan by quercetin on the human leukaemia cell line K562. *Br J Cancer* 59: 347–348, 1989.

11. Varma SD, et al. Diabetic cataracts and flavonoids. *Science* 195: 205–206, 1977.

12. Kaul TN, et al. Antiviral effect of flavonoids on human viruses. *J Med Virol* 15: 71–79, 1985.

13. Musci I and Pragai BM. Inhibition of virus multiplication and alteration of cyclic AMP level in cell cultures by flavonoids. *Experientia* 41: 930–931, 1985.

14. Stavric B. Quercetin in our diet: From potent mutagen to probable anticarcinogen. *Clin Biochem* 27: 245–248, 1994.

15. Friedman M and Smith GA. Factors which facilitate inactivation of quercetin mutagenicity. *Adv Exp Med Biol* 177: 527–544, 1984.

## Red Clover

1. Newall C, et al. Herbal medicines: A guide for healthcare professionals. London: Pharmaceutical Press, 1996: 227.

2. Yanagihara K, et al. Antiproliferative effects of isoflavones on human cancer cell lines established from the gastrointestinal tract. *Cancer Res* 53: 5815–5821, 1993.

## Red Raspberry

1. Bamford DS, et al. Raspberry leaf tea: A new aspect to an old problem. *Br J Pharmacol* 40: 161–162, 1970.

## Resveratrol

1. Goldberg DM. More on antioxidant activity of resveratrol in red wine. *Clin Chem* 42: 113–114, 1996.

2. Siemann EH and Creasy LL. Concentration of the phytoalexin resveratrol in wine. *Am J Enol Vitic* 43: 49–52, 1992.

3. Kopp P. Resveratrol, a phytoestrogen found in red wine. A possible explanation for the conundrum of the 'French paradox'? *Eur J Endocrinol* 138: 619–620, 1998.

4. Rotondo S, Rajtar G, Manarini S, et al. Effect of trans-resveratrol, a natural polyphenolic compound, on human polymorphonuclear leukocyte function. *Br J Pharmacol* 123: 1691–1699, 1998.

5. Turrens JF, Lariccia J, and Nair MG. Resveratrol has no effect on lipoprotein profile and does not prevent peroxidation of serum lipids in normal rats. *Free Radic Res* 27: 557–562, 1997.

6. Pace-Asciak CR, Rounova O, Hahn SE, et al. Wines and grape juices as modulators of platelet aggregation in healthy human subjects. *Clin Chim Acta* 246: 163–182, 1996.

7. Wilson T, Knight TJ, Beitz DC, et al. Resveratrol promotes atherosclerosis in hypercholesterolemic rabbits: *Life Sci* 59: PL15–PL21, 1996.

8. Jang M, Cai L, Udeani GO, et al. Cancer chemopreventive activity of resveratrol, a natural product derived from grapes. *Science* 275: 218–220, 1997.

9. Mgbonyebi OP, Russo J, and Russo IH. Antiproliferative effect of synthetic resveratrol on human breast epithelial cells. *Int J Oncol* 12: 865–869, 1998.

10. Subbaramaiah K, Chung WJ, and Michaluart P. Resveratrol inhibits cyclooxygenase-2 transcription and activity in phorbol ester-treated human mammary epithelial cells. *J Biol Chem* 273: 21875–21882, 1998.

11. Clement MV, Hirpara JL, and Chawdhury SH. Chemopreventive agent resveratrol, a natural product derived from grapes, triggers CD95 signaling-dependent apoptosis in human tumor cells. *Blood* 92: 996–1002, 1998.

12. Johnson JL and Maddipati KR. Paradoxical effects of resveratrol on the two prostaglandin H synthases. *Prostaglandins Other Lipid Mediat* 56: 131–143, 1998.

## SAMe (S-adenosylmethionine)

1. di Padova C. S-adenosylmethionine in the treatment of osteoarthritis. Review of the clinical studies. *Am J Med* 83(Supp5A): 60–65, 1989.

2. Bressa GM. S-adenosyl-l-methionine (SAMe) as antidepressant: meta-analysis of clinical studies. *Acta Neurol Scand* (Suppl. 154): 7–14, 1994.

3. Frezza M, et al. Oral S-adenosyl-methionine in the symptomatic treatment of intrahepatic cholestasis: A double-blind, placebo-controlled study. *Gastroenterology* 99: 211–215, 1990.

4. Bombardieri G, et al. Effects of S-adenosyl-L-methionine (SAMe) in the treatment of Gilbert's syndrome. *Curr Ther Res* 37: 580–585. 1985.

5. di Padova C. S-adenosylmethionine in the treatment of osteoarthritis. Review of the clinical studies. *Am J Med* 83(Supp5A): 60–65, 1989.

6. Nicastri P, Diaferia A, Tartagni M, et al. A randomised placebo-controlled trial of ursodeoxycholic acid and S-adenosylmethionine in the treatment of intrahepatic cholestasis of pregnancy. Br J Obstet Gynaecol 105(11): 1205–1207, 1998.

7. Jacobsen S, et al. Oral S-adenosylmethionine in primary fibromyalgia. Double-blind clinical evaluation. *Scand J Rheumatol* 20: 294–302, 1991.

8. Volkmann H, Norregaard J, Jacobsen S, et al. Double-blind, placebo-controlled cross-over study of intravenous S- adenosyl-L-methionine in patients with fibromyalgia. *Scand J Rheumatol* 26: 206–211, 1997.

9. Liu X, Lamango N, and Charlton C. L-dopa depletes S-adenosylmethionine and increases S-adenosyl homocysteine: Relationship to the wearing-off effects. *Society of Neuroscience Abstracts* 24(1–2): 1469, 1998.

10. di Padova C. S-adenosylmethionine in the treatment of osteoarthritis. Review of the clinical studies. *Am J Med* 83(Supp5A): 60–65, 1989.

11. Caruso I, et al. Italian double-blind multicenter study comparing S-adenosylmethionine, naproxen and placebo in the treatment of degenerative joint disease. *Am J Med* 83(Suppl. 5A): 66–71, 1987.

12. Maccagno A. Double-blind controlled clinical trial of oral S-adenosylmethionine versus piroxicam in knee osteoarthritis. *Am J Med* 83(Suppl. 5A): 72–77, 1987.

13. Glorioso S, et al. Double-blind multicentre study of the activity of S-adenosylmethionine in hip and knee osteoarthritis. *Int J Clin Pharmacol Res* 5: 39–49, 1985.

14. Muller-Fassbender H. Double-blind clinical trial of S-adenosylmethionine versus ibuprofen in the treatment of osteoarthritis. *Am J Med* 83(Suppl. 5A): 81–83, 1987.

15. Vetter G. Double-blind comparative clinical trial with S-adenosylmethionine and indomethacin in the treatment of osteoarthritis. *Am J Med* 83(Suppl. 5A): 78–80, 1987.

16. Agnoli A, et al. Effect of S-adenosyl-L-methionine upon depressive symptoms. *J Psychiatry Res* 13: 43–54, 1976.

17. De Vanna M, et al. Oral S-adenosyl-L-methionine in depression. *Curr Ther Res* 52: 478–485, 1992.

18. Bell MB, et al. Oral s-adenosylmethionine in the treatment of depression: a double-blind comparison with desipramine. Study Report BioResearch file, 1990. In Bressa GM. S-adenosyl-L-methionine (SAMe) as antidepressant: meta-analysis of clinical studies. *Acta Neurol Scand* (Suppl.)154: 7–14, 1994.

19. Kagan BL, et al. Oral S-adenosylmethionine in depression: A randomized, double-blind placebo-controlled trial. *Am J Psychiatry* 147: 591–595, 1990.

20. Salmaggi P, et al. Double-blind, placebo-controlled study of s-adenosylmethionine in depressed postmenopausal women. *Psychother Psychosom* 59: 34–40, 1993.

21. Fava M, et al. The thyrotropin response to thyrotropin-releasing hormone as a predictor of response to treatment in depressed outpatients. *Acta Psychiatr Scand* 86: 42–45. Additional 39 patients reported in Bressa GM. (S-adenosyl-l-methionine (SAMe) as antidepressant: meta-analysis of clinical studies. *Acta Neurol Scand* (Suppl.) 154: 7–14, 1992.

22. Bressa GM. S-adenosyl-l-methionine (SAMe) as antidepressant: meta-analysis of clinical studies. *Acta Neurol Scand* (Suppl. 154): 7–14, 1994.

23. Cozens DD, et al. Reproductive toxicity studies of ademetionine. *Arzneimittelforschung* 38(11): 1625–1629, 1988.

24. Berger R, et al. A new medical approach to the treatment of osteoarthritis: Report of an open phase IV study with ademetionine (Gumbaral). *Am J Med* 83 (Suppl. 5A): 84–88, 1987.

25. Konig B. A long-term (two years) clinical trial with S-adenosylmethionine for the treatment of osteoarthritis. *Am J Med* 83(Suppl. 5A): 89–94, 1987.

26. Caruso I, et al. Italian double-blind multicenter study comparing S-adenosylmethionine, naproxen and placebo in the treatment of degenerative joint disease. *Am J Med* 83(Suppl. 5A): 66–71, 1987.

27. di Padova C. S-adenosylmethionine in the treatment of osteoarthritis. Review of the clinical studies. *Am J Med* 83 (Supp5A): 60–65, 1989.

28. Carney MWP, et al. The switch mechanism and the bipolar/unipolar dichotomy. *Br J Psychiatry* 154: 48–51.

29. Carney. MWP, et al. Switch and S-adenosylmethionine. *Ala J Med Sci* 25(3): 316–319, 1988.

30. Kagan BL, et al. Oral S-adenosylmethionine in depression: A randomized, double-blind placebo-controlled trial. *Am J Psychiatry* 147: 591–595, 1990.

31. Iruela LM, et al. Toxic interaction of S-adenosylmethionine and clomipramine. *Am J Psych* 150: 522, 1993.

32. Reicks M, et al. Effects of methionine and other sulfur compounds on drug conjugations. *Pharmacol Ther* 37: 67–79, 1988.

## Saw Palmetto

1. Nickel JC. Placebo therapy of benign prostatic hyperplasia: A 25-month study. *Br J Urol* 81: 383–387, 1988.

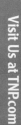

2. Braeckman J. The extract of *Serenoa repens* in the treatment of benign prostatic hyperplasia: A multicenter open study. *Curr Ther Res* 55: 776–785, 1994.

3. Romics I, Schmitz H, and Frang D. Experience in treating benign prostatic hypertrophy with *Sabal serrulata* for one year. *Int Urol Nephrol* 25: 565–569, 1993.

4. Emili E, et al. Clinical trial of a new drug for treating hypertrophy of the prostate (Permixon). *Urologia* 50: 1042–1048, 1983.

5. Champault G, et al. A double-blind trial of an extract of the plant *Serenoa repens* in benign prostatic hyperplasia. *Br J Clin Pharmacol* 18(3): 461–462, 1984.

6. Tasca A, et al. Treatment of obstructive symptomatology caused by prostatic adenoma with an extract of *Serenoa repens*. Double-blind clinical study vs. placebo. *Minerva Urol Nefrol* 37(1): 87–91, 1985.

7. Boccafoschi S, et al. Comparison of *Serenoa repens* extract with placebo by controlled clinical trial in patients with prostatic adenomatosis. *Urologia* 50: 1257–1268, 1983.

8. Smith RH, et al. The value of Permixon in benign prostatic hypertrophy. *Br J Urol* 58:36–40, 1986.

9. Descotes JL, et al. Placebo-controlled evaluation of the efficacy and tolerability of Permixon in benign prostatic hyperplasia after exclusion of placebo responders. *Clin Drug Invest* 9: 291–297, 1995.

10. Mattei FM, et al. *Serenoa repens* extract in the medical treatment of benign prostatic hypertrophy. *Urologia* 55: 547–552, 1988.

11. Plosker GL, et al. *Serenoa repens* (Permixon). A review of its pharmacology and therapeutic efficacy in benign prostatic hyperplasia. *Drugs Aging* 9(5): 379–395, 1996.

12. Carraro J, et al. Comparison of phytotherapy (Permixon) with finasteride in the treatment of benign prostate hyperplasia: A randomized international study of 1,098 patients. *Prostate* 29(4): 231–240, 241–242, 1996.

13. Bach D. Medikamentosse Langzeitbehandlung der BPH. Ergebnisse einer prospektiven 3-Jahresstudie mit dem Sabal extrakt IDS 89. *Urologe B* 35: 178–183, 1995.

14. Bach D, et al. Phytopharmaceutical and synthetic agents in the treatment of benign prostatic hyperplasia (BPH). *Phytomedicine* 3(4): 309–313, 1997.

15. Braeckman J, et al. Efficacy and safety of the extract of *Serenoa repens* in the treatment of benign prostatic hyperplasia: The therapeutic equivalence between twice and once daily dosage forms. *Phytother Res* 11(8): 558–563, 1997.

16. Plosker GL, et al. *Serenoa repens* (Permixon). A review of its pharmacology and therapeutic efficacy in benign prostatic hyperplasia. *Drugs Aging* 9(5): 379–395, 1996.

17. Plosker GL, et al. *Serenoa repens* (Permixon). A review of its pharmacology and therapeutic efficacy in benign prostatic hyperplasia. *Drugs Aging* 9(5): 379–395, 1996.

18. Bach D, et al. Phytopharmaceutical and synthetic agents in the treatment of benign prostatic hyperplasia (BPH). *Phytomedicine* 3(4): 309–313, 1997.

## Selenium

1. Gallegos A, Berggren M, Gasdaska JR, and Powis G. Mechanisms of the regulation of thioredoxin reductase activity in cancer cells by the chemopreventive agent selenium. *Cancer Res* 57: 4965–4970, 1997.

2. Harrison PR, Lanfear J, Wu L, Fleming J, McGarry L, and Blower L. Chemopreventive and growth inhibitory effects of selenium. *Biomed Environ Sci* 10: 235–245, 1997.

3. Tolonen M. Finnish studies on antioxidants with special reference to cancer, cardiovascular diseases and aging. *Int Clin Nutr Rev* 9(2): 68–75, 1989.

4. Stewart MS, Spalholz JE, Neldner KH, and Pence BC. Selenium compounds have disparate abilities to impose oxidative stress and induce apoptosis. *Free Radic Biol Med* 26: 42–48, 1999.

5. Shiobara Y, Yoshida T, and Suzuki KT. Effects of dietary selenium species on Se concentrations in hair, blood, and urine. *Toxicol Appl Pharmacol* 152: 309–314, 1998.

6. Wen HY, Davis RL, and Shi B. Bioavailability of selenium from veal, chicken, beef, lamb, flounder, tuna, selenomethionine, and sodium selenite assessed in selenium-deficient rats. *Biol Trace Elem Res* 58: 43–53, 1997.

7. Neve J. Human selenium supplementation as assessed by changes in blood selenium concentration and glutathione peroxidase activity. *J Trace Elem Med Biol* 9: 65–73, 1995.

8. Peretz A, et al. Selenium in rheumatic diseases. *Semin Arth Rheum* 20: 305–316, 1991.

9. Clark LC, Combs GF Jr, Turnbull BW, Slate EH, Chalker DK, et al. Effects of selenium supplementation for cancer prevention in patients with carcinoma of the skin. A randomized controlled trial. Nutritional Prevention of Cancer Study Group. *JAMA* 276: 1957–1963, 1996.

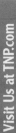

10. Yu SY, et al. Protective role of selenium against hepatitis B virus and primary liver cancer in Qidong. *Biol Trace Elem Res* 56: 117–124, 1997.

11. National Research Council, Diet and Health. Implications for reducing chronic disease risk. Washington, DC: National Academy Press, 1989: 376–379.

12. Hocman G. Chemoprevention of cancer: Selenium. *Int J Biochem* 20: 123–132, 1988.

13. Tanaka T, Makita H, Kawabata K, Mori H, and El-Bayoumy K. 1,4-phenylenebis(methylene)selenocyanate exerts exceptional chemopreventive activity in rat tongue carcinogenesis. *Cancer Res* 57: 3644–3648, 1997.

14. Yan L, Yee JA, McGuire MH, and Graef GL. Effect of dietary supplementation of selenite on pulmonary metastasis of melanoma cells in mice. *Nutr Cancer* 28: 165–169, 1997.

15. Tarp U. Selenium in rheumatoid arthritis. A review. *Analyst* 120: 877–881, 1995.

16. Clark LC, Combs GF Jr, Turnbull BW, Slate EH, Chalker DK, et al. Effects of selenium supplementation for cancer prevention in patients with carcinoma of the skin. A randomized controlled trial. Nutritional Prevention of Cancer Study Group. *JAMA* 276: 1957–1963, 1996.

17. Yu SY, et al. Protective role of selenium against hepatitis B virus and primary liver cancer in Qidong. *Biol Trace Elem Res* 56: 117–124, 1997.

18. National Research Council, Diet and Health. Implications for reducing chronic disease risk. Washington, DC: National Academy Press, 1989: 376–379.

19. Hocman G. Chemoprevention of cancer: Selenium. *Int J Biochem* 20: 123–132, 1988.

20. Tanaka T, Makita H, Kawabata K, Mori H, and El-Bayoumy K. 1,4-phenylenebis(methylene)selenocyanate exerts exceptional chemopreventive activity in rat tongue carcinogenesis. *Cancer Res* 57: 3644–3648, 1997.

21. Yan L, Yee JA, McGuire MH, and Graef GL. Effect of dietary supplementation of selenite on pulmonary metastasis of melanoma cells in mice. *Nutr Cancer* 28: 165–169, 1997.

## Sitosterol

1. Schulz V, et al. Rational phytotherapy. New York: Springer-Verlag, 1998: 231.

2. Pegel K. The importance of sitosterol and sitosterolin in human and animal nutrition. *S African J Science* 93: 263–268, 1997.

3. Berges B, et al. Randomised, placebo-controlled, double-blind clinical trial of beta-sitosterol in patients with benign prostatic hyperplasia. *Lancet* 345: 1529–1532, 1995.

4. Schulz V, et al. Rational phytotherapy. New York: Springer-Verlag, 1998: 231.

5. Berges B, et al. Randomised, placebo-controlled, double-blind clinical trial of beta-sitosterol in patients with benign prostatic hyperplasia. *Lancet* 345: 1529–1532, 1995.

## Skullcap

1. Newall C, et al. Herbal medicines: A guide for healthcare professionals. London: Pharmaceutical Press, 1996: 239.

## Slippery Elm

1. Castleman M. The healing herbs. Emmaus, PA: Rodale Press, 1991: 342–344.

## Soy Protein

1. Potter SM, Baum JA, Teng H, et al. Soy protein and isoflavones: their effects on blood lipids and bone density in postmenopausal women. *Am J Clin Nutr* 68(Suppl.): 1375S–1379S, 1998.

2. Anderson JW, et al. Meta-analysis of the effects of soy protein intake on serum lipids. *N Engl J Med* 33: 276–282, 1995.

3. Albertazzi P, Pansini F, Bonaccorsi G, et al. The effect of dietary soy supplementation on hot flashes. *Obstet Gynecol* 91: 6–11, 1998.

4. Goodman MT, et al. Association of soy and fiber consumption with the risk of endometrial cancer. *Am J Epidemiol* 146: 294–306, 1997.

5. Messina MJ, Persky V, Setchell KDR, and Barnes S. Soy intake and cancer risks: a review of the in vitro and in vivo data. *Nutr Cancer* 21: 113–131, 1994.

6. Anderson JW, et al. Meta-analysis of the effects of soy protein intake on serum lipids. *N Engl J Med* 33: 276–282, 1995.

7. Baum JA, Teng H, Erdman JW Jr, et al. Long-term intake of soy protein improves blood lipid profiles and increases mononuclear cell low-density-lipoprotein receptor messenger RNA in hypercholesterolemic, postmenopausal women. *Am J Clin Nutr* 68: 545–551, 1998.

8. Anderson JW, et al. Meta-analysis of the effects of soy protein intake on serum lipids. *N Engl J Med* 33: 276–282, 1995.

9. Albertazzi P, Pansini F, Bonaccorsi G, et al. The effect of dietary soy supplementation on hot flashes. *Obstet Gynecol* 91: 6–11, 1998.

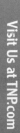

10. Werbach M. Foundations of nutritional medicine. Tarzana, CA: Third Line Press, 1997: 202.

11. Hallberg L, et al. Phytates and the inhibitory effects of bran on iron absorption in man. *Am J Clin Nutr* 45: 988–996, 1987.

12. Heaney RP, et al. Soybean phytate content effects on calcium absorption. *Am J Clin Nutr* 53: 745–747, 1991.

## Stevia

1. Leung A, et al. Encyclopedia of common natural ingredients used in foods, drugs, and costmetics. New York: John Wiley and Sons, 1996.

2. Kinghorn D, et al. Current status of stevioside as a sweetening agent for human use. Economics and medicinal plant research. Vol. I. London: Academic Press, Inc. Ltd, 1985.

3. Leung A, et al. Encyclopedia of common natural ingredients used in foods, drugs, and cosmetics. New York: John Wiley and Sons, 1996.

## St. John's Wort

1. Erdelmeier CA. Hyperforin, possibly the major non-nitrogenous secondary metabolite of *Hypericum perforatum. Pharmacopsychiat* 31(Suppl.): 2–6, 1998.

2. Schulz V. Hyperforin-Werte keinesfalls nur "Spuren." *Deutsche Apotheker Zeitung* 138: 65, 1998. As cited in Chatterjee S, Noldner M, Koch E, et al. Antidepressant activity of *Hypericum perforatum* and hyperforin: the neglected possibility. *Pharmacopsychiat* 31(Suppl.): 7–15, 1998.

3. Suzuki O, et al. Inhibition of monoamine oxidase by hypericin. *Planta Med* 50: 2722–2724, 1984.

4. Bladt S, et al. Inhibition of MAO by fractions and constituents of hypericum extract. *J Geriatr Psychiatry Neurol* 7(Suppl. 1): S57–S59, 1994.

5. Thiede B, et al. Inhibition of MAO and COMT by hypericum extracts and hypericin. *J Geriatr Psychiatry Neurol* 7(Suppl. 1): 54–56, 1994.

6. Muller WEG, et al. Effects of hypericum extract on the expression of serotonin receptors. *J Geriatry Psychiatry Neurol* 7(Suppl. 1): S63–S64, 1994.

7. Muller WE, et al. Hypericum extract (LI160) as an herbal antidepressant. *Pharmacopsychiatry* 30(Suppl. 2): 71–134, 1997.

8. Muller WE, Siner A, Wonnemann M, et al. Hyperforin represents the neurotransmitter reuptake inhibiting constituent of hypericum extract. *Pharmacopsychiatry* 31(Suppl.): 16–21, 1998.

9. Ghattacharya SK, Chakrabareti A, and Chatterjee SS. Activity profiles of two hyperforin-containing hypericum extracts in behavioural models. *Pharmacopsychiatry* 31(Suppl.): 22–29, 1998.

10. Laakman G, et al. St. John's wort in mild to moderate depression: The relevance of hyperforin for the clinical efficacy. *Pharmacopsychiatry* 31(Suppl.): 54–59, 1998.

11. Dipfel W, Schober F, and Mannel M. Effects of a methanolic extract and a hyperforin-enriched $CO_2$ extract of St. John's wort (*Hypericum perforatum*) on intracerebral field potentials in the freely moving rat (tele-stereo-EEG). *Pharmacopsychiatry* 31(Suppl.): 30–35, 1998.

12. Hansgen KD, et al. Multicenter double-blind study examining the antidepressant effectiveness of the hypericum extract LI 160. *J Geriatr Psychiatry Neurol* 7(Suppl. 1): S15–S18, 1994.

13. Laakman G, et al. St. John's wort in mild to moderate depression: The relevance of hyperforin for the clinical efficacy. *Pharmacopsychiatry* 31(Suppl.): 54–59, 1998.

14. Linde K, et al. St. John's wort for depression—An overview and meta-analysis of randomized clinical trials. *BMJ* 313: 253–258, 1996.

15. Ernst E. St. John's wort, an anti-depressant? A systematic, criteria-based review. *Phytomedicine* 2(1): 67–71, 1995.

16. Schulz V, et al. Rational phytotherapy. New York: Springer-Verlag, 1998: 59.

17. Linde K, et al. St. John's wort for depression—An overview and meta-analysis of randomized clinical trials. *BMJ* 313: 253–258, 1996.

18. Ernst E. St. John's wort, an anti-depressant? A systematic, criteria-based review. *Phytomedicine* 2(1): 67–71, 1995.

19. Vorbach EU, et al. Efficacy and tolerability of St. John's wort extract LI 160 vs. imipramine in patients with severe depressive episodes according to ICD-10. *Pharmacopsychiatry* 30(Suppl. 2): 81–85, 1997.

20. Martinez B, et al. Hypericum in the treatment of seasonal affective disorders. *J Geriatr Psychiatry Neurol* 7(Suppl. 1): 29–33, 1994.

21. Woelk H, et al. Benefits and risks of the hypericum extract LI 160: Drug monitoring study with 3,250 patients. *J Geriatr Psychiatry Neurol* 7(Suppl 1): S34–S38, 1994.

22. Smet P and Nolen W. St. John's wort as an anti-depressant. *BMJ* 3: 241–242, 1996.

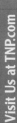

23. Schulz V, et al. Rational phytotherapy. New York: Springer-Verlag, 1998: 56.

24. Seigers CP, et al. Phototoxicity caused by hypericum. *Nervenhielkunde* 12: 320–322, 1993.

25. Brockmoller J, et al. Hypericin and pseudohypericin: Pharmacokinetics and effects on photosensitivity in humans. *Pharmacopsychiatry* 30(Suppl. 2): 94–101, 1997.

26. Roberts J. 1999 meeting of the American Society for Photobiology.

27. Suzuki O, et al. Inhibition of monoamine oxidase by hypericin. *Planta Med* 50: 2722–2724, 1984.

28. Bladt S, et al. Inhibition of MAO by fractions and constituents of hypericum extract. *J Geriatr Psychiatry Neurol* 7(Suppl. 1): S57–S59, 1994.

29. Thiede B, et al. Inhibition of MAO and COMT by hypericum extracts and hypericin. *J Geriatr Psychiatry Neurol* 7(Suppl. 1): 54–56, 1994.

30. Demott K. St. John's wort tied to serotonin syndrome. *Clin Psychiatr News* 26: 28, 1998.

31. Gordon JB. SSRIs and St. John's wort: possible toxicity? *Am Fam Phys* 57: 950, 1998.

32. Nebel A, Baker RK, and Kroll DJ. Potential metabolic interaction between theophylline and St. John's wort. Submitted to *Ann Pharmacother* 1998.

33. Baker RK, Sampey B, and Kroll DJ. Catalytic inhibition of human DNA topoisomerase II alpha by hypericin, a naphthodianthone from St. John's wort (*Hypericum perforatum*). Manuscript in preparation.

## Suma

1. De Oliveira F. *Pfaffia paniculata* (Martius) Kuntze-Brazilian ginseng. *Rev Bras Farmacog* 1(1): 86–92, 1986.

## Taurine

1. Azuma J, Sawamura A, and Awata N. Usefulness of taurine in chronic congestive heart failure and its prospective application. *Jpn Circ J* 56: 95–99, 1992.

2. Matsuyama Y, Morita T, Higuchi M, and Tsujii T. The effect of taurine administration on patients with acute hepatitis. As cited in K Kuriyama, RJ Huxtable, H Iwata, eds. Sulfur amino acids: biochemical and clinical aspects. New York: Alan R. Liss, Inc., 1983: 461–468.

3. Yamori Y, et al. Studies on stroke prevention in animal models, and their supportable epidemiological evidence. As cited in H Barnett, et al., eds. Cerebrovascular diseases: new trends in surgical and medical aspects. Amsterdam: Elsevier/North Holland, 1981: 47–62.

4. Franconi F, Bennardini F, Mattana A, et al. Plasma and platelet taurine are reduced in subjects with insulin-dependent diabetes mellitus: effects of taurine supplementation. *Am J Clin Nutr* 61: 1115–1119, 1995.

5. Marchesi GF, Quattrini A, Scarpino O, and Dellantonio R. Therapeutic effects of taurine in epilepsy: a clinical and polyphysiographic study. *Riv Patol Nerv Ment* 96: 166–184, 1975.

6. Fukuyama Y and Ochiai Y. Therapeutic trial by taurine for intractable childhood epilepsies. *Brain Dev* 4: 63–69, 1982.

7. Podda M, et al. Effects of ursodeoxycholic acid and taurine on serum liver enzymes and bile acids in chronic hepatitis. *Gastroenterology* 98: 1044–1050, 1990.

8. Azuma J, et al. Double-blind randomized crossover trial of taurine in congestive heart failure. *Curr Ther Res* 34: 543–557, 1983.

9. Azuma J, Sawamura A, Awata N, et al. Therapeutic effect of taurine in congestive heart failure: a double-blind crossover trial. *Clin Cardiol* 8: 276–282, 1985.

10. Azuma J, Takihara K, Awata N, et al. Taurine and failing heart: experimental and clinical aspects. *Prog Clin Biol Res* 179: 195–213, 1985.

11. Azuma J, et al. Therapy of congestive heart failure with orally administered taurine. *Clin Ther* 5: 398–408, 1983.

12. Takihara K, et al. Beneficial effect of taurine in rabbits with chronic congestive heart failure. *Am Heart J* 112: 1278, 1986.

13. Azuma J, et al. Beneficial effect of taurine on congestive heart failure induced by chronic aortic regurgitation in rabbits. *Res Comm Chem Pathol Pharmacol* 435: 261, 1984.

14. Azuma J, Sawamura A, and Awata N. Usefulness of taurine in chronic congestive heart failure and its prospective application. *Jpn Circ J* 56: 95–99, 1992.

15. Matsuyama Y, Morita T, Higuchi M, and Tsujii T. The effect of taurine administration on patients with acute hepatitis. As cited in K Kuriyama, RJ Huxtable, H Iwata, eds. Sulfur amino acids: biochemical and clinical aspects. New York: Alan R. Liss, Inc., 1983: 461–468.

16. Podda M, et al. Effects of ursodeoxycholic acid and taurine on serum liver enzymes and bile acids in chronic hepatitis. *Gastroenterology* 98: 1044–1050, 1990.

## Tea Tree

1. Williams LR, et al. The composition and bactericidal activity of oil of *Melaleuca alternifolia* (tea tree oil). *Int J Aromather* 1(3): 15, 1989.

2. Bassett IB, et al. *Med J Aust* 153: 455–458, 1990.

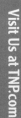

## TMG (Trimethylglycine)

1. Wilcken DE, Dudman NP, and Tyrrell PA. Homocystinuria due to cystathionine beta-synthase deficiency—the effects of betaine treatment in pyridoxine-responsive patients. *Metabolism* 34: 1115–1121, 1985.

2. Barak AJ, Beckenhauer HC, and Tuma DJ. Betaine, ethanol and the liver: a review. *Alcohol* 4: 395–398, 1996.

3. Barak AJ, Beckenhauer HC, Junnila M, and Tuma DJ. Dietary betaine promotes generation of hepatic S-adenosylmethionine and protects the liver from ethanol-induced fatty infiltration. *Alcohol Clin Exp Res* 17: 552–555, 1993.

4. Gray ME and Titlow LW. The effect of pangamic acid on maximal treadmill performance. *Med Sci Sports Exerc* 14: 424–427, 1982.

## Turmeric

1. Ammon HPT, et al. Pharmacology of *Curcuma longa*. *Planta Med* 57: 1–7, 1991.

2. Sreejayan N, et al. Free radical scavenging activity of curcuminoids. *Arzneimittelforschung Drug Res* 46: 169–171, 1996.

3. Deodhar SD, et al. Preliminary studies on antirheumatic activity of curcumin. *Indian J Med Res* 71: 632–634, 1980.

4. Brinker F. Herb contraindications and drug interactions, 2nd ed. Sandy, Oregon: Eclectic Medical Publications, 1998: 133.

5. Ravindranath V, et al. Absorption and tissue distribution of curcumin in rats. *Toxicology* 16: 259–265, 1980.

6. Ammon HPT, et al. Pharmacology of *Curcuma longa*. *Planta Med* 57: 1–7, 1991.

7. Shankar TNB, et al. Toxicity studies on turmeric (*Cucurma longa*): Acute toxicity studies in rats, guinea pigs and monkeys. *Indian J Exp Biol* 18: 73–75, 1980.

## Tyrosine

1. Neri DF, et al. The effects of tyrosine on cognitive performance during extended wakefulness. *Avit Space Environ Med* 66: 313–319, 1995.

2. Eisenberg J, et al. Effect of tyrosine on attention deficit disorder with hyperactivity. *J Clin Psychiatry* 49(5): 193–195, 1988.

3. Reimherr FW, et al. An open trial of L-tyrosine in the treatment of attention deficit disorder, residual type. *Am J Psychiatry* 144(8): 1071–1073, 1987.

4. Wender PH, et al. Amino acid precursors for the treatment of ADD-residual type. *Psychopharmacol Bull* 21: 146–149, 1985.

5. Gibson C and Gelenberg A. Tyrosine for depression. *Adv Biol Psychiat* 10: 148–159, 1983.

6. Gelenberg AJ, Wojcik JD, Falk WE, et al. Tyrosine for depression: a double-blind trial. *J Affect Disord* 19: 125–132, 1990.

7. Neri DF, et al. The effects of tyrosine on cognitive performance during extended wakefulness. *Avit Space Environ Med* 66: 313–319, 1995.

8. Gibson C and Gelenberg A. Tyrosine for depression. *Adv Biol Psychiat* 10: 148–159, 1983.

9. Gelenberg AJ, Wojcik JD, Falk WE, et al. Tyrosine for depression: a double-blind trial. *J Affect Disord* 19: 125–132, 1990.

## Uva Ursi

1. Frohne V, et al. Untersuchungen zur Frage der harndesifizierenden Wirkungen von Barentraubenblatt-extracten. *Planta Med* 18: 1–25, 1970.

2. Tyler V. Herbs of choice. New York: Pharmaceutical Products Press, 1994: 79.

3. Leung A, et al. Encyclopedia of common natural ingredients used in food, drugs, and cosmetics, 2nd ed. New York: John Wiley and Sons, 1996: 505.

4. ESCOP monographs. Fascicule 5: *Uvae Ursi Folium*. Exeter, UK: European Scientific Cooperative on Phytotherapy, 1997.

5. Schulz V, et al. Rational phytotherapy. New York: Springer-Verlag, 1998: 223.

6. Frohne V, et al. Untersuchungen zur Frage der harndesifizierenden Wirkungen von Barentraubenblatt-extracten. *Planta Med* 18: 1–25, 1970.

7. Kedzia B, et al. Antibacterial action of urine containing arbutin metabolic products. *Med Dosw Mikrobiol* 27: 305–314, 1975.

8. Larsson B, et al. Prophylactic effect of UVA-E in women with recurrent cystitis: A preliminary report. *Curr Ther Res* 53: 441–443, 1993.

9. ESCOP monographs. Fascicule 5: *Uvae Ursi Folium*. Exeter, UK: European Scientific Cooperative on Phytotherapy, 1997.

10. Tyler V. Herbs of choice. New York: Pharmaceutical Products Press, 1994: 79.

11. Schulz V, et al. Rational phytotherapy. New York: Springer-Verlag, 1998: 224.

12. Nowak AK, et al. Darkroom hepatitis after exposure to hydroquinone. *Lancet* 345: 1187, 1995.

13. U.S. Environmental Protection Agency. Extremely hazardous substances. Superfund chemical profiles.

Park Ridge, NJ: Noyes Data Corporation, 1988: 1906–1907.

14. Lewis RJ. Sax's dangerous properties of industrial materials, 8th ed. New York: Van Nostrand Reinhold, 1989: 1906–1907.

15. Schulz V, et al. Rational phytotherapy. New York: Springer-Verlag, 1998: 223.

16. ESCOP monographs. Fascicule 2: *Urticae radix*. Exeter, UK: European Scientific Cooperative on Phytotherapy, 1997.

## Valerian

1. Houghton PF. The biological activity of valerian and related plants. *J Ethnopharmacol* 22(2): 121–142, 1988.

2. Krieglstein J, et al. Valepotriate, valenrensaure, valeranon und atherisches 01 sind jedoch unwirksam. Zentraldampfende inhaltsstoffe im baldrian. *Deutsch Apoth Z* 128: 2041–2046, 1988.

3. Holzl J, et al. Receptor binding studies with *Valeriana officinalis* on the benzodiazepine receptor. *Planta Med* 55: 642, 1989.

4. Mennini T, et al. In vitro study on the interaction of extracts and pure compounds from *Valeriana officinalis* roots with GABA, benzodiazepine, and barbiturate receptors in rat brain. *Fitoterapia* 54: 291–300, 1993.

5. Schulz V, et al. Rational phytotherapy. New York: Springer-Verlag, 1998: 75–76.

6. Cavadas C, et al. In vitro study on the interaction of *Valeriana officinalis* L. Extracts and their amino acids on GABA(A) receptor in rat brain. *Arzneimittelforschung* 45(7): 753–755, 1995.

7. Schulz V, et al. Rational phytotherapy. New York: Springer-Verlag, 1998: 81.

8. Schulz V, et al. Rational phytotherapy. New York: Springer-Verlag, 1998: 78–80.

9. Lindahl O, et al. Double blind study of a valerian preparation. *Pharmacol Biochem Behav* 32(4): 1065–1066, 1989.

10. ESCOP monographs. Fascicule 4: *Valerianae radix*. Exeter, UK: European Scientific Cooperative on Phytotherapy, 1997: 5–6.

11. Leathwood PD, et al. Aqueous extract of valerian root (*Valeriana officinalis* L.) improves sleep quality in man. *Pharmacol Biochem Behav* 17(1): 65–71, 1982.

12. Dressing H, et al. Insomnia: Are valerian/balm combinations of equal value to benzodiazepine? *Therapiewoche* 42: 726-736, 1992.

13. Kohnen R, et al. The effects of valerian, propranolol, and their combination on activation, performance and mood of healthy volunteers under social stress conditions. *Pharmacopsychiatry* 21: 447–448, 1988.

14. Hendriks H, et al. Central nervous depressant activity of valerenic acid in the mouse. *Planta Med* 51: 28–31, 1985.

15. Leuschner J, et al. Characterization of the central nervous depressant activity of a commercially available valerian root extract. *Arzneimittelforschung* 43(6): 638–641, 1993.

16. Krieglstein J, et al. Valepotriate, valenrensaure, valeranon und atherisches 01 sind jedoch unwirksam. Zentraldampfende inhaltsstoffe im baldrian. *Deutsch Apoth Z* 128: 2041–2046, 1988.

17. ESCOP monographs. Fascicule 4: *Valerianae radix*. Exeter, UK: European Scientific Cooperative on Phytotherapy, 1997: 3–4.

18. Schulz V, et al. Rational phytotherapy. New York: Springer-Verlag, 1998: 77, 81.

19. Rosecrans JA, et al. Pharmacological investigation of certain *Valeriana officinalis* L. extracts. *J Pharmacol Sci* 50: 240–244, 1996.

20. Tyler V. Herbs of choice. New York: Pharmaceutical Products Press, 1994: 118.

21. ESCOP monographs. Fascicule 4: *Valerianae radix*. Exeter, UK: European Scientific Cooperative on Phytotherapy, 1997: 1.

22. Schulz V, et al. Rational phytotherapy. New York: Springer-Verlag, 1998: 77, 81.

23. Albrecht M, et al. Psychopharmaceuticals and safety in traffic. *Z Allg Med* 71: 1215–1221, 1995.

24. Gerhard U, et al. Vigilance-decreasing effects of two plant-derived sedatives. *Schweiz Rundsch Med Prax* 85(15): 473–481, 1996.

25. ESCOP monographs. Fascicule 4: *Valerianae radix*. Exeter, UK: European Scientific Cooperative on Phytotherapy, 1997: 2.

26. ESCOP monographs. Fascicule 4: *Valerianae radix*. Exeter, UK: European Scientific Cooperative on Phytotherapy, 1997: 2.

27. Albrecht M, et al. Psychopharmaceuticals and safety in traffic. *Z Allg Med* 71: 1215–1221, 1995.

28. Sakamoto T, et al. Psychotropic effects of Japanese valerian root extract. *Chem Pharm Bull* (Tokyo) 40(3): 758–761, 1992.

## Vanadium

1. Harland BF and Harden-Williams BA. Is vanadium of human nutritional importance yet? *J Am Diet Assoc* 94: 891–894, 1994.

2. Harland BF and Harden-Williams BA. Is vanadium of human nutritional importance yet? *J Am Diet Assoc* 94: 891–894, 1994.

3. Boden G, et al. Effects of vanadyl sulfate on carbohydrate and lipid metabolism in patients with non-insulin-dependent diabetes mellitus. *Metabolism* 45: 1130–1135, 1996.

4. Halberstam M. Oral vanadyl sulfate improves insulin sensitivity in NIDDM but not in obese diabetic subjects. *Diabetes* 45: 659–666, 1996.

5. Fawcett JP, Farquhar SJ, Walker RJ, et al. The effect of oral vanadyl sulfate on body composition and performance in weight-training athletes. *Int J Sport Nutr* 6: 382–390, 1996.

6. Amano R, Enomoto S, and Nobuta M. Bone uptake of vanadium in mice: simultaneous tracing of V, Se, Sr, Y, Zr, Ru and Rh using a radioactive multitracer. *J Trace Elm Med Biol* 10: 145–148, 1996.

7. Matsumoto J. Vanadate, molybdate and tungstate for orthomolecular medicine. *Med Hypotheses* 43(3): 177–182, 1994.

8. Shamberger RJ. The insulin-like effects of vanadium *Journal of Advances in Medicine* 9: 121–131, 1996.

9. Ramanadham S, Mongold J, Brownsey R, et al. Oral vanadyl sulfate in treatment of diabetes mellitus in rats. *Am J Physiol* 257: 904–911, 1989.

10. Brichard SM, Okitolonda W, and Henquin JC. Long-term improvement of glucose homeostasis by vanadate treatment in diabetic rats. *Endocrinology* 123: 2048–2053, 1988.

11. Kanthasamy A, Sekar N, and Govindasamy S. Vanadate substitutes insulin role in chronic experimental diabetes. *Indian J Exp Biol* 26: 778–780, 1988.

12. Shechter Y. Insulin-mimetic effects of vanadate. Possible implications for future treatment of diabetes. *Diabetes* 39(1): 1–5, 1990.

13. Challiss RAJ, Leighton B, Lozeman FJ, et al. Effects of chronic administration of vanadate to the rat on the sensitivity of glycolysis and glycogen synthesis in skeletal muscle to insulin. *Biochem Pharmacol* 36: 357–361, 1987.

14. Sakurai H, Tsuchiya K, Nakatsuka M, et al. Insulin-like effect of vanadyl ion on streptozocin-induced diabetic rats. *J Endocrinology* 126: 451–459, 1990.

15. Pederson RA, Ramanadham S, Buchan A, and McNeil JH. Long-term effects of vanadyl treatment on streptozocin-induced diabetes in rats. *Diabetes* 38: 1390–1395, 1989.

16. Myerovitch J, Farfel A, Sack J, and Schecter Y. Oral administration of vanadate normalizes blood glucose levels in streptozocin-treated rats. *J Biol Chem* 262: 6658–6662, 1987.

17. Heylinger C, Tahiliani A, and McNeil J. Effect of vanadate on elevated blood glucose and depressed cardiac performance of diabetic rats. *Science* 227: 1474–1476, 1985.

18. Boden G, et al. Effects of vanadyl sulfate on carbohydrate and lipid metabolism in patients with non-insulin-dependent diabetes mellitus. *Metabolism* 45: 1130–1135, 1996.

19. Cohen N, Halberstam M, Shlimovich P, et al. Oral vanadyl sulfate improves hepatic and peripheral insulin sensitivity in patients with non-insulin-dependent diabetes mellitus. *J Clin Invest* 95: 2501–2509, 1995.

20. Goldfine AB, Folli F, Patti PE, et al. Effects of sodium vanadate and in vitro insulin action in diabetes. *Clin Res* 42: 116A, 1994.

21. Halberstam M. Oral vanadyl sulfate improves insulin sensitivity in NIDDM but not in obese diabetic subjects. *Diabetes* 45: 659–666, 1996.

22. Fawcett JP, Farquhar SJ, Walker RJ, et al. The effect of oral vanadyl sulfate on body composition and performance in weight-training athletes. *Int J Sport Nutr* 6: 382–390, 1996.

23. Domingo JL, Gomez M, Llobet JM, et al. Oral vanadium administration to streptozotocin-diabetic rats has marked negative side effects which are independent of the form of vanadium used. *Toxicology* 66: 279–287, 1991.

24. Domingo JL, Gomez M, Llobet JM, et al. *Toxicology* 68: 249–253, 1991.

25. Sanchez DJ, Colomina MT, and Domingo JL. Effects of vanadium on activity and learning in rats. *Physiol Behav* 63: 345–350, 1998.

26. Domingo JL. Vanadium: a review of the reproductive and developmental toxicity. *Reprod Toxicol* 10: 175–182, 1996.

## Vitamin A

1. Combs G. The vitamins, 2nd ed. New York: Academic Press, 1998: 5–6.

2. Holt GA. Food and drug interactions. Chicago: Precept Press, 1998: 49.

3. Glasziou PP and Mackerras DEM. Vitamin A supplementation in infectious diseases: a meta-analysis. *BMJ* 306: 366—370, 1993.

4. Lithgow DM and Politzer WM. Vitamin A in the treatment of menorrhagia. *Afr Med J* 51: 191–193, 1977.

5. Wright JP, et al. Vitamin A therapy in patient's with Crohn's disease. *Gastroenterology* 88(2): 512–514, 1985.

6. Glasziou PP and Mackerras DEM. Vitamin A supplementation in infectious diseases: a meta-analysis. *BMJ* 306: 366–370, 1993.

7. Bresee JS, Fischer M, Dowell SF, et al. Vitamin A therapy for children with respiratory syncytial virus infection: a multicenter trial in the United States. *Pediatr Infect Dis J* 15: 777–782, 1996.

8. Neuzil KM, et al. Safety issues and pharmacokinetics of vitamin A therapy for infants with respiratory syncytial virus infections. *Antimicrob Agents Chemother* 39: 1191–1193, 1995.

9. Martinoli L, Di Felice M, Seghieri G, et al. Plasma retinol and alpha-tocopherol concentrations in insulin-dependent diabetes mellitus: their relationship to microvascular complications. *Int J Vitam Nutr Res* 63(2): 87–92, 1993.

10. Singh RB, Niaz MA, Ghosh S, et al. Dietary intake and plasma levels of antioxidant vitamins in health and disease: a hospital-based case-control study. *J Nutr Environ Med* 5: 235–242, 1995.

11. Basualdo CG, Wein EE, and Basu TK. Vitamin A (retinol) status of First Nation adults with non-insulin-dependent diabetes mellitus. *J Am Coll Nutr* 16(1): 39–45, 1997.

12. Straub RH, Rokitzki L, Schumacher T, et al. No evidence of deficiency of vitamins A, E, beta-carotene, $B_1$, $B_2$, $B_6$, $B_{12}$ and folate in neuropathic non-insulin-dependent diabetic women. *Int J Vitam Nutr Res* 63(3): 239–240, 1993.

13. Facchini F, Coulston AM, and Reaven GM. Relation between dietary vitamin intake and resistance to insulin-mediated glucose disposal in healthy volunteers. *Am J Clin Nutr* 63: 946–949, 1996.

14. Strosser AV and Nelson LS. Synthetic vitamin A in the treatment of eczema in children. *Ann Allergy* 10: 703–704, 1952.

15. Kligman AM, et al. Oral vitamin A in acne vulgaris. *Int J Dermatol* 20(4): 278–285, 1981.

16. Marrakchi S, Kim I, Delaporte E, et al. Vitamin A and E blood levels in erythrodermic and pustular psoriasis associated with chronic alcoholism. *Acta Derm Venereol* 74: 298–301, 1994.

17. Brenner S and Horwitz C. Possible nutrient mediators in psoriasis and seborrheic dermatitis. *Wld Rev Nutr Diet* 55: 165–182, 1988.

18. Lithgow DM and Politzer WM. Vitamin A in the treatment of menorrhagia. *Afr Med J* 51: 191–193, 1977.

19. Wright JP, et al. Vitamin A therapy in patient's with Crohn's disease. *Gastroenterology* 88(2): 512–514, 1985.

## Vitamin B₁

1. Gold M, Hauser RA, and Chen MF. Plasma thiamine deficiency associated with Alzheimer's disease but not Parkinson's disease. *Metab Brain Dis* 13: 43–53, 1998.

2. Bettendorff L, Mastrogiacomo F, Wins P, et al. Low thiamine diphosphate levels in brains of patients with frontal lobe degeneration of the non-Alzheimer's type. *J Neurochem* 69: 2005–2010, 1997.

3. Mimori Y, Katsuoka H, and Nakamura S. Thiamine therapy in Alzheimer's disease. *Metab Brain Dis* 11: 89–94, 1996.

4. Meador K, Loring D, Nichols M, et al. Preliminary findings of high-dose thiamine in dementia of Alzheimer's type. *J Geriatr Psychiatry Neurol* 6: 222–229, 1993.

5. Nolan KA, Black RS, Sheu KF, et al. A trial of thiamine in Alzheimer's disease. *Arch Neurol* 48: 81–83. 1991.

6. Holt GA. Food and drug interactions. Chicago: Precept Press, 1998: 59.

## Vitamin B₂

1. Powers H and Thronham D. (No title.) *Br J Nutr* 46: 257, 1981.

2. Elsborg L, et al. The intake of vitamins and minerals by the elderly at home. *Int J Vitam Nutr Res* 53: 321–329, 1983.

3. Lopez R, et al. Riboflavin deficiency in an adolescent population in New York City. *Am J Clin Nutr* 33: 1283–1286, 1980.

4. Southon S, et al. Micronutrient undernutrition in British schoolchildren. *Pro Nutr Soc* 52: 155–163, 1993.

5. Schoenen J, Jacquy J, and Lenaerts M. Effectiveness of high-dose riboflavin in migraine prophylaxis. A randomized controlled trial. *Neurology* 50: 466–470, 1998.

6. Sperduto RD, Hu TS, Milton RC, et al. The Linxian cataract studies. Two nutrition intervention trials. *Arch Ophthalmol* 111: 1246–1253, 1993.

7. Ajayi OA, George BO, and Ipadeola T. Clinical trial of riboflavin in sickle-cell disease. *East Afr Med J* 70: 418–421, 1993.

8. Nolan A, McIntosh WB, Allam BF, et al. Recurrent aphthous ulceration: vitamin $B_1$, $B_2$ and $B_6$ status and response to replacement therapy. *J Oral Pathol Med* 20: 389–391, 1991.

9. Schoenen J, Jacquy J, and Lenaerts M. Effectiveness of high-dose riboflavin in migraine prophylaxis. A randomized controlled trial. *Neurology* 50: 466–470, 1998.

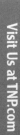

10. Sperduto RD, Hu TS, Milton RC, et al. The Linxian cataract studies. Two nutrition intervention trials. *Arch Ophthalmol* 111: 1246–1253, 1993.

## Vitamin B₃ (Niacin)

1. DiLorenzo PA. Pellagra-like syndrome associated with isoniazid therapy. *Acta Dermatol Venereol* 47: 318–322, 1967.

2. Vague P, et al. Effect of nicotinamide treatment on residual insulin secretion in type 1 (insulin-dependent) patients. *Diabetologia* 32: 316–321, 1989.

3. Illingworth DR, et al. Comparative effects of lovastatin and niacin in primary hypercholesterolemia. *Arch Intern Med* 154: 1586–1595, 1994.

4. Guyton JR, Goldberg AC, Kreisberg RA, et al. Effectiveness of once-nightly dosing of extended-release niacin alone and in combination for hypercholesterolemia. *Am J Cardiol* 82: 737–743, 1998.

5. Vega GL and Grundy SM. Lipoprotein responses to treatment with lovastatin, gemfibrozil, and nicotinic acid in normolipidemic patients with hypoalphalipoproteinemia. *Arch Intern Med* 154: 73–82, 1994.

6. Lal SM, et al. Effects of nicotinic acid and lovastatin in renal transplant patients: A prospective, randomized, open-label crossover trial. *Am J Kidney Dis* 25: 616–622, 1995.

7. Canner PL, et al. Fifteen year mortality in Coronary Drug Project patients: Long-term benefit with niacin. *J Am Coll Cardiol* 8: 1245–1255, 1986.

8. Elliott RB, Pilcher CC, Fergusson DM, et al. A population based strategy to prevent insulin-dependent diabetes using nicotinamide. *J Pediatr Endocrinol Metab* 9: 501–509, 1996.

9. Pozzilli P, Visalli N, Signore A, et al. Double blind trial of nicotinamide in recent-onset IDDM (the IMDIAB III study). *Diabetologia* 38: 848–852, 1995.

10. Polo V, Saibene A, and Pontiroli AE. Nicotinamide improves insulin secretion and metabolic control in lean type 2 diabetic patients with secondary failure to sulphonylureas. *Acta Diabetol* 35: 61–64, 1998.

11. Head KA. Inositol hexaniacinate: A safer alternative to niacin. *Alt Med Rev* 1: 176–184, 1996.

12. Sunderland GT, Belch JJF, Sturrock RD, et al. A double blind randomised placebo controlled trial of Hexopal in primary Raynaud's disease. *Clin Rheumatol* 7: 46–49, 1988.

13. Jonas WB, Rapoza CP, and Blair WF. The effect of niacinamide on osteoarthritis: a pilot study. *Inflamm Res* 45: 330–334, 1996.

14. Kellman M. Bursitis: A new chemotherapeutic approach. *J Am Osteopathic Assoc* 61: 896–903, 1962.

15. Sperduto RD, Hu TS, Milton RC, et al. The linxian cataract studies. *Arch Ophtlamol* 111: 1246–1253, 1993.

16. Doyle W, et al. The association between maternal diet and birth dimensions. *J Nutr Med* 1: 9–17, 1990.

17. Illingworth DR, et al. Comparative effects of lovastatin and niacin in primary hypercholesterolemia. *Arch Intern Med* 154: 1586–1595, 1994.

18. Guyton JR, Goldberg AC, Kreisberg RA, et al. Effectiveness of once-nightly dosing of extended-release niacin alone and in combination for hypercholesterolemia. *Am J Cardiol* 82: 737–743, 1998.

19. Vega GL and Grundy SM. Lipoprotein responses to treatment with lovastatin, gemfibrozil, and nicotinic acid in normolipidemic patients with hypoalphalipoproteinemia. *Arch Intern Med* 154: 73–82, 1994.

20. Lal SM, et al. Effects of nicotinic acid and lovastatin in renal transplant patients: A prospective, randomized, open-label crossover trial. *Am J Kidney Dis* 25: 616–622, 1995.

21. Canner PL, et al. Fifteen year mortality in Coronary Drug Project patients: Long-term benefit with niacin. *J Am Coll Cardiol* 8: 1245–1255, 1986.

22. Elliott RB, Pilcher CC, Fergusson DM, et al. A population based strategy to prevent insulin-dependent diabetes using nicotinamide. *J Pediatr Endocrinol Metab* 9: 501–509, 1996.

23. Lampeter EF, et al. The Deutsche Nicotinamide Intervention Study: an attempt to prevent type 1 diabetes. DENIS Group. *Diabetes* 47: 980–984, 1998.

24. Pozzilli P, Visalli N, Signore A, et al. Double blind trial of nicotinamide in recent-onset IDDM (the IMDIAB III study). *Diabetologia* 38: 848–852, 1995.

25. Polo V, Saibene A, and Pontiroli AE. Nicotinamide improves insulin secretion and metabolic control in lean type 2 diabetic patients with secondary failure to sulphonylureas. *Acta Diabetol* 35: 61–64, 1998.

26. O'Hara J, Jolly PN, and Nicol CG. The therapeutic efficacy of inositol nicotinate (Hexopal) in intermittent claudication: a controlled trial. *Br J Clin Pract* 42(9): 377–383, 1988.

27. Kiff RS. Does inositol nicotinate (Hexopal) influence intermittent claudication? A controlled trial. *Br J Clin Pract* 42(4): 141–145, 1988.

28. Head A. Treatment of intermittent claudication with inositol nicotinate. *Practitioner* 230: 49–54, 1986.

29. O'Hara J. A double-blind placebo-controlled study of Hexopal in the treatment of intermittent claudication. *J Int Med Res* 13: 322–327, 1985.

30. Tyson VCH. Treatment of intermittent claudication. *Practitioner* 223: 121–126, 1979.

31. O'Hara J, Jolly PN, and Nicol CG. The therapeutic efficacy of inositol nicotinate (Hexopal) in intermittent claudication: a controlled trial. *Br J Clin Pract* 42(9): 377–383, 1988.

32. Jonas WB, Rapoza CP, and Blair WF. The effect of niacinamide on osteoarthritis: a pilot study. *Inflamm Res* 45: 330–334, 1996.

33. Sunderland GT, Belch JJF, Sturrock RD, et al. A double blind randomised placebo controlled trial of Hexopal in primary Raynaud's disease. *Clin Rheumatol* 7: 46–49, 1988.

34. Gibbons LW, at al. The prevalence of side effects with regular and sustained-released nicotinic acid. *Am J Med* 99: 378–385, 1995.

35. Physicians' desk reference. Montvale, NJ: Medical Economics Company, 1999: 1507.

36. Physicians' desk reference. Montvale, NJ: Medical Economics Company, 1999: 1508.

## Vitamin B$_6$ (Pyridoxine)

1. Kant AK and Block G. Dietary vitamin B$_6$ intake and food sources in the U.S. population: NHANES II, 1976–80. *Am J Clin Nutr* 52: 707–716, 1990.

2. van der Wielen, et al. Dietary intake of water soluble vitamins in elderly people living in a Western society (1980–1993). *Nutr Res* 14(4): 605–638, 1994.

3. Albertson AM, et al. Nutrient intakes of 2- to 10-year-old American children: 10 year trends. *J Am Diet Assoc* 92(12):1492–1496, 1992.

4. Roe DA. Drug-induced nutritional deficiencies, 2d ed. Westport, CT: AVI Publishing, 1985: 178–179, 281–287.

5. Robinson C and Weigly E. Basic nutrition and diet therapy. New York: Macmillan, 1984: 46–54.

6. Goodhart R and Shils M, eds. Modern nutrition in health and disease. Philadelphia: Lea and Febiger, 1980.

7. Rumsby PC and Shepherd DM. The effect of penicillamine on vitamin B$_6$ function in man. *Biochem Pharmacol* 30: 3051–3053, 1981.

8. Delport R, et al. Vitamin B$_6$ nutritional status in asthma: the effect of theophylline therapy on plasma pyridoxal-5-phosphate and pyridoxal levels. *Int J Vitam Nutr Res* 58(1): 67–72, 1988.

9. Ubbink JB, et al. The relationship between vitamin B$_6$ metabolism, asthma, and theophylline therapy. *Ann N Y Acad Sci* 585: 285–294, 1990.

10. Holt GA. Food and drug interactions. Chicago: Precept Press, 1998.

11. Goodman L and Gilman A. The pharmacological basis of therapeutics, 9th ed. Hardman J, et al (eds.). New York: McGraw-Hill, 1996.

12. Rimm EB, et al. Folate and vitamin B$_6$ from diet and supplements in relation to risk of coronary heart disease among women. *JAMA* 279(5): 359–364, 1998.

13. Vutyananich T, Wongtra-ngan S, and Rung-aroon R. Pyridoxine for nausea and vomiting of pregnancy. A randomized, double-blind, placebo-controlled trial. *Am J Obstet Gynecol* 173: 881–884, 1995.

14. Keniston RC, Nathan PA, Leklem JE, et al. Vitamin B$_6$, vitamin C, and carpal tunnel syndrome. A cross-sectional study of 441 adults. *J Occup Environ Med* 39: 949–959, 1997.

15. Phalen GS. The birth of a syndrome, or carpal tunnel syndrome revisited. *J Hand Surg* 6: 109–110, 1981.

16. Diegoli MS, da Fonseca AM, Diegoli CA, and Pinotti JA. A double-blind trial of four medications to treat severe premenstrual syndrome. *Int J Gynaecol Obstet* 62: 63–67, 1998.

17. Cohen KL, Gorecki GA, Silverstein SB, et al. Effect of pyridoxine (vitamin B$_6$) on diabetic patients with peripheral neuropathy. *J Am Podiatry Assoc* 74(8): 394–397, 1984.

18. McCann VJ and Davis RE. Pyridoxine and diabetic neuropathy: a double-blind controlled study. Letter. *Diabetes Care* 6(1): 102–103, 1983.

19. Levin ER, Hanscom TA, Fisher M, et al. The influence of pyridoxine in diabetic peripheral neuropathy. *Diabetes Care* 4(6): 606–609, 1981.

20. Bell IR, Edman JS, Morrow FD, et al. Brief communication. Vitamin B$_1$, B$_2$, and B$_6$ augmentation of tricyclic antidepressant treatment in geriatric depression with cognitive dysfunction. *J Am Coll Nutr* 11: 159–163, 1992.

21. Collipp PJ. Pyridoxine treatment of childhood bronchial asthma. *Ann Allergy* 35: 93–97, 1975.

22. Sur S, Camara M, Buchmeier A, et al. Double-blind trial of pyridoxine (vitamin B$_6$) in the treatment of steroid-dependent asthma. *Ann Allergy* 70: 147–152, 1993.

23. Bennink HJ, et al. Improvement of oral glucose tolerance in gestational diabetes by pyridoxine. *BMJ* 3: 13–15, 1975.

24. Murthy MS, Talwar HS, Thind SK, and Nath R. Vitamin $B_6$ deficiency as related to oxalate-synthesizing enzymes in growing rats. *Ann Nutr Metab* 26: 201–208, 1982.

25. Murthy MS, Farooqui S, Talwar HS, et al. Effect of pyridoxine supplementation on recurrent stone formers. *Int J Clin Pharmacol Ther Toxicol* 20: 434–437, 1982.

26. Gershoff S and Prien E. Effect of daily MgO and vitamin $B_6$ administration to patients with recurring calcium oxalate stones. *Am J Clin Nutr* 20: 393–399, 1967.

27. Martineau J, Barthelemy C, Garreau B, et al. Vitamin $B_6$, magnesium, and combined $B_6$-Mg: therapeutic effects in childhood autism. *Biol Psychiatry* 20: 467–478, 1985.

28. Rimm EB, et al. Folate and vitamin $B_6$ from diet and supplements in relation to risk of coronary heart disease among women. *JAMA* 279(5): 359–364, 1998.

29. Folsom AR, et al. Prospective study of coronary heart disease incidence in relation to fasting total homocysteine, related genetic polymorphisms, and B vitamins: the Atherosclerosis Risk in Communities (ARIC) study. *Circulation* 98(3): 204–210, July 21, 1998.

30. Sermet A, et al. Effect of oral pyridoxine hydrochloride supplementation on in vitro platelet sensitivity to different agonists. *Arzneim Forsch* 45: 19–21, 1995.

31. Ayback M, et al. Effect of oral pyridoxine hydrochloride supplementation on arterial blood pressure in patients with essential hypertension. *Arzneim Forsch* 45: 19–21, 1995.

32. Vutyananich T, Wongtra-ngan S, and Rung-aroon R. Pyridoxine for nausea and vomiting of pregnancy. A randomized, double-blind, placebo-controlled trial. *Am J Obstet Gynecol* 173: 881–884, 1995.

33. Kleijnen J, Ter Riet G, and Knipschild P. Vitamin $B_6$ in the treatment of premenstrual syndrome—a review. *Br J Obstet Gynaecol* 97: 847–852, 1990.

34. Diegoli MS, da Fonseca AM, Diegoli CA, and Pinotti JA. A double-blind trial of four medications to treat severe premenstrual syndrome. *Int J Gynaecol Obstet* 62: 63–67, 1998.

35. Martineau J, Barthelemy C, Garreau B, et al. Vitamin $B_6$, magnesium, and combined $B_6$-Mg: therapeutic effects in childhood autism. *Biol Psychiatry* 20: 467–478, 1985.

36. Collipp PJ. Pyridoxine treatment of childhood bronchial asthma. *Ann Allergy* 35: 93–97, 1975.

37. Sur S, Camara M, Buchmeier A, et al. Double-blind trial of pyridoxine (vitamin $B_6$) in the treatment of steroid-dependent asthma. *Ann Allergy* 70: 147–152, 1993.

38. Parry G and Bredesen DE. Sensory neuropathy with low-dose pyridoxine. *Neurology* 35: 1466–1468, 1985.

39. Zempleni J. Pharmacokinetics of vitamin $B_6$ supplements in humans. *J Am Coll Nutr* 14: 579–586, 1995.

40. Sheretz EF. Acneform eruption due to megadose vitamins $B_6$ and $B_{12}$. *Cutis* 48: 19–20, 1991.

41. Braun-Falco O and Lincke H. The problem of vitamin $B_6$/$B_{12}$ acne. A contribution on acne medicamentosa. *MMW* 118(6): 155–160, 1976.

42. Lim D and McKay M. Food-drug interactions. *Drug Information Bulletin* 15(2): UCLA Dept. of Pharmaceutical Services, 1995.

## Vitamin $B_{12}$

1. Saltzman JR, et al. Effect of hypochlorhydria due to omeprazole treatment or atrophic gastritis on protein-bound $B_{12}$ absorption. *J Am Coll Nutr* 13(6): 584–591, 1994.

2. Van Goor L. et al. Review. Cobalamin deficiency and mental impairment in elderly people. *Age Ageing* 24: 536–542, 1995.

3. Pennypacker C, et al. High prevalence of cobalamin deficiency in elderly outpatients. *J Am Gerontol Soc* 40: 1197–1204, 1992.

4. Yao Y, et al. Prevalence of vitamin $B_{12}$ deficiency among geriatric outpatients. *J Fam Pract* 35: 524–528, 1992.

5. Marcuard SP, et al. Omeprazole therapy causes malabsorption of cyanocobalamin (vitamin $B_{12}$). *Ann Intern Med* 120: 211–215, 1994.

6. Saltzman JR, et al. Effect of hypochlorhydria due to omeprazole treatment or atrophic gastritis on protein-bound $B_{12}$ absorption. *J Am Coll Nutr* 13(6): 584–591, 1994.

7. Streeter AM, et al. Cimetidine and malabsorption of cobalamin. *Dig Dis Sci* 27: 13–16, 1982.

8. Roe DA. Drug-induced nutritional deficiencies, 2d ed. Westport, CT: AVI Publishing, 1985: 249–259.

9. Robison C and Weigly E. Basic nutrition and diet therapy. New York: Macmillan, 1984: 46–54.

10. Hodges R. Drug-nutrient interaction. As cited in Nutrition in medical practice. Philadelphia: W.B. Saunders, 1980: 323–331.

11. Coronato A and Glass GBJ. Depression of the intestinal uptake of radio-vitamin B12 by cholestyramine. *Proc Soc Exp Biol Med* 142: 1341–1344, 1973.

12. Holt GA. Food and drug interactions. Chicago: Precept Press, 1998.

13. Drug evaluations subscription, vol. 3 (section 19, chapter 5). Chicago: American Medical Association, Spring 1993.

14. Elia M. Oral parenteral therapy for B$_{12}$ deficiency. *Lancet* 352: 1721–1722, 1998.

15. McIntyre PA, et al. Treatment of pernicious anemia with orally administered cyanocobalamin (vitamin B$_{12}$). *Arch Intern Med* 106: 280–292, 1960.

16. Waife SO, et al. Oral vitamin B$_{12}$ without intrinsic factor in the treatment of pernicious anemia. *Ann Intern Med* 58: 810–817, 1963.

17. Berlin H, Berlin R, and Brante G. Oral treatment of pernicious anemia with high doses of vitamin B$_{12}$ without intrinsic factor. *Acta Med Scand* 184: 247–248, 1968.

18. Kumamoto Y, et al. Clinical efficacy of mecobalamin in treatment of oligozoospermia: Results of double-blind comparative clinical study. *Acta Urol Jpn* 34: 1109–1132, 1988.

19. Sandler B and Faragher B. Treatment of oligospermia with vitamin B$_{12}$. *Infertility* 7: 133–138, 1984.

20. Wright J. Vitamin B$_{12}$: Powerful protection against asthma. *Int Clin Nutr Rev* 9: 185–188, 1989.

21. Rule SA, Hooker M, Costello C, et al. Serum vitamin B$_{12}$ and transcobalamin levels in early HIV disease. *Am J Hematol* 47: 167–171, 1994.

22. Richman DD, Fischl MA, Grieco MH, et al. The toxicity of azidothymidine (AZT) in the treatment of patients with AIDS and AIDS-related complex. A double-blind, placebo-controlled trial. *N Engl J Med* 317: 192–197, 1987.

23. Ide H, Fujiya S, Asanuma Y, et al. Clinical usefulness of intrathecal injection of methylcobalamin in patients with diabetic neuropathy. *Clin Ther* 9: 183–192, 1987.

24. Yaqub BA, Siddique A, and Sulimani R. Effects of methylcobalamin on diabetic neuropathy. *Clin Neurol Neurosurg* 94: 105–111, 1992.

25. Kira J, Tobimatsu S, and Goto I. Vitamin B$_{12}$ metabolism and massive-dose methyl vitamin B$_{12}$ therapy in Japanese patients with multiple sclerosis. *Int Med* 33: 82–86, 1994.

26. Goodkin DE, Jacobsen DW, Galvez N. Serum cobalamin deficiency is uncommon in multiple sclerosis. *Arch Neurol* 51: 1110–1114, 1994.

27. Shemish A, et al. Vitamin B$_{12}$ deficiency in patients with chronic tinnitus and noise-induced hearing loss. *Am J Otolarygol* 14: 94–99, 1994.

28. Martin DC, Francis J, Protetch J, and Huff FJ. Time dependency of cognitive recovery with cobalamin replacement: report of a pilot study. *J Am Geriatr Soc* 40: 168–172, 1992.

29. Kwok T, Tang C, Woo J, et al. Randomized trial of the effect of supplementation on the cognitive function of older people with subnormal cobalamin levels. *Int J Geriatr Psychiatry* 13: 611–616, 1998.

30. Teunisse S, Bollen AE, van Gool WA, and Walstra GJ. Dementia and subnormal levels of vitamin B$_{12}$: effects of replacement therapy on dementia. *J Neurol* 243: 522–529, 1996.

31. Kumamoto Y, et al. Clinical efficacy of mecobalamin in treatment of oligozoospermia: Results of double-blind comparative clinical study. *Acta Urol Jpn* 34: 1109–1132, 1988.

32. Sandler B and Faragher B. Treatment of oligospermia with vitamin B$_{12}$. *Infertility* 7: 133–138, 1984.

33. Sheretz EF. Acneform eruption due to megadose vitamins B$_6$ and B$_{12}$. *Cutis* 48: 19–20, 1991.

34. Braun-Falco O and Lincke H. The problem of vitamin B$_6$/B$_{12}$ acne. A contribution on acne medicamentosa. *MMW* 118(6): 155–160, 1976.

## Vitamin C

1. Hercberg S, et al. Vitamin status of a healthy French population: dietary intakes and biochemical markers. *Int J Vitam Nutr Res* 64(3): 220–232, 1994.

2. Lowik MR, et al. Assessment of the adequacy of vitamin C intake in the Netherlands. Abstract. *J Am Coll Nutr* 10(5): 544, 1991.

3. U.S. Department of Agriculture. National Food Consumption Survey, 1985.

4. Baker B. Vitamin C deficiency common in hospitalized. *Fam Pract News* 25: March 15, 1995.

5. Holt GA. Food and drug interactions. Chicago: Precept Press, 1998: 83.

6. Coffey G and Wilson SWM. Ascorbic acid deficiency and aspirin-induced haematemesis. *BMJ* I: 208, 1975.

7. Hodges R. Drug-nutrient interaction. As cited in Nutrition in medical practice, Philadelphia: W. B. Saunders, 1980: 323–331.

8. Holt GA. Food and drug interactions. Chicago: Precept Press, 1998: 258.

9. Blanchard J, Tozar T, et al. Pharmacokinetic perspective on megadoses of ascorbic acid. *Am J Clin Nutr* 66: 1165–1171, 1997.

10. Dawson E, et al. Effect of ascorbic acid on male fertility. *Ann N Y Acad Sci* 498: 312–323, 1987.

11. Hemilä H. Does vitamin C alleviate symptoms of the common cold? A review of current evidence. *Scand J Infect Dis* 26: 1–6, 1994.

12. Hemilä H. Vitamin C and the common cold. *Br J Nutr* 67: 3–16, 1992.

13. Hemilä H. Vitamin C intake and susceptibility to the common cold. *Br J Nutr* 77: 1–14, 1997.

14. Hankinson S, Stampfer M, Seddon J, et al. Nutrient intake and cataract extraction in women: A prospective study. *BMJ* 305: 335–339, 1992.

15. Jacques PF, Taylor A, Hankinson SE, et al. Long-term vitamin C supplement use and prevalence of early age-related lens opacities. *Am J Clin Nutr* 66: 911–916. 1997.

16. Will JC, et al. Does diabetes mellitus increase the requirement for vitamin C? *Nutr Rev* 54: 193–202, 1996.

17. Mares-Perlman J, Klein R, Klein B, et al. Relationship between age-related maculopathy and intake of vitamin and mineral supplements. Abstract. *Invest Ophthalmol Vis Sci* 34: 1133, 1993.

18. Mares-Perlman JA, et al. Association of zinc and antioxidant nutrients with age-related maculopathy. *Arch Ophthalmol* 114: 991–997, 1996.

19. Age-Related Macular Degeneration Study Group. Multicenter ophthalmic and nutritional age-related macular degeneration study—Part 2: antioxidant intervention and conclusions. *J Am Optom Assoc* 67: 30–49, 1996.

20. Bielory L and Gandhi R. Asthma and vitamin C. *Ann Allergy* 73: 89–96, 1994.

21. Taylor TV, Rimmer S, Day B, et al. Ascorbic acid supplementation in the treatment of pressure-sores. *Lancet* 2: 544–546, 1974.

22. Dawson EB, et al. Effect of ascorbic acid on male fertility. *Ann N Y Acad Sci* 498: 312–323, 1987.

23. Bucca C, et al. Effect of vitamin C on histamine bronchial responsiveness of patients with allergic rhinitis. *Ann Allergy* 65: 311–314, 1990.

24. Bellioni P, et al. La provocazione istaminica in soggetti allergici. Il ruolo dell'acido ascorbico. *Eur Rev Med Pharm Sci* 9: 419–422, 1987.

25. Fortner BR Jr, et al. The effect of ascorbic acid on cutaneous and nasal response to histamine and allergen. *J Allergy Clin Immunol* 69: 484–488, 1982.

26. McAlindon TE, et al. Do antioxidant micronutrients protect against the development and progression of knee OA. *Arth Rheum* 39: 648–656, 1996.

27. Schwartz ER. The modulation of osteoarthritic development by vitamins C and E. *Int J Vit Nutr Res*(Suppl. 26): 141–146, 1984.

28. Hemilä H. Does vitamin C alleviate symptoms of the common cold? A review of current evidence. *Scand J Infect Dis* 26: 1–6, 1994.

29. Hemilä H. Vitamin C and the common cold. *Br J Nutr* 67: 3–16, 1992.

30. Hemilä H. Vitamin C intake and susceptibility to the common cold. *Br J Nutr* 77: 1–14, 1997.

31. Peters EM, Goetzsche JM, Grobbelaar B, and Noakes TD. Vitamin C supplementation reduces the incidence of postrace symptoms of upper-respiratory-tract infection in ultramarathon runners. *Am J Clin Nutr* 57(2): 170–174, 1993.

32. Hemilä H. Vitamin C and common cold incidence: a review of studies with subjects under heavy physical stress. *Int J Sports Med* 17(5): 379–383, July 1996.

33. Chalmers TC. Effects of ascorbic acid on the common cold. An evaluation of the evidence. *Am J Med* 58: 532–536, 1975.

34. Hemilä H, et al. Vitamin C and the common cold: a retrospective analysis of Chalmers' review. *J Am Coll Nutr* 14: 116–123, 1995.

35. Hankinson S, Stampfer M, Seddon J, et al. Nutrient intake and cataract extraction in women: A prospective study. *BMJ* 305: 335–339, 1992.

36. Jacques PF, Taylor A, Hankinson SE, et al. Long-term vitamin C supplement use and prevalence of early age-related lens opacities. *Am J Clin Nutr* 66: 911–916. 1997.

37. Will JC, et al. Does diabetes mellitus increase the requirement for vitamin C? *Nutr Rev* 54: 193–202, 1996.

38. Mares-Perlman J, Klein R, Klein B, et al. Relationship between age-related maculopathy and intake of vitamin and mineral supplements. Abstract. *Invest Ophthalmol Vis Sci* 34: 1133, 1993.

39. Mares-Perlman JA, et al. Association of zinc and antioxidant nutrients with age- related maculopathy. *Arch Ophthalmol* 114: 991–997, 1996.

40. Age-Related Macular Degeneration Study Group. Multicenter ophthalmic and nutritional age-related macular degeneration study—Part 2: antioxidant intervention and conclusions. *J Am Optom Assoc* 67: 30–49, 1996.

41. Bruemmer B, et al. Nutrient intake in relation to bladder cancer among middle-aged men and women. *Am J Epidemiol* 144: 485–495, 1996.

42. Otoole P and Lombard M. Vitamin C and gastric cancer: supplements for some or fruit for all. *Gut* 39: 345–347, 1996.

43. Greenberg ER, Baron JA, Tosteson TD, et al. A clinical trial of antioxidant vitamins to prevent colorectal adenoma. *N Engl J Med* 331: 141–147, 1994.

44. Kushi L, Fee R, Sellers T, et al. Intake of vitamins A, C, and E and postmenopausal breast cancer: the Iowa Women's Health Study. *Am J Epidemiol* 144(2): 165–174, 1996.

45. Hunter DJ, Manson JE, Colditz GA, et al. A prospective study of the intake of vitamins C, E, and A and the risk of breast cancer. *N Engl J Med* 329(4): 234–240, 1993.

46. Cameron E and Pauling L. Supplemental ascorbate in the supportive treatment of cancer: Prolongation of survival times in terminal human cancer. *Proc Natl Acad Sci USA* 73: 3685–3689, 1976.

47. Cameron E and Campbell A. Innovation vs. quality control: an "unpublishable" clinical trial of supplemental ascorbate in incurable cancer. *Med Hypotheses* 36: 185–189, 1991.

48. Creagan ET, Moertel CG, O'Fallon JR, et al. Failure of high-dose vitamin C (ascorbic acid) therapy to benefit patients with advanced cancer. A controlled trial. *N Engl J Med* 301: 687–690, 1979.

49. Moertel CG, Fleming TR, Creagan ET, et al. High-dose vitamin C versus placebo in the treatment of patients with advanced cancer who have had no prior chemotherapy. A randomized double-blind comparison. *N Engl J Med* 312: 137–141, 1985.

50. Weijl, M et al. Free radicals and antioxidants in chemotherapy-induced toxicity. *Cancer Treatment Res* 23: 209–240, 1997.

51. Ness AR. Vitamin C and cardiovascular disease. *Nutrition Report* 15: May/June 1997.

52. Simon JA. Vitamin C and cardiovascular disease: a review. *J Am Coll Nutr* 11: 107–125, 1992.

53. Trout DL. Vitamin C and cardiovascular risk factors. *Am J Clin Nutr* 53: 322S–325S, 1991.

54. Losonczy KG, Harris TB, and Havlik RJ. Vitamin E and vitamin C supplement use and risk of all-cause and coronary heart disease mortality in older persons: the Established Populations for Epidemiologic Studies of the Elderly. *Am J Clin Nutr* 64: 190–196, 1996.

55. Feldman E, Gold S, Greene J, et al. Ascorbic acid supplements and blood pressure. *Ann N Y Acad Sci* 669: 342–344, 1992.

56. Ghosh S, Ekpo E, and Shah I. A double-blind, placebo-controlled parallel trial of vitamin C treatment in elderly patients with hypertension. *Gerontology* 40: 268–272, 1994.

57. Osilesi O, et al. Blood pressure and plasma lipids during ascorbic acid supplementation in borderline hypertensive and normotensive adults. *Nutr Res* 11: 405–412, 1991.

58. Austin S. Vitamin C and mutagenesis—much ado about nothing? *Quart Rev Nat Med*: 227, Fall 1998. (Health Notes, Inc., Portland, OR).

59. Aves BL, et al. Relative hyperoxaluria, crystalluria, and hematuria after mega-dose ingestion of vitamin C. *Eur J Clin Invest* 28: 695–700, 1998.

60. Gerster H. No contribution of ascorbic acid to renal calcium oxalate stones. *Ann Nutr Metab* 41: 269–282, 1997.

61. Aves BL, et al. Relative hyperoxaluria, crystalluria, and hematuria after mega-dose ingestion of vitamin C. *Eur J Clin Invest* 28: 695–700, 1998.

62. Owen CA Jr, et al. Heparin-ascorbic acid antagonism. *Mayo Clin Proc* 45: 140, 1970.

63. Rosenthal G. Interaction of ascorbic acid and warfarin. *JAMA* 215: 1671, 1971.

## Vitamin D

1. Utiger R. The need for more vitamin D. *N Engl J Med* 338(12): 828–829, 1998.

2. Werbach M. Foundations of nutritional medicine. Tarzana, CA: Third Line Press, 1997: 74–75.

3. Holmes R and Kummerow F. The relationship of adequate and excessive intake of vitamin D to health and disease. *J Am Coll Nutr* 2: 173–199, 1983.

4. Roe DA. Drug-induced nutritional deficiencies, 2d ed. Westport, CT: AVI Publishing, 1985: 164–166, 249.

5. Roe D. Risk factors in drug-induced nutritional deficiencies. As cited in D Roe and T Campbell (eds.). Drugs and nutrients: the interactive effects. New York: Marcel Decker, 1984: 505–523.

6. Hodges R. Drug-nutrient interaction. As cited in Nutrition in medical practice. Philadelphia: WB Saunders, 1980: 323–331.

7. Bengoa JM, et al. Hepatic vitamin D 25-hydroxylase inhibition by cimetidine and isoniazid. *J Lab Clin Med* 104: 546–552, 1984.

8. Brodie MJ, et al. Effect of isoniazid on vitamin D metabolism and hepatic homooxygenase activity. *Clin Pharmacol Ther* 30: 363–367, 1981.

9. Holt GA. Food and drug interactions. Chicago: Precept Press, 1998.

10. Dawson-Hughes B, Harris S, Krall E, et al. Effect of calcium and vitamin D supplementation on bone density

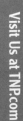

in men and women 65 years of age or older. *N Engl J Med* 337(10): 670–673, 1997.

11. Dawson-Hughes B, Dallal GE, and Krall EA. The effect of vitamin D supplementation on wintertime and overall bone loss in healthy postmenopausal women. *Ann Intern Med* 115(7): 505–512, 1991.

12. Garland FC, et al. Geographic variation in breast cancer mortality in the United States: a hypothesis involving exposure to solar radiation. *Prev Med* 19(6): 614–622, November 1990.

13. Key SW and Marble M. Studies link sun exposure to protection against cancer. *Cancer Weekly Plus:* 5–6, November 17, 1997.

14. Martinez ME, et al. Calcium, vitamin D, and the occurrence of colorectal cancer among women. *J Natl Cancer Inst* 88(19): 1375–1382, 1996.

15. Kearney J, et al. Calcium, vitamin D, and dairy foods and the occurrence of colon cancer in men. *Am J Epidemiol* 143(9): 907–917, 1996.

16. James SY, et al. Effects of 1,25 dihydroxyvitamin D$_3$ and its analogues on induction of apoptosis in breast cancer cells. *J Steroid Biochem Mol Biol* 58(4): 395–401, July 1996.

17. Taylor JA, et al. Association of prostate cancer with vitamin D receptor gene polymorphism. *Cancer Res* 56(18): 4108–4110, September 15, 1996.

18. Douglas WC. Vitamin D scores again. *Second Opinion* 7(7): 4–5, July 1997.

19. Kragballe K. Vitamin D$_3$ analogues in psoriasis. *Dermatologica* 180: 110–111.1990.

20. Dawson-Hughes B, Dallal GE, and Krall EA. The effect of vitamin D supplementation on wintertime and overall bone loss in healthy postmenopausal women. *Ann Intern Med* 115(7): 505–512, 1991.

21. Dawson-Hughes B, Harris S, Krall E, et al. Effect of calcium and vitamin D supplementation on bone density in men and women 65 years of age or older. *N Engl J Med* 337(10): 670–673, 1997.

22. Lips P, Graafmans WC, Ooms ME, et al. Vitamin D supplementation and fracture incidence in elderly persons. A randomized, placebo-controlled clinical trial. *Ann Intern Med* 124: 400–406, 1996.

## Vitamin E

1. Hercberg S, et al. Vitamin status of a healthy French population: dietary intakes and biochemical markers. *Int J Vitamin Nutr Res* 64(3): 220–232, 1994.

2. Murphy SP, et al. Vitamin E intakes and sources in the United States. *Am J Clin Nutr* 52: 361–367, 1990.

3. Elinder LS, et al. Probucol treatment decreases serum concentrations of diet-derived antioxidants. *Arteriscler Thromb Basc Biol* 15(8): 1057–1063, 1995.

4. West RJ and Lloyd JK. The effect of cholestyramine on intestinal absorption. *Gut* 16: 93, 1975.

5. Vitamin E fact book. LaGrange, IL: VERIS (Vitamin E Research and Information Service, 5325 S. 9th Ave., LaGrange, IL 60525), 1994.

6. Roe D. Risk factors in drug-induced nutritional deficiencies. As cited in D Roe, T Campbell, eds. Drugs and nutrients: the interactive effects. New York: Marcel Decker, 1984: 505–523.

7. Christen S, et al. Gamma-tocopherol traps mutagenic electrophiles such as NOX and complements alpha-tocopherol: physiological implications. *Proc Natl Acad Sci USA* 94: 3217–3222, 1997.

8. Kiyose C, et al. Biodiscrimination of alpha-tocopherol stereoisomers in humans after oral administration. *Am J Clin Nutr* 65(3): 785–789, March 1997.

9. Burton GW, et al. Human plasma and tissue alpha-tocopherol concentrations in response to supplementation with deuterated natural and synthetic vitamin E. *Am J Clin Nutr* 67(4): 669–684, April 1998.

10. Stephens NG, Parsons A, Schofield PM, et al. Randomized controlled trial of vitamin E in patients with coronary disease: Cambridge Heart Antioxidant Study (CHAOS). *Lancet* 347: 781–786, 1996.

11. Rimm EB, Stampfer MJ, Ascherio A, et al. Vitamin E consumption and the risk of coronary heart disease in men. *N Engl J Med* 328: 1450–1456, 1993.

12. Stampfer M, Hennekens C, Manson J, et al. Vitamin E consumption and the risk of coronary heart disease in women. *N Engl J Med* 328: 1444–1449, 1993.

13. Losonczy KG, Harris TB, and Havlik RJ. Vitamin E and vitamin C supplement use and risk of all-cause and coronary heart disease mortality in older persons: the Established Populations for Epidemiologic Studies of the Elderly. *Am J Clin Nutr* 64: 190–196, 1996.

14. Heinonen OP, et al. Prostate cancer and supplementation with alpha-tocopherol and beta-carotene: incidence and mortality in a controlled trial. *Natl Cancer Inst* 90: 440–446, 1998.

15. White E, et al. Relationship between vitamin and calcium supplement use and colon cancer. *Cancer Epidemiol Biomarkers Prev* 10: 769–774, 1997.

16. Adler LA, Edson R, Lavori P, et al. Long-term treatment effects of vitamin E for tardive dyskinesia. *Biol Psychiatry* 43: 868–872, 1998.

17. Lohr JB and Caligiuri MP. A double-blind placebo-controlled study of vitamin E treatment of tardive dyskinesia. *J Clin Psychiatry* 57: 167–173, 1996.

18. Rotrosen J, et al. Antioxidant treatment of tardive dyskinesia. *Prostaglandins Leukot Essent Fatty Acids* 55 (1&2): 77–81, 1996.

19. Adler LA, Peselow E, Rotrosen J, et al. Vitamin E treatment of tardive dyskinesia. *Am J Psychiatry* 150: 1405–1407, 1993.

20. Hashim S and Sajjad A. Vitamin E in the treatment of tardive dyskinesia: A preliminary study over 7 months at different doses. *Interrat Clin Psychopharmacol* 13: 147–155, 1998.

21. Meydani SM, et al. Vitamin E supplementation and in vivo immune response in healthy elderly subjects: A randomized controlled trial. *JAMA* 277: 1380–1386, 1997.

22. Sano M, Ernesto C, Thomas RG, et al. A controlled trial of selegiline, alpha-tocopherol, or both as treatment for Alzheimer's disease. *N Engl J Med* 336: 1216–1222, 1997.

23. Suleiman SA, Ali ME, Zaki ZM, et al. Lipid peroxidation and human sperm motility: protective role of vitamin E. *J Androl* 17: 530–537, 1996.

24. Paolisso G, D'Amore A, Galzerano D, et al. Daily vitamin E supplements improve metabolic control but not insulin secretion in elderly non-insulin-dependent diabetic patients. *Diabetes Care* 16: 1433–1437, 1993.

25. Paolisso G, et al. Pharmacological doses of vitamin E and insulin action in elderly subjects. *Am J Clin Nutr* 59: 1291–1296, 1994.

26. Paolisso G, D'Amore A, Giugliano D, et al. Pharmacologic doses of vitamin E improve insulin action in healthy subjects and non-insulin-dependent diabetic patients. *Am J Clin Nutr* 57: 650–656, 1993.

27. London RS, et al. Efficacy of alpha-tocopherol in the treatment of the premenstrual syndrome. *J Reprod Med* 32: 400–404, 1987.

28. London RS, Sundaram GS, Murphy L, and Goldstein PJ. The effect of alpha-tocopherol on premenstrual symptomatology: a double-blind study. *J Am Coll Nutr* 2: 115–122, 1983.

29. Tavani A, et al. Food and nutrient intake and risk of cataract. *Ann Epidemiol* 6: 41–46, 1996.

30. Leske MC, Chylack LT, Jr, He Q, et al. Antioxidant vitamins and nuclear opacities: the longitudinal study of cataract. *Ophthalmology* 105(5): 831–836, 1998.

31. Teikari JM, Rautalahti M, Haukka J, et al. Incidence of cataract operations in Finnish male smokers unaffected by alpha tocopherol or beta carotene supplements. *J Epidemiol Community Health* 52: 468–472, 1998.

32. Seddon JM, Christen WG, Manson JE, et al. The use of vitamin supplements and the risk of cataract among U.S. male physicians. *Am J Public Health* 84: 788–792, 1994.

33. McAlindon TE, et al. Do antioxidant micronutrients protect against the development and progression of knee OA. *Arth Rheum* 39: 648–656, 1996.

34. London RS, Sundaram GS, Murphy L, et al. The effect of vitamin E on mammary dysplasia: a double-blind study. *Obstet Gynecol* 65: 104–106, 1985.

35. Kachel DL, et al. Amiodarone-induced injury of human pulmonary artery endothelial cells: protection by alpha-tocopherol. *J Pharmacol Exp Ther* 254: 1107–1112, 1990.

36. Stephens NG, Parsons A, Schofield PM, et al. Randomized controlled trial of vitamin E in patients with coronary disease: Cambridge Heart Antioxidant Study (CHAOS). *Lancet* 347: 781–786, 1996.

37. Rimm EB, Stampfer MJ, Ascherio A, et al. Vitamin E consumption and the risk of coronary heart disease in men. *N Engl J Med* 328: 1450–1456, 1993.

38. Stampfer M, Hennekens C, Manson J, et al. Vitamin E consumption and the risk of coronary heart disease in women. *N Engl J Med* 328: 1444–1449, 1993.

39. Losonczy KG, Harris TB, and Havlik RJ. Vitamin E and vitamin C supplement use and risk of all-cause and coronary heart disease mortality in older persons: the Established Populations for Epidemiologic Studies of the Elderly. *Am J Clin Nutr* 64: 190–196, 1996.

40. Rapola JM, Virtamo J, Ripatti S, et al. Randomized trial of a-tocopherol and b-carotene supplements on incidence of major coronary events in men with previous myocardial infarction. *Lancet* 349: 1715–1720, 1997.

41. Albanes D, Heinonen OP, Huttunen JK, et al. Effects of a-tocopherol and b-carotene supplements on cancer incidence in the Alpha-Tocopherol Beta-Carotene Cancer Prevention Study. *Am J Clin Nutr* 62(suppl.): 1427S–1430S, 1995.

42. Jialal I and Fuller CJ. Effect of vitamin E, vitamin C and beta-carotene on LDL oxidation and atherosclerosis. *Can J Cardiol* 1(Suppl. G): 97G–103G, 1995.

43. Calzada C, Bruckdorfer K, and Rice-Evans C. The influence of antioxidant nutrients on platelet function in healthy volunteers. *Atherosclerosis* 128: 97–105, 1997.

44. Heinonen OP, et al. Prostate cancer and supplementation with alpha-tocopherol and beta-carotene: inci-

dence and mortality in a controlled trial. *Natl Cancer Inst* 90: 440–446, 1998.

45. White E, et al. Relationship between vitamin and calcium supplement use and colon cancer. *Cancer Epidemiol Biomarkers Prev* 10: 769–774, 1997.

46. Losonczy KG, Harris TB, and Havlik RJ. Vitamin E and vitamin C supplement use and risk of all-cause and coronary heart disease mortality in older persons: the Established Populations for Epidemiologic Studies of the Elderly. *Am J Clin Nutr* 64: 190–196, 1996.

47. Adler LA, Edson R, Lavori P, et al. Long-term treatment effects of vitamin E for tardive dyskinesia. *Biol Psychiatry* 43: 868–872, 1998.

48. Lohr JB and Caligiuri MP. A double-blind placebo-controlled study of vitamin E treatment of tardive dyskinesia. *J Clin Psychiatry* 57: 167–173, 1996.

49. Rotrosen J, et al. Antioxidant treatment of tardive dyskinesia. *Prostaglandins Leukot Essent Fatty Acids* 55 (1&2): 77–81, 1996.

50. Adler LA, Peselow E, Rotrosen J, et al. Vitamin E treatment of tardive dyskinesia. *Am J Psychiatry* 150: 1405–1407, 1993.

51. Adler LA, Edson R, Lavori P, et al. Long-term treatment effects of vitamin E for tardive dyskinesia. *Biol Psychiatry* 43: 868–872, 1998.

52. Shriqui CL, Bradwejn J, Annable L, and Jones BD. Vitamin E in the treatment of tardive dyskinesia: a double-blind placebo-controlled study. *Am J Psychiatry* 149: 391–393, 1992.

53. Hashim S and Sajjad A. Vitamin E in the treatment of tardive dyskinesia: A preliminary study over 7 months at different doses. *Interrat Clin Psychopharmacol* 13: 147–155, 1998.

54. Meydani SM, et al. Vitamin E supplementation and in vivo immune response in healthy elderly subjects: A randomized controlled trial. *JAMA* 277: 1380–1386, 1997.

55. Sano M, Ernesto C, Thomas RG, et al. A controlled trial of selegiline, alpha-tocopherol, or both as treatment for Alzheimer's disease. *N Engl J Med* 336: 1216–1222, 1997.

56. Suleiman SA, Ali ME, Zaki ZM, et al. Lipid peroxidation and human sperm motility: protective role of vitamin E. *J Androl* 17: 530–537, 1996.

57. Albanes D, Heinonen OP, Huttunen JK, et al. Effects of a-tocopherol and b-carotene supplements on cancer incidence in the Alpha-Tocopherol Beta-Carotene Cancer Prevention Study. *Am J Clin Nutr* 62(suppl.): 1427S–1430S, 1995.

58. Steiner M, Glantz M, and Lekos A. Vitamin E plus aspirin compared with aspirin alone in patients with transient ischemic attacks. *Am J Clin Nutr* 62(Suppl.): 1381S–1384S, 1995.

59. Kim JM and White RH. Effect of vitamin E on the anticoagulant response to warfarin. *Am J Cardiol* 77: 545–546, 1996.

60. Holt GA. Food and drug interactions. Chicago: Precept Press, 1998: 143.

61. Bieri JG, et al. Medical uses of vitamin E. *N Engl J Med* 308(18): 1063 –1071, 1983.

62. Roe D. Risk factors in drug-induced nutritional deficiencies, in D Roe, T Campbell, eds. Drugs and nutrients: the interactive effects: New York: Marcel Decker, 1984, 505–523.

## Vitamin K

1. Feskanich D, Weber P, Willett WC, et al. Vitamin K intake and hip fractures in women: a prospective study. *Am J Clin Nutr* 69: 74–79, 1999.

2. *Family Practice News* 14(5): 27, 1984.

3. Block CA, et al. Mother-infant prothrombin precursor status at birth. *J Pediatr Gastroenterol Nutr* 3(1): 101–103, 1984.

4. Ferland G. Subclinical vitamin K deficiency: a recent development. *Nutr Rep* 12(1): January 1994.

5. Bieri JG, et al. Medical uses of vitamin E. *N Engl J Med* 308(18): 1063–1071, 1983.

6. Roe D. Risk factors in drug-induced nutritional deficiencies. As cited in D Roe, T Campbell, eds. Drugs and nutrients: the interactive effects. New York: Marcel Decker, 1984: 505–523.

7. Crowther MA, Donovan D, Harrison L, et al. Low-dose oral vitamin K reliably reverses over-anticoagulation due to warfarin. *Thromb Haemost* 79: 1116–1118, 1998.

8. Avery RA, Duncan WE, and Alving BM. Severe vitamin K deficiency induced by occult celiac disease BR96-026. *Am J Hematol* 53(1): 55, 1996.

9. Benitez L, Hernandez Hernandez L, Sanchez Arcos E, and Jimenez-Alonso J. Changes in the prothrombin complex as clinical manifestation of celiac sprue in adults. *Rev Clin Esp* 196(7): 492–493, 1996.

10. Krasinski SD, et al. The prevalence of vitamin K deficiency in chronic gastrointestinal disorders. *Am J Clin Nutr* 41(3): 639–643, 1985.

11. Krejs GJ. Diarrhea. As cited in JB Wyngaarden and LH Smith, Jr, eds. Cecil Textbook of medicine. 18th ed. Philadelphia: W. B. Saunders, 1988.

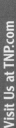

12. Iber FL, Shamszad M, Miller PA, and Jacob R. Vitamin K deficiency in chronic alcoholic males. *Alcohol Clin Exp Res* 10(6): 679–681, 1986.

13. Binkley N and Suttie J. Vitamin K nutrition and osteoporosis. *J Nutr* 125: 1812–1821, 1995.

14. Vermeer C, Gijsbers BL, Craciun AM, et al. Effects of vitamin K on bone mass and bone metabolism. *J Nutr* 126: 1187S–1191S, 1996.

15. Kanai T, Takagi T, Masuhiro K, et al. Serum vitamin K level and bone mineral density in post-menopausal women. *Int J Gynecol Obstet* 56: 25–30, 1997.

16. Hart JP. Electrochemical detection of depressed circulating levels of vitamin K in osteoporosis. *J Clin Endocrinol Metab* 60: 1268–1269, 1985.

17. Hart JP, et al. Circulation vitamin K levels in patients with fractures. *J Bone Joint Surg* 70-B: 663, 1998.

18. Hodges SJ, Pilkington MJ, Stamp TCB, et al. Depressed levels of circulating menaquinones in patients with osteoporotic fractures of the spine and femoral neck. *Bone* 12: 387–389, 1991.

19. Feskanich D, Weber P, Willett WC, et al. Vitamin K intake and hip fractures in women: a prospective study. *Am J Clin Nutr* 69: 74–79, 1999.

20. Jie K-SG et al. Effects of vitamin K and oral anticoagulants on urinary calcium excretion. *Br J Haematol* 83: 100–104, 1993.

21. Knapen MHJ, et al. The effect of vitamin K supplementation on circulating osteocalcin (bone Gla protein) and urinary calcium excretion. *Ann Intern Med* 111: 1001–1005, 1989.

22. Tomita A. Postmenopausal osteoporosis 47 Ca study with vitamin K$_2$. *Clin Endocrinol* (Jpn) 19: 731–736, 1971.

23. Suttie JW. Vitamin K and human nutrition. *J Am Diet Assoc* 92: 585–590, 1992.

24. Gubner R and Ungerleider HE. Vitamin K therapy in menorrhagia. *South Med* 37: 556–558, 1944.

25. Kanai T, Takagi T, Masuhiro K, et al. Serum vitamin K level and bone mineral density in post-menopausal women. *Int J Gynecol Obstet* 56: 25–30, 1997.

26. Hart JP. Electrochemical detection of depressed circulating levels of vitamin K in osteoporosis. *J Clin Endocrinol Metab* 60: 1268–1269, 1985.

27. Hart JP, et al. Circulation vitamin K levels in patients with fractures. *J Bone Joint Surg* 70-B: 663, 1998.

28. Hodges SJ, Pilkington MJ, Stamp TCB, et al. Depressed levels of circulating menaquinones in patients with osteoporotic fractures of the spine and femoral neck. *Bone* 12: 387–389, 1991.

29. Feskanich D, Weber P, Willett WC, et al. Vitamin K intake and hip fractures in women: a prospective study. *Am J Clin Nutr* 69: 74–79, 1999.

30. Jie K-SG et al. Effects of vitamin K and oral anticoagulants on urinary calcium excretion. *Br J Haematol* 83: 100–104, 1993.

31. Knapen MHJ, et al. The effect of vitamin K supplementation on circulating osteocalcin (bone Gla protein) and urinary calcium excretion. *Ann Intern Med* 111: 1001–1005, 1989.

32. Tomita A. Postmenopausal osteoporosis 47 Ca study with vitamin K$_2$. *Clin Endocrinol* (Jpn) 19: 731–736, 1971.

33. Golding J, Paterson M and Kinlon LJ. Factors associated with childhood cancer in a national cohort study. *Br J Cancer* 62: 304–308, 1990.

34. Ekelund H, Finnstrom O, Gunnerskog J, et al. Administration of vitamin K to newborn infants and childhood cancer. *BMJ* 305: 109, 1993.

35. Klebanoff MA, Read JS, Mills JL, and Shiono PH. The risk of childhood cancer after neonatal exposure to vitamin K. *N Engl J Med* 329: 905–908, 1993.

## White Willow

1. Newall C, et al. Herbal medicines: A guide for healthcare professionals. London: Pharmaceutical Press, 1996: 268.

2. Lininger S, et al. The natural pharmacy. Rocklin, CA: Prima Publishing, 1998: 319.

## Wild Yam

1. Lininger S, et al. The natural pharmacy. Rocklin, CA: Prima Publishing, 1998: 320.

2. Tierra M. The way of herbs. New York: Pocket Books, 1990: 246.

3. Tyler V, et al. Pharmacognosy, 8th ed. Philadelphia, PA: Lea & Febiger, 1981.

4. Hudson TND. *Townsend Letter for Doctors and Patients*. Port Townsend, WA, 1996, Issue No. 156.

## Yarrow

1. Newall C, et al. Herbal medicines: A guide for healthcare professionals. London: Pharmaceutical Press, 1996: 272.

## Yerba Santa

1. Lawrence Review of Natural Products. Yerba santa monograph. St. Louis, MO: Facts and Comparisons, Division, J.B. Lipincott Company, 1991.

2. Tierra M. The way of herbs. New York: Pocket Books, 1990: 254.

3. Lawrence Review of Natural Products. Yerba santa monograph. St. Louis, MO: Facts and Comparisons, Division, J.B. Lipincott Company, 1991.

### Yohimbe

1. Riley AJ. Yohimbine in the treatment of erectile disorder. *Br J Clin Pract* 48(3): 133–136, 1994.

2. Riley AJ. Yohimbine in the treatment of erectile disorder. *Br J Clin Pract* 48(3): 133–136, 1994.

3. Lawrence Review of Natural Products. Yohimbe monograph. St. Louis, MO: Facts and Comparisons Division, J.B. Lipincott Company, 1993.

4. Brinker F. Herb contraindications and drug interactions, 2nd ed. Sandy, Oregon: Eclectic Medical Publications, 1998: 140–141.

### Yucca

1. Bingham R, et al. Yucca plant saponin in the management of arthritis. *J Appl Nutr* 27(2–3): 45–51, 1975.

### Zinc

1. Sanstead H. Zinc nutrition in the United States. *Am J Clin Nutr* B26: 1251–1260, 1973.

2. Prasad AS. Role of zinc in human health. *Contemp Nutr* 16(5): 1991.

3. Baum MK, et al. Zidovudine-associated adverse reactions in a longitudinal study of asymptomatic HIV-1 infected homosexual males. *J Acquir Immune Defic Syndr* 4(12): 1218–1226, 1991.

4. Sandstrom B, et al. Oral iron, dietary ligands and zinc absorption. *J Nutr* 115(3): 411–414, 1985.

5. Scott KC and Turnlund JR. A compartmental model of zinc metabolism in adult men used to study effects of three levels of dietary copper. *Am J Physiol* 267(1 Pt. 1): E165–E173, 1994.

6. Werbach M. Foundations of nutritional medicine. Tarzana, CA: Third Line Press, 1997: 202.

7. Freeland-Graves JH. Manganese: An essential nutrient for humans. *Nutr Today* 23: 10–13, 1989.

8. Holt, GA. Food and drug interactions. Chicago: Precept Press. 1998.

9. Butterworth CE Jr and Tamura T. Folic acid safety and toxicity: A brief review. *Am J Clin Nutr* 50: 353–358, 1989.

10. Butterworth CE Jr and Tamura T. Folic acid safety and toxicity: A brief review. *Am J Clin Nutr* 50: 353–358, 1989.

11. Spencer H, et al. Effect of calcium and phosphorus on zinc metabolism in man. *Am J Clin Nutr* 40: 1213–1218, 1984.

12. Holt GA. Food and drug interactions. Chicago: Precept Press, 1998: 265.

13. Navert B, et al. A reduction of the phytate content of bran by leavening in bread and its effect on zinc absorption in man. *Br J Nutr* 53: 47–53, 1985.

14. Vohra P, et al. Phytic acid-metal complexes. *Proc Soc Exp Biol Med* 120: 447–449, 1965.

15. Hoffman HN II, et al. Zinc-induced copper deficiency. *Gastroenterology* 94: 508–512, 1988.

16. Sandstead HH. Requirements and toxicity of essential trace elements, illustrated by zinc and copper. *Am J Clin Nutr* 61(suppl.): 621S–624S, 1995.

17. Spencer H, Norris C, and Williams D. Inhibitory effects of zinc on magnesium balance and magnesium adsorption in man. *J Am Coll Nutr* 13(5): 479–484, 1994.

18. Werbach M. Foundations of nutritional medicine. Tarzana, CA: Third Line Press, 1997: 179.

19. Yadrick MK, et al. Iron, copper, and zinc status: response to supplementation with zinc or zinc and iron in adult females. *Am J Clin Nutr* 49: 145–150, 1989.

20. Marshall S. Zinc gluconate and the common cold. Review of randomized controlled trials. *Can Fam Physician* 44: 1037–1042, 1998.

21. Eby GA. Zinc ion availability—the determinant of efficacy in zinc lozenge treatment of common colds. *H Antimicrob Chemother* 40: 483–493, 1997.

22. Marshall S. Zinc gluconate and the common cold. Review of randomized controlled trials. *Can Fam Physician* 44: 1037–1042, 1998.

23. Girodon F, Lombard M, Galan P, et al. Effect of micronutrient supplementation on infection in institutionalized elderly subjects: a controlled trial. *Ann Nutr Metab* 41(2): 98–107, 1997.

24. Dreno B, et al. Low doses of zinc gluconate for inflammatory acne. *Acta Derm Venereol* 69: 541–543, 1989.

25. Gupta VL and Chaubey BS. Efficacy of zinc therapy in prevention of crisis in sickle-cell anemia: a double-blind, randomized controlled clinical trial. *J Assoc Physicians India* 43: 467–469, 1995.

26. Frommer DJ. The healing of gastric ulcers by zinc sulphate. *Med J Aust* 2: 793–796, 1975.

27. Garcia-Plaza A, Arenas JI, Belda O, et al. A multicenter clinical trial. Zinc acexamate versus famotidine in the treatment of acute duodenal ulcer. *Rev Esp Enferm Dig* 88: 757–762, 1996.

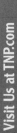

28. Simkin PA. Treatment of rheumatoid arthritis with oral zinc sulfate. *Agents Actions* 8: 587–595, 1981.

29. Pandley SP, Bhattacharya SK, and Sundar S. Zinc in rheumatoid arthritis. *Ind J Med Res* 81: 618–620, 1985.

30. Mattingly PC, et al. Zinc sulphate in rheumatoid arthritis. *Ann Rheum Dis* 41: 456–457, 1982.

31. Rasker JJ and Kardaun SH. Lack of beneficial effect of zinc sulphate in rheumatoid arthritis. *Scand J Rheumatol* 11: 168 –170, 1982.

32. Dixon JS, et al. Biochemical and clinical changes occurring during the treatment of rheumatoid arthritis with novel antirheumatoid drugs. *Int J Clin Pharmacol Res* 5(1): 25–33, 1985.

33. Job C, et al. Zinc sulphate in the treatment of rheumatoid arthritis. *Arthritis Rheum* 23: 1408, 1980.

34. Simkin PA. Treatment of rheumatoid arthritis with oral zinc sulfate. *Agents Actions* 8 (Suppl.): 587–596, 1981.

35. Netter A, et al. Effect of zinc administration on plasma testosterone, dihydrotestosterone and sperm count. *Arch Androl* 7: 69–73, 1981.

36. Stur M, Tittl M, Reitner A, and Meisinger V. Oral zinc and the second eye in age-related macular degeneration. *Invest Ophthalmol Vis Sci* 37: 1225–1235, 1993.

37. Newsome DA, Swartz M, Leone NC, et al. Oral zinc in macular degeneration. *Arch Ophthalmol* 106(2): 192–198, 1988.

38. Bandlish U, Prabhakar BR, and Wadehra PL. Plasma zinc level estimation in enlarged prostate. *Indian J Pathol Microbiol* 31(3): 231–234, 1988.

39. Gonick P, et al. Atomic absorption spectrophotometric determination of zinc in the prostate. *Invest Urol* 6: 345–347, 1969.

40. Schrodt GR, et al. The concentration of zinc in diseased human prostate glands. *Cancer* 17: 1555–1566, 1964.

41. Gyorkey F, et al. Zinc and magnesium in human prostate gland: Normal, hyperplastic and neoplastic. *Cancer Res* 27: 1348–1353, 1967.

42. Gyorkey F and Sato CS. In vitro 65 zinc-binding capacities of normal hyperplastic and carcinomatous human prostate gland. *Exp Mol Pathol* 8: 216–224, 1968.

43. Judd AM, et al. Zinc acutely, selectively and reversibly inhibits pituitary prolactin secretion. *Brain Res* 294: 190–192, 1984.

44. Leake A, et al. Interaction between prolactin and zinc in the human prostate gland. *J Endocrinol* 102(1): 73–76, 1984.

45. Leake A, Chisholm GD, and Habib FK. The effect of zinc on the 5-alpha-reduction of testosterone by the hyperplastic human prostate gland. *J Steroid Biochem* 20: 651–655, 1984.

46. Leake A, et al. Subcellular distribution of zinc in the benign and malignant human prostate: Evidence for a direct zinc androgen interaction. *Acta Endocrinol* 105: 281–288, 1984.

47. Neal DE, Kaack MB, Fussell EN, and Roberts JA. Changes in seminal fluid zinc during experimental prostatitis. *Urol Res* 21: 71–74, 1993.

48. Rodger RS, Sheldon WL, Watson MJ et al. Zinc deficiency and hyperprolactinaemia are not reversible causes of sexual dysfunction in uraemia. *Nephrol Dial Transplant* 4: 888–892, 1989.

49. Goldenberg RL, Tamura T, Neggers Y, et al. The effect of zinc supplementation on pregnancy outcome. *JAMA* 274: 463–468, 1995.

50. Sustrova M, et al. Thyroid function and plasma immunoglobulins in subjects with Down's syndrome (DS) during ontogenesis and zinc therapy. *J Endocrinol Invest* 17: 385–390, 1994.

51. Licastro F, et al. Modulation of the neuroendocrine system and immune functions by zinc supplementation in children with Down's syndrome. *J Trace Elem Electrolytes Health Dis* 7: 237–239, 1993.

52. Lockitch G, et al. Infection and immunity in Down syndrome: a trial of long-term low oral doses of zinc. *J Pediatr* 114: 781–787, 1989.

53. Constantinidis J. Alzheimer's disease and the zinc theory. *Encephale* 16: 231–239, 1990.

54. Constantinidis J. The hypothesis of zinc deficiency in the pathogenesis of neurofibrillary tangles. *Med Hypotheses* 35: 319–323, 1991.

55. Cuajungco MP and Lees GJ. Zinc metabolism in the brain: relevance to human neurodegenerative disorders. *Neurobiol Dis* 4: 137–169, 1997.

56. Lovell MA, Robertson JD, Teesdale W, et al. Copper, iron and zinc in Alzheimer's disease senile plaques. *J Neurol Sci* 158: 47–52, 1998.

57. Han CM. Changes in body zinc and copper levels in severely burned patients and the effects of oral administration of $ZnSO_4$ by a double-blind method. *Chung Hua Cheng Hsing Shao Shang Wai Ko Tsa Chih* 6: 83–86, 155, 1990.

58. Agren MS, et al. Selenium, zinc, iron and copper levels in serum of patients with arterial and venous leg ulcers. *Acta Derm Venereol* 66: 237–240, 1986.

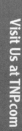

59. Floersheim GL and Lais E. Lack of effect of oral zinc sulfate on wound healing in leg ulcer. *Schweiz Med Wochenschr* 110: 1138–1145, 1980.

60. Sjogren A, Floren CH, and Nilsson A. Evaluation of zinc status in subjects with Crohn's disease. *J Am Coll Nutr* 7: 57–60, 1988.

61. Van de Wal Y, Van der Sluys Veer A, Verspaget HW, et al. Effect of zinc therapy on natural killer cell activity in inflammatory bowel disease. *Aliment Pharmacol Ther* 7: 281–286, 1993.

62. Mulder TP, van der Sluys Veer A, Verspaget HW, et al. Effect of oral zinc supplementation on metallothionein and superoxide dismutase concentrations in patients with inflammatory bowel disease. *J Gastroenterol Hepatol* 9: 472–477, 1994.

63. Dronfield MW, Malone JD, Langman MJ. Zinc in ulcerative colitis: a therapeutic trial and report on plasma levels. *Gut* 18: 33–36, 1977.

64. Gersdorff M, et al. The zinc sulfate overload test in patients suffering from tinnitus associated with low serum zinc. Preliminary report. *Acta Otorhinolaryngol Belg* 41: 498–505, 1987.

65. Paaske PB, et al. Zinc therapy of tinnitus. A placebo-controlled study. *Ugeskr Laeger* 152: 2473–2475, 1990.

66. Relea P, Revilla M, Ripoll E, et al. Zinc, biochemical markers of nutrition, and type-I osteoporosis. *Age Ageing* 24: 303–307, 1995.

67. Schmidt LE, Arfken CL, and Heins JM. Evaluation of nutrient intake in subjects with non-insulin-dependent diabetes mellitus. *J Am Diet Assoc* 94: 773–774, 1994.

68. Blostein-Fujii A, DeSilvestro RA, Frid D, et al. Short-term zinc supplementation in women with non-insulin-dependent diabetes mellitus: effects on plasma 5'-nucleotidase activities, insulin-like growth factor I concentrations, and lipoprotein oxidation rates in vitro. *Am J Clin Nutr* 66: 639–642, 1997.

69. Rauscher AM, Fairweather-Tait SJ, Wilson PD, et al. Zinc metabolism in non-insulin-dependent diabetes mellitus. *J Trace Elem Med Biol* 11: 65–70, 1997.

70. Mocchegiani E, Veccia S, Ancarani F, et al. Benefit of oral zinc supplementation as an adjunct to zidovudine (AZT) therapy against opportunistic infections in AIDS. *Int J Immunopharmacol* 17: 719–727, 1995.

71. Birmingham CL, Goldner EM, and Bakan R. Controlled trial of zinc supplementation in anorexia nervosa. *Int J Eat Disord* 15: 251–255, 1994.

72. Katz RL, Keen CL, Litt IF, et al. Zinc deficiency in anorexia nervosa. *J Adolesc Health Care* 8: 400–406, 1987.

73. Lask B, Fosson A, Rolfe U, and Thomas S. Zinc deficiency and childhood-onset anorexia nervosa. *J Clin Psychiatry* 54: 63–66, 1993.

74. Roijen SB, Worsaae U, and Zlotnik G. Zinc in patients with anorexia nervosa. *Ugeskr Laeger*, 153: 721–723, 1991.

75. Marshall S. Zinc gluconate and the common cold. Review of randomized controlled trials. *Can Fam Physician* 44: 1037–1042, 1998.

76. Eby GA. Linearity in dose-response from zinc lozenges in treatment of common colds. *J Pharmacy Technol* 11: 110–122, 1995.

77. Mossad SB, et al. Zinc gluconate lozenges for treating the common cold: a randomized, double-blind placebo-controlled study. *Ann Int Med* 125: 142–144, 1996.

78. Marshall S. Zinc gluconate and the common cold. Review of randomized controlled trials. *Can Fam Physician* 44: 1037–1042, 1998.

79. Petrus EJ, Lawson KA, and Bucci LR. Randomized, double-masked, placebo-controlled clinical study of the effectiveness of zinc acetate lozenges on common cold symptoms in allergy-tested subjects. *Curr Ther Res* 59: 595–607, 1998.

80. Marshall S. Zinc gluconate and the common cold. Review of randomized controlled trials. *Can Fam Physician* 44: 1037–1042, 1998.

81. Macknin ML, et al. Zinc gluconate lozenges for treating the common cold in children: a randomized controlled trial. *JAMA* 279: 1962–1967, 1998.

82. Girodon F, Lombard M, Galan P, et al. Effect of micronutrient supplementation on infection in institutionalized elderly subjects: a controlled trial. *Ann Nutr Metab* 41(2): 98–107, 1997.

83. Sugarman B. Zinc and infection. *Rev Infect Dis* 5(1): 137–147, 1983.

84. Pohit J, et al. Zinc status of acne vulgaris patients. *J Appl Nutr* 37: 18–25, 1985.

85. Amer M, et al. Serum zinc in acne vulgaris. *Int J Dermatol* 21: 481, 1982.

86. Michaelsson G, et al. Serum zinc and retinol-binding protein in acne. *Br J Dermatol* 96: 283–286, 1977.

87. Liden S, et al. Clinical evaluation of acne. *Acta Derm Venereol* 89: 49–52, 1980.

88. Goransson K, et al. Oral zinc in acne vulgaris: A clinical and methodological study. *Acta Derm Venereol (Stockh)* 58(5): 443–448, 1978.

89. Dreno B, et al. Low doses of zinc gluconate for inflammatory acne. *Acta Derm Venereol* 69: 541–543, 1989.

90. Verma KC, et al. Oral zinc sulfate therapy in acne vulgaris: a double blind trial. *Acta Dermatovener* 60: 337, 1980.

91. Weimar VM, et al. Zinc sulfate in acne vulgaris. *Arch Dermatol* 114(12): 1776–1778, 1978.

92. Hillstrom L, Pettersson L, Hellbe L, et al. Comparison of oral treatment with zinc sulphate and placebo in acne vulgaris. *Br J Dermatol* 97(6): 679–684, 1977.

93. Michaelsson G, Johlin L, and Ljunghall K. A double blind study of the effect of zinc and vitamin A in acne vulgaris. *Arch Dermatol* 113: 31, 1977.

94. Weissman K, Wadskov S, and Sondergaard J. Oral zinc sulphate therapy for acne vulgaris. *Acta Derm Venereol* (Stockh) 57(4): 357–60, 1977.

95. Orris L, et al. Oral zinc therapy of acne. Absorption and clinical effect. *Arch Dermatol* 114(7): 1018–1020, 1978.

96. Michaelsson G, Johlin L, and Ljunghall K. A double-blind study of the effect of zinc and oxytetracycline in acne vulgaris. *Br J Dermatol* 97: 56–566, 1977.

97. Cunliffe WJ, et al. A double-blind trial of a zinc sulphate/citrate complex and tetracycline in the treatment of acne vulgaris. *Br J Dermatol* 101: 321–325, 1979.

98. Gupta VL and Chaubey BS. Efficacy of zinc therapy in prevention of crisis in sickle-cell anemia: a double-blind, randomized controlled clinical trial. *J Assoc Physicians India* 43: 467–469, 1995.

99. Newsome DA, Swartz M, Leone NC, et al. Oral zinc in macular degeneration. *Arch Ophthalmol* 106(2): 192–198, 1988.

100. Stur M, Tittl M, Reitner A, and Meisinger V. Oral zinc and the second eye in age-related macular degeneration. *Invest Ophthalmol Vis Sci* 37: 1225–1235, 1993.

101. Hoffman HN II, et al. Zinc-induced copper deficiency. *Gastroenterology* 94: 508–512, 1988.

102. Sandstead HH. Requirements and toxicity of essential trace elements, illustrated by zinc and copper. *Am J Clin Nutr* 61(suppl.): 621S–624S, 1995.

103. Fosmire GJ. Zinc toxicity. *Am J Clin Nutr* 51: 225–227, 1990.

104. Lim D and McKay M. Food-drug interactions. *Drug Information Bulletin* (UCLA Dept. of Pharmaceutical Services) 15(2): 1995.

105. Drug evaluations subscription, vol. 2 (section 13, chapter 5 Chicago: American Medical Association): Winter 1993.

106. Holt GA. Food and drug interactions. Chicago: Precept Press, 1998: 275, 284.

# INDEX

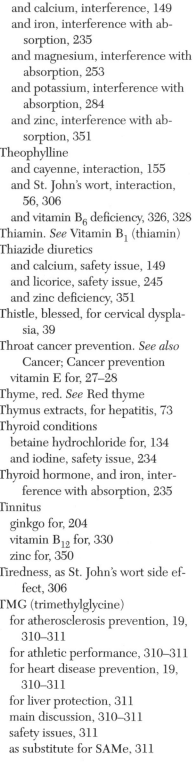

Index

Visit Us at TNP.com